Clinical Coding Workout:

Practice Exercises for Skill Development

With Answers

2012 Edition

Melanie Endicott, MBA/HCM, RHIA, CCS, CCS-P,

Kathy Giannangelo, MA, RHIA, CCS, CPHIMS, FAHIMA,

Anita C. Hazelwood, MLS, RHIA, FAHIMA,

Karen Kostick, RHIT, CCS, CCS-P, and

Carol A. Venable, MPH, RHIA, FAHIMA

AHIMA

PRESS

ISBN: 978-1-58426-333-3
AHIMA Product No. AC201612

AHIMA Staff:
Claire E. Blondeau, MBA, Senior Editor
Katherine Greenock, Editorial and Production Coordinator
Ashley Sullivan, Assistant Editor
Ken Zielske, CAE, Director of Publications

American Health Information Management Association
233 North Michigan Avenue, 21st Floor
Chicago, Illinois 60601-5800

http://www.ahima.org

Contents

Preface

The *Clinical Coding Workout* is designed to challenge coding professionals and students alike to develop expert skills in the assignment of clinical codes required for administrative use.

The coding process requires a range of skills that combines knowledge and practice. Someone new to this discipline must conquer the basic principles of using the required code sets. A student at the intermediate level learns to apply code set conventions, guidelines, and principles in various combinations, settings, and scenarios. A person with advanced coding skills analyzes complex health data and determines what needs to be reported to accurately reflect each patient's condition and treatment. Like a violinist or a gymnast, the coding professional develops virtuosity step-by-step through systematic exercise. At each level of skill development, practice enhances performance.

The AHIMA Practice Resources team has gathered coding scenarios and case studies together to create a resource for skill development and review of guidelines and conventions applied in code selection. Practice exercises take the user from beginning concepts and selection of codes, through intermediate applications using short code assignment scenarios, to advanced case studies that are based on excerpts from health records and that require complex clinical analysis skills and multiple code assignments. The user is encouraged to reference the American Hospital Association's *Coding Clinic*, National Center for Health Statistics' *ICD-9-CM Official Guidelines for Coding and Reporting*, and American Medical Association's *CPT Assistant* cited within select case scenarios to further enhance learning. Not all cases include a reference and not all references are cited for a particular case or topic. Coding challenges in the final chapter include exercises for ICD-10-CM and ICD-10-PCS, CPT modifiers, HCPCS Level II modifiers, home health, LTAC coding, and rehabilitation and SNF cases. A CD-ROM resource contains tables that link each exercise to the AHIMA certifications and competencies to which it pertains. Lastly, the annotated answer key serves as a unique instructional guide not only providing the correct answer to each question, but also explaining why the answer is correct and why the incorrect answers are not appropriate.

Ways in which this valuable resource can be used include the following:

- Health information management (HIM) educators and coding program trainers can use the exercises to supplement basic- and intermediate-level course materials for students seeking extra credit or advanced preparation.

- HIM students can use the exercises for self-directed learning.

- Coding professionals can use the exercises to gain additional coding experience in a variety of specialties and settings that may not be available to them in their current workplace.

- Employers can use this resource to challenge new coding professionals who are ready to sharpen their skills to the intermediate and advanced levels of coding performance.

- Coding managers can use this material as a tool to assess the competency of coding staff for complex coding practice.

- Employers seeking high-level competency in the more difficult coding practice areas can use the case studies as a means of screening for advanced coding skills.

Clinical Coding Workout is also an excellent tool for:

- Preparing to sit for the mastery-level coding exams offered by AHIMA (CCS and CCS-P) to gain additional insight into a variety of specialty coding topics.

- Evaluating or instructing coding professionals as part of ongoing compliance initiatives.

How to Use This Book

Unlike coding instructional books that are based on one coding classification system, *Clinical Coding Workout* uses the full range of administrative code sets applicable in today's healthcare environment for reporting diagnoses, procedures, and services in various settings and specialty practice areas.

The actual codes used in the exercises and answer key for this book are those that were confirmed or already in effect at the time of publication, as follows:

- *International Classification of Diseases, 9th Revision, Clinical Modification (ICD-9-CM),* 2012 edition, codes effective October 1, 2011

- *International Classification of Diseases, 10th Revision, Clinical Modification (ICD-10-CM),* 2011 draft edition

- *International Classification of Diseases, 10th Revision, Procedure Coding System (ICD-10-PCS),* 2011 draft edition

- *Current Procedural Terminology (CPT),* 2011 edition, codes effective January 1, 2012

- *Healthcare Common Procedural Coding System Level II (HCPCS),* 2011 edition, codes effective January 1, 2012

Use of different versions of coding books with this resource will require attention to the code changes after the effective date. Revised answer keys will be created that are consistent with coding changes for the upcoming year soon after the effective date of the new codes. All answer keys are available to instructors in online format from the individual book page in the AHIMA Bookstore (http://imis.ahima.org/orders), and also are posted on the AHIMA Assembly on Education Community of Practice (AOE CoP) Web site. Instructors who are AHIMA members can sign up for this private community by clicking on the help icon within the CoP home page and requesting additional information on becoming an AOE CoP member. An instructor who is not an AHIMA member or a member who is not an instructor may contact the publisher at publications@ahima.org.

As in actual practice, ICD-9-CM codes are used for diagnoses and inpatient procedures for hospital reporting in this book; whereas for ambulatory facility and physician service reporting, ICD-9-CM codes are used for diagnoses and HCPCS/CPT codes are used for procedures and services.

The Centers for Medicare and Medicaid Services (CMS) and the National Center for Health Statistics (NCHS) provide the *ICD-9-CM and ICD-10-CM/PCS Official Guidelines for Coding and Reporting*, which should be used as a companion document to the official version. The guidelines have been approved by the four organizations that make up the Cooperating Parties for the ICD-9-CM: the American Hospital Association (AHA), the American Health Information Management Association (AHIMA), CMS, and NCHS.

The guidelines are a set of rules that have been developed to accompany and complement the official conventions and instructions provided within ICD-9-CM and ICD-10-CM/PCS. The guidelines are based upon the coding and sequencing instructions found in ICD-9-CM and ICD-10-CM/PCS, and they provide additional instruction. Adherence to the guidelines is required under the Health Insurance Portability and Accountability Act (HIPAA). The guidelines for ICD-9-CM and ICD-10-CM are organized into sections. Section I includes the structure and conventions of the classification, general guidelines that apply to the entire classification, and chapter-specific guidelines that correspond to the chapters as they are arranged in the classification. This section is applicable to all healthcare settings unless otherwise indicated. Section II includes guidelines for selecting principal diagnoses for non-outpatient settings. Section III includes guidelines for reporting additional diagnoses in non-outpatient settings. Section IV is for outpatient coding (including physician) and reporting. The guidelines for ICD-10-PCS are organized into three sections. Section A includes the structure and conventions of the classification. Section B includes the Medical and Surgical section guidelines. Section C includes Obstetrics section guidelines.

The ICD-9-CM and ICD-10-CM guidelines are regularly updated and are available at: http://www.cdc.gov/nchs/icd.htm. The ICD-10-PCS guidelines are available at http://www.cms.gov/ICD10/.

Federal Register notices and other regulatory updates are available from the Centers for Medicare and Medicaid Services at http://www.cms.gov. HCPCS Level II codes are updated each quarter and are available by download from https://www.cms.gov/HCPCSRelease CodeSets/. CPT code sets are generally released in mid-September for implementation by January 1 of the following year.

Refer to the instructions in each chapter for additional information. Please report any potential inconsistencies or inaccuracies in this book to publications@ahima.org.

Part I
Beginning Coding Exercises

Chapter 1

Basic Principles of ICD-9-CM and ICD-10-CM/PCS Coding

The following exercises are designed to review ICD-9-CM and ICD-10-CM/PCS coding guidelines and to provide practice in assigning ICD-9-CM and ICD-10-CM/PCS codes. Because ICD-9-CM and ICD-10-CM/PCS index diagnoses and procedures in many different ways, the rationale for the selection of a particular code may be different from the approach that you use. The information included in the rationale is not meant to describe the only way to obtain an appropriate code but to represent one possible way.

Note: The exercises in this chapter are based on the 2012 edition of ICD-9-CM and the 2011 draft editions of ICD-10-CM and ICD-10-PCS but are suitable for other editions in most instances.

Instructions: Circle the correct answer, fill in the blank, or assign the correct code(s) for each of the following exercise items.

Characteristics and Conventions of the ICD-9-CM Classification System

1.1. Nonessential modifiers are enclosed in:

    a. Brackets
    b. Parentheses
    c. Slanted brackets
    d. Boxes

1.2. A diagnostic descriptor that is listed in italics is a(n):

    a. Manifestation code
    b. Inappropriate principal diagnosis
    c. CC exclusion
    d. Code that must be reported first

1.3. The abbreviation UHDDS refers to the _____.

1.4. Diagnoses described as "suspected," "possible," "probable," "likely," and "still to be ruled out" are reported if present for _____ records.

1.5. For patients receiving therapeutic services in the outpatient setting for chemotherapy, radiation therapy, or rehabilitation, the first listed reported diagnosis is:

a. The diagnosis toward which the treatment is directed
b. The appropriate V code
c. Either a or b
d. The diagnosis that the physician lists first on the order

1.6. When multiple burns are present, the first sequenced diagnosis is the:

a. Burn that is treated surgically
b. Burn that is closest to the head
c. Highest-degree burn
d. Any of the above

1.7. A coding professional may assume a cause-and-effect relationship between hypertension and which of the following complications?

a. Hypertension and heart disease
b. Hypertension and chronic kidney disease
c. Hypertension and heart and chronic kidney disease
d. None of the above

1.8. ICD-9-CM Codes that describe the behavior of cells in neoplasms are called _____.

1.9. New ICD-9-CM codes go into effect on _____ of each year.

1.10. Supplementary classifications include:

a. V codes
b. V codes and E codes
c. V codes, E codes, and M codes
d. None of the above

1.11. The neoplasm table includes:

a. The nature and status (primary, secondary, in situ) for malignancies
b. A listing of the morphology codes
c. The stage of benign neoplasms
d. E codes for reactions to chemotherapy

1.12. V codes can be used as:

a. Principal diagnosis only
b. Secondary diagnosis only
c. Either principal diagnosis or secondary diagnosis, depending on the code and the circumstances of the admission
d. Secondary diagnosis only on inpatient stays and principal diagnosis only on outpatient visits

1.13. Terms listed in the Alphabetic Index in boldface type are known as

_____.

1.14. Manifestation codes:

a. Can never be reported first
b. Are printed in italics in the Tabular List
c. Describe a condition that results from another, underlying condition
d. All of the above

1.15. Codes that contain the descriptive abbreviation NOS are to be used:

a. When the record itself is not available for review
b. When the coder lacks sufficient information to assign a more specific code
c. When only outpatient diagnostic records are being coded
d. All the time

Infectious and Parasitic Diseases

1.16. Meningitis due to ECHO virus

ICD-9-CM Code(s): _____

ICD-10-CM Code(s): _____

1.17. Chickenpox

ICD-9-CM Code(s): _____

ICD-10-CM Code(s): _____

1.18. Pulmonary anthrax

ICD-9-CM Code(s): _____

ICD-10-CM Code(s): _____

1.19. *Aerobacter aerogenes* is an example of a gram-_____ bacterial organism.

1.20. Genital herpes

ICD-9-CM Code(s): _____

ICD-10-CM Code(s): _____

1.21.   Patients with any known prior diagnosis of an HIV-related illness should be reported with this ICD-9-CM code: _____.

ICD-10-CM Code(s): _____

1.22.   Acute salpingitis due to gonococcal infection

ICD-9-CM Code(s): _____

ICD-10-CM Code(s): _____

1.23.   A patient with known AIDS is admitted to the hospital for treatment of *Pneumocystis carinii* pneumonia. Assign the principal ICD-9-CM diagnosis code.

a. 042
b. 486
c. 136.3
d. Any of the above

1.24.   A patient with known chronic hepatitis C is seen in the outpatient department for interferon treatment. Assign the primary diagnosis.

ICD-9-CM Code(s):

a. 070.51
b. 070.44
c. 070.54
d. 070.32

ICD-10-CM Code(s): _____

1.25.   Paratyphoid fever A

ICD-9-CM Code(s): _____

ICD-10-CM Code(s): _____

1.26.   Food poisoning due to *Staphylococcus* organism

ICD-9-CM Code(s): _____

ICD-10-CM Code(s): _____

1.27.   Infectious diarrhea

ICD-9-CM Code(s): _____

ICD-10-CM Code(s): _____

1.28.   Pulmonary tuberculosis, bacilli identified with microscopy

ICD-9-CM Code(s): _____

ICD-10-CM Code(s): _____

1.29. Scarlatina

ICD-9-CM Code(s): _____

ICD-10-CM Code(s): _____

1.30. Pneumococcal septicemia

ICD-9-CM Code(s): _____

ICD-10-CM Code(s): _____

1.31. Dermatophytosis of scalp

ICD-9-CM Code(s): _____

ICD-10-CM Code(s): _____

1.32. Pneumonia as a complication of measles

ICD-9-CM Code(s): _____

ICD-10-CM Code(s): _____

1.33. Mumps

ICD-9-CM Code(s): _____

ICD-10-CM Code(s): _____

1.34. Plantar wart

ICD-9-CM Code(s): _____

ICD-10-CM Code(s): _____

1.35. Infectious mononucleosis

ICD-9-CM Code(s): _____

ICD-10-CM Code(s): _____

1.36. Condyloma acuminata

ICD-9-CM Code(s): _____

ICD-10-CM Code(s): _____

1.37. Infection with Shiga toxin-producing *Escherichia coli*

ICD-9-CM Code(s): _____

ICD-10-CM Code(s): _____

Neoplasms

1.38. Hodgkin's sarcoma of thoracic lymph nodes

ICD-9-CM Code(s): _____

ICD-10-CM Code(s): _____

1.39.   Malignant neoplasm of bronchus

ICD-9-CM Code(s): _____

ICD-10-CM Code(s): _____

1.40.   When a patient is admitted to the hospital for radiation therapy for a primary malignancy that is still present, what code is reported as the principal diagnosis?

ICD-9-CM Code(s): _____

ICD-10-CM Code(s): _____

1.41.   A patient is admitted as an inpatient to receive radiation and chemotherapy for distal esophageal carcinoma. What is the appropriate principal diagnosis?

ICD-9-CM Code(s):

a. V58.0
b. V58.11
c. 150.5
d. Either a or b

ICD-10-CM Code(s): _____

1.42.   Carcinoma of the broad ligament (confined to this location)

ICD-9-CM Code(s): _____

ICD-10-CM Code(s): _____

1.43.   Adenoma of the islet cells of the pancreas

ICD-9-CM Code(s): _____

ICD-10-CM Code(s): _____

1.44.   Neoplasms at the cellular level that are incapable of spreading to distant sites are called _____ neoplasms.

1.45.   Malignant melanoma of the skin of the chest wall

ICD-9-CM Code(s): _____

ICD-10-CM Code(s): _____

1.46.   Adenocarcinoma of the lesser curvature of the stomach

ICD-9-CM Code(s): _____

ICD-10-CM Code(s): _____

1.47.   Secondary carcinoma of the submandibular salivary gland

ICD-9-CM Code(s): _____

ICD-10-CM Code(s): _____

1.48. Benign neoplasm of the appendix

ICD-9-CM Code(s): _____

ICD-10-CM Code(s): _____

1.49. Carcinoma in situ of breast

ICD-9-CM Code(s): _____

ICD-10-CM Code(s): _____

1.50. Which of the following neoplasm types is correct for sympathicoblastoma?

a. Benign
b. Malignant
c. Uncertain behavior
d. Unspecified

1.51. Myxofibrosarcoma is a malignant neoplasm that affects what type of tissue?

_____

1.52. The site at which a malignant neoplasm originated is known as the
_____ site.

1.53. Bronchogenic carcinoma

ICD-9-CM Code(s): _____

ICD-10-CM Code(s): _____

1.54. Carcinoma in situ of the uterine cervix

ICD-9-CM Code(s): _____

ICD-10-CM Code(s): _____

1.55. In ICD-9-CM, neoplasm coding of the lymphatic and hematopoietic systems
(200–202), a fifth digit of 4–5 refers to which organs?

a. Lymph nodes of inguinal region and lower limb
b. Lymph nodes of head, face, and neck
c. Lymph nodes of axilla and upper limb
d. Intrapelvic lymph nodes

1.56. Merkel cell carcinoma of the neck

ICD-9-CM Code(s): _____

ICD-10-CM Code(s): _____

1.57. Acute myelogenous leukemia in relapse

ICD-9-CM Code(s): _____

ICD-10-CM Code(s): _____

1.58.   Carcinoma of the bladder trigone

ICD-9-CM Code(s): _____

ICD-10-CM Code(s): _____

1.59.   Squamous cell carcinoma of skin of the left ear

ICD-9-CM Code(s): _____

ICD-10-CM Code(s): _____

Endocrine, Nutritional, and Metabolic Diseases and Immunity Disorders

1.60.   Hereditary hemochromatosis

ICD-9-CM Code(s): _____

ICD-10-CM Code(s): _____

1.61.   Hyponatremia

ICD-9-CM Code(s): _____

ICD-10-CM Code(s): _____

1.62.   Primary hypercholesterolemia

ICD-9-CM Code(s): _____

ICD-10-CM Code(s): _____

1.63.   Bartter's syndrome is a form of which of the following?

a. Diabetic neuropathy
b. Hyperaldosteronism
c. Hypertriglyceridemia
d. Polycystic ovarian disease

1.64.   Type I diabetes mellitus with diabetic renal nephrosis, out of control

ICD-9-CM Code(s): _____

ICD-10-CM Code(s): _____

1.65.   Secondary diabetes mellitus

ICD-9-CM Code(s): _____

ICD-10-CM Code(s): _____

1.66.   Type I diabetes mellitus with proliferative retinopathy

ICD-9-CM Code(s): _____

ICD-10-CM Code(s): _____

1.67. Type I diabetes mellitus with ketoacidosis

ICD-9-CM Code(s): _____

ICD-10-CM Code(s): _____

1.68. Type I diabetes mellitus with ophthalmic manifestations

ICD-9-CM Code(s): _____

ICD-10-CM Code(s): _____

1.69. Hypoinsulinemia following total pancreatectomy

ICD-9-CM Code(s): _____

ICD-10-CM Code(s): _____

1.70. ICD-9-CM code 255.2 (adrenogenital disorders) includes which of the following?

a. Achard-Thiers syndrome
b. Macrogenitosomia praecox in the male
c. Congenital adrenal hyperplasia
d. All of the above

1.71. Hypophyseal dwarfism

ICD-9-CM Code(s): _____

ICD-10-CM Code(s): _____

1.72. Hypopotassemia

ICD-9-CM Code(s): _____

ICD-10-CM Code(s): _____

1.73. Cystic fibrosis with pulmonary manifestations

ICD-9-CM Code(s): _____

ICD-10-CM Code(s): _____

1.74. Hurler's syndrome, gargoyle syndrome, and Sanfilippo's syndrome are all forms of _____.

1.75. Adult morbid obesity with a BMI of 40.0

ICD-9-CM Code(s): _____

ICD-10-CM Code(s): _____

1.76. Polycystic ovaries

ICD-9-CM Code(s): _____

ICD-10-CM Code(s): _____

1.77.   Renal glycosuria

ICD-9-CM Code(s): _____

ICD-10-CM Code(s): _____

1.78.   Nodular goiter with hyperthyroidism

ICD-9-CM Code(s): _____

ICD-10-CM Code(s): _____

1.79.   Congenital hypothyroidism

ICD-9-CM Code(s): _____

ICD-10-CM Code(s): _____

1.80.   Agammaglobulinemia

ICD-9-CM Code(s): _____

ICD-10-CM Code(s): _____

Disorders of the Blood and Blood-Forming Organs

1.81.   Iron-deficiency anemia secondary to chronic blood loss

ICD-9-CM Code(s): _____

ICD-10-CM Code(s): _____

1.82.   Sickle cell anemia and thalassemia are both types of:

a. Iron-deficiency anemias
b. Hereditary hemolytic anemias
c. Aplastic anemia
d. Coagulation defects

1.83.   Sickle cell trait

ICD-9-CM Code(s): _____

ICD-10-CM Code(s): _____

1.84.   Anemia due to acute blood loss

ICD-9-CM Code(s): _____

ICD-10-CM Code(s): _____

1.85.   Anemia due to antineoplastic chemotherapy

ICD-9-CM Code(s): _____

ICD-10-CM Code(s): _____

1.86. Which of the following is (are) not an example(s) of constitutional red blood cell aplasia?

    a. Fanconi's anemia
    b. Familial hypoplastic anemia
    c. Blackfan-Diamond syndrome
    d. All of the above

1.87. von Willebrand's disease

ICD-9-CM Code(s): _____

ICD-10-CM Code(s): _____

1.88. Agranulocytosis is a disease of the _____ blood cells.

1.89. Aplastic anemia

ICD-9-CM Code(s): _____

ICD-10-CM Code(s): _____

1.90. Folate deficiency anemia due to drugs

ICD-9-CM Code(s): _____

ICD-10-CM Code(s): _____

1.91. Refractory megaloblastic anemia

ICD-9-CM Code(s): _____

ICD-10-CM Code(s): _____

1.92. Osteosclerotic anemia

ICD-9-CM Code(s): _____

ICD-10-CM Code(s): _____

1.93. Posttransfusion purpura

ICD-9-CM Code(s): _____

ICD-10-CM Code(s): _____

1.94. Thrombocytopenic purpura

ICD-9-CM Code(s): _____

ICD-10-CM Code(s): _____

1.95. Thrombocytopenia following massive blood transfusions

ICD-9-CM Code(s): _____

ICD-10-CM Code(s): _____

1.96.   Anemia

ICD-9-CM Code(s): _____

ICD-10-CM Code(s): _____

1.97.   Congenital aplastic anemia

ICD-9-CM Code(s): _____

ICD-10-CM Code(s): _____

1.98.   Eosinophilic leukocytosis

ICD-9-CM Code(s): _____

ICD-10-CM Code(s): _____

1.99.   Anemia secondary to vitamin B_{12} deficiency

ICD-9-CM Code(s): _____

ICD-10-CM Code(s): _____

1.100. Hemophilia

ICD-9-CM Code(s): _____

ICD-10-CM Code(s): _____

1.101. Fe deficiency anemia

ICD-9-CM Code(s): _____

ICD-10-CM Code(s): _____

1.102. Aplastic anemia due to antineoplastic chemotherapy, initial encounter

ICD-9-CM Code(s): _____

ICD-10-CM Code(s): _____

Mental Disorders

> Because the code assignment for mental disorders can have significant impact on the patient, coding professionals must take special care to ensure that codes are based on diagnostic statements clearly provided in physician documentation.

1.103. In ICD-9-CM coding, to report Jakob-Creutzfeldt disease with dementia, you would need:

a. One code
b. Two codes
c. Either one or two codes
d. More than two codes

1.104. Alcoholic dependent chronic brain syndrome

ICD-9-CM Code(s): _____

ICD-10-CM Code(s): _____

1.105. Chronic paranoid schizophrenia with acute exacerbation

ICD-9-CM Code(s): _____

ICD-10-CM Code(s): _____

1.106. Hypomanic personality disorder

ICD-9-CM Code(s): _____

ICD-10-CM Code(s): _____

1.107. Panic attack

ICD-9-CM Code(s): _____

ICD-10-CM Code(s): _____

1.108. Which of the following is a synonym for multiple personality disorder?

a. Dissociative identity disorder
b. Factitious illness
c. Adjustment reaction
d. Multiple psychoses

1.109. Childhood autism

ICD-9-CM Code(s): _____

ICD-10-CM Code(s): _____

1.110. Which of the following is a sexual deviation or disorder per ICD-9-CM?

a. Bestiality
b. Pedophilia
c. Voyeurism
d. All of the above

1.111. Alcoholism with acute intoxication

ICD-9-CM Code(s): _____

ICD-10-CM Code(s): _____

1.112. Morphine addiction, in remission

ICD-9-CM Code(s): _____

ICD-10-CM Code(s): _____

1.113. Heroin and diazepam addiction

ICD-9-CM Code(s): _____

ICD-10-CM Code(s): _____

1.114. Psychogenic torticollis

ICD-9-CM Code(s): _____

ICD-10-CM Code(s): _____

1.115. Gilles de la Tourette's syndrome

ICD-9-CM Code(s): _____

ICD-10-CM Code(s): _____

1.116. Major depression, recurrent

ICD-9-CM Code(s): _____

ICD-10-CM Code(s): _____

1.117. Separation anxiety disorder

ICD-9-CM Code(s): _____

ICD-10-CM Code(s): _____

1.118. Moderate intellectual disabilities, measured IQ of 42

ICD-9-CM Code(s): _____

ICD-10-CM Code(s): _____

1.119. Attention deficit/hyperactivity disorder

ICD-9-CM Code(s): _____

ICD-10-CM Code(s): _____

1.120. Alcoholic paranoia

ICD-9-CM Code(s): _____

ICD-10-CM Code(s): _____

1.121. DTs due to alcohol withdrawal

ICD-9-CM Code(s): _____

ICD-10-CM Code(s): _____

1.122. Multi-infarct dementia with depression

ICD-9-CM Code(s): _____

ICD-10-CM Code(s): _____

1.123. Passive-aggressive personality disorder

ICD-9-CM Code(s): _____

ICD-10-CM Code(s): _____

1.124. Multi-infarct dementia with behavioral disturbance

ICD-9-CM Code(s): _____

ICD-10-CM Code(s): _____

Nervous System and Sense Organs

1.125. Acute endophthalmitis

ICD-9-CM Code(s): _____

ICD-10-CM Code(s): _____

1.126. Duchenne muscular dystrophy

ICD-9-CM Code(s): _____

ICD-10-CM Code(s): _____

1.127. Which of the following are the correct ICD-9-CM codes for proliferative type 1 diabetic retinopathy?

a. 250.53, 362.01
b. 362.02, 250.50
c. 250.51, 362.02
d. 362.02, 250.01

1.128. Central retinal artery occlusion

ICD-9-CM Code(s): _____

ICD-10-CM Code(s): _____

1.129. Acanthamoeba keratitis

ICD-9-CM Code(s): _____

ICD-10-CM Code(s): _____

1.130. Bilateral retinal detachment, traction type

ICD-9-CM Code(s): _____

ICD-10-CM Code(s): _____

1.131. Senile cataract, posterior subcapsular

ICD-9-CM Code(s): _____

ICD-10-CM Code(s): _____

1.132. Angle closure glaucoma, acute

ICD-9-CM Code(s): _____

ICD-10-CM Code(s): _____

1.133. Tritan defect

ICD-9-CM Code(s): _____

ICD-10-CM Code(s): _____

1.134. Bullous keratopathy, bilateral

ICD-9-CM Code(s): _____

ICD-10-CM Code(s): _____

1.135. Temporal sclerosis

ICD-9-CM Code(s): _____

ICD-10-CM Code(s): _____

1.136. All but one of the following conditions are examples of strabismus (ICD-9-CM category 378). Identify the condition that is not a form of strabismus.

a. Esotropia
b. Exotropia
c. Presbyopia
d. Heterotropia

1.137. Chronic serous otitis media

ICD-9-CM Code(s): _____

ICD-10-CM Code(s): _____

1.138. Acute suppurative otitis media with eardrum rupture due to pressure

ICD-9-CM Code(s): _____

ICD-10-CM Code(s): _____

1.139. Cholesteatoma involving left middle ear and mastoid

ICD-9-CM Code(s): _____

ICD-10-CM Code(s): _____

1.140. Hyperactive labyrinth, right side

ICD-9-CM Code(s): _____

ICD-10-CM Code(s): _____

1.141. Anisocoria

ICD-9-CM Code(s): _____

ICD-10-CM Code(s): _____

1.142. Malignant otitis externa

ICD-9-CM Code(s): _____

ICD-10-CM Code(s): _____

1.143. Poorly controlled epilepsy

ICD-9-CM Code(s): _____

ICD-10-CM Code(s): _____

1.144. Reflex sympathetic dystrophy, both arms

ICD-9-CM Code(s): _____

ICD-10-CM Code(s): _____

1.145. Alzheimer's disease with behavioral disturbance, early onset

ICD-9-CM Code(s): _____

ICD-10-CM Code(s): _____

1.146. Brain death

ICD-9-CM Code(s): _____

ICD-10-CM Code(s): _____

Circulatory System

1.147. Pulmonary aneurysm

ICD-9-CM Code(s): _____

ICD-10-CM Code(s): _____

1.148. Malignant hypertension with hypertensive heart disease and congestive heart failure is coded:

ICD-9-CM Code(s):

a. 402.01
b. 402.01, 428.9
c. 428.0, 402.11
d. 402.01, 428.0

ICD-10-CM Code(s): _____

1.149. Mitral valve stenosis and aortic valve insufficiency

ICD-9-CM Code(s): _____

ICD-10-CM Code(s): _____

1.150. Hospital discharge diagnosis: Acute inferolateral myocardial infarction

ICD-9-CM Code(s): _____

ICD-10-CM Code(s): _____

1.151. In ICD-9-CM, a myocardial infarction is considered to be acute when it is less than _____ weeks old.

ICD-10-CM Answer: _____

1.152. Hypertension

ICD-9-CM Code(s): _____

ICD-10-CM Code(s): _____

1.153. Identify the main term and codes in the diagnostic statement "idiopathic hypertrophic subaortic stenosis (IHSS)."

ICD-9-CM Main Term and Code(s): _____

ICD-10-CM Main Term and Code(s): _____

1.154. Atrial flutter

ICD-9-CM Code(s): _____

ICD-10-CM Code(s): _____

1.155. Ventricular fibrillation

ICD-9-CM Code(s): _____

ICD-10-CM Code(s): _____

1.156. Acute diastolic heart failure

ICD-9-CM Code(s): _____

ICD-10-CM Code(s): _____

1.157. Preinfarction angina

ICD-9-CM Code(s): _____

ICD-10-CM Code(s): _____

1.158. Pulmonary infarction

ICD-9-CM Code(s): _____

ICD-10-CM Code(s): _____

1.159. ASHD of transplanted heart (native artery)

ICD-9-CM Code(s): _____

ICD-10-CM Code(s): _____

1.160. Atherosclerosis of left internal mammary artery bypass graft

ICD-9-CM Code(s): _____

ICD-10-CM Code(s): _____

1.161. Dysarthria secondary to old stroke (cerebrovascular disease)

ICD-9-CM Code(s): _____

ICD-10-CM Code(s): _____

1.162. Cerebral infarct due to stenosis of the vertebral artery

ICD-9-CM Code(s): _____

ICD-10-CM Code(s): _____

1.163. Chronic pulmonary embolism

ICD-9-CM Code(s): _____

ICD-10-CM Code(s): _____

1.164. Orthostatic hypotension

ICD-9-CM Code(s): _____

ICD-10-CM Code(s): _____

1.165. Varicose veins of the left leg with ulceration

ICD-9-CM Code(s): _____

ICD-10-CM Code(s): _____

1.166. Abdominal aortic aneurysm, ruptured

ICD-9-CM Code(s): _____

ICD-10-CM Code(s): _____

1.167. Chronic diastolic heart failure

ICD-9-CM Code(s): _____

ICD-10-CM Code(s): _____

1.168. Saddle embolus of abdominal aorta

ICD-9-CM Code(s): _____

ICD-10-CM Code(s): _____

Respiratory System

1.169. Acute bronchitis

ICD-9-CM Code(s): _____

ICD-10-CM Code(s): _____

1.170. Acute laryngitis with airway obstruction

ICD-9-CM Code(s): _____

ICD-10-CM Code(s): _____

1.171. Hypertrophy of tonsils and adenoids

ICD-9-CM Code(s): _____

ICD-10-CM Code(s): _____

1.172. Maxillary sinus polyp(s)

ICD-9-CM Code(s): _____

ICD-10-CM Code(s): _____

1.173. The correct code assignment(s) for pneumonia due to the RSV organism is (are):

ICD-9-CM Code(s):

a. 486 and 079.6
b. 480.1
c. 466.11
d. 079.6

ICD-10-CM Code(s): _____

1.174. Methicillin resistant pneumonia due to Staphylococcus aureus

ICD-9-CM Code(s): _____

ICD-10-CM Code(s): _____

1.175. Acute exacerbation of chronic obstructive pulmonary disease

ICD-9-CM Code(s): _____

ICD-10-CM Code(s): _____

1.176. Emphysema

ICD-9-CM Code(s): _____

ICD-10-CM Code(s): _____

1.177. Bilateral granulomatous hemorrhagic septic pneumonia

ICD-9-CM Code(s): _____

ICD-10-CM Code(s): _____

1.178. Influenza A due to identified 2009 H1N1 influenza virus with pneumonia

ICD-9-CM Code(s): _____

ICD-10-CM Code(s): _____

1.179. Chronic obstructive asthma with status asthmaticus

ICD-9-CM Code(s): _____

ICD-10-CM Code(s): _____

1.180. Postoperative pneumothorax

ICD-9-CM Code(s): _____

ICD-10-CM Code(s): _____

1.181. Chronic respiratory failure

ICD-9-CM Code(s): _____

ICD-10-CM Code(s): _____

1.182. Tracheostomy stenosis

ICD-9-CM Code(s): _____

ICD-10-CM Code(s): _____

1.183. Postinfective bronchiectasis

ICD-9-CM Code(s): _____

ICD-10-CM Code(s): _____

1.184. What is the correct code assignment for extrinsic asthma with acute exacerbation and status asthmaticus?

ICD-9-CM Code(s):

a. 493.02
b. 493.00
c. 493.01
d. 493.02, 493.01

ICD-10-CM Code(s): _____

1.185. Spontaneous pneumothorax

ICD-9-CM Code(s): _____

ICD-10-CM Code(s): _____

1.186. Childhood asthma

ICD-9-CM Code(s): _____

ICD-10-CM Code(s): _____

1.187. Radiation pneumonitis due to radioactive isotope

ICD-9-CM Code(s): _____

ICD-10-CM Code(s): _____

1.188. Common cold

ICD-9-CM Code(s): _____

ICD-10-CM Code(s): _____

1.189. Aspiration pneumonia

ICD-9-CM Code(s): _____

ICD-10-CM Code(s): _____

1.190. Methicillin susceptible pneumonia due to Staphylococcus aureus

ICD-9-CM Code(s): _____

ICD-10-CM Code(s): _____

1.191. Respiratory bronchiolitis interstitial lung disease

ICD-9-CM Code(s): _____

ICD-10-CM Code(s): _____

Digestive System

1.192. Dental caries

ICD-9-CM Code(s): _____

ICD-10-CM Code(s): _____

1.193. Acute duodenal ulcer with bleeding

ICD-9-CM Code(s): _____

ICD-10-CM Code(s): _____

1.194. Gastric ulcer

ICD-9-CM Code(s): _____

ICD-10-CM Code(s): _____

1.195. Leukoplakia of tongue

ICD-9-CM Code(s): _____

ICD-10-CM Code(s): _____

1.196. Identify the appropriate code for reflux esophagitis.

ICD-9-CM Code(s):

a. 530.81
b. 530.11
c. 530.10
d. 530.89

ICD-10-CM Code(s): _____

1.197. Select the correct code for acute peptic ulcer of stomach with perforation.

ICD-9-CM Code(s):

a. 533.10
b. 531.50
c. 533.60
d. 531.10

ICD-10-CM Code(s): _____

1.198. Angiodysplasia of the stomach

ICD-9-CM Code(s): _____

ICD-10-CM Code(s): _____

1.199. Alcoholic gastritis with hemorrhage

ICD-9-CM Code(s): _____

ICD-10-CM Code(s): _____

1.200. Acute obstructive appendicitis

ICD-9-CM Code(s): _____

ICD-10-CM Code(s): _____

1.201. Incisional hernia

ICD-9-CM Code(s): _____

ICD-10-CM Code(s): _____

1.202. Bilateral inguinal hernia, recurrent

ICD-9-CM Code(s): _____

ICD-10-CM Code(s): _____

1.203. Incarcerated right femoral hernia

ICD-9-CM Code(s): _____

ICD-10-CM Code(s): _____

1.204. Crohn's disease of the large bowel

ICD-9-CM Code(s): _____

ICD-10-CM Code(s): _____

1.205. Ulcerative colitis

ICD-9-CM Code(s): _____

ICD-10-CM Code(s): _____

1.206. Ileus due to gallstones impacting the intestine

ICD-9-CM Code(s): _____

ICD-10-CM Code(s): _____

1.207. Select the correct code for diverticulosis of the colon.

ICD-9-CM Code(s):

a. 562.11
b. 562.00
c. 562.10
d. 562.12

ICD-10-CM Code(s): _____

1.208. Postoperative peritoneal adhesions

ICD-9-CM Code(s): _____

ICD-10-CM Code(s): _____

1.209. Cholelithiasis with acute and chronic cholecystitis

ICD-9-CM Code(s): _____

ICD-10-CM Code(s): _____

1.210. Chronic pancreatitis

ICD-9-CM Code(s): _____

ICD-10-CM Code(s): _____

1.211. Pouchitis

ICD-9-CM Code(s): _____

ICD-10-CM Code(s): _____

1.212. Reflux esophagitis

ICD-9-CM Code(s): _____

ICD-10-CM Code(s): _____

Genitourinary System

1.213. Acute renal failure with lesion of tubular necrosis

ICD-9-CM Code(s): _____

ICD-10-CM Code(s): _____

1.214. Ureterolithiasis

ICD-9-CM Code(s): _____

ICD-10-CM Code(s): _____

1.215. Acute pyelonephritis

ICD-9-CM Code(s): _____

ICD-10-CM Code(s): _____

1.216. Urethrolithiasis

ICD-9-CM Code(s): _____

ICD-10-CM Code(s): _____

1.217. Hydronephrosis

ICD-9-CM Code(s): _____

ICD-10-CM Code(s): _____

1.218. UTI

ICD-9-CM Code(s): _____

ICD-10-CM Code(s): _____

1.219. Overactive bladder

ICD-9-CM Code(s): _____

ICD-10-CM Code(s): _____

1.220. Gross hematuria

ICD-9-CM Code(s): _____

ICD-10-CM Code(s): _____

1.221. Select the appropriate code for urethral stricture.

ICD-9-CM Code(s):

a. 598
b. 598.9
c. 598.00
d. 598.8

ICD-10-CM Code(s): _____

1.222. In the diagnostic statement "urinary tract infection due to *Escherichia coli*," which condition is coded as the principal diagnosis?

a. The *E coli*
b. The urinary tract infection
c. Either may be coded as the principal diagnosis.
d. The circumstances of the admission determine which condition is coded as the principal diagnosis.

1.223. Select the appropriate code for benign prostatic hypertrophy.

ICD-9-CM Code(s):

a. 222.2
b. 600.20
c. 600.00
d. 600.90

ICD-10-CM Code(s): _____

1.224. PIN II

ICD-9-CM Code(s): _____

ICD-10-CM Code(s): _____

1.225. In the diagnostic statement "tuberculous prostatitis," which condition is coded as the principal diagnosis in ICD-9-CM?

a. The tuberculosis
b. The prostatitis
c. Either may be coded as the principal diagnosis.
d. The circumstances of the admission determine which condition is coded as the principal diagnosis.

1.226. Micromastia

ICD-9-CM Code(s): _____

ICD-10-CM Code(s): _____

1.227. Acute PID

ICD-9-CM Code(s): _____

ICD-10-CM Code(s): _____

1.228. Endometriosis of the broad ligament

ICD-9-CM Code(s): _____

ICD-10-CM Code(s): _____

1.229. Corpus luteum cyst of ovary

ICD-9-CM Code(s): _____

ICD-10-CM Code(s): _____

1.230. Dysmenorrhea

ICD-9-CM Code(s): _____

ICD-10-CM Code(s): _____

1.231. Postmenopausal atrophic vaginitis

ICD-9-CM Code(s): _____

ICD-10-CM Code(s): _____

1.232. CIN II

ICD-9-CM Code(s): _____

ICD-10-CM Code(s): _____

1.233. Priapism due to trauma

ICD-9-CM Code(s): _____

ICD-10-CM Code(s): _____

1.234. Stenosis of cystostomy

ICD-9-CM Code(s): _____

ICD-10-CM Code(s): _____

Pregnancy, Childbirth, and the Puerperium

1.235. Contracted pelvis, infant delivered vaginally

ICD-9-CM Code(s): _____

ICD-10-CM Code(s): _____

1.236. Gestational diabetes, admitted for control, not delivered

ICD-9-CM Code(s): _____

ICD-10-CM Code(s): _____

1.237. Maternal hypotension syndrome, onset 10 minutes after delivery

ICD-9-CM Code(s): _____

ICD-10-CM Code(s): _____

1.238. In ICD-9-CM, the postpartum period begins immediately following delivery and lasts for _____ weeks following delivery.

1.239. By ICD-9-CM definition, an "elderly primigravida" is a woman who is _____ years or older at the time of her first delivery.

1.240. Large-for-dates baby, delivered this admission (maternal record)

ICD-9-CM Code(s): _____

ICD-10-CM Code(s): _____

1.241. Primary uterine inertia, delivered this admission

ICD-9-CM Code(s): _____

ICD-10-CM Code(s): _____

1.242. Vaginal delivery with third-degree perineal laceration

ICD-9-CM Code(s): _____

ICD-10-CM Code(s): _____

1.243. Postpartum puerperal sepsis, patient readmitted 2 weeks after delivery

ICD-9-CM Code(s): _____

ICD-10-CM Code(s): _____

1.244. Hyperemesis gravidarum at 16 weeks, with dehydration, not delivered

ICD-9-CM Code(s): _____

ICD-10-CM Code(s): _____

1.245. False labor, 39 weeks, not delivered

ICD-9-CM Code(s): _____

ICD-10-CM Code(s): _____

1.246. Pregnancy in bicornuate uterus, 20 weeks, undelivered this admission

ICD-9-CM Code(s): _____

ICD-10-CM Code(s): _____

1.247. Dehiscence of cesarean section wound requiring readmission 1 week after delivery

ICD-9-CM Code(s): _____

ICD-10-CM Code(s): _____

1.248. Postpartum amniotic fluid embolism occurring while patient is still in the hospital

ICD-9-CM Code(s): _____

ICD-10-CM Code(s): _____

1.249. In ICD-9-CM the fifth digit to describe a delivery that was accompanied by a postpartum complication while the patient was still in the hospital is

_____.

1.250. In ICD-9-CM if a patient is admitted for treatment of a postpartum condition following delivery that occurred during a previous episode of care, the appropriate fifth digit is _____.

1.251. Oligohydramnios, reported with ICD-9-CM code 658.0X, is:

    a. Infection of the amniotic fluid
    b. Excessive amount of amniotic fluid
    c. Deficient amount of amniotic fluid
    d. Embolism of amniotic fluid

1.252. Missed abortion

    ICD-9-CM Code(s): _____

    ICD-10-CM Code(s): _____

1.253. In ICD-9-CM when an abortion is complicated by septic shock, the appropriate fourth digit is _____.

1.254. Ectopic pregnancies include which of the following types?

    a. Tubal
    b. Abdominal
    c. Septic
    d. a and b

1.255. Classical hydatidiform mole

    ICD-9-CM Code(s): _____

    ICD-10-CM Code(s): _____

1.256. Spontaneous abortion at 21 weeks of gestation, complete

    ICD-9-CM Code(s): _____

    ICD-10-CM Code(s): _____

Skin and Subcutaneous Tissue

1.257. Carbuncle of the hand

    ICD-9-CM Code(s): _____

    ICD-10-CM Code(s): _____

1.258. Paronychia of right finger

    ICD-9-CM Code(s): _____

    ICD-10-CM Code(s): _____

1.259. Sunburn

    ICD-9-CM Code(s): _____

    ICD-10-CM Code(s): _____

1.260. Cellulitis of chin

ICD-9-CM Code(s): _____

ICD-10-CM Code(s): _____

1.261. Pilonidal cyst with abscess

ICD-9-CM Code(s): _____

ICD-10-CM Code(s): _____

1.262. Poison ivy

ICD-9-CM Code(s): _____

ICD-10-CM Code(s): _____

1.263. Dermatitis due to cat dander

ICD-9-CM Code(s): _____

ICD-10-CM Code(s): _____

1.264. Lupus erythematosus

ICD-9-CM Code(s): _____

ICD-10-CM Code(s): _____

1.265. Keloid scar

ICD-9-CM Code(s): _____

ICD-10-CM Code(s): _____

1.266. Actinic keratosis

ICD-9-CM Code(s): _____

ICD-10-CM Code(s): _____

1.267. Alopecia areata

ICD-9-CM Code(s): _____

ICD-10-CM Code(s): _____

1.268. Hidradenitis suppurativa

ICD-9-CM Code(s): _____

ICD-10-CM Code(s): _____

1.269. Select the correct code(s) for a stage II pressure ulcer of heel.

ICD-9-CM Code(s):

a. 707.15
b. 707.14
c. 707.07, 707.22
d. 707.09, 707.20

ICD-10-CM Code(s): _____

1.270. In the diagnostic statement "diabetic foot ulcer," what condition should be assigned as the principal diagnosis in ICD-9-CM?

    a. The ulcer

    b. The diabetes mellitus

    c. Either condition

    d. The circumstances of the admission will determine which condition is classified as the principal diagnosis.

1.271. Lichen planus, generalized

    ICD-9-CM Code(s): _____

    ICD-10-CM Code(s): _____

1.272. Contact dermatitis due to new detergent

    ICD-9-CM Code(s): _____

    ICD-10-CM Code(s): _____

1.273. Abscess of right axilla

    ICD-9-CM Code(s): _____

    ICD-10-CM Code(s): _____

1.274. Ammonia dermatitis from soiled diapers

    ICD-9-CM Code(s): _____

    ICD-10-CM Code(s): _____

1.275. Erythema multiforme

    ICD-9-CM Code(s): _____

    ICD-10-CM Code(s): _____

1.276. Second-degree sunburn

    ICD-9-CM Code(s): _____

    ICD-10-CM Code(s): _____

1.277. Dermatitis due to base metals in jewelry

    ICD-9-CM Code(s): _____

    ICD-10-CM Code(s): _____

1.278. Pressure ulcer of the right heel, stage II

    ICD-9-CM Code(s): _____

    ICD-10-CM Code(s): _____

1.279. Pilar cyst

ICD-9-CM Code(s): _____

ICD-10-CM Code(s): _____

1.280. Trichilemmal cyst

ICD-9-CM Code(s): _____

ICD-10-CM Code(s): _____

Musculoskeletal System and Connective Tissue

1.281. Pyogenic arthritis of the hip

ICD-9-CM Code(s): _____

ICD-10-CM Code(s): _____

1.282. Rheumatoid arthritis involving the hands

ICD-9-CM Code(s): _____

ICD-10-CM Code(s): _____

1.283. Aseptic necrosis of femoral head

ICD-9-CM Code(s): _____

ICD-10-CM Code(s): _____

1.284. Osteoarthritis of the knees

ICD-9-CM Code(s): _____

ICD-10-CM Code(s): _____

1.285. DJD, generalized

ICD-9-CM Code(s): _____

ICD-10-CM Code(s): _____

1.286. Chronic bucket handle tear of the lateral meniscus of the knee

ICD-9-CM Code(s): _____

ICD-10-CM Code(s): _____

1.287. Chondromalacia patellae

ICD-9-CM Code(s): _____

ICD-10-CM Code(s): _____

1.288. Hemarthrosis of the elbow, chronic

ICD-9-CM Code(s): _____

ICD-10-CM Code(s): _____

1.289. Ankylosing spondylitis

ICD-9-CM Code(s): _____

ICD-10-CM Code(s): _____

1.290. Osteoarthritis of the cervical spine with cord compression documented at surgery

ICD-9-CM Code(s): _____

ICD-10-CM Code(s): _____

1.291. HNP L4–5, with left lower extremity sciatica

ICD-9-CM Code(s): _____

ICD-10-CM Code(s): _____

1.292. Degenerative disk disease of lumbar spine

ICD-9-CM Code(s): _____

ICD-10-CM Code(s): _____

1.293. Low back pain

ICD-9-CM Code(s): _____

ICD-10-CM Code(s): _____

1.294. Synovial cyst of wrist

ICD-9-CM Code(s): _____

ICD-10-CM Code(s): _____

1.295. SLE

ICD-9-CM Code(s): _____

ICD-10-CM Code(s): _____

1.296. Osteomyelitis, acute, of first and second metatarsi

ICD-9-CM Code(s): _____

ICD-10-CM Code(s): _____

1.297. Postmenopausal osteoporosis

ICD-9-CM Code(s): _____

ICD-10-CM Code(s): _____

1.298. Pathologic fracture of neck of femur, initial encounter

ICD-9-CM Code(s): _____

ICD-10-CM Code(s): _____

1.299. Hallux valgus

ICD-9-CM Code(s): _____

ICD-10-CM Code(s): _____

1.300. Kyphosis

ICD-9-CM Code(s): _____

ICD-10-CM Code(s): _____

Newborn/Congenital Disorders

1.301. Spina bifida of lumbar region with congenital hydrocephalus

ICD-9-CM Code(s): _____

ICD-10-CM Code(s): _____

1.302. Branchial cleft cyst

ICD-9-CM Code(s): _____

ICD-10-CM Code(s): _____

1.303. VSD

ICD-9-CM Code(s): _____

ICD-10-CM Code(s): _____

1.304. Coarctation of the aorta

ICD-9-CM Code(s): _____

ICD-10-CM Code(s): _____

1.305. Bilateral complete cleft palate

ICD-9-CM Code(s): _____

ICD-10-CM Code(s): _____

1.306. Hypospadias

ICD-9-CM Code(s): _____

ICD-10-CM Code(s): _____

1.307. Polycystic kidney disease

ICD-9-CM Code(s): _____

ICD-10-CM Code(s): _____

1.308. Congenital dislocation of left hip, with subluxation of right hip

ICD-9-CM Code(s): _____

ICD-10-CM Code(s): _____

1.309. Syndactyly of fingers involving soft tissues only

ICD-9-CM Code(s): _____

ICD-10-CM Code(s): _____

1.310. Spondylolisthesis, L5–S1

ICD-9-CM Code(s): _____

ICD-10-CM Code(s): _____

1.311. Congenital rectouterine fistula

ICD-9-CM Code(s): _____

ICD-10-CM Code(s): _____

1.312. Klinefelter's syndrome

ICD-9-CM Code(s): _____

ICD-10-CM Code(s): _____

1.313. Osteogenesis imperfecta

ICD-9-CM Code(s): _____

ICD-10-CM Code(s): _____

1.314. Congenital CMV infection

ICD-9-CM Code(s): _____

ICD-10-CM Code(s): _____

1.315. Meconium aspiration syndrome

ICD-9-CM Code(s): _____

ICD-10-CM Code(s): _____

1.316. Hemolytic disease of newborn due to Rh maternal/fetal incompatibility

ICD-9-CM Code(s): _____

ICD-10-CM Code(s): _____

1.317. Omphalocele

ICD-9-CM Code(s): _____

ICD-10-CM Code(s): _____

1.318. Drug withdrawal syndrome in newborn

ICD-9-CM Code(s): _____

ICD-10-CM Code(s): _____

1.319. In the diagnostic statement "newborn male with meconium aspiration syndrome, subarachnoid hemorrhage, and neonatal jaundice due to prematurity," what is the ICD-9-CM principal diagnosis?

a. 772.2
b. V30.00
c. 770.1
d. 774.2

1.320. Necrotizing enterocolitis of the newborn

ICD-9-CM Code(s): _____

ICD-10-CM Code(s): _____

1.321. Supernumerary cervical rib

ICD-9-CM Code(s): _____

ICD-10-CM Code(s): _____

1.322. Pulmonary artery coarctation and atresia

ICD-9-CM Code(s): _____

ICD-10-CM Code(s): _____

1.323. Pulmonary arteriovenous malformation

ICD-9-CM Code(s): _____

ICD-10-CM Code(s): _____

1.324. Hemolytic disease in newborn due to ABO antibodies; baby has jaundice

ICD-9-CM Code(s): _____

ICD-10-CM Code(s): _____

1.325. Crack baby

ICD-9-CM Code(s): _____

ICD-10-CM Code(s): _____

Symptoms, Signs, and Ill-Defined Conditions

1.326. Anorexia

ICD-9-CM Code(s): _____

ICD-10-CM Code(s): _____

1.327. Failure to thrive, 35-year-old patient

ICD-9-CM Code(s): _____

ICD-10-CM Code(s): _____

1.328. Fussy infant

ICD-9-CM Code(s): _____

ICD-10-CM Code(s): _____

1.329. Posttransfusion fever

ICD-9-CM Code(s): _____

ICD-10-CM Code(s): _____

1.330. Syncope

ICD-9-CM Code(s): _____

ICD-10-CM Code(s): _____

1.331. Chronic fatigue syndrome

ICD-9-CM Code(s): _____

ICD-10-CM Code(s): _____

1.332. Chest pain

ICD-9-CM Code(s): _____

ICD-10-CM Code(s): _____

1.333. Post-traumatic seizure

ICD-9-CM Code(s): _____

ICD-10-CM Code(s): _____

1.334. Concentration deficit

ICD-9-CM Code(s): _____

ICD-10-CM Code(s): _____

1.335. Abnormal GTT

ICD-9-CM Code(s): _____

ICD-10-CM Code(s): _____

1.336. Nausea and vomiting

ICD-9-CM Code(s): _____

ICD-10-CM Code(s): _____

1.337. Infant colic

ICD-9-CM Code(s): _____

ICD-10-CM Code(s): _____

1.338. Urinary frequency

ICD-9-CM Code(s): _____

ICD-10-CM Code(s): _____

1.339. RUQ abdominal pain

ICD-9-CM Code(s): _____

ICD-10-CM Code(s): _____

1.340. Abnormal EEG

ICD-9-CM Code(s): _____

ICD-10-CM Code(s): _____

1.341. Nonvisualization of gallbladder on x-ray examination

ICD-9-CM Code(s): _____

ICD-10-CM Code(s): _____

1.342. Abnormal mammogram

ICD-9-CM Code(s): _____

ICD-10-CM Code(s): _____

1.343. SIDS

ICD-9-CM Code(s): _____

ICD-10-CM Code(s): _____

1.344. Cachexia

ICD-9-CM Code(s): _____

ICD-10-CM Code(s): _____

1.345. Hyperventilation

ICD-9-CM Code(s): _____

ICD-10-CM Code(s): _____

1.346. Dysphagia, pharyngeal phase

ICD-9-CM Code(s): _____

ICD-10-CM Code(s): _____

1.347. Altered mental status

ICD-9-CM Code(s): _____

ICD-10-CM Code(s): _____

1.348. Acute idiopathic pulmonary hemorrhage in a 2-month-old infant

ICD-9-CM Code(s): _____

ICD-10-CM Code(s): _____

1.349. Fecal incontinence

ICD-9-CM Code(s): _____

ICD-10-CM Code(s): _____

1.350. Abnormality of gait

ICD-9-CM Code(s): _____

ICD-10-CM Code(s): _____

1.351. Elevated blood pressure reading without diagnosis of hypertension

ICD-9-CM Code(s): _____

ICD-10-CM Code(s): _____

Trauma/Poisoning

1.352. Open skull fracture with subarachnoid and subdural hemorrhage, expired without regaining consciousness, initial encounter

ICD-9-CM Code(s): _____

ICD-10-CM Code(s): _____

1.353. Fracture of C3 with complete transection of spinal cord at that level, initial encounter

ICD-9-CM Code(s): _____

ICD-10-CM Code(s): _____

1.354. Fracture ribs 2 to 4 right and 2 to 5 left, initial encounter

ICD-9-CM Code(s): _____

ICD-10-CM Code(s): _____

1.355. Multiple fractures of pelvis with loss of continuity of pelvic circle, initial encounter

ICD-9-CM Code(s): _____

ICD-10-CM Code(s): _____

1.356. Comminuted, impacted fracture of surgical neck of right humerus, initial encounter

ICD-9-CM Code(s): _____

ICD-10-CM Code(s): _____

1.357. Torus fracture of radius and ulna, left arm, initial encounter

ICD-9-CM Code(s): _____

ICD-10-CM Code(s): _____

1.358. Nursemaid's elbow, initial encounter

ICD-9-CM Code(s): _____

ICD-10-CM Code(s): _____

1.359. Missile fracture of patella due to bullet, initial encounter

ICD-9-CM Code(s): _____

ICD-10-CM Code(s): _____

1.360. Dislocation of jaw, initial encounter

ICD-9-CM Code(s): _____

ICD-10-CM Code(s): _____

1.361. Sprained wrist, initial encounter

ICD-9-CM Code(s): _____

ICD-10-CM Code(s): _____

1.362. Pneumothorax with knife wound of chest wall, initial encounter

ICD-9-CM Code(s): _____

ICD-10-CM Code(s): _____

1.363. Mosquito bite, buttocks, with secondary infection, initial encounter

ICD-9-CM Code(s): _____

ICD-10-CM Code(s): _____

1.364. Third-degree burns of palm of hand, initial encounter

ICD-9-CM Code(s): _____

ICD-10-CM Code(s): _____

1.365. Poisoning by salicylate ingestion, initial encounter

ICD-9-CM Code(s): _____

ICD-10-CM Code(s): _____

1.366. Anaphylactic shock due to ingestion of pecans, initial encounter

ICD-9-CM Code(s): _____

ICD-10-CM Code(s): _____

1.367. Frostbite of face, initial encounter

ICD-9-CM Code(s): _____

ICD-10-CM Code(s): _____

1.368. Leakage of prosthetic heart valve, initial encounter

ICD-9-CM Code(s): _____

ICD-10-CM Code(s): _____

1.369. Rejection of transplanted liver

ICD-9-CM Code(s): _____

ICD-10-CM Code(s): _____

1.370. Accidental laceration of aorta during laminectomy procedure

ICD-9-CM Code(s): _____

ICD-10-CM Code(s): _____

1.371. Confirmed battered spouse (wife seeking care), initial encounter

ICD-9-CM Code(s): _____

ICD-10-CM Code(s): _____

1.372. Retained cholelithiasis following cholecystectomy

ICD-9-CM Code(s): _____

ICD-10-CM Code(s): _____

1.373. Anaphylactic reaction due to vaccination, initial encounter

ICD-9-CM Code(s): _____

ICD-10-CM Code(s): _____

1.374. Aspiration pneumonia following surgery

ICD-9-CM Code(s): _____

ICD-10-CM Code(s): _____

1.375. Multiple closed pelvic fractures without disruption of pelvic circle, initial encounter

ICD-9-CM Code(s): _____

ICD-10-CM Code(s): _____

ICD-9-CM and ICD-10-CM External Causes of Morbidity

1.376. A patient was injured due to a tackle in a football game. The injury occurred on a football field, and the patient is a student who is on a recreational football team, initial encounter.

Assign the applicable ICD-9-CM and ICD-10-CM External Cause, Place of Occurrence, Activity, and Status Codes.

ICD-9-CM Code(s): _____

ICD-10-CM Code(s): _____

1.377. A patient fell from a ladder inside a building construction site. Patient is an employed construction worker, initial encounter.

Assign the applicable ICD-9-CM and ICD-10-CM External Cause, Place of Occurrence, Activity, and Status Codes.

ICD-9-CM Code(s): _____

ICD-10-CM Code(s): _____

1.378. Assign the appropriate main external cause code for burns due to ignition of clothing from fireplace in restaurant, initial encounter.

ICD-9-CM Code(s): _____

ICD-10-CM Code(s): _____

1.379. Assign the appropriate main external cause code for injury from rattlesnake bite, initial encounter.

ICD-9-CM Code(s): _____

ICD-10-CM Code(s): _____

1.380. Assign the appropriate main external cause code for injury in an avalanche, initial encounter.

ICD-9-CM Code(s): _____

ICD-10-CM Code(s): _____

1.381. A patient injured her toe due to bumping into a table while performing household maintenance in the kitchen of her home. The patient is an unemployed homeowner, initial encounter.

Assign the applicable ICD-9-CM and ICD-10-CM main External Cause, Place of Occurrence, Activity, and Status Codes.

ICD-9-CM Code(s): _____

ICD-10-CM Code(s): _____

1.382. Assign the appropriate main external cause code for drowning in the bathtub, initial encounter.

ICD-9-CM Code(s): _____

ICD-10-CM Code(s): _____

1.383. Assign the appropriate main external cause code for injury from fireworks, initial encounter.

ICD-9-CM Code(s): _____

ICD-10-CM Code(s): _____

1.384. Assign the appropriate activity code involving rappelling.

ICD-9-CM Code(s): _____

ICD-10-CM Code(s): _____

1.385. Laceration of hand from assault with knife. Assign both the diagnosis code and the main external cause code, initial encounter.

ICD-9-CM Code(s): _____

ICD-10-CM Code(s): _____

1.386. Cervical strain due to motor vehicle accident, secondary to loss of control and collision with tree. Patient was the restrained driver. Assign both the diagnosis code and the main external cause code, initial encounter.

ICD-9-CM Code(s): _____

ICD-10-CM Code(s): _____

1.387. Fracture of ulna due to fall from motorcycle. Patient was a passenger on the back of the motorcycle, initial encounter. Assign both the diagnosis code and the main external cause code.

ICD-9-CM Code(s): _____

ICD-10-CM Code(s): _____

1.388. Assign the appropriate activity code for an injury that occurred while riding a roller coaster.

ICD-9-CM Code(s): _____

ICD-10-CM Code(s): _____

1.389. Assign the appropriate main external cause code for injury from dog bite, initial encounter.

ICD-9-CM Code(s): _____

ICD-10-CM Code(s): _____

1.390. What is the appropriate place of occurrence code for an accident occurring on a street or highway?

ICD-9-CM Code(s): _____

ICD-10-CM Code(s): _____

1.391. Assign the appropriate main external cause code for clamp left inside a patient during a surgical procedure.

ICD-9-CM Code(s): _____

ICD-10-CM Code(s): _____

1.392. Assign the appropriate main external cause code for injury during earthquake, initial encounter.

ICD-9-CM Code(s): _____

ICD-10-CM Code(s): _____

1.393. Assign the appropriate main external cause code for injury from a lathe, initial encounter.

ICD-9-CM Code(s): _____

ICD-10-CM Code(s): _____

1.394. While at work, a patient was shot by another person, with the intent to injure using a shotgun. The accident occurred on the employer factory premises, initial encounter.

Assign the applicable ICD-9-CM and ICD-10-CM External Cause, Place of Occurrence, Activity, and Status Codes.

ICD-9-CM Code(s): _____

ICD-10-CM Code(s): _____

1.395. Laceration of pinna of the ear from accidental human bite, with secondary infection. Assign both the diagnosis code and the main external cause code, initial encounter.

ICD-9-CM Code(s): _____

ICD-10-CM Code(s): _____

ICD-9-CM V Codes/ICD-10-CM Z Codes

1.396. Encounter for artificial insemination

ICD-9-CM Code(s): _____

ICD-10-CM Code(s): _____

1.397. Hepatitis B carrier

ICD-9-CM Code(s): _____

ICD-10-CM Code(s): _____

1.398. History of carcinoma of the breast

ICD-9-CM Code(s): _____

ICD-10-CM Code(s): _____

1.399. History of colonic polyps

ICD-9-CM Code(s): _____

ICD-10-CM Code(s): _____

1.400. Family history of ovarian cancer

ICD-9-CM Code(s): _____

ICD-10-CM Code(s): _____

1.401. Well-baby visit, baby is 30 days old

ICD-9-CM Code(s): _____

ICD-10-CM Code(s): _____

1.402. Incidental pregnancy

ICD-9-CM Code(s): _____

ICD-10-CM Code(s): _____

1.403. Liveborn male twin, delivered by cesarean section

ICD-9-CM Code(s): _____

ICD-10-CM Code(s): _____

1.404. Encounter for amniocentesis for screening for chromosomal anomalies

ICD-9-CM Code(s): _____

ICD-10-CM Code(s): _____

1.405. Body mass index (BMI) 47.0 adult

ICD-9-CM Code(s): _____

ICD-10-CM Code(s): _____

1.406. Renal dialysis status

ICD-9-CM Code(s): _____

ICD-10-CM Code(s): _____

1.407. Cardiac pacemaker status, without complications

ICD-9-CM Code(s): _____

ICD-10-CM Code(s): _____

1.408. Encounter for reprogramming of AICD

ICD-9-CM Code(s): _____

ICD-10-CM Code(s): _____

1.409. Aftercare for pathological fracture of L4 vertebra, routine healing

ICD-9-CM Code(s): _____

ICD-10-CM Code(s): _____

1.410. Admission for change of tracheostomy tube and stoma revision

ICD-9-CM Code(s): _____

ICD-10-CM Code(s): _____

1.411. Admission for planned colostomy closure

ICD-9-CM Code(s): _____

ICD-10-CM Code(s): _____

1.412. Admission for chemotherapy

ICD-9-CM Code(s): _____

ICD-10-CM Code(s): _____

1.413. Patient status is "do not resuscitate (DNR)"

ICD-9-CM Code(s): _____

ICD-10-CM Code(s): _____

1.414. Observation of child post-MVA with no apparent injury and no complaints

ICD-9-CM Code(s): _____

ICD-10-CM Code(s): _____

1.415. Encounter for screening mammogram

ICD-9-CM Code(s): _____

ICD-10-CM Code(s): _____

1.416. History of gestational diabetes

ICD-9-CM Code(s): _____

ICD-10-CM Code(s): _____

1.417. Exposure to uranium

ICD-9-CM Code(s): _____

ICD-10-CM Code(s): _____

1.418. Homicidal ideation

ICD-9-CM Code(s): _____

ICD-10-CM Code(s): _____

ICD-9-CM Procedure Coding

1.419. Vasectomy

ICD-9-CM Code(s): _____

1.420. Stapling of left atrial appendage (LAA)

ICD-9-CM Code(s): _____

1.421. Right thyroid lobectomy

ICD-9-CM Code(s): _____

1.422. Lamellar keratoplasty with donor corneal tissue

ICD-9-CM Code(s): _____

1.423. Myringotomy with placement of pressure equalization tube

ICD-9-CM Code(s): _____

1.424. Cleft palate repair

ICD-9-CM Code(s): _____

1.425. Lung volume reduction surgery

ICD-9-CM Code(s): _____

1.426. Open-heart surgery for repair of atrial septal defect with mesh

ICD-9-CM Code(s): _____

1.427. Right coronary artery PTCA

ICD-9-CM Code(s): _____

1.428. Coronary artery bypass grafting using left and right internal mammary arteries

ICD-9-CM Code(s): _____

1.429. Bilateral radical neck dissection

ICD-9-CM Code(s): _____

1.430. Total intra-abdominal colectomy performed by laparoscope

ICD-9-CM Code(s): _____

1.431. Whipple procedure

ICD-9-CM Code(s): _____

1.432. Right direct inguinal herniorrhaphy with mesh

ICD-9-CM Code(s): _____

1.433. Transplant nephrectomy

ICD-9-CM Code(s): _____

1.434. Paraurethral suspension utilizing Pereyra suture

ICD-9-CM Code(s): _____

1.435. Pelvic exenteration for ovarian cancer

ICD-9-CM Code(s): _____

1.436. Repair of fourth-degree laceration of rectum during delivery

ICD-9-CM Code(s): _____

1.437. Right total hip replacement

ICD-9-CM Code(s): _____

1.438. Reattachment of arm amputated through humerus

ICD-9-CM Code(s): _____

1.439. Mid-forceps extraction with episiotomy

ICD-9-CM Code(s): _____

1.440. Retropubic prostatectomy

ICD-9-CM Code(s): _____

1.441. Subtotal jejunectomy with end-to-end anastomosis

ICD-9-CM Code(s): _____

1.442. Percutaneous transmyocardial revascularization

ICD-9-CM Code(s): _____

1.443. Insertion of drug-eluting coronary artery stent

ICD-9-CM Code(s): _____

ICD-10-PCS Coding

1.444. Bilateral vasectomy, open.

ICD-10-PCS Code(s): _____

1.445. Ventriculoperitoneostomy: The operative report indicates that a synthetic shunt is placed to allow passage of the cerebral spinal fluid to the peritoneal cavity.

ICD-10-PCS Code(s): _____

1.446. Right thyroid lobectomy: The operative report indicates that the entire right thyroid lobe was excised using an open approach.

ICD-10-PCS Code(s): _____

1.447. Percutaneous lamellar keratoplasty, left cornea, with donor corneal tissue.

ICD-10-PCS Code(s): _____

1.448. Right myringotomy with placement of pressure equalization tube.

ICD-10-PCS Code(s): _____

1.449. Left below knee amputation, proximal tibia and fibula.

ICD-10-PCS Code(s): _____

1.450. Mitral valve replacement using porcine tissue, open.

ICD-10-PCS Code(s): _____

1.451. Right coronary artery PTCA.

ICD-10-PCS Code(s): _____

1.452. Fulguration of sigmoid colon polyp, endoscopic.

ICD-10-PCS Code(s): _____

1.453. Thrombectomy of arteriovenous dialysis graft. The operative report indicates that the AV graft is located in the right upper arm with the right cephalic vein being obstructed with the thrombus. An incision was performed as the approach to the procedure.

ICD-10-PCS Code(s): _____

1.454. Bilateral direct inguinal herniorrhaphy, open.

ICD-10-PCS Code(s): _____

1.455. Right kidney transplant, organ donor match.

ICD-10-PCS Code(s): _____

1.456. Laparoscopic left carpal tunnel release.

ICD-10-PCS Code(s): _____

1.457. Open reduction with internal fixation, left fibula.

ICD-10-PCS Code(s): _____

1.458. Right total hip replacement. The operative report indicated that the procedure was performed via an incision and the devices implanted were ceramic-on-ceramic.

ICD-10-PCS Code(s): _____

1.459. Posterior spinal fusion of the posterior column at L2–L4 with Bak cage interbody fusion device, open.

ICD-10-PCS Code(s): _____

1.460. Diagnostic arthroscopy of the right knee.

ICD-10-PCS Code(s): _____

1.461. Revision of left knee replacement with readjustment of prosthesis, open.

ICD-10-PCS Code(s): _____

1.462. EGD with duodenal biopsy.

ICD-10-PCS Code(s): _____

1.463. Laparoscopic-assisted total vaginal hysterectomy.

ICD-10-PCS Code(s): _____

1.464. Hysteroscopy with diagnostic D&C.

ICD-10-PCS Code(s): _____

1.465. Extracorporeal shockwave lithotripsy (EWSL) of right ureter.

ICD-10-PCS Code(s): _____

Chapter 2

Basic Principles of CPT Coding

The following exercises are designed to review CPT coding guidelines and to provide practice in assigning CPT codes. Because CPT indexes procedures in many different ways, the rationale for the selection of a particular code may be different from the approach that you use. The information included in the rationale is not meant to describe the only way to obtain an appropriate code but to represent one possible way. Unless the coder is specifically instructed to assign modifiers, no modifiers will appear in the rationale.

Note: These exercises were developed to be used with the 2011 edition of CPT but are suitable for other editions in most cases.

Instructions: Circle the correct answer, fill in the blank, or assign the correct code(s) for each of the following exercise items.

CPT Organization, Structure, and Guidelines

2.1.   Category II codes cover all but one of the following topics. Which is not addressed by Category II codes?

   a. Patient management
   b. New technology
   c. Therapeutic, preventive, or other interventions
   d. Patient safety

2.2.   In CPT, the symbols ▶◀ are used to indicate:

   a. Changes in verbiage within code descriptions
   b. A new code
   c. Changes in verbiage other than that in code descriptions; for example, changes in coding guidelines or parenthetical notes
   d. A code for which there is a corresponding HCPCS Level II code

2.3.   During the performance of a femoral angioplasty, a patient develops additional areas of occlusion. A diagnostic angiogram of the affected artery is performed. Is it appropriate to code this diagnostic study in addition to the therapeutic procedure?

a. No. All diagnostic procedures are included in therapeutic interventional procedures.
b. Yes. Per revised coding guidelines, if there is a clinical change during an interventional procedure that requires further diagnostic study, the diagnostic angiogram may be reported in addition to the therapeutic procedure.

2.4.   Per CPT coding guidelines, a "complete" diagnostic ultrasound of the retroperitoneum includes at least the following organs:

a. Kidneys, abdominal aorta, common iliac artery origins, inferior vena cava
b. Kidneys, abdominal aorta, common iliac artery origins, inferior vena cava, urinary bladder
c. Liver, gallbladder, common bile duct, pancreas, spleen, kidneys, upper aorta, inferior vena cava
d. Kidneys, abdominal aorta, common iliac artery origins

2.5.   A list of codes describing procedures that include conscious sedation, if administered by the same surgeon as performs the procedure, can be found in:

a. Appendix E
b. Appendix F
c. Appendix G
d. Appendix H

2.6.   True or false? Category II codes may be used as the first-listed CPT code when the patient is seen only for counseling.

a. True
b. False

2.7.   Which of the appendices would a neurologist's practice consult to determine the nerve conduction code to assign for a study of the suprascapular motor nerve to the infraspinatus?

a. Appendix I
b. Appendix J
c. Appendix K
d. Appendix L

2.8.   In order to be included in the CPT manual, a procedure must meet which of the following criteria?

a. It must be commonly performed by many physicians across the country.
b. It must be consistent with contemporary medical practice.
c. It must be covered by Medicare.
d. Both a and b

2.9. Which of the following statements about CPT Category III codes is false?

    a. They are updated only once every 2 years.
    b. They were developed to reflect emerging technologies and procedures.
    c. They are archived after 5 years if the code has not been accepted for inclusion in the main body of CPT.
    d. Reimbursement for these services is dependent on individual payer policy.

2.10. Per CPT guidelines, a separate procedure:

    a. Is coded when it is performed as a part of another, larger procedure
    b. Is considered to be an integral part of another, larger service
    c. Is never coded under any circumstances
    d. Both a and b above

2.11. Which of the following statements is (are) true of CPT codes?

    a. They are numeric.
    b. They describe nonphysician services.
    c. They are updated annually by CMS.
    d. All of the above

2.12. What does the symbol ▲ before a code in the CPT manual signify?

    a. The code is new for this year.
    b. The code is exempt from bundling requirements.
    c. The code can only be used as an add-on code, never reported alone or first.
    d. The code has been revised in some way this year.

2.13. What does the symbol ● before a code in the CPT manual signify?

    a. The code is new for this year.
    b. The code is exempt from bundling requirements.
    c. The code can only be used as an add-on code, never reported alone or first.
    d. The code has been revised in some way this year.

2.14. CPT was developed and is maintained by:

    a. CMS
    b. AMA
    c. The Cooperating Parties
    d. WHO

2.15. CPT is updated:

    a. Annually for the main body of codes and every 6 months for Category III codes
    b. Annually
    c. Every 6 months
    d. As often as required by new technology

2.16.   The Alphabetic Index to CPT includes listings for:

    a. Procedures/services
    b. Examinations/tests
    c. Anatomic sites
    d. All of the above

2.17.   The use of the term "for" followed by a diagnosis in CPT means that:

    a. The procedure must be reported for that diagnosis.
    b. The procedure can only be reported for that diagnosis.
    c. The diagnosis is an example of the types of diagnoses for which this procedure could be done.
    d. None of the above

2.18.   If a surgeon performs a procedure for which there is no CPT code and no HCPCS Level II code, what code should be reported on the CMS 1500 form?

    a. CPT code 99999
    b. An unlisted procedure code from the appropriate chapter of CPT
    c. An ICD-9-CM procedure code
    d. A procedure that does not have a valid CPT code should not be reported.

2.19.   There are six sections to CPT: E/M, anesthesia, surgery, radiology, medicine, and _____.

2.20.   The symbol + before a code in CPT means that:

    a. This code can never be reported alone.
    b. This code can never be reported first.
    c. This is an add-on code.
    d. All of the above

2.21.   A listing of all current modifiers is found in which appendix of CPT?

    a. Appendix A
    b. Appendix B
    c. Appendix C
    d. Appendix D

2.22.   The codes in the musculoskeletal section of CPT may be used by:

    a. Orthopedic surgeons only
    b. Orthopedic surgeons and emergency department physicians
    c. Any physician
    d. Orthopedic surgeons and neurosurgeons

Evaluation and Management (E/M) Services

2.23. A nursing facility patient develops an acute illness and is seen by her attending physician. He performs a detailed interval history and a detailed physical examination and performs medical decision making of moderate complexity. What code should the physician use to report these services?

a. 99304
b. 99305
c. 99309
d. 99310
e. 99318

2.24. For reporting of physician services, E/M codes are usually based on:

a. Documentation of history, physical examination, and medical decision making
b. The final diagnosis for the visit
c. The amount of time spent with the patient
d. Documentation of medical decision making

2.25. Select the appropriate E/M code for a new patient office visit in which a comprehensive history and comprehensive physical examination were performed and medical decision making was of high complexity.

_____

2.26. Select the appropriate E/M code for a new patient office visit in which a comprehensive history and comprehensive physical examination were performed and medical decision making was of straightforward complexity. _____

2.27. Select the appropriate E/M code for an established patient visit in which a comprehensive history and expanded problem-focused physical examination were performed and medical decision making was of low complexity.

_____

2.28. When counseling consumes more than half the total visit time, _____ may be used as the criterion for assigning the E/M code.

2.29. Observation E/M codes (99218–99220) are used when:

a. A patient is admitted and discharged on the same date.
b. A patient is admitted for routine nursing care following surgery.
c. A patient does not meet admission criteria.
d. A patient is placed in designated observation status.

2.30. A physician sees a patient in his office in the morning, then again in the early afternoon, at which time he sends the patient to the hospital in observation status. Later that day he visits the patient in the hospital and admits him as a full inpatient. What E/M codes should be assigned for this day of care?

    a. Two E/M codes for the office visits, one for the observation care, and one for the inpatient admission

    b. One code combining the two office visits, one for the observation care, and one for the inpatient admission

    c. One code for the observation care and one for the inpatient admission

    d. One code for the inpatient admission only

2.31. History, physical examination, and medical decision making are the _____ components considered in assigning an E/M code.

2.32. Which of the following are considered components of the social history?

    a. Occupational history

    b. Marital history

    c. Allergic history

    d. a and b above

2.33. Documentation in history of use of drugs, alcohol, and/or tobacco is considered part of the_____.

    a. Past medical history

    b. Social history

    c. Systems review

    d. History of present illness

2.34. Per CPT guidelines, a presenting problem of moderate severity is one that:

    a. May not require the presence of a physician, but for which care is provided under the supervision of a physician

    b. Runs a definite and prescribed course, is transient in nature and is not likely to permanently alter health status, or has a good prognosis with management and compliance

    c. Has a low risk of morbidity without treatment, little or no risk of mortality without treatment, with full recovery expected without functional impairment

    d. Has a moderate risk of morbidity without treatment, a moderate risk of mortality without treatment, uncertain prognosis, or increased probability of functional impairment

2.35. Pediatric inpatient critical care, patient 6 months of age, first day

    Code(s): _____

2.36. Dr. Smith sees a patient in consultation in the hospital at the request of Dr. Jones. He renders an opinion. He then takes over the management of a portion of the patient's care. What codes should Dr. Smith use to bill for his subsequent hospital visits?

   a. Inpatient consultation codes
   b. Initial inpatient hospital care codes
   c. Subsequent hospital care codes
   d. No codes; the initial consultation includes all subsequent visits

2.37. Assign the appropriate E/M code for an outpatient office consultation in which the physician performed a detailed history, a comprehensive physical examination, and medical decision making of moderate complexity.

   _____

2.38. Per CPT guidelines, a concise statement describing the symptom, problem, condition, diagnosis, or other factor that is the reason for the encounter, usually stated in the patient's words, is the definition of the:

   a. History of present illness
   b. Chief complaint
   c. Admission diagnosis
   d. Past history

2.39. Which of the following are parts of medical decision making?

   a. Number of possible diagnoses or management options that must be considered
   b. Amount or complexity of medical record, diagnostic tests, or other information that must be obtained, reviewed, and analyzed
   c. Risk of significant complications, morbidity, and/or mortality associated with the patient's presenting problem, the diagnostic procedures, and/or the management options
   d. All of the above

2.40. Which E/M codes are used to report services to patients in a facility that provides room, board, and other personal assistance services, generally on a long-term basis?

   a. Outpatient services
   b. Nursing facility care
   c. Domiciliary, rest home, or custodial care services
   d. Care plan oversight services

2.41. Preventive medicine services are based on which of the following criteria?

   a. Documentation of history, physical examination, and medical decision making
   b. Age of the patient
   c. Amount of time spent with the patient
   d. The final diagnosis for the visit

2.42. AHIMA Hospital has a "fast-track" department attached to the emergency department. This area is staffed by emergency department physicians on a rotating basis, treats minor problems, and is open from 5:00 a.m. until 8:00 p.m. What codes should be used to report services rendered in this department?

a. Emergency department services codes
b. Office or other outpatient services codes
c. These are not codable services because the department is not open 24 hours per day.
d. Either office or emergency department codes may be used.

2.43. In order to report a critical care code, a physician must spend at least _____ minutes with a critically ill patient.

Anesthesia Services

2.44. Per CPT guidelines, anesthesia time begins when the anesthesiologist begins to prepare the patient for induction, and ends:

a. When the patient leaves the operating room
b. When the anesthesiologist is no longer in personal attendance
c. When the patient has fulfilled postanesthesia care unit criteria for recovery
d. When the patient leaves the postanesthesia care unit

2.45. A physical status anesthesia modifier of P3 means that a patient:

a. Has a mild systemic disease
b. Has a severe systemic disease
c. Has a severe systemic disease that is a constant threat to life
d. Is moribund

2.46. Qualifying circumstances anesthesia codes are used:

a. In addition to the anesthesia codes
b. To describe provision of anesthesia under particularly difficult circumstances
c. To describe circumstances that impact the character of the anesthesia
d. All of the above

2.47. The qualifying circumstance code to assign when anesthesia services are provided under emergency circumstances is _____.

2.48. Anesthesia for total repair of cleft palate, patient 4 years of age

Code(s): _____

2.49. Anesthesia for tracheal reconstruction, patient 6 months of age

Code(s): _____

2.50. Anesthesia for permanent transvenous pacemaker insertion

Code(s): _____

2.51. Anesthesia for lumbar laminectomy with fusion and insertion of rods and hooks

Code(s): _____

2.52. Anesthesia for ventral hernia repair, patient a 76-year-old female

Code(s): _____

2.53. Anesthesia for donor nephrectomy

Code(s): _____

2.54. Anesthesia for left knee arthroscopy with medial meniscectomy

Code(s): _____

2.55. Anesthesia for total hip replacement

Code(s): _____

2.56. Anesthesia for vasectomy

Code(s): _____

2.57. Anesthesia for cesarean section following failed attempt at vaginal delivery under spinal anesthesia

Code(s): _____

2.58. Anesthesia for emergency completion of near-total amputation through the midthigh with laceration of femoral artery with imminent exsanguination

Code(s): _____

2.59. Anesthesia for ORIF of fracture of the distal tibia and fibula

Code(s): _____

2.60. Anesthesia for left ventricular reduction surgery with heart–lung bypass and systemic hypothermia

Code(s): _____

2.61. Anesthesia for Whipple procedure

Code(s): _____

2.62. Anesthesia for direct coronary artery bypass grafting with pump oxygenator

Code(s): _____

2.63. Anesthesia for laparoscopically assisted vaginal hysterectomy

Code(s): _____

Integumentary System

2.64.   A patient undergoes placement of brachytherapy after loading of catheters into her right breast under conscious sedation. The physician who performs the procedure administers the Versed himself, and a nurse is present throughout the procedure to monitor the patient. Is it appropriate for the surgeon to report the conscious sedation for this procedure?

   a. Yes
   b. No

2.65.   Tissue transplanted from one individual to another of the same species but different genotype is called a(n):

   a. Autograft
   b. Xenograft
   c. Allograft or allogeneic graft
   d. Heterograft

2.66.   True or false? Per coding guidelines, skin grafting codes cannot be used unless there is surgical fixation of the graft to the recipient tissue.

   a. True
   b. False

2.67.   When a malignant lesion is excised and the resultant skin defect is closed with a Z-plasty, what code(s) should be reported?

   a. A code for the Z-plasty only (14000–14061)
   b. A code for the malignant lesion excision (11600–11646) and a code for the Z-plasty (14000–14061)
   c. A code for the malignant lesion excision only (11600–11646)
   d. A code for the complex repair only (13100–13160)

2.68.   When lesions are excised from multiple sites, which of the following is the correct coding protocol?

   a. Add all the dimensions and assign one code based on the total area.
   b. Code each lesion separately.
   c. Code only the largest lesion.
   d. Add all the dimensions for each body part, such as arms, legs, and so on, and assign as many codes as there are body parts treated.

2.69.   A patient presents with a palpable lump in the left breast. The surgeon dissects down to the mass and removes it entirely. The procedure is described as "Biopsy of mass of left breast." Assign the appropriate CPT code (omitting modifiers).

   a. 19120
   b. 19101
   c. 19125
   d. 19301

2.70. When calculating dimensions for assigning a lesion excision code, which of the following is the appropriate method?

    a. Measurement of the lesion documented by the surgeon preexcision

    b. Measurement of the lesion plus circumferential margins documented by the surgeon preexcision

    c. Measurement of the lesion documented by the pathologist postexcision

    d. Measurement of the lesion plus circumferential margins documented by the pathologist postexcision

2.71. "The sharp removal by transverse incision or horizontal slicing to remove epidermal and dermal lesions without a full-thickness dermal excision" is the CPT definition of_____.

2.72. Debridement of skin, subcutaneous tissue, muscle, and bone. A total surface area of 18 sq cm was debrided down to and including removal of subcutaneous tissue.

    Code(s): _____

2.73. Excision of 2.5-cm solar keratosis of the cheek with no significant margins

    Code(s): _____

2.74. Excision of basal cell carcinoma, abdominal wall, 1.2 cm in diameter, with 1-cm skin margin all around

    Code(s): _____

2.75. Excision of skin and subcutaneous tissue from the right groin for hidradenitis, with layered closure

    Code(s): _____

2.76. Insertion and injection of tissue expander, scalp

    Code(s): _____

2.77. Repair of 5.2-cm laceration of the left hand, dorsum, with layered closure

    Code(s): _____

2.78. Repair of 3.4-cm laceration of the left forearm, single-layer closure with 4-0 Dexon; repair of 2.0-cm laceration of the left upper arm, single-layer closure

    Code(s): _____

2.79. Repair of 3.0-cm laceration of the scalp, 2.5-cm laceration of the left foot, and 6.0-cm laceration of the left lower leg

    Code(s): _____

2.80.   Repair of 5.0-cm laceration of the left cheek, 3.2-cm laceration of the forehead, and 16.0-cm complex laceration of the left chest wall, utilizing multilayered closure

Code(s): _____

2.81.   Incision and drainage of complicated pilonidal cyst

Code(s): _____

2.82.   A wound repair that involves layered closure of one or more of the deeper layers of subcutaneous tissue and superficial (nonmuscle) fascia or extensive cleaning of heavily contaminated wounds is a (an) _____ repair.

2.83.   Open excisional biopsy of breast lesion identified by preoperative placement of radiological marker

Code(s): _____

2.84.   Mohs micrographic surgery involves the surgeon acting as:

a. Both plastic surgeon and general surgeon
b. Both surgeon and pathologist
c. Both plastic surgeon and dermatologist
d. Both dermatologist and pathologist

2.85.   Excision of nonpalpable suspicious area of possible microcalcification identified on mammogram (needle identifying the site placed at an outside radiologist's suite)

Code(s): _____

2.86.   Excision of 2-cm squamous cell carcinoma from left chest with repair of resultant 8-cm^2 defect using V-Y plasty

Code(s): _____

2.87.   Insertion of breast expander in post-mastectomy patient

Code(s): _____

2.88.   Debridement down to and including removal of muscle and subcutaneous system; total surface area is 22 sq cm.

Code(s): _____

2.89.   Complex wound repair (13100–13160) may require extensive undermining, placement of stents, or retention sutures.

a. True
b. False

2.90. Debridement is always considered a separate procedure and should always be reported.

    a. True
    b. False

2.91. Simple repair of a 3.0-cm laceration cheek with extensive removal of gravel and debris.

    Code(s): _____

Musculoskeletal System

2.92. Per coding guidelines, the type of fracture does not have a coding correlation to the type of treatment provided.

    a. True
    b. False

2.93. True or false? If a bone biopsy is performed in conjunction with a kyphoplasty procedure, it is separately coded.

    a. True
    b. False

2.94. Per the description of code 22523, fracture reduction and bone biopsy, if performed, are included in the procedure and are not separately coded. 3D reconstruction is not to be reported with which of the following base modalities?

    a. CT angiography
    b. MR angiography
    c. PET scans
    d. All of the above

2.95. Which of the following terms does not describe an open fracture?

    a. Missile
    b. Comminuted
    c. Infected
    d. Compound

2.96. Open fracture treatment includes which of the following scenarios?

    a. The fractured bone is exposed to the environment.
    b. The bone ends are visualized and internal fixation inserted.
    c. The fractured bone is opened remote from the fracture site and an intramedullary nail is inserted across the fracture site.
    d. All of the above

2.97. If an orthopedic surgeon attempted to reduce a fracture but was unsuccessful in obtaining acceptable alignment, what type of code should be assigned for the procedure?

    a. A "with manipulation" code
    b. A "without manipulation" code
    c. An unlisted procedure code
    d. An E/M code only

2.98. Keller bunionectomy

    Code(s): _____

2.99. Diagnostic arthroscopy, left knee, with medial and lateral meniscectomy

    Code(s): _____

2.100. Open reduction of knee dislocation with repair of the anterior cruciate ligament by anchor suture

    Code(s): _____

2.101. Percutaneous vertebroplasty, T10. (Do not assign radiological supervision and interpretation code.)

    Code(s): _____

2.102. Incision and drainage of infected shoulder bursa

    Code(s): _____

2.103. Putti-Platt procedure, left shoulder

    Code(s): _____

2.104. Open reduction, internal fixation humerus shaft fracture with cast application

    Code(s): _____

2.105. Wrist fusion with bone graft from iliac crest

    Code(s): _____

2.106. Closed reduction of distal radial wrist fracture

    Code(s): _____

2.107. Total hip arthroplasty

    Code(s): _____

2.108. Casting is separately reported:

    a. When applied to stabilize or for comfort, by a separate physician
    b. For initial application by a physician who does not perform the fracture care
    c. When recasting is done during fracture follow-up
    d. All of the above

2.109. Anterior removal of artificial cervical disc

Code(s): _____

2.110. Bone biopsy obtained from iliac crest

Code(s): _____

2.111. Application of short leg walking cast for severe sprain of ankle

Code(s): _____

2.112. Arthroscopy of shoulder with complete rotator cuff repair

Code(s): _____

2.113. Midthigh amputation of leg

Code(s): _____

2.114. Closed reduction, temporomandibular joint dislocation

Code(s): _____

2.115. Which of the following terms is used to describe the reduction of a fracture?

a. Manipulation
b. Traction
c. Percutaneous fixation
d. External fixation

2.116. Hip arthroscopy to perform a femoroplasty

Code(s): _____

2.117. Open treatment of 2 lumbar vertebral fractures, posterior approach

Code(s): _____

2.118. Non-segmental instrumentation is defined as fixation at each end of the construct and at least one additional interposed bony attachment.

a. True
b. False

2.119. Cranial halo application with seven pins placed for thin skull osteology

Code(s): _____

2.120. Excision of a 2.3-cm soft tissue tumor of the hand

Code(s): _____

2.121. Incision and drainage of infected bursa of the left shoulder.

Code(s): _____

2.122. Removal of 19 skin tags.

Code(s): _____

Respiratory System

2.123. A pulmonologist performed a diagnostic bronchoscopy with biopsy. The endoscope was introduced into the bronchus, and attachments were used to perforate the bronchial wall. Tissue was obtained and submitted to the pathologist, who identified it as "lung parenchyma." What type of biopsy was performed?

    a. Transbronchial lung biopsy
    b. Bronchial biopsy
    c. Bronchoalveolar lavage
    d. Protected specimen brush biopsy

2.124. Submucous resection of nasal turbinates

Code(s): _____

2.125. Control of epistaxis, anterior, by packing and silver nitrate cautery

Code(s): _____

2.126. Nasal sinus endoscopy with total ethmoidectomy

Code(s): _____

2.127. Total laryngectomy with left radical neck dissection

Code(s): _____

2.128. Direct laryngoscopy with vocal cord stripping using the operating microscope

Code(s): _____

2.129. Bronchoscopy with transbronchial lung biopsy

Code(s): _____

2.130. Thoracentesis with placement of tube

Code(s): _____

2.131. Thoracoscopy of the mediastinal space

Code(s): _____

2.132. Open Caldwell-Luc procedure of maxillary sinuses

Code(s): _____

2.133. Emergency endotracheal intubation

Code(s): _____

2.134. Flexible bronchoscopy with placement of catheters for afterloading of radiotherapeutic agents

Code(s): _____

2.135. Right lung middle lobectomy

Code(s): _____

2.136. Double-lung transplant

Code(s): _____

2.137. Functional endoscopic sinus surgery (FESS) with frontal sinus polyp removal

Code(s): _____

2.138. Endoscopic control of nasal hemorrhage

Code(s): _____

2.139. When a bronchoscopy is performed under fluoroscopic guidance, how are the codes assigned per CPT coding guidelines?

    a. The fluoroscopy guidance code is assigned as a secondary procedure code with the bronchoscopy code.

    b. The fluoroscopy guidance code is assigned as the first procedure code.

    c. The fluoroscopy is included in the bronchoscopy and no code is assigned for it.

    d. Individual hospital coding guidelines determine whether the fluoroscopy is separately coded.

2.140. Talc pleurodesis for pneumothorax

Code(s): _____

2.141. Laryngoplasty for reconstruction following third-degree chemical burns of the larynx

Code(s): _____

2.142. Anterovertical hemilaryngectomy

Code(s): _____

2.143. A surgical thoracoscopy always includes a diagnostic thoracoscopy.

    a. True

    b. False

2.144. Nasal endoscopy with dilation of frontal sinus ostium

Code(s): _____

2.145. Thoracotomy with removal of foreign body in the lung

Code(s): _____

2.146. Clagett procedure of chest wall

Code(s): _____

Cardiovascular System

2.147. Codes describing endovascular repair of the descending thoracic aorta include all of the following procedures except one. Which procedure is not included in the repair code?

a. Arterial embolization
b. Angiography of the thoracic aorta
c. Fluoroscopic guidance in delivery of the endovascular components
d. Preprocedure diagnostic imaging

2.148. True or false? A combination code exists for ligation and stripping of the long saphenous vein and ligation and stripping of the short saphenous vein.

a. True
b. False

2.149. In coding arterial catheterizations, when the tip of the catheter is manipulated from the insertion into the aorta and then out into another artery, this is called:

a. Selective catheterization
b. Nonselective catheterization
c. Manipulative catheterization
d. Radical catheterization

2.150. Complete pericardiectomy with cardiopulmonary bypass

Code(s): _____

2.151. Insertion of permanent pacemaker with ventricular transvenous leads

Code(s): _____

2.152. When coding a selective catheterization, how are codes assigned?

    a. One code for each vessel entered

    b. One code for the point of entry vessel

    c. One code for the final vessel entered

    d. One code for the vessel of entry and one for the final vessel, with intervening vessels not coded

2.153. Replacement of the mitral valve with cardiopulmonary bypass

    Code(s): _____

2.154. CABG using saphenous vein to the LAD

    Code(s): _____

2.155. LIMA graft to the circumflex coronary artery and sequentially to the right coronary artery

    Code(s): _____

2.156. Removal of intra-aortic balloon pump, percutaneous

    Code(s): _____

2.157. Introduction of catheter into the aorta

    Code(s): _____

2.158. Venipuncture by cutdown, patient 32 years of age

    Code(s): _____

2.159. A 4-year-old patient required implantation of a tunneled central venous catheter with insertion of a Life-Port vascular access device (VAD).

    Code(s): _____

2.160. Creation of Brescia-Cimino fistula for chronic hemodialysis

    Code(s): _____

2.161. Ligation and stripping of long and short saphenous veins

    Code(s): _____

2.162. Laparoscopic splenectomy

    Code(s): _____

2.163. Injection for identification of sentinel node

Code(s): _____

2.164. Temporal artery biopsy

Code(s): _____

2.165. A tunneled centrally-inserted central venous catheter is placed in a 57-year-old patient.

Code(s): _____

2.166. Blood transfusion

Code(s): _____

2.167. Aortobifemoral bypass graft

Code(s): _____

2.168. Percutaneous transluminal popliteal angioplasty

Code(s): _____

2.169. The physician documents that he replaced the cardiac pacemaker "battery." The physician is actually referring to the:

a. Lead
b. Generator
c. Electrode
d. Cardioverter

2.170. Replacement of a peripherally inserted central venous catheter (through same access)

Code(s): _____

2.171. Percutaneous endovascular revascularization of the right femoral vessel with transluminal stent placement and atherectomy

Code(s): _____

2.172. Application of right and left pulmonary artery bands

Code(s): _____

Digestive System

2.173. Primary repair of bilateral cleft lip, one-stage procedure

Code(s): _____

2.174. Laparoscopical repair of paraesophageal hernia with mesh

Code(s): _____

2.175. Uvulopalatopharyngoplasty for sleep apnea

Code(s): _____

2.176. T&A, 16-year-old patient

Code(s): _____

2.177. Upper gastrointestinal endoscopy with biopsy of lesion of esophagus

Code(s): _____

2.178. Per CPT coding guidelines, if a lesion is biopsied and then the remainder of the lesion is removed, what code(s) is (are) assigned?

    a. A code for the biopsy and one for the lesion excision
    b. A code for the lesion excision only
    c. A code for the biopsy only
    d. Hospital-specific coding procedures determine what is coded.

2.179. Rigid esophagoscopy with removal of impacted food

Code(s): _____

2.180. EGD with esophageal dilation over guidewire

Code(s): _____

2.181. When the physician does not specify the method used to remove a lesion during an endoscopy, what is the appropriate procedure?

    a. Assign the removal by snare technique code.
    b. Assign the removal by hot biopsy forceps code.
    c. Assign the ablation code.
    d. Query the physician as to the method used.

2.182. ERCP with sphincterotomy

Code(s): _____

2.183. Laparoscopic Nissen fundoplication

Code(s): _____

2.184. Laparoscopic gastric banding

Code(s): _____

2.185. Endoscopic percutaneous gastrostomy tube placement

Code(s): _____

2.186. Incision and drainage perianal abscess

Code(s): _____

2.187. Laparoscopic partial colectomy with end colostomy (Hartmann procedure)

Code(s): _____

2.188. Placement of seton

Code(s): _____

2.189. Small bowel endoscopy with control of hemorrhagic site in ileum using bipolar cautery

Code(s): _____

2.190. Colonoscopy with removal of five colonic polyps using hot biopsy forceps

Code(s): _____

2.191. Flexible sigmoidoscopy with decompression of volvulus

Code(s): _____

2.192. Laparoscopic cholecystectomy with cholangiography duct

Code(s): _____

2.193. Destruction of 2 groups of internal hemorrhoids with the use of infrared coagulation

Code(s): _____

2.194. Proctosigmoidoscopy with multiple biopsies and removal of foreign body

Code(s): _____

2.195. Complete esophagogastric fundoplasty via thoracotomy

Code(s): _____

Urinary System

2.196. Percutaneous needle biopsy of kidney

Code(s): _____

2.197. Donor nephrectomy, live donor

Code(s): _____

2.198. Surgical laparoscopy with ablation of renal cysts

Code(s): _____

2.199. Extracorporeal sound wave lithotripsy of large kidney stone

Code(s): _____

2.200. Change of ureterostomy tube

Code(s): _____

2.201. Cystometrogram with voiding pressure studies

Code(s): _____

2.202. Placement of indwelling bladder catheter

Code(s): _____

2.203. Cystourethroscopy with fulguration of three bladder tumors ranging in size from 0.4 to 1.6 cm

Code(s): _____

2.204. Cystourethroscopy with insertion of urethral stent

Code(s): _____

2.205. Cystourethroscopy with insertion of double-J ureteral stent

Code(s): _____

2.206. Percutaneous cryoablation of two moderate-sized renal tumors

Code(s): _____

2.207. Transurethral resection of prostate with control of postoperative bleeding

Code(s): _____

2.208. Insertion of inflatable urethra–bladder neck sphincter

Code(s): _____

2.209. Repeat dilation of urethral stricture with filiforms and followers, male patient

Code(s): _____

2.210. Laparoscopic ureterolithotomy

Code(s): _____

2.211. Insertion of temporary prostatic urethral stent

Code(s): _____

2.212. Anterior vesicourethropexy by Marshall-Marchetti-Krantz procedure

Code(s): _____

2.213. Cystourethroscopy with biopsy of bladder wall

Code(s): _____

2.214. Cystourethroscopy with diagnostic ureteroscopy and removal of ureteral stones

Code(s): _____

2.215. Repeat transurethral resection of prostate tissue 4 years after original procedure

Code(s): _____

2.216. Transurethral radiofrequency micro-remodeling of the female bladder neck and proximal urethra

Code(s): _____

2.217. Closure of nephrovisceral fistula via thoracic approach

Code(s): _____

2.218. Backbench preparation of cadaver renal donor prior to transplantation including dissection of fat and other attachments, excision of adrenal gland, and preparation of ureters and vascular structures

Code(s): _____

Male/Female Genital System and Laparoscopy

2.219. Laser destruction of condylomata of penis

Code(s): _____

2.220. Insertion of inflatable penile prosthesis

Code(s): _____

2.221. Removal and replacement of semi-rigid penile prosthesis from infected site, with irrigation and debridement of infected and necrotic tissue

Code(s): _____

2.222. Laparoscopic orchiopexy for undescended (intra-abdominal) testicle

Code(s): _____

2.223. Vasectomy

Code(s): _____

2.224. Needle biopsy of prostate

Code(s): _____

2.225. Radical retropubic prostatectomy

Code(s): _____

2.226. Incision and drainage of Bartholin's abscess

Code(s): _____

2.227. Colposcopy of cervix with cervical curettage

Code(s): _____

2.228. Total abdominal hysterectomy with concurrent Marshall-Marchetti-Krantz urethropexy

Code(s): _____

2.229. Vaginal hysterectomy (weight of uterus, 283 g) with bilateral salpingo-oophorectomy

Code(s): _____

2.230. Biopsy of right ovary

Code(s): _____

2.231. Laparoscopic myomectomy with removal of eight intramural myomas

Code(s): _____

2.232. Ligation of fallopian tubes for elective sterilization

Code(s): _____

2.233. Laparoscopic sterilization procedure with Falope-rings, bilateral

Code(s): _____

2.234. Bilateral salpingo-oophorectomy for ovarian malignancy with pelvic lymph node and peritoneal biopsies

Code(s): _____

2.235. Catheterization with dye injection for hysterosalpingogram

Code(s): _____

2.236. Eight-day-old male infant surgically circumcised per parents' request

Code(s): _____

2.237. Testicular torsion repair

Code(s): _____

2.238. Laparoscopic fulguration of endometrial implants on the peritoneum and broad ligament

Code(s): _____

2.239. What is the correct CPT code assignment for hysteroscopy with lysis of intrauterine adhesions?

   a. 58559
   b. 58558, 58559
   c. 58559, 58558, 58740
   d. 58559, 58740

2.240. Insertion of a radiation afterloading apparatus into the vagina for brachytherapy

Code(s): _____

2.241. Repair of an incomplete circumcision

Code(s): _____

2.242. One stage urethroplasty using local skin flaps; patient has hypospadias

Code(s): _____

2.243. Excision of hydrocele, bilateral

Code(s): _____

2.244. Incision and drainage of a vulvar abscess

Code(s): _____

2.245. Hysteroscopy, with sampling of endometrium

Code(s): _____

Endocrine System

2.246. Incision and drainage of infected thyroglossal duct cyst

Code(s): _____

2.247. Percutaneous needle biopsy of thyroid gland

Code(s): _____

2.248. Excision of adenoma of thyroid

Code(s): _____

2.249. Partial right-sided thyroidectomy

Code(s): _____

2.250. Partial right-sided thyroid lobectomy with isthmusectomy and subtotal resection of left thyroid

Code(s): _____

2.251. Left total thyroid lobectomy

Code(s): _____

2.252. Total right-sided thyroid lobectomy with isthmusectomy and subtotal resection of left thyroid

Code(s): _____

2.253. Total thyroidectomy

Code(s): _____

2.254. Total thyroidectomy for thyroid carcinoma with partial neck dissection

Code(s): _____

2.255. Thyroidectomy for thyroid carcinoma with radical neck dissection

Code(s): _____

2.256. Parathyroidectomy

Code(s): _____

2.257. Thyroidectomy (with sternal portion of thyroid) via cervical approach

Code(s): _____

2.258. Excision of recurrent thyroglossal duct cyst

Code(s): _____

2.259. Parathyroidectomy with mediastinal exploration

Code(s): _____

2.260. Transthoracic thymectomy

Code(s): _____

2.261. Exploration and biopsy of adrenal glands, transabdominal

Code(s): _____

2.262. Laparoscopic adrenalectomy

Code(s): _____

2.263. Excision of carotid body tumor and carotid artery

Code(s): _____

2.264. Thymectomy with radical mediastinal dissection

Code(s): _____

2.265. Aspiration of thyroid gland cyst

Code(s): _____

2.266. Repair of an intracranial AV malformation, dural, simple

Code(s): _____

2.267. Injection of a combination anesthetic and cortisone into the cervical spine

Code(s): _____

Nervous System

2.268. Cranial burr holes for drainage of subdural hematoma

Code(s): _____

2.269. Decompression craniectomy for treatment of intracranial hypertension

Code(s): _____

2.270. Excision of posterior fossa meningioma tumor via craniectomy

Code(s): _____

2.271. Percutaneous transcatheter embolization, spinal cord

Code(s): _____

2.272. Stereotactic radiosurgery for eradication of a 2.0-cm pituitary tumor

Code(s): _____

2.273. Ventriculoperitoneal shunt procedure

Code(s): _____

2.274. Diagnostic lumbar spinal tap

Code(s): _____

2.275. Implantation of cranial neurostimulator pulse generator

Code(s): _____

2.276. Excision neuroma, digital nerve, right fourth finger. Assign the CPT code and appropriate modifier.

Code(s): _____

2.277. Subtemporal decompression procedure for pseudotumor cerebri

Code(s): _____

2.278. Repair of 20-mm aneurysm, vertebrobasilar circulation

Code(s): _____

2.279. Stereotactic biopsy of intracranial lesion with magnetic resonance (MR) guidance. (Do not assign the radiological supervision and interpretation code.)

Code(s): _____

2.280. Intracranial neuroendoscopy with excision of pituitary tumor

Code(s): _____

2.281. Reprogramming of programmable cerebrospinal fluid shunt

Code(s): _____

2.282. Anterior diskectomy, T2–3 interspace

Code(s): _____

2.283. Injection of lidocaine, brachial plexus

Code(s): _____

2.284. Suture of digital nerves to the left third and fourth fingers. Assign the appropriate modifier(s) in addition to the CPT code.

Code(s): _____

2.285. Phenol injection for destruction of the infraorbital branch of the trigeminal nerve

Code(s): _____

Eye/Ocular Adnexa

2.286. Removal of corneal foreign body using slit lamp

Code(s): _____

2.287. Penetrating keratoplasty, aphakic eye

Code(s): _____

2.288. Removal ocular implant

Code(s): _____

2.289. Extracapsular cataract extraction by phacoemulsification with placement of posterior chamber IOL

Code(s): _____

2.290. Scleral buckle for retinal detachment

Code(s): _____

2.291. YAG laser photocoagulation of diabetic retinopathy

Code(s): _____

2.292. Strabismus surgery with recession of lateral and medial rectus muscles

Code(s): _____

2.293. Strabismus surgery with recession of superior oblique muscle

Code(s): _____

2.294. Strabismus surgery with 6-mm recession of superior rectus muscle and 3-mm recession of inferior rectus muscle, with placement of adjustable suture at inferior rectus

Code(s): _____

2.295. Repair of blepharoptosis by frontalis muscle fascial sling

Code(s): _____

2.296. Repair of entropion by thermocauterization

Code(s): _____

2.297. Dacryocystorhinostomy

Code(s): _____

2.298. Probing of nasolacrimal duct with stent placement

Code(s): _____

2.299. Excision of chalazions (three) from left upper and left lower eyelids

Code(s): _____

2.300. Laser photocoagulation of retina for prophylaxis of retinal detachment

Code(s): _____

2.301. Trabeculectomy ab externo

Code(s): _____

2.302. Enucleation of eyeball with implant, muscle controlled

Code(s): _____

2.303. Removal of foreign body from posterior chamber using magnet

Code(s): _____

2.304. Excision of pterygium with normal conjunctival tissue graft

Code(s): _____

2.305. Subtotal vitrectomy with endolaser panretinal photocoagulation

Code(s): _____

2.306. Placement of amniotic membrane on the eye for wound healing; a single-level suture is used.

Code(s): _____

2.307. Excision of 1.3-cm conjunctival lesion

Code(s): _____

2.308. Photocoagulation, iridoplasty, 3 sessions

Code(s): _____

Auditory System

2.309. Removal of exostosis, external ear canal

Code(s): _____

2.310. Myringotomy with aspiration under general anesthesia

Code(s): _____

2.311. Myringotomy with PE tube insertion

Code(s): _____

2.312. Tympanoplasty with mastoidectomy with ossicular chain reconstruction

Code(s): _____

2.313. Decompression of internal auditory canal

Code(s): _____

2.314. Drainage of abscess of external ear canal

Code(s): _____

2.315. Removal of bead from a toddler's external ear canal using conscious sedation

Code(s): _____

2.316. Biopsy external ear

Code(s): _____

2.317. Removal of impacted cerumen, bilateral

Code(s): _____

2.318. Tympanoplasty without mastoidectomy, with placement of PORP

Code(s): _____

2.319. Tympanostomy with ventilation tube insertion under general anesthesia

Code(s): _____

2.320. Transmastoid excision of glomus tumor of ear

Code(s): _____

2.321. Repair of tympanic membrane perforation using synthetic patch

Code(s): _____

2.322. Stapedotomy with footplate drillout

Code(s): _____

2.323. Implantation of cochlear device

Code(s): _____

2.324. Oval window fistula repair

Code(s): _____

2.325. Transcanal labyrinthectomy with mastoidectomy

Code(s): _____

2.326. Removal and replacement of electromagnetic hearing aid in temporal bone

Code(s): _____

2.327. Debridement of mastoid cavity under general anesthesia

Code(s): _____

2.328. Removal of ventilation tubes under general anesthesia

Code(s): _____

Radiology Services

2.329. True or false? Code 76856 Ultrasound, pelvic (nonobstetrical), real time with image documentation, complete, can be used to describe examinations of either the male or female pelvis.

a. True
b. False

2.330. X-ray of mandible, three views

Code(s): _____

2.331. X-ray, including fluoroscopy, of pharynx for foreign body

Code(s): _____

2.332. CT scan of the brain, with and without contrast

Code(s): _____

2.333. Chest x-ray, AP and lateral

Code(s): _____

2.334. Whole-body PET scan

Code(s): _____

2.335. X-ray, neck, six views, including oblique and flexion

Code(s): _____

2.336. Cervical myelogram, radiological supervision and interpretation

Code(s): _____

2.337. Shoulder arthrogram, radiological supervision and interpretation

Code(s): _____

2.338. X-ray of fractured hip in the operating room to confirm reduction

Code(s): _____

2.339. Barium enema with KUB

Code(s): _____

2.340. Percutaneous transhepatic cholangiography, radiological supervision and interpretation

Code(s): _____

2.341. Intravenous pyelogram with KUB and tomograms

Code(s): _____

2.342. Left external carotid angiography, selective, radiological supervision and interpretation

Code(s): _____

2.343. Ultrasound, pregnant uterus, second trimester

Code(s): _____

2.344. Nonselective pulmonary angiography, radiological supervision and interpretation

Code(s): _____

2.345. SPECT bone scan

Code(s): _____

2.346. Mammographic guidance for preoperative needle placement in breast, radiological supervision and interpretation

Code(s): _____

2.347. Retroperitoneal ultrasound

Code(s): _____

2.348. Acute gastrointestinal blood loss imaging scan

Code(s): _____

2.349. CT scan of the abdomen and pelvis without contrast material would be coded:

a. 72192, 74176
b. 74178
c. 74176
d. 74178, 74177

2.350. A physician administers the injection for a retrograde urethrocystogram. He also provided supervision and interpretation services. What is the correct code(s)?

Code(s): _____

2.351. Ultrasonic guidance for amniocentesis, imaging supervision and interpretation

Code(s): _____

Pathology/Laboratory Services

2.352. The symbol ⟋ added to the Laboratory and Pathology section means:

    a. This is an add-on laboratory code.
    b. The code is sex specific.
    c. This code should only be reported for Medicare patients.
    d. FDA approval of the vaccine is pending.

2.353. Mr. Smith is seen in his primary care physician's office for his annual physical examination. He has a digital rectal examination and is given three small cards to take home and return with fecal samples to screen for colorectal cancer. Assign the appropriate CPT code to report this occult blood sampling.

    a. 82270
    b. 82271
    c. 82272
    d. 82274

2.354. True or false? Code 80048, basic metabolic panel, can be assigned with a modifier of 52, reduced services, if only seven of the eight tests are performed.

    a. True
    b. False

2.355. Code 87900, infectious agent drug susceptibility phenotype prediction using regularly updated genotypic bioinformatics, is used in the management of patients with what disease?

    a. Cancer patients on toxic chemotherapy agents
    b. HIV patients on antiretroviral therapy
    c. Tuberculosis patients on rifampin therapy
    d. Organ transplant patients on immunosuppressive therapy

2.356. Creatine phosphokinase isoenzymes

    Code(s): _____

2.357. Homocysteine

    Code(s): _____

2.358. Free prostate-specific antigen

    Code(s): _____

2.359. Spinal fluid pH

    Code(s): _____

2.360. Hepatic function panel

    Code(s): _____

2.361. Urine sodium

Code(s): _____

2.362. Automated CBC with automated differential

Code(s): _____

2.363. Urine pregnancy test

Code(s): _____

2.364. Protime

Code(s): _____

2.365. Antinuclear antibody titer

Code(s): _____

2.366. VDRL

Code(s): _____

2.367. HBsAb

Code(s): _____

2.368. Chlamydia antibody, IgM

Code(s): _____

2.369. Erythrocyte sedimentation rate, automated

Code(s): _____

2.370. Surgical pathology, examination (gross and microscopic) of arterial biopsy

Code(s): _____

2.371. Surgical pathology, examination (gross and microscopic) of breast and regional lymph nodes

Code(s): _____

2.372. Lyme disease antibody

Code(s): _____

2.373. Automated urinalysis by dip stick with microscopy

Code(s): _____

2.374. Annual Pap test, smear manually obtained under physician supervision and examined by independent laboratory, test results reported using the Bethesda system

Code(s): _____

2.375. Blood culture

Code(s): _____

2.376. Antigen testing of donor blood using reagent serum

Code(s): _____

2.377. Infectious agent genotype analysis by nucleic acid, HIV-1, integrase regions

Code(s): _____

Medicine

2.378. An infusion that lasts less than 15 minutes would be reported with a(n) _____ code.

    a. Intravenous infusion
    b. Intravenous piggyback
    c. Intravenous push
    d. Intravenous hydration

2.379. Codes 96360 and 96361 are used to report infusion of:

    a. Chemotherapeutic agents
    b. Sequential drugs of the same drug family
    c. Hormonal antineoplastics
    d. Prepackaged fluids and/or electrolytes

2.380. A 7-year-old patient is seen for a minor routine therapeutic service that required the administration of moderate sedation for 40 minutes performed by a physician other than the physician performing the therapeutic service. Assign the appropriate CPT code(s).

    a. 99143
    b. 99144
    c. 99149
    d. 99149, 99150

2.381. A prostate cancer patient is seen in the office for infusion of luteinizing hormone-releasing hormone agonist therapy, given subcutaneously. Assign the appropriate CPT code.

    a. 96401
    b. 96402
    c. 96413
    d. 96405

2.382. True or false? When reported by the physician, the "initial service" code under Hydration, Infusions and Chemotherapy is chosen based on the first substance infused.

    a. True
    b. False

2.383. Select the appropriate code(s) to report an injection of rabies immune globulin performed under direct physician supervision.

    a. 96372
    b. 90471
    c. 90375, 96372
    d. 90375, 90473

2.384. Psychotherapy that involves the use of physical aids and nonverbal communication to overcome barriers to therapeutic intervention is called _____ psychotherapy.

2.385. Individual psychotherapy, inpatient hospital, 50 minutes

    Code(s): _____

2.386. Gastric manometry

    Code(s): _____

2.387. Fluorescein angiography

    Code(s): _____

2.388. Reprogramming of cochlear implant device, patient 11 years of age

    Code(s): _____

2.389. Transcatheter placement of coronary artery stent, right coronary artery

    Code(s): _____

2.390. EKG, physician interpretation and report, using hospital equipment

    Code(s): _____

2.391. Combined right heart catheterization and retrograde left heart catheterization for congenital cardiac anomalies

    Code(s): _____

2.392. Electronic analysis of pacing cardioverter-defibrillator, dual chamber, with reprogramming

    Code(s): _____

2.393. Duplex scan of left lower extremity arteries

Code(s): _____

2.394. Pulmonary stress testing with measurements of CO2 production, O2 uptake, and electrocardiographic recordings

Code(s): _____

2.395. EEG, awake and asleep

Code(s): _____

2.396. Therapeutic exercises, 35 minutes

Code(s): _____

2.397. Chiropractic manipulation of the spine, cervical, thoracic, lumbar, and sacral regions

Code(s): _____

2.398. EMG testing of both upper extremities and related paraspinal musculature

Code(s): _____

2.399. Bronchospasm provocation evaluation

Code(s): _____

2.400. Lymphatic drainage (15 minutes of manual traction)

Code(s): _____

2.401. Chemotherapy administration via IV push

Code(s): _____

2.402. Comprehensive electrophysiologic testing with induction of arrhythmia

Code(s): _____

2.403. Vaccine for influenza virus, pandemic formulation, split virus for IM use; patient is 20 years old

Code(s): _____

2.404. Computerized ophthalmic diagnostic imaging, posterior segment, of the right retina

Code(s): _____

2.405. A cardiac clinic performs several cardiac catheterization procedures. Which of the following would be correct to report a right heart catheterization with measurement of oxygen saturation?

    a. 93451, 93455
    b. 93456
    c. 93453
    d. 93451

2.406. Coronary angiography, left ventriculography through left heart catheterization

Code(s): _____

2.407. Chemotherapy administered into the peritoneal cavity via indwelling port

Code(s): _____

Modifiers

2.408. In physician professional fee coding, when multiple procedures other than E/M services are provided on the same date by the same provider, modifier _____ should be appended to the second and all subsequent procedures.

2.409. The modifier used to report therapeutic interventional procedures on the right coronary artery is_____.

2.410. Which of the following circumstances can be described by the use of a HCPCS modifier?

    a. A service has been increased or reduced.
    b. Only part of a service was performed.
    c. A service was provided more than once.
    d. All of the above

2.411. A radiologist interprets x-rays for a community hospital. The equipment belongs to the hospital. What modifier should the radiologist append to his CPT codes? _____

2.412. A patient underwent repair of an ectropion of the left upper eyelid by tarsal wedge technique. Assign the appropriate CPT code and modifier(s).

_____

2.413. A pediatric thoracic and cardiovascular surgeon performs a curative procedure on an infant but does not see the child again. Instead, a pediatric cardiologist does all follow-up. What modifier should the surgeon append to his CPT procedure code? _____

2.414. A surgeon performs a palmar fasciotomy for Dupuytren's contracture of the right hand by open technique. Assign the appropriate CPT code(s) and modifier(s). _____

2.415. A patient is scheduled for a colonoscopy, but due to a sudden drop in blood pressure, the procedure is canceled just as the scope is introduced into the rectum. Because of moderately severe mental retardation, the patient is given a general anesthetic prior to the procedure. How should this procedure be coded by the hospital?

    a. Assign the code for a colonoscopy with modifier -74.
    b. Assign the code for a colonoscopy with modifier -52.
    c. Assign no code because no procedure was performed.
    d. Assign an anesthesia code only.

2.416. When clinical laboratory tests are repeated on the same day, what modifier should be assigned? _____

2.417. When a surgeon performs a procedure and a separately identifiable E/M service on the same date, how should codes and modifiers be assigned?

    a. Assign a code for the procedure only.
    b. Assign a code for the procedure and one for the E/M service without any modifiers.
    c. Assign a code for the procedure and one for the E/M service, with modifier -25 appended to the E/M code.
    d. Assign a code for the procedure and one for the E/M service, with modifier -25 appended to both the E/M code and the procedure code.

2.418. When absolutely identical procedures are performed on both members of a set of paired organs, such as kidneys, what modifier is assigned?

_____

2.419. Planned rigid proctosigmoidoscopy with removal of foreign body under conscious sedation, procedure not completed due to hypotension. How would the physician report this?

Code(s): _____

2.420. When a separately identifiable evaluation and management service is performed by the same physician on the same day of a procedure of their service, what modifier should be reported with the E/M code?

_____

2.421. When a physician performs a consultation as a required second opinion for an HMO, what modifier should be appended to the consultation code?

_____

2.422. When a patient is seen in two hospital outpatient departments in 1 day, what modifier should be appended to the second E/M code to ensure appropriate reimbursement? _____

2.423. When a hospital provides ambulance services by arrangement with a transport company, what modifier should be appended to the codes for ambulance services? _____

2.424. When a procedure or service is performed on the same day as other non-E/M services that are not normally reported together, but are appropriate under certain circumstances, modifier _____ should be appended to indicate that the procedure/service was distinct or independent.

2.425. In addition to the claim submitted by the surgeon, the assistant surgeon also bills for his or her services. What modifier does the assistant surgeon attach to the procedure code? _____

2.426. When two surgeons work together as primary surgeons performing distinct parts of a procedure, each surgeon should report which modifier to the procedure code(s)? _____

2.427. Some reconstructive plastic surgical procedures are performed in multiple stages. What modifier should the surgeon report when the patient is returned to surgery for a planned-staged procedure? _____

Category III Codes

2.428. Which of the following statements about Category III CPT codes is true?

    a. They are temporary.
    b. They are updated more frequently than the rest of CPT.
    c. They are intended to allow for the coding of new technologies, services, and procedures.
    d. All of the above

2.429. Both a regular CPT unlisted procedure code and a Category III code may exist to report the same procedure. Which code(s) should be reported?

    a. Report the CPT unlisted procedure code.
    b. Report the Category III code.
    c. Report both the CPT unlisted procedure code and the Category III code.
    d. Report the Category III code with modifier -59.

2.430. After 5 years, all Category III codes:

    a. Will be archived unless there is evidence that a temporary code is still needed
    b. Will be automatically renewed for another 5 years
    c. Will be automatically retired
    d. Will be replaced with a regular CPT code

2.431. Fistulization of sclera for glaucoma, through ciliary body

    Code(s): _____

2.432. Holotranscobalamin, quantitative

    Code(s): _____

2.433. Excision of rectal tumor via TEMS approach

Code(s): _____

2.434. Lumbar discectomy and arthrodesis utilizing pre-sacral interbody fusion technique

Code(s): _____

2.435. How frequently are Category III codes updated?

    a. Annually
    b. Semiannually
    c. Every two years
    d. Every four months

2.436. Antiprothrombin antibody

Code(s): _____

2.437. Remote real-time interactive video-conferenced critical care, evaluation, and management of a critically ill patient for 60 minutes

Code(s): _____

2.438. Suprachoroidal delivery of pharmacologic agent

Code(s): _____

2.439. Anterior diskectomy and total arthroplasty, utilizing artificial disk, of C3 and C4

Code(s): _____

2.440. Category III codes can be used by what groups of providers?

    a. Hospital outpatient providers only
    b. Physicians only
    c. Hospitals, physicians, insurers, health services researchers
    d. Medicare-approved providers only

2.441. 64-lead electrocardiogram with tracing and graphics, without interpretation and report

Code(s): _____

2.442. Antiprothrombin (phospholipid cofactor) antibody, each Ig class

Code(s): _____

2.443. Laparoscopic removal of gastric stimulation electrodes of the lesser curvature

Code(s): _____

2.444. Speech audiometry threshold, automated

Code(s): _____

2.445. Cerebral perfusion study using CT with contrast

Code(s): _____

2.446. Open treatment of 3 rib fractures using internal fixation

Code(s): _____

2.447. Automated Comprehensive Audiometry threshold evaluation and speech recognition

Code(s): _____

Chapter 3

HCPCS Level II Coding

> **Note:** These exercises are intended for use with the 2011 version of the Healthcare Common Procedure Coding System (HCPCS) Level II codes. HCPCS codes are revised annually by the Centers for Medicare and Medicaid Services (CMS) and become effective January 1 each calendar year. Books are available from a variety of publishers. An electronic file is available for downloading from the Internet at https://www.cms.gov/HCPCSReleaseCodeSets/ANHCPCS/list.asp#TopOfPage.
>
> **Instructions:** Circle the correct answer, fill in the blank, or assign the correct code(s) for each of the following exercise items.

Drugs

3.1. HCPCS Level II contains codes for drugs that are administered:

    a. Subcutaneously
    b. Intramuscularly
    c. Intravenously
    d. All of the above

3.2. Injection Unasyn, 1.5 g

    Code(s): _____

3.3. Injection baclofen, 50 mcg intrathecal trial

    Code(s): _____

3.4. Injection Botox, three units

    Code(s): _____

3.5. Injection Dilaudid, 2 mg

    Code(s): _____

3.6.   Injection RhoGam, 300 mcg

Code(s): _____

3.7.   Injection Cytosar-U, 100 mg

Code(s): _____

3.8.   Injection mitomycin, 5 mg

Code(s): _____

3.9.   Injection digoxin, 0.3 mg

Code(s): _____

3.10.   Intra-articular injection of Synvisc, 16 mg, left knee

Code(s): _____

3.11.   Injection adrenalin, 0.1 mg

Code(s): _____

3.12.   Injection Bicillin CR, 200,000 mg

Code(s): _____

3.13.   Injection ARZERRA, 10 mg

Code(s): _____

Supplies

3.14.   CPAP device

Code(s): _____

3.15.   Blood tubing, venous, for hemodialysis

Code(s): _____

3.16.   Urinary ostomy pouch with barrier attached

Code(s): _____

3.17.   Alginate dressing, 36-in^2 pad

Code(s): _____

3.18.   Radiopharmaceutical technetium medronate (Tc-99m), 30 millicuries

Code(s): _____

3.19. Three-way Foley catheter

Code(s): _____

3.20. Tracheal suction, closed system, for 72 or more hours of use

Code(s): _____

3.21. Blood glucose reagent strips for home glucose monitor, bottle of 50 strips

Code(s): _____

3.22. Distilled water used with nebulizer, 1,000 mL

Code(s): _____

3.23. Surgical trays used in physician-office surgery

Code(s): _____

Ambulance

3.24. Advanced life support IV drug therapy disposable supplies

Code(s): _____

3.25. The two-character modifier to indicate that a patient was taken from the acute hospital to a skilled nursing facility by ambulance is:

Code(s): _____

3.26. Basic life support ambulance services

Code(s): _____

3.27. Ground ambulance transport services are reported:

a. Per trip
b. Per mile
c. Per minute of travel time
d. Per hour of travel time

3.28. Helicopter transport, per mile

Code(s): _____

3.29. Because of the patient's condition, an additional EMT is required for the transport. What is the code for the presence of the extra attendant?

Code(s): _____

3.30. Ambulance waiting time is measured in:

    a. Minutes

    b. Hours

    c. Half hours

    d. 10-minute increments

3.31. Routine disposable supplies used during a basic life support transport

Code(s): _____

3.32. Neonatal transport

Code(s): _____

3.33. Oxygen administered during advanced life support transport

Code(s): _____

3.34. Advanced life support defibrillation

Code(s): _____

Durable Medical Equipment

3.35. Rental of portable liquid oxygen system

Code(s): _____

3.36. Totally electric hospital bed, without mattress, and alternating pressure mattress for hospital bed

Code(s): _____

3.37. Cycler dialysis machine for peritoneal dialysis

Code(s): _____

3.38. Portable whirlpool

Code(s): _____

3.39. Wheelchair, amputee, with detachable arms and detachable, swing-away footrests

Code(s): _____

3.40. Adult transport chair

Code(s): _____

3.41. Pulse oximeter

Code(s): _____

3.42. Eggcrate dry pressure pad

Code(s): _____

3.43. Four-lead TENS unit

Code(s): _____

3.44. Recording apnea monitor

Code(s): _____

3.45. Skin protection wheelchair seat cushion, adjustable, 28 inches in width

Code(s): _____

3.46. Breast pump, electric

Code(s): _____

Procedures/Services

3.47. True or false? Code G0118 should be assigned when an ophthalmologist screens a high-risk patient for glaucoma.

    a. True
    b. False

3.48. Colorectal cancer screening by barium enema

Code(s): _____

3.49. Diagnostic mammography, unilateral

Code(s): _____

3.50. PET scanning, whole body, for diagnosis of esophageal carcinoma, for restaging

Code(s): _____

3.51. Direct hospital observation referral for a patient with diagnosis of congestive heart failure (CHF), chest pain, or asthma

Code(s): _____

3.52. Transcatheter placement of drug-eluting stent, coronary artery, percutaneous

Code(s): _____

3.53.   Sacroiliac joint injection for arthrography

Code(s): _____

3.54.   Diabetes self-management training, group session, per 30 minutes

Code(s): _____

3.55.   Trimming of dystrophic nails

Code(s): _____

3.56.   Influenza virus vaccine

Code(s): _____

3.57.   Implantable silicone breast prosthesis

Code(s): _____

3.58.   Auditory osseointegrated device abutment, replacement

Code(s): _____

3.59.   Screening for prostate cancer, digital rectal examination

Code(s): _____

Part II
Intermediate Coding Exercises

Chapter 4

Case Studies from Inpatient Health Records

> **Note:** Even though the specific cases are divided by setting, most of the information pertaining to the diagnosis is applicable to most settings. If you practice or apply codes in a particular type of setting, you may find additional information in other sections of this publication that may be pertinent to you.
>
> Every effort has been made to follow current recognized coding guidelines and principles, as well as nationally recognized reporting guidelines. The material presented may differ from some health plan requirements for reporting. The ICD-9-CM codes used are effective October 1, 2011, through September 30, 2012. The current standard transactions and code sets named in HIPAA have been utilized, which require ICD-9-CM Volume III procedure codes for inpatients. The 2011 draft editions of ICD-10-CM and ICD-10-PCS are utilized in this chapter.
>
> **Instructions:** Cases are presented as either multiple choice or fill in the blank.
>
> - For multiple-choice cases:
>   —Select the letter of the appropriate code set.
> - For the fill-in-the-blank cases:
>   —Assign the MS-DRG, where indicated.
>   —Assign present on admission (POA) indicator for each ICD-9-CM diagnosis code.
>   - Y: Yes (POA)
>   - N: No (Not POA)
>   - U: Unknown (Documentation is insufficient to determine if condition is POA.)
>   - W: Clinically undetermined (Provider is unable to clinically determine whether or not the condition was POA.)
>   - Leave blank for the exercises in this book all codes that are exempt from POA reporting. See the Exempt List as published in the *ICD-9-CM Official Guidelines for Coding and Reporting*. These codes are exempt because they represent circumstances regarding healthcare encounters or factors influencing health status that do not represent a current disease or injury, or are always present on admission.

ICD-9-CM Coding Instructions:

- Sequence the ICD-9-CM principal diagnosis in the first diagnosis position.
- Assign all reportable secondary diagnosis codes including V codes and E codes (both cause of injury and place of occurrence).
- Sequence the ICD-9-CM principal procedure code in the first procedure position.
- Assign all reportable secondary ICD-9-CM procedure codes.

ICD-10-CM and ICD-10-PCS Coding Instructions:

- Sequence the ICD-10-CM principal diagnosis code in the first diagnosis position.
- Assign all reportable secondary ICD-10-CM codes.
- Sequence the principal ICD-10-PCS code in the first procedure position.
- Assign all reportable secondary ICD-10-PCS codes.

The scenarios are based on selected excerpts from health records. In practice, the coding professional should have access to and refer to the entire health record. Health records are analyzed and codes assigned based on physician documentation. Documentation for coding purposes must be assigned based on medical record documentation. A physician may be queried when documentation is ambiguous, incomplete, or conflicting. The queried documentation must be a permanent part of the medical record.

The objective of the cases and scenarios reproduced in this publication is to provide practice in assigning correct codes, not necessarily to emulate complete coding, which can be achieved only with the complete medical record. For example, the reader may be asked to assign codes based on only an operative report when in real practice, a coder has access to the entire medical record.

The *ICD-9-CM Official Guidelines for Coding and Reporting*, published by the National Center for Health Statistics (NCHS), includes Present on Admission (POA) Reporting Guidelines in Appendix I. These guidelines supplement the official conventions and instructions provided within ICD-9-CM. Adherence to these guidelines when assigning ICD-9-CM diagnosis codes is required under the Health Insurance Portability and Accountability Act (HIPAA) of 1996. Additional official coding guidance can be found in the American Hospital Association (AHA)'s *Coding Clinic for ICD-9-CM* publication.

Disorders of the Blood and Blood-Forming Organs

4.1.   This 45-year-old man underwent colon resection for carcinoma of the transverse colon. The physician progress note on postoperative day 2 states anemia. Hemoglobin and hematocrit levels dropped significantly after surgery, and a blood transfusion was ordered. How is the anemia coded?

ICD-9-CM Code(s):

a. 285.1
b. 998.11
c. 998.11, 285.1
d. Query the physician because opportunity exists to improve documentation of etiology of anemia

ICD-10-CM Code(s): _____

4.2. This 82-year-old female was admitted for acute exacerbation of chronic obstructive pulmonary disease. The progress notes indicate that the patient received a transfusion for anemia. The discharge diagnoses state acute exacerbation of chronic obstructive pulmonary disease and pancytopenia. Transfusion of nonautologous packed red blood cells was given via peripheral vein. What codes are assigned for this case?

ICD-9-CM Code(s):

a. 491.21, 284.19, 99.04
b. 491.21, 284.19, 285.9, 99.04
c. 496, 284.19, 99.04
d. 491.21, 284.19, 285.9, 99.02

ICD-10-CM Code(s): _____

ICD-10-PCS Code(s): _____

4.3. This 35-year-old female patient has carcinoma of the upper-outer left breast. She had a lumpectomy performed and a sentinel lymph node biopsy of the axillary lymph node. The pathology report for the lymph node states no pathological change. What codes are assigned in this case?

ICD-9-CM Diagnosis Code(s) with POA Indicator: _____

ICD-9-CM Procedure Code(s): _____

ICD-10-CM Code(s): _____

ICD-10-PCS Code(s): _____

ICD-10-PCS Note: Assign only the procedure codes for the lumpectomy and excision of left axillary lymph node for biopsy.

4.4. An 8-year-old male hemophiliac is admitted with acute blood loss anemia following uncontrolled bleeding. He was given 4 units of packed red blood cells via the peripheral vein. While in the hospital he also received his regular preventive infusion of clotting factors. Which of the following answers would be correct?

ICD-9-CM Code(s):

a. 286.0, 99.06, 99.03
b. 285.1, 286.0, 99.04, 99.06
c. 286.0, 285.1, 99.06, 99.03
d. 285.1, 99.06, 99.03

ICD-10-CM Code(s): _____

ICD-10-PCS Code(s): _____

4.5. What code(s) is/are assigned for a patient admitted for an azathioprine I drug-induced aplastic anemia? The patient has peripheral neuropathy of multiple joints of the lower extremities secondary to severe rheumatoid arthritis.

ICD-9-CM Diagnosis Code(s) with POA Indicator and MS-DRG:

_____

ICD-9-CM Procedure Code(s): _____

ICD-10-CM Code(s): _____

ICD-10-PCS Code(s): _____

Disorders of the Cardiovascular System

4.6. When a diagnostic statement lists hypertension and chronic kidney disease, which of the following coding guidelines applies?

ICD-9-CM

a. The conditions are reported with two separate codes unless the physician specifically states that there is a cause-and-effect relationship.
b. Code 403.9X is assigned, with an additional code to identify the stage of chronic kidney disease.
c. A cause-and-effect relationship is never assumed.
d. Code 403.9X is assigned, with an additional code to specify the type of hypertension.

ICD-10-CM

a. The conditions are reported with two separate codes unless the physician specifically states that there is a cause-and-effect relationship.
b. A code from category I12.9 is assigned, with an additional code from category N18 to identify the stage of chronic kidney disease.
c. A cause-and-effect relationship is never assumed.
d. Code I12.9 is assigned, with an additional code to specify the type of hypertension.

4.7. This 52-year-old male stayed one week in Hospital A for an ST elevation lateral wall myocardial infarction (STEMI) and was then transferred to Hospital B for further treatment. A cardiac catheterization was performed at Hospital B, which revealed severe occlusive disease, and a coronary bypass grafting was carried out. The physician's final diagnostic statement at Hospital B listed, "Acute lateral wall STEMI due to severe coronary atherosclerosis." What is the appropriate principal diagnosis for Hospital B?

ICD-9-CM Diagnosis Code(s): _____

ICD-10-CM Code(s): _____

4.8. A patient is readmitted to the acute care hospital from a long-term care facility for treatment of heart failure. She had an acute non-ST anterior wall myocardial infarction (MI) 4 weeks ago. She was placed in the intensive care unit and monitored on telemetry. She was also found to have urinary tract infection (UTI) due to *Escherichia coli*. After intense drug therapy, she continued to improve and was transferred back to the long-term care facility. The acute systolic and diastolic heart failure was improved, but she will be monitored. What codes are assigned in this case?

ICD-9-CM Code(s):

a. 428.21, 428.31, 410.12, 599.0, 041.49, 89.54
b. 428.41, 410.72, 599.0, 041.49, 89.54
c. 428.0, 412, 599.0, 041.49, 89.54
d. 428.41, 410.11, 599.0, 041.49, 89.54

ICD-10-CM Code(s): _____

ICD-10-PCS Code(s): _____

4.9. A patient with severe arteriosclerotic heart disease (ASHD) of native arteries and severe chronic obstructive pulmonary disease (COPD) was admitted for coronary artery bypass graft (CABG) with cardiopulmonary bypass for two hours. An open 3-vessel CABG with the left internal mammary artery anastomosed to the left anterior descending coronary artery and separate greater saphenous vein grafts, harvested endoscopically from the left leg, to the obtuse marginal branch and posterior descending coronary artery. Postoperatively, the patient developed pulmonary arterial embolus that required treatment and extended the inpatient stay.

ICD-9-CM Diagnosis Code(s) with POA Indicator and MS-DRG:

_____

ICD-9-CM Procedure Code(s): _____

ICD-10-CM Code(s): _____

ICD-10-PCS Code(s): _____

4.10. The following was documented in the history and physical:

This patient was admitted with a diagnosis of acute myocardial infarction. He was hospitalized for pneumonia last year and 2 years ago had surgery for a bleeding gastric ulcer. Additional history is that he was diagnosed 5 years ago with Parkinson's disease, which is getting progressively worse. He is being treated with levodopa. History also notes emphysema being treated with bronchodilators and corticosteroids.

Discharge Summary: The discharge summary repeats the information in the history and physical examination (H&P), plus adds the following information. During the hospital stay, the patient developed congestive heart failure confirmed by x-ray and started Lasix p.o.

Discharge Diagnoses: Acute ST elevation myocardial infarction, Parkinson's disease, congestive heart failure, emphysema, history of pneumonia, and history of bleeding gastric ulcer. What conditions are coded in this example?

a. Acute ST elevation myocardial infarction, congestive heart failure, Parkinson's disease, emphysema
b. Acute ST elevation myocardial infarction, congestive heart failure
c. Acute ST elevation myocardial infarction, congestive heart failure, Parkinson's disease, emphysema, pneumonia, bleeding ulcer
d. Acute ST elevation myocardial infarction, pneumonia, congestive heart failure, emphysema

4.11. The following documentation is from the health record of a cardiac service patient.

Discharge Summary

Admit Date:	1/9/XX
Discharge Date:	1/12/XX
Final Diagnoses:	1. Coronary artery disease (CAD)
	2. Sick sinus syndrome
Procedures:	1. Permanent dual chamber pacemaker insertion
	2. Percutaneous transluminal coronary angioplasty (PTCA) with stent insertion

History of Present Illness: The patient is a 60-year-old female who was admitted to another hospital on 1/8/XX, after experiencing tachycardia. There she underwent a cardiac catheterization, showing the presence of severe single-vessel coronary artery disease. The patient does not have any history of a CABG in the past. The patient has a history of sick sinus syndrome. She was transferred to our hospital to undergo a percutaneous transluminal angioplasty.

Physical Examination: No physical abnormalities were found on the cardiovascular examination. Pulse 50, blood pressure 100/66. HEENT: PERRLA, faint carotid bruits. Lungs: Clear to percussion and auscultation. Heart: Normal sinus rhythm with a 2.6 systolic ejection murmur. Extremities and abdomen were negative.

Laboratory Data: Unremarkable

Hospital Course: To manage the patient's sick sinus syndrome, a permanent dual chamber pacemaker with atrial and ventricular leads was implanted on 1/9. An incision was made into the left chest wall with the dual chamber pacemaker being placed in the subcutaneous pocket. Next, a small incision was made in the skin and the leads were percutaneously passed into the right ventricle and right atrium.

On 1/10, the patient underwent a PTCA with insertion of a drug-eluting stent in the right coronary artery without complications, and good results were obtained.

Postoperatively, the patient was stable and was subsequently discharged. Patient was discharged on the following medications: Cardizem, 30 mg p.o. q. 6 hours; ASA, 5 grains q. a.m.; Metamucil and Colace p.r.n.; Nitro paste 1/2 inch q. 6 hours.

ICD-9-CM Diagnosis Code(s) with POA Indicator and MS-DRG:

_____

ICD-10-CM Code(s): _____

4.12.   This 62-year-old male patient was admitted to the hospital with progressive episodes of chest pain determined to be crescendo angina. He had myocardial infarction 5 years ago and progressively has been having more frequent episodes of chest pain. During the hospital stay, he was given IV nitroglycerin and was subsequently placed on Cardizem for further treatment of his angina. He is scheduled for cardiac catheterization next week because he refused to have it performed during this admission. No other complications arose during the hospitalization. What is the code assignment?

ICD-9-CM Diagnosis Code(s): _____

ICD-9-CM Procedure Code(s): _____

ICD-10-CM Code(s): _____

ICD-10-PCS Code(s): _____

4.13. This 55-year-old female patient is admitted with occlusion of the cerebral arteries resulting in an infarction. The patient suffered a stroke 2 years ago with residual hemiplegia affecting her left dominant side. What would be the correct code assignment for this case?

ICD-9-CM Diagnosis Code(s) with POA Indicator and MS-DRG:

_____

ICD-10-CM Code(s): _____

4.14. A 75-year-old male patient was admitted for an acute exacerbation of chronic systolic congestive heart failure and severe mitral regurgitation and aortic stenosis. What would be the correct code assignment for this case?

ICD-9-CM Code(s):

a. 428.23, 396.2
b. 428.23, 428.0, 396.2
c. 428.0, 394.1, 424.1
d 391.8, 396.2

ICD-10-CM Code(s): _____

4.15. What code(s) is/are assigned for percutaneous transluminal coronary angioplasty of two arteries, RCA with bare metal stent and LAD without stent?

ICD-9-CM Procedure Code(s): _____

ICD-10-PCS Code(s): _____

Disorders of the Digestive System

4.16. This 44-year-old male patient was admitted for evaluation of melena. This patient is known to have diverticulitis of the colon. He has noticed melena occasionally for the past week. The initial impression was that this is bleeding from diverticulitis. Patient was scheduled for colonoscopy. Colonoscopy identified the cause of the bleeding to be angiodysplasia of the ascending colon. What are the codes assigned for this case?

ICD-9-CM Diagnosis Code(s) with POA Indicator:

_____

ICD-9-CM Procedure Code(s): _____

ICD-10-CM Code(s): _____

ICD-10-PCS Code(s): _____

4.17. The patient was admitted because of severe abdominal pain. There has been a history of abdominal pain and some bleeding, but never this severe. Because of the symptoms, the patient underwent emergency laparotomy to repair the perforation in the antrum of the stomach by suturing. The physician states: acute peptic ulcer with perforation and bleeding. What codes are assigned for this case?

ICD-9-CM Diagnosis Code(s) with POA Indicator and MS-DRG:

_____

ICD-9-CM Procedure Code(s): _____

ICD-10-CM Code(s): _____

ICD-10-PCS Code(s): _____

4.18. This patient with chronic systolic congestive heart failure was admitted because of melena. Patient had EGD with biopsy of the stomach and duodenum. No findings were found to determine the source of the melena. What codes are assigned in this case?

ICD-9-CM Diagnosis Code(s) with POA Indicator and MS-DRG:

_____

ICD-9-CM Procedure Code(s): _____

ICD-10-CM Code(s): _____

ICD-10-PCS Code(s): _____

4.19. The patient is a 44-year-old male who started having abdominal pain the day before yesterday. Subsequently he had diarrhea. He had 4 episodes of diarrhea last night and then 4 episodes in the morning. The stools have turned to fairly frank blood. Also the abdominal pain got worse, and he said he felt dizzy when he stood up. Patient admitted for treatment of dehydration. Patient has frank blood coming out from his bowels. Stool culture and sensitivity revealed *Salmonella*. Physician documented that the abdominal pain, diarrhea, and bleeding were due to Salmonella gastroenteritis. Patient put on Levaquin IV and also rehydrated. Patient responded well and was discharged. What codes are assigned?

ICD-9-CM Code(s):

a. 003.0, 276.51
b. 558.9, 003.0, 276.51
c. 003.0, 578.9, 276.51, 787.91
d. 276.51, 003.0

ICD-10-CM Code(s): _____

4.20. A patient with diabetes and osteoarthritis of the knee is admitted for bilateral direct inguinal hernia repair. The operative report states the repair is done laparoscopically with Marlex mesh. What is the correct code assignment?

ICD-9-CM Diagnosis Code(s) with POA Indicator and MS-DRG:

_____

ICD-9-CM Procedure Code(s): _____

ICD-10-CM Code(s): _____

ICD-10-PCS Code(s): _____

4.21. An 80-year-old patient with hypertension was admitted to the hospital for cholecystectomy. The patient underwent an open cholecystectomy with exploration of the common duct and choledocholithotomy. Final diagnostic statement: 1. Acute and chronic cholecystitis with choledocholithiasis and cholelithiasis. 2. Hypertension. Correct code assignment would be:

ICD-9-CM Diagnosis Code(s) with POA Indicator and MS-DRG:

_____

ICD-9-CM Procedure Code(s): _____

ICD-10-CM Code(s): _____

ICD-10-PCS Code(s): _____

4.22. A 5-month-old patient presents with vomiting, diarrhea, and growth failure. The discharge diagnosis was eosinophilic allergic gastroenteritis and colitis. What is the correct code assignment?

ICD-9-CM Diagnosis Code(s) with POA Indicator:

_____

ICD-10-CM Code(s): _____

4.23. **Preoperative Diagnoses:** Extensive diverticulitis of sigmoid colon with perforation; obstruction of right colon and proximal transverse colon Crohn's disease

Postoperative Diagnosis: Same

Procedures: Exploratory laparotomy sigmoid colectomy; extended right hemicolectomy; permanent colostomy

Procedure Description: After consent was obtained for the procedure, risks and benefits were described at length. The patient was taken to the operating room and placed supine on the operating room table. Preoperatively the patient received 3 g of IV Unasyn. The patient was placed under general endotracheal anesthesia. PAS stockings were applied to both extremities. The patient's abdomen was then prepped and draped in the standard surgical fashion.

A midline laparotomy incision was made from just around the umbilicus to the pubic symphysis. The midline of the fascia was divided, and the abdomen was entered. With exploration of the abdomen, extensive diverticular disease of the distal sigmoid colon was noted.

First order of business was to mobilize the sigmoid colon for a sigmoid colectomy. The left ureter was identified and was far from the area of the sigmoid colon. The sigmoid colon was mobilized laterally to include the area of the diverticulitis. The sigmoid colon was mobilized down to the peritoneal reflection. The medial aspect of the sigmoid colon was also mobilized. The colon was then completely mobilized. A point of transaction was chosen at the proximal sigmoid colon. The mesentery was then taken down across the sacrum. The vessels were tied with 2-0 silk sutures. The sigmoid colon was mobilized down to the proximal rectum. Once the proximal rectum was identified, the sigmoid colon was again transected, this time using a contour Ethicon stapler with a blue load. Both the right and left ureters were identified prior to any transection of the sigmoid colon. A 3-0 Prolene suture was then tagged to either edge of the rectal staple line.

The right colon was then inspected. Multiple perforations with sites of deserosalization with exposed mucosa were identified in the right colon. The right colon was mobilized by taking down the white line of Toldt all the way up to and including the hepatic flexure. The omentum was taken off the transverse colon with electrocautery. Once the colon was completely mobilized and became a medial structure, the terminal ileum was transected this time also using a 45-mm GIA stapler with a blue load. A point of transaction was chosen in the mid transverse colon just proximal to the middle colic artery where the last site of deserosalization was identified. The mid transverse colon was divided with a GIA 45-mm stapler with a blue load. The mesentery to the right colon and transverse colon were then taken down with Pean clamps and tied with 2-0 silk sutures. The specimen was then passed off the field.

The abdomen was then irrigated. Hemostasis was assured. The ileocolic anastomosis was then created between the terminal ileum and the mid transverse colon. The bowel were positioned to lie along side each other, and a side-to-side functional end-to-end anastomosis was created using a 45-mm GIA stapler with a blue load. The enterostomes were then closed together with a running 3-0 PDS suture followed by interrupted 3-0 GI silks in a Lembert fashion. A stitch was placed at the crotch of each of the bowel connections. A finger was palpated at the anastomosis, and it was widely patent. Mesenteric defect was then closed using 3-0 Vicryl suture in a running fashion.

Attention then turned toward formation of the end-descending colostomy. The descending colon had already been mobilized enough to make it to the anterior abdominal wall without any difficulty. A point on the anterior abdominal wall on the left-hand side just below the umbilicus was chosen for the colostomy. A small 1.5- to 2-cm circular incision was made on the anterior abdominal wall midway through the rectus muscle. The anterior fascia was divided in a cruciate fashion. The rectus muscles were split, and two fingers were palpated through the defect into the abdominal cavity. The descending colon was then grasped with an Allis clamp and passed through the defect and exteriorized. There was no tension on the colon.

On the undersurface of the peritoneum, the colon was tagged with 3-0 GI silk sutures ×2.

The midline fascial incision was then closed with a running #1 looped PDS ×2. The surgical incision was then irrigated with copious saline. The skin was then closed with surgical staples. The ostomy was then matured by removing the staple line and sewing the ostomy in place with 3-0 Vicryl sutures. The sutures were sown in circumferentially. An ostomy appliance was applied.

Sterile dressings were applied, and the patient was awakened from general anesthesia and transported to the recovery room in stable condition.

ICD-9-CM Diagnosis Code(s) with POA Indicator and MS-DRG:

_____

ICD-9-CM Procedure Code(s): _____

ICD-10-CM Code(s): _____

ICD-10-PCS Code(s): _____

Endocrine, Nutritional, and Metabolic Diseases and Immunity Disorders

4.24. This 75-year-old female admitted because of chronic diarrhea and dehydration. History of herpes zoster, right upper extremity, leading to monoparesis, right upper extremity, with postherpetic neuralgia on the right side of the chest. She has been treated with heavy doses of Neurontin with no significant relief. On admission her chest x-ray showed resolving lingular and left lower lobe pneumonia and pneumonia in the right perihilar region. The patient is being treated with Levaquin for the pneumonia. She had colonoscopy in the hospital to determine a cause of her iron deficiency anemia. Colonoscopy with biopsies taken of the small bowel as well as the rectosigmoid area showed no specific etiology. What codes are assigned?

ICD-9-CM Diagnosis Code(s) with POA Indicator and MS-DRG:

_____

ICD-9-CM Procedure Code(s): _____

ICD-10-CM Code(s): _____

ICD-10-PCS Code(s): _____

4.25. A 55-year-old female was admitted with diabetic gastroparesis documented as due to steroid-induced diabetes. The patient is on long-term use of systemic corticosteroids, which are properly taken. What codes would be assigned?

ICD-9-CM Diagnosis Code(s) with POA Indicator and MS-DRG:

_____

ICD-10-CM Code(s): _____

4.26.   The following information is contained in the health record.

Chief Complaint: History of nausea with severe vomiting for the past 2 to 3 days. Diabetes mellitus diagnosed at the age of 12 years.

Hospital Course: This 31-year-old male patient has a history of type I diabetes mellitus and is on 15 units of NPH and 10 of Regular in the morning, and 10 units of NPH and 5 of Regular in the evening. The patient started having symptoms of nausea. The patient at the same time had increased frequency of urination and polydipsia with evidence of uncontrolled diabetes. The patient was severely dehydrated on admission. There was no evidence of thrombophlebitis, varicosities, or edema on examination of the extremities. The patient was hydrated and, as a result, his blood sugar decreased from more than 600 to normal levels. The patient was discharged with the diagnosis of diabetic ketoacidosis, type 1.

What code(s) are assigned for this admission?

ICD-9-CM Diagnosis Code(s) with POA Indicator and MS-DRG:

_____

ICD-10-CM Code(s): _____

4.27.   From the health record of a patient requiring thyroid surgery:

History: Patient is a 50-year-old female who noted a swelling in the neck. Outpatient workup was done. Thyroid scan and thyroid sonogram revealed moderate enlargement of the left lobe of the thyroid gland measuring 1.1 × 2.2 cm, a solid nodule at the anterior aspect of the mid of the left lobe of thyroid measuring approximately 1 × 1.9 cm, a small cyst in the middle of the left lobe of the thyroid measuring 2.4 cm, normal right lobe of the thyroid, and a small cyst in the mid of the right lobe measuring 2.3 mm. Thyroid scan showed hot nodule, which is usually negative for malignancy. The fine-needle aspiration was strongly suspicious for papillary carcinoma.

Impression: Papillary carcinoma of the thyroid

Report of Operation:

Preoperative Diagnosis: Steroid nodule left lobe, rule out papillary carcinoma

Postoperative Diagnosis: Papillary carcinoma of thyroid

Procedure: Left thyroid lobectomy with isthmectomy and frozen section. Subsequently, patient underwent total thyroid right lobectomy.

Anesthesia: General endotracheal

Estimated Blood Loss: 50 cc. Replacement: IV fluids, sponge count, needle count times two correct

Technique: After patient was well anesthetized with general endotracheal anesthesia, a sand bag was placed underneath the shoulder blades. The neck was extended and stabilized and placed on a foam head pillow. Entire neck and anterior chest was prepped and draped in the usual manner. The skin incision site was marked with 2-0 VICRYL suture with pressure. Preempt analgesia was obtained with infiltration of .25 percent

Marcaine. Transverse skin incision was made in the anterior part of the neck, which was deepened through the subcutaneous tissue and the platysma. Upper and lower flaps were raised, upper flap up to the thyroid cartilage, lower flap up to the sternal notch. Hemostasis obtained with cautery as well as 3-0 VICRYL sutures. Midline fascia was incised. Strap muscles on the left side were separated from the underlying thyroid gland. Strap muscles were retracted laterally with a Green retractor. Middle thyroid veins were identified, divided between the clamps, ligated with 3-0 VICRYL suture. Patient was noted to have palpable thyroid nodule on the left lower part of the thyroid gland. Superior thyroid vessels were identified. External of the superior laryngeal nerve was identified and protected. Superior thyroid vessels were divided close to the thyroid clamp between the Mixter clamp and ligated with 2-0 VICRYL suture. Recurrent laryngeal nerve was identified and protected throughout the procedure. Superior and inferior parathyroids were identified, protected with their vasculature. Inferior thyroid vessels were divided close to the thyroid capsule after its branching to preserve the blood supply to the parathyroid gland. Isthmus was divided between the clamps, and the entire thyroid lobe was removed and sent for frozen section, which was reported to be a papillary carcinoma. After the pathology report, the decision was made to proceed with the total thyroidectomy, which was carried out in the following manner:

Strap muscles on the right side were separated from the right thyroid gland. Middle thyroid vessels were divided between the clamps, ligated with 3-0 VICRYL suture. Superior and inferior thyroid poles were identified. Superior thyroid vessels were divided close to the upper pole. During the procedure, the external branch of the superior laryngeal nerve was identified and protected. The divided vessels were ligated with 2-0 VICRYL suture. Recurrent laryngeal nerve was identified and protected. Inferior and superior parathyroid glands were identified and protected with vasculature. Inferior thyroid vessel branches were divided between the clamps; thereby the blood supply to the parathyroid glands was preserved. Care was taken to protect the recurrent laryngeal nerve throughout the procedure. The right lobe of the thyroid was completely removed after satisfactory hemostasis. No drains were placed. The strap muscles were approximated with interrupted 3-0 VICRYL suture. Platysma and subcutaneous tissue was approximated with interrupted 4-0 VICRYL suture. Skin approximated with subcuticular 4-0 Dexon. Sterile dressings were applied. At the end of the procedure the vocal cords were inspected. They were moving equally well. The patient tolerated the entire procedure well and was discharged in stable condition to the recovery room.

Discharge Information: Patient discharged after 2 days, with no complications.

Diagnosis: Papillary carcinoma of the thyroid, left and right lobes, with follicular pattern. Papillary carcinoma positive in one cervical lymph node. Will follow up with me in the office.

What are the correct codes in this case?

ICD-9-CM Diagnosis Code(s) with POA Indicator and MS-DRG:

_____

ICD-9-CM Procedure Code(s): _____

ICD-10-CM Code(s): _____

ICD-10-PCS Code(s): _____

4.28.   This 51 year-old male is a Type I insulin-dependent diabetic admitted for treatment of a grade III foot ulcer which involved necrosis of the muscle on the left foot with gangrenous changes resulting from diabetic neuropathy, atherosclerosis, and chronic peripheral vascular insufficiency. Excisional debridement of the ulcer to the muscle is accomplished.

Which of the following answers would be correct?

ICD-9-CM Code(s):

a. 250.71, 440.23, 250.61, 357.2, 86.22
b. 250.71, 440.24, 250.61, 357.2, 707.15, 83.45
c. 250.01, 440.20, 785.4, 357.2, 707.15, 86.28
d. 250.71, 440.24, 250.61, 357.2, 707.15, 86.28

ICD-10-CM Code(s): _____

ICD-10-PCS Code(s): _____

Disorders of the Genitourinary System

4.29.   From the health record of a patient with urinary retention admitted through the emergency department:

Discharge Summary

Pertinent History: The patient is a 34-year-old female admitted through the ER with severe, stabbing, low back pain and inability to urinate. The patient has a long history of pelvic inflammatory disease, with three surgical episodes to remove implants. CT scan revealed a mass in the area of the kidneys.

Hospital Course: The patient was admitted, prepped, and taken to surgery. Exploratory laparotomy revealed an area of pelvic inflammatory disease involving both kidneys in dense adhesions. Cultures indicate chlamydia. Both ureters were almost totally blocked. Dense adhesions were painstakingly taken down. This was done very carefully and required several hours of surgery. Care was taken not to sever the kidneys or ureters. INTERCEED adhesion barrier was applied.

Postoperatively, the patient was pain free.

Discharge Instructions: The patient was discharged home to return to see me in the office in 1 week.

Diagnosis: Severe pelvic adhesions, chlamydia infection.

Which of the following code sets would be reported for this admission?

ICD-9-CM Code(s):

a. 614.9, 079.98, 59.02
b. 614.6, 079.98, 59.02, 99.77
c. 614.6, 079.88, 54.59, 99.77
d. 614.3, 079.98, 59.02, 99.77

ICD-10-CM Code(s): _____

ICD-10-PCS Code(s): _____

4.30. From the health record of a patient requiring radical surgery:

Discharge Summary

Pertinent History: The patient is a 68-year-old female admitted through the ER. The patient's abdomen is enlarged to about 18-week size; however, the patient states she has actually lost 22 pounds over the past few weeks. Patient says her appetite has disappeared. Patient is admitted for workup and definitive treatment.

Hospital Course: The patient's CT scan and MRI revealed a suspicious mass in the pelvis. Patient was taken to surgery, where exploration revealed and pathology report later confirmed right ovarian cancer. A radical abdominal hysterectomy was performed, which in this case included removal of the uterus and upper vagina. Also performed were regional pelvic lymph nodes dissection and bilateral salpingo-oophorectomy. The patient tolerated the procedure well.

Discharge Instructions: The patient was discharged home to see me in the office in 1 week for removal of staples and scheduling for oncologist consultation.

Which of the following code sets should be reported for this admission?

ICD-9-CM Code(s):

a. 183.0, 68.41, 65.61, 40.3
b. 183.0, 68.69, 65.61, 40.3
c. 198.6, 68.61, 65.61, 40.3
d. 183.0, 68.69, 65.61, 40.59

ICD-10-CM Code(s): _____

ICD-10-PCS Code(s): _____

4.31. This 80-year-old female patient was admitted with fever, malaise, and left flank pain. A urinalysis was performed and showed bacteria more than 100,000/mL. This was followed by a culture, showing *Escherichia coli* growth documented as *E. coli* urinary tract infection (UTI). On day 2 the patient had an exacerbation of chronic obstructive pulmonary disease (COPD) and was treated with inhaler. This resolved the same day. Patient is also on current medication therapy for hypertension and arteriosclerotic heart disease (ASHD) of the native vessels. What codes are assigned for this encounter?

ICD-9-CM Diagnosis Code(s) with POA Indicator and MS-DRG:

_____

ICD-10-CM Code(s): _____

4.32. This is a 47-year-old female admitted to the hospital for a scheduled total abdominal hysterectomy and bilateral salpingo-oophorectomy due to submucous leiomyoma of the uterus. The patient also has extensive endometriosis of the uterus, ovaries, and pelvic peritoneum. On the day of admission the patient was taken to surgery and, in addition to the scheduled procedure, lysis of extensive pelvic adhesions was also carried out. In the process of removing the adhesions, the physician accidently punctured the small bowel. This small puncture was quickly repaired. The patient was diagnosed with acute blood-loss anemia with a documented loss of 1,500 ml of blood during surgery. The remainder of the postoperative course was uneventful and the patient was discharged on day 4. Assign the codes for the diagnoses only.

ICD-9-CM Diagnosis Code(s) with POA Indicator:

_____

ICD-10-CM Code(s): _____

4.33. This 38-year-old mother of four children has been treated for nearly 20 years for severe cystic breast disease. The patient has elected to have her breasts removed to relieve the pain. She is also very worried about developing breast cancer because her mother died from breast cancer at age 42 years. She has had numerous breast biopsies, and each time they are benign. She may consider plastic reconstruction later, but is not interested in it now. She is in good health. She was taken to surgery, and bilateral simple mastectomies were performed. The pathology report shows severe cystic disease of both breasts. What codes are assigned?

ICD-9-CM Diagnosis Code(s) with POA Indicator and MS-DRG:

_____

ICD-9-CM Procedure Code(s): _____

ICD-10-CM Code(s): _____

ICD-10-PCS Code(s): _____

4.34. This elderly patient has been treated for hypertension for many years. Otherwise he is in relatively good condition considering his age. He was brought to the ER and admitted in acute renal failure due to severe dehydration with hyponatremia. What code(s) are assigned for this case?

ICD-9-CM Diagnosis Code(s) with POA Indicator and MS-DRG:

_____

ICD-10-CM Code(s): _____

4.35. The 56-year-old patient who has type I diabetes mellitus is admitted with acute renal failure. Past medical history includes: hypertension, diabetic nephropathy, and chronic kidney disease stage IV. What codes are assigned?

ICD-9-CM Diagnosis Code(s) with POA Indicator and MS-DRG:

_____

ICD-10-CM Code(s): _____

4.36. A 56-year-old patient with end-stage renal failure has a bloodstream infection due to the central dialysis catheter. He is admitted for replacement of the catheter. What diagnosis code(s) are assigned?

ICD-9-CM Diagnosis Code(s) with POA Indicator:

_____

ICD-10-CM Code(s): _____

Infectious Diseases

4.37. This is a 35-year-old HIV-positive male with progressive lymphadenopathy and unexplained fevers, night sweats, and chills. Low osmolar CT scan of the chest, abdomen, pelvis, and neck showed extensive lymphadenopathy involving mediastinum and left hilum, paratracheal nodal chains, retroperitoneum, right iliac nodal chains, and right inguinal nodes. There were several areas of atelectasis evident in the right lung. Lymph node biopsy suspicious for tuberculosis and in fact was AFB-positive. The patient was placed on respiratory isolation and serial sputums were obtained. The patient's sputum contained positive AFB on concentrated specimen. Also during the course of hospitalization, the patient complained of swelling in the bilateral lower extremities. Dopplers were negative for DVT. The patient was diagnosed with tuberculosis of intrathoracic, retroperitoneum, and inguinal lymph nodes, tubercle bacilli found by microscopy. The patient will be referred to the clinic for management of his HIV disease and associated tuberculosis. What diagnosis codes are assigned?

ICD-9-CM Diagnosis Code(s) with POA Indicator:

_____

ICD-10-CM Code(s): _____

4.38. The discharge diagnosis for a patient admitted with urosepsis due to streptococcus and white blood cell count of 15,000. Urine culture and blood cultures were positive for streptococcus. After query to the physician regarding the meaning of the term *urosepsis*, an addendum was added to the record: Sepsis with streptococcal septicemia and urinary tract infection (UTI), both due to streptococcus B. What codes are assigned?

ICD-9-CM Diagnosis Code(s) with POA Indicator and MS-DRG:

_____

ICD-10-CM Code(s): _____

4.39. This 25-year-old patient was admitted with difficulty breathing. She has AIDS and is in the 21st week of pregnancy. Workup shows *Pneumocystis carinii* pneumonia. What codes are assigned in this case?

ICD-9-CM Diagnosis Code(s) with POA Indicator and MS-DRG:

_____

ICD-10-CM Code(s): _____

4.40. This 53-year-old male with emphysema, previous lung transplant 2 years ago, was admitted with history of elevated temperature of 101 degrees with associated malaise, fatigue, and headache. The patient continued to have temperature elevations after admission. He was started on intravenous ganciclovir and intravenous Imipenem. Blood and urine cultures were basically nondiagnostic. He underwent a bronchoscopy for bronchoalveolar lavage from his left transplanted lung, which did not show any evidence of viral or bacterial pathogens. The BAL was performed by washing out the alveolar tissue in order to obtain alveolar tissue for diagnosis. Blood CMV antigen test was positive and hence he was diagnosed with CMV infection. He has had a persistent cough, and microscopy confirmed the presence of pulmonary tuberculosis. The physician documentation shows the infiltrating pulmonary tuberculosis and CMV are HIV-related. Patient was treated with ethambutol. What codes are assigned?

ICD-9-CM Diagnosis Code(s) with POA Indicator and MS-DRG:

_____

ICD-9-CM Procedure Code(s): _____

ICD-10-CM Code(s): _____

ICD-10-PCS Code(s): _____

4.41. This 23-year-old female is admitted with pneumonia. She also has multiple bilateral lesions of the vulva and vagina with fluid-filled blisters. The history includes fever, and pain for 2 days. Sputum cultures show group A streptococcus. History also includes pain, particularly with urination, and itching of the genitals. Physician documents group A streptococcus pneumonia, vulvovaginitis due to herpes. What codes are assigned?

ICD-9-CM Diagnosis Code(s) with POA Indicator:

_____

ICD-10-CM Code(s): _____

Disorders of the Skin and Subcutaneous Tissue

4.42. An elderly nursing home patient was admitted for pneumonia. He has frequent aspiration because of difficulty swallowing due to a previous stroke. This pneumonia was documented as aspiration pneumonia. He was also found on admission to have stage one decubitus ulcer on the hip. The patient received skin care by the nursing staff for this ulcer. What codes are assigned in this case?

ICD-9-CM Diagnosis Code(s) with POA Indicator and MS-DRG:

_____

ICD-9-CM Procedure Code(s): _____

ICD-10-CM Code(s): _____

ICD-10-PCS Code(s): _____

4.43. This patient had surgery 2 weeks ago for appendicitis. She is admitted now because of fever, pain, and redness at the operative site. There is evidence of cellulitis of the operative wound, and cultures confirm *Staphylococcus aureus* as the cause. She received IV antibiotics. She also has type II diabetes mellitus and is on oral antidiabetic medication. What codes are assigned?

ICD-9-CM Diagnosis Code(s) with POA Indicator:

_____

ICD-10-CM Code(s): _____

4.44. This nursing home patient was admitted to the hospital with severe cellulitis in the leg. The cultures grew streptococcus B, and this was documented by the physician as the cause of the cellulitis. Patient was given IV antibiotics. He also has dominant right-sided hemiplegia from an old cerebrovascular accident (CVA) and was found to have decubitus ulcers in the left gluteal region. What code(s) are assigned?

ICD-9-CM Diagnosis Code(s) with POA Indicator and MS-DRG:

_____

ICD-10-CM Code(s): _____

4.45. This 85-year-old patient, who is a resident at the skilled nursing facility, was admitted with a severe decubitus ulcer on the right buttock, stage II, and a small chronic ulcer on the left heel limited to the skin area. Patient also has Alzheimer's disease. The treatment was an excisional debridement of the skin of the heel and an open excisional debridement into the muscle of the buttock. What is the code assignment?

ICD-9-CM Diagnosis Code(s) with POA Indicator and MS-DRG:

_____

ICD-9-CM Procedure Code(s): _____

ICD-10-CM Code(s): _____

ICD-10-PCS Code(s): _____

4.46. This 29-year-old female patient is admitted for wide local excision of melanoma on the back. She also has a history of asthma. The melanoma is a 2-mm lesion so a margin of 2 cm of normal skin was removed as well. After surgery, she had an acute exacerbation of her asthma treated with two nebulizer treatments with Alupent. The wide excision was performed and a full-thickness skin graft from the left thigh was applied. The donor site was sutured closed directly. What codes are assigned?

ICD-9-CM Diagnosis Code(s) with POA Indicator:

_____

ICD-9-CM Procedure Code(s): _____

ICD-10-CM Code(s): _____

ICD-10-PCS Code(s): _____

Behavioral Health Conditions

4.47. **Case Scenario:** A patient in a state of acute intoxication presented for care. The patient's 12-year alcohol dependence is consistent with a high level of daily alcohol consumption. The patient was admitted for alcohol detoxification and rehabilitation. On the second day of admission, he began experiencing withdrawal symptoms of sweating and nausea. On the third day, the sweating became more profuse, and he developed irregular tremors and tachycardia. The delirium tremors were managed medically. The patient did not experience any seizures. Hallucinations abated by day 4. By day 5, the patient was resting more comfortably, and plans for rehabilitation were initiated. The patient expressed a desire to reduce his alcohol abuse to a "controlled" level. A motivational treatment plan was developed and implemented, with the short-term goal of assisting the patient in reaching a stable level of use; that is, controlled drinking and a long-range goal of motivating the patient to accept a goal of total abstinence. Initially, the patient actively participated in the program, but his motivation waned, and he left the program after signing out AMA without meeting any of the rehabilitation goals.

Which of the following code sets most accurately reflects this case scenario?

ICD-9-CM Code(s):

a. 291.81, 303.01, 94.63, 94.39
b. 291.81, 303.90, 94.62, 94.39
c. 291.0, 303.01, 94.63, 94.39
d. 291.0, 303.90, 94.62, 94.39

ICD-10-CM Code(s): _____

ICD-10-PCS Code(s): _____

4.48. This 30-year-old male was admitted after being transferred from the outpatient therapy services because of severe major depressive disorder with psychotic features. After a complete neuropsychological, personality, and behavioral psychological evaluation, the risks and benefits of ECT were reviewed and explained to the patient and his family. Single seizure unilateral ECT was administered three times per week. The patient tolerated the therapy well and responded quickly with overall improvement in the acute phase of his depressive disorder. After establishing adequate therapeutic levels of lithium, the patient was discharged to be managed as an outpatient. What codes are assigned?

ICD-9-CM Diagnosis Code(s) with POA Indicator and MS-DRG:

_____

ICD-9-CM Procedure Code(s): _____

ICD-10-CM Code(s): _____

ICD-10-PCS Code(s): _____

4.49. This patient has been living at home, but his dementia has been getting progressively worse. He was diagnosed with Alzheimer's disease over 2 years ago. The family called the police because he was missing from home. A search was conducted and an observant passerby called in a report of an elderly man who seemed to be disoriented at a nearby public park. He was found after several hours and brought to the hospital. He had fallen in the park and had a laceration on his right knee that required suturing of the subcutaneous tissue and skin. What codes are reported in this case?

ICD-9-CM Diagnosis Code(s) with POA Indicator and MS-DRG:

_____

ICD-9-CM Procedure Code(s): _____

ICD-10-CM Code(s): _____

ICD-10-PCS Code(s): _____

4.50. The patient was brought to the ER and then admitted because of acute alcohol inebriation. The discharge diagnosis is acute and chronic alcoholism, continuous. What codes are assigned?

ICD-9-CM Diagnosis Code(s) with POA Indicator:

_____

ICD-10-CM Code(s): _____

4.51. This 65-year-old chronic cigarette smoker for the past 40 years was admitted to the hospital with acute exacerbation of her chronic obstructive pulmonary disease. She has a history of anxiety syndrome due to hypothyroidism, and is maintained on medications for both the anxiety and the hypothyroidism. No symptomatology at the time of admission. On hospital day 2, she developed extreme anxiety and a psychiatric consultation was ordered. What codes are assigned in this case?

ICD-9-CM Diagnosis Code(s) with POA Indicator and MS-DRG:

_____

ICD-10-CM Code(s): _____

Disorders of the Musculoskeletal System and Connective Tissue

4.52. This patient was admitted for treatment of a traumatic left second metatarsal fracture. The fracture site was opened and reduced, followed by placement of three internal Kirschner wires. Two pins were then placed, and an external fixator frame was connected to the pins to provide pressure and hold them in reduction. What codes are assigned in this case?

ICD-9-CM Diagnosis Code(s) with POA Indicator and MS-DRG:

_____

ICD-9-CM Procedure Code(s): _____

ICD-10-CM Code(s): _____

ICD-10-PCS Code(s): _____

4.53. A patient is admitted with an infected right partial hip prosthesis. The prosthesis was removed, and the patient underwent a total hip titanium-polyethylene arthroplasty. What are the correct code assignments?

ICD-9-CM Diagnosis Code(s) with POA Indicator and MS-DRG:

_____

ICD-9-CM Procedure Code(s): _____

ICD-10-CM Code(s): _____

ICD-10-PCS Code(s): _____

4.54. A patient was admitted for recurrent dislocation of the left shoulder. The operation included debridement of the acromion, subacromial bursectomy, division of the coracoacromial ligament, and an abrasion acromioplasty with Mitek suture placement. Which of the following is the correct code assignment?

ICD-9-CM Code(s):

a. 718.31, 81.82
b. 718.31, 81.82, 83.5
c. 831.00, 81.82, 83.5
d. 831.00, 81.82, 83.5, 80.41

ICD-10-CM Code(s): _____

ICD-10-PCS Code(s): _____

4.55. This is a 65-year-old lady with complaints of low-back pain with radiation down her right leg to her foot. This pain has been progressively worse over the last several months. MRI scan of the lumbar spine showed degenerative disc disease at L2–3, L3–4, and L4–5; L3–L4 with mild central canal stenosis; and facet arthropathy at L3–L4 and L4–L5. Past medical history includes coronary artery disease, hypertension, and lumbar osteoarthritis. Her current medications include Lipitor, Avapro, Ecotrin, Imdur, Lasix, K-Dur, calcium, and Vioxx. She had a CABG two years ago and PTCA with cardiac stents placed three years ago. Patient admitted for lumbar epidural steroid injections for her lumbar radiculopathy due to degenerative disc disease as noted on MRI results. Which of the following answers would be correct?

ICD-9-CM Code(s):

a. 722.52, 721.3, 414.00, 401.9, V45.81, V45.82, 03.92, 99.23, 88.93
b. 722.52, 721.3, 724.02, 724.4, 414.00, 401.9, V45.81, V45.82, 03.92, 99.23, 88.93
c. 724.4, 414.00, 401.9, V45.81, V45.82, 03.92, 99.23, 88.93
d. 722.52, 721.3, 414.00, 401.9, V45.81, V45.82, 03.91, 88.93

ICD-10-CM Code(s): _____

ICD-10-PCS Code(s): _____

4.56. This 70-year-old female has been treated for progressive increasing pain in her back. She is to the point that she is unable to move. She was brought to the ER and admitted after x-ray shows severe compression fractures of the lumbar vertebrae due to her senile osteoporosis. An injection of local anesthetic was done into the spinal canal. What codes are assigned?

ICD-9-CM Diagnosis Code(s) with POA Indicator and MS-DRG:

_____

ICD-9-CM Procedure Code(s): _____

ICD-10-CM Code(s): _____

ICD-10-PCS Code(s): _____

4.57. This 45-year-old male patient in whom conservative treatment for degenerative disk disease of the lumbar spine has failed came to the hospital. The discectomy was performed at L5 and total spinal disk prosthesis inserted to restore disk function and anatomy. What procedure code(s) are assigned?

ICD-9-CM Code(s):

a. 80.51
b. 80.51, 84.65
c. 84.65, 80.51
d. 84.65

ICD-10-PCS Code(s):

a. 0ST20ZZ
b. 0ST20ZZ, 0SR20JZ
c. 0SR20JZ, 0ST20ZZ
d. 0SR20JZ

4.58. What procedure code(s) is/are assigned for open osteotomy of the capitates and lunate bones, right hand?

ICD-9-CM Procedure Code(s): _____

ICD-10-PCS Code(s): _____

4.59. ## Discharge Summary

Date of Admission: 06/28/XX

Date of Discharge: 07/07/XX

Diagnoses: 1. Status post fractured right femoral neck.
2. Chronic obstructive pulmonary disease.
3. Rheumatoid arthritis, steroid dependent.
4. Osteoporosis.

Pertinent History: The patient was admitted on the 28th of June after a fall. She did not pass out but just fell and fractured her hip. She fell off of a stool at home. She underwent surgery for this. She had a hemiarthroplasty. She tolerated the procedure well and was transferred to A Pavilion for continued physical therapy and rehabilitation.

Pertinent Laboratory: CBC initially showed a white count of 15,400, subsequently the white count is 10,900 with 78 neutrophils. H&H was stable at 12.2 and 36.9. Theophylline level was 10.3, therapeutic.

Hospital Course: The patient tolerated physical therapy well. She was able to give her own Lovenox shots. She was anxious to go home on Saturday. Orthopedics had planned for 14 more days of Lovenox, and that will be given by the patient and prescribed by Dr. Thomas's group. She will be back in about 3 weeks. She will continue with her current medications, which are proventil 2 puffs q.i.d., Fosamax 10 mg q.a.m., Soma 350 mg q.i.d., Lovenox 30 mg q. 12 hours, folic acid 1 mg q. day, Lasix 40 mg b.i.d., Atrovent 2 puffs q. 6 hours, synthroid

0.075 q day, potassium 20 mEq b.i.d., prednisone 20 mg a day, Theo-Dur 100 mg in the morning and 200 mg in the evening. She takes Sonata and she will continue with 5 mg q.h.S. She will continue with her laxative of choice. She will restart her Nasonex, Celebrex, Vicodin, and Vanceril when she gets home. She will stay on a regular diet. Activities per her primary care physician. She will see me back in 3 weeks.

History and Physical Examination

Admission Date: 6/28

Chief Complaint: Hip fracture.

Present Illness: The patient is a 79-year-old white female who slipped off of a stool in the apartment's kitchen while talking to her daughter. She was apparently trying to do too many things at one time, trying to clean some books or something like that and then just slipped and fell off and fractured her hip. She lives alone, had to call for help. She denies any type of passing out, no head injury, and no history of falling a lot before.

Past Medical History: The patient denies any kind of past history of chest pains, exertional chest pain. She stopped smoking some time ago but continues to be mildly short of breath and that has been stable.

She has no gastrointestinal (GI) symptoms, only occasionally some mild stress incontinence.

Medications:
1. Nasonex nasal spray
2. Soma 350 mg 1 q.i.d.
3. Potassium 10 mEq. 2 b.i.d.
4. Celebrex 200 mg q.d.
5. Synthroid 0.075 q.d.
6. Vicodin p.r.n.
7. Fosamax 10 mg q.a.m.
8. Theo-Dur 200 mg ~ in the morning and 1 in the evening
9. Folic acid 1 q.d.
10. Lasix 40 mg b.i.d.
11. Prednisone 10 mg. 2 g.d.
12. Vanceril inhaler
13. Atrovent inhaler
14. Albuterol inhaler

Allergies: Halcion, which causes her to hallucinate.

Medical History: Her medical history includes rheumatoid arthritis, chronic obstructive pulmonary disease (COPD), osteoporosis, and congestive heart failure (CHF).

Social History: She is a widow, stopped smoking 12 years ago. Does not use any alcohol.

Family History: Noncontributory.

Physical Examination: Finds her alert and oriented in no acute distress. Her blood pressure is 140/68, pulse 74, respirations 18. She was afebrile. HEENT: Examination was negative. Neck: Supple without any adenopathy, no bruit was heard. Chest: Clear to auscultation. Heart: Sounds regular without any murmur or gallop. Abdomen: Soft, positive bowel sounds, nontender, no bruits heard. Extremities: Showed normal vascular status.

Laboratory and X-Ray Data: She has a complete blood count (CBC) and urinalysis essentially normal. EKG shows no acute changes. Chest x-ray is pending at this time. If that is normal, she will be able to go on to surgery; that is decided on by Dr. Rowan.

Impression(s):   1. Fracture right femoral neck.
2. Chronic obstructive pulmonary disease and rheumatoid arthritis. She is steroid dependent so we are going to increase the amount of steroids that she is taking right now. Continue her on her inhalers and restart her oral medications as directed later.

Operative Report

Date: 06/28

Preoperative Diagnosis: Displaced right femoral neck hip fracture.

Postoperative Diagnosis: Displaced right femoral neck hip fracture.

Operation: Right hip hemiarthroplasty (Zimmer LD/Fx cemented monopolar metal prosthesis).

Anesthesia: Spinal.

Indications: This is a 79-year-old, previously ambulatory female with a history of rheumatoid arthritis, osteoporosis, steroid-dependent, and emphysema, with the above diagnosis. Risks, benefits, and alternatives of the above procedure were explained to the patient in detail, and she consented to proceed.

Operative Procedure: The patient was taken to the operating room and placed in the lateral position on the transfer bed, where spinal anesthesia was administered. She was transferred to the left lateral decubitus position on a beanbag on the operative table. Padded all bony prominences. Peritoneum was sealed off with Steri-Drape. The right hip was prepped and draped in the usual sterile fashion. Longitudinal incision over the greater trochanter and proximal femur was performed curving posteriorly proximally along the gluteus maximus. Sharp dissection to the skin, Bovie dissection to the subcutaneous tissues down to tensor fascia lata, identifying the greater trochanter. Besides the tensor fascia lata and along with the incision splitting the fibrous gluteus maximus, controlling bleeders with Bovie cautery. Piriformis was identified and short external rotators were tagged with a #5 Tycron suture. These are moved from their insertion. T capsulotomy was performed. Displaced hip fracture was identified, femoral head was removed and measured, copious irrigation was performed, acetabular was visibly and palpable normal appearing. Sagittal saw was used to make cut in the femoral neck. Box osteotome was used to gain lateral entrance to the canal. The canal finder was used, easily locating the femoral canal. Sequential broaching was performed up to a 14, which fit well. Stating the appropriate anteversion. Trawled with an endofemoral head. Had full range of motion without instability and grossly equal leg lengths. I could bring the hip and knee up to 90 degrees of flexion, neutral adduction, start to internally rotate to 30 degrees before it would become unstable. Hip was redislocated, trial components were removed. Measured the canal for a centralizer. I placed a distal cement restrictor 2 cm distal to the component. Copious lavage of the canal was performed and brushed. Acetabulum was irrigated clean; palpable and visibly free of loose fragments. It was packed off with lap sponge. Dried the femoral canal. Placed cement in the femoral canal with retrograde manor using proximal pressurizer. Placed the 14-mm Zimmer LD/Fx with a distal centralizer in the appropriate anteversion, held in place with a cement set. Copious irrigation was performed. After the cement set, placed the final endo head, tapped into position with Morris taper, reduced the head. Could take the hip through the same range of motion without any instability. The short external rotator is in the drill holes in the greater trochanter. The tensor fascia lata closed with interrupted 0-0 VICRYL suture. We copiously irrigated each layer. Subcutaneous tissue closed with interrupted 2-0 VICRYL sutures, skin was closed with staples. Sterile dressing was applied.

ICD-9-CM Diagnosis Code(s) with POA Indicator and MS-DRG:

_____

ICD-9-CM Procedure Code(s): _____

ICD-10-CM Code(s): _____

ICD-10-PCS Code(s): _____

Neoplasms

4.60. The following documentation is from the health record of a terminally ill oncology patient.

Discharge Summary

History of Present Illness: The patient is an 80-year-old white female with a known history of advanced metastatic carcinoma of the breast, widely metastatic. The patient was admitted because of increasing shortness of breath and severe pain. The pain, which was worse in her left chest, was associated with increasing shortness of breath. At the time of admission, the patient was in so much pain that she was unable to remember her history. The patient initially presented for congestive heart failure over 1 year ago. This was subsequently found to be secondary to metastatic breast cancer, post left mastectomy, 3 years ago. The patient had previously been on chemotherapy.

Laboratory Data and Hospital Course: The patient was treated initially with IV pain medication to control her pain. Subsequently, she became able to be stable on oral medication. By the time of discharge, the patient was stable on oral Vicodin, and she was able to eat. Blood sugars were improved, and her Tolinase was withheld. Laboratory results at time of discharge included BUN 17, creatinine 1, sodium 141, potassium 4.5, chloride 105, CO_2 25, alkaline phosphatase elevated at 170 with

GGT 267, SGOT 68. Admission BUN was up to 38 with creatinine 1.3 secondary to dehydration. By the time of discharge, these had improved. Admission glucose 225, down to 110 at discharge. Patient treated with Lanoxin and Lasix for CHF.

Medications at Discharge Include: Aldactone, 25 mg twice a day; Lanoxin, 0.125 mg daily; Metamucil, 5 cc in 4 ounces of juice twice a day; Tolinase, 250 mg half tablet b.i.d. (but hold if preceding Accu-Chek is less than 125); Reglan, 10 mg p.o. a.c.; Pepcid, 20 mg b.i.d.; Lasix, 40 mg daily (only if pedal edema is present); Vicodin tablets, 1 every 3 hours p.r.n. for pain.

Discharge Diagnoses: 1. Uncontrolled pain, secondary to widely metastatic breast carcinoma
2. Dehydration
3. Type II diabetes mellitus, uncontrolled
4. Congestive heart failure

Which of the following is the correct ICD-9-CM code assignment?

ICD-9-CM Code(s):

a. 338.3, 199.1, V10.3, 276.51, 250.02, 428.0
b. 174.9, 276.51, 250.02, 428.0
c. 199.1, V10.3, 276.51, 250.02, 428.0
d. 786.59, 199.1, 276.51, 250.02, 428.0

ICD-10-CM Code(s): _____

4.61.   This 60-year-old male had bronchoscopy with brushings, washings, and fine-needle aspiration due to left lung tumor. The bronchoscope was advanced into the left upper lobe. Brushings were taken followed by transbronchial lavage to the area and then two fine-needle aspirations. The pathology report describes tissue from the fine-needle biopsy of the left upper lobe of the lung, bronchoalveolar lavage and bronchial brushings of the left upper lobe as well as bronchus brushing. Final diagnosis was oat cell carcinoma of the left upper lobe of the lung and emphysema. What are the code assignments for this patient?

ICD-9-CM Diagnosis Code(s) with POA Indicator and MS-DRG:

_____

ICD-9-CM Procedure Code(s): _____

ICD-10-CM Code(s): _____

ICD-10-PCS Code(s): _____

4.62.   This female patient with terminal carcinoma of the breast, metastatic to the liver and brain, was admitted with dehydration. Patient rehydrated with IVs and discharged, with no treatment given to the cancer. What are the codes assigned?

ICD-9-CM Diagnosis Code(s) with POA Indicator and MS-DRG:

_____

ICD-10-CM Code(s): _____

4.63. This 45-year-old female patient was diagnosed with right breast carcinoma 3 years ago, at which time she had a mastectomy performed with chemotherapy administration. She has been well since that time with no further treatment but yearly checkups. She has metastasis in 3 axillary lymph nodes. She is admitted now with visual disturbances, dizziness, headaches, and blurred vision. Workup was done that revealed metastasis to the brain. What is the correct code assignment for this admission?

ICD-9-CM Diagnosis Code(s) with POA Indicator:

_____

ICD-10-CM Code(s): _____

4.64. This patient was admitted for chemotherapy due to a primary hepatocellular carcinoma of the transplanted liver. What codes are assigned?

ICD-9-CM Code(s):

a. V58.11, 155.0
b. V58.11, 155.0, 199.2
c. V58.11, 996.82, 199.2, 155.0
d. 996.82, 199.2, 155.0

ICD-10-CM Code(s): _____

4.65. This patient was admitted with a large pelvic mass and underwent an exploratory laparotomy. Pathology confirmed carcinoma of the left ovary with extensive metastasis to the omentum. A total greater omentectomy, excision of left ovarian mass, and radical abdominal hysterectomy were performed, which in this case included removal of the uterus and upper vagina. Bilateral salpingo-oophorectomy was also performed. What codes are assigned?

ICD-9-CM Diagnosis Code(s) with POA Indicator and MS-DRG:

_____

ICD-9-CM Procedure Code(s): _____

ICD-10-CM Code(s): _____

ICD-10-PCS Code(s): _____

4.66. A patient with known carcinoma of the pancreatic head is admitted with an Hgb of 9.1. She has been receiving Docetaxel chemotherapy and the physician determines this new anemia as an adverse effect of the chemotherapy. The patient is treated with darbepoetin alpha and IV iron. The patient is discharged with an improvement in the Hgb to 11.3. Assign the correct diagnostic code(s).

ICD-9-CM Diagnosis Code(s) with POA Indicator:

_____

ICD-10-CM Code(s): _____

Disorders of the Nervous System and Sense Organs

4.67.   This is one of multiple hospital admissions for this 37-year-old white male with a history of meningoencephalitis 20 years ago. He developed obstructive hydrocephalus as a late effect/sequela and underwent ventriculoperitoneal shunting of the right lateral ventricle using a high-pressure valve. The patient is now complaining of numbness in his right leg, headaches, and diplopia. The patient had a low osmolar CT head scan which showed a slight increase in the hydrocephalus involving the fourth ventricle. Cisternogram was done. The dye went into the fourth ventricle but never into the lateral ventricles. Impression was shunt malfunction. He is admitted this time for VP shunt revision. Ventricular shunt was replaced via open approach and was functioning well at the time of discharge. Which of the following is the correct code assignment?

ICD-9-CM Code(s):

a. 996.2, 331.4, 326, 02.42, 87.02, 87.03
b. 331.4, 326, 02.42, 87.02, 87.03
c. 996.63, 331.4, 02.42
d. 996.2, 02.42, 87.03

ICD-10-CM Code(s): _____

ICD-10-PCS Code(s): _____

4.68.   This 32-year-old female patient was admitted with intractable partial epilepsy after an MRI showed mesial temporal sclerosis on the right side with hippocampal atrophy. The neurosurgeon carried out a selective amygdalohippocampectomy with intraoperative electrocorticography. The rest of her hospital stay was uneventful. What codes are assigned?

ICD-9-CM Diagnosis Code(s) with POA Indicator:

_____

ICD-9-CM Procedure Code(s): _____

ICD-10-CM Code(s): _____

ICD-10-PCS Code(s): _____

4.69.   This 19-year-old college student was brought to the ER and admitted with high fever, stiff neck, chest pain, cough, and nausea. A lumbar puncture was performed, and results were positive for meningitis. Chest x-ray revealed pneumonia. Sputum cultures grew *Pneumococcus*. Patient was treated with IV antibiotics and was discharged with the diagnosis of pneumococcal meningitis and pneumococcal pneumonia. What codes are assigned?

ICD-9-CM Diagnosis Code(s) with POA Indicator and MS-DRG:

_____

ICD-9-CM Procedure Code(s): _____

ICD-10-CM Code(s): _____

ICD-10-PCS Code(s): _____

4.70. This patient was admitted when MRI revealed cerebral aneurysm. After admission, a cerebral angiogram was performed and showed nonruptured arteriosclerotic aneurysm of the anterior cerebral artery. An aneurysmectomy by anastomosis was performed using Marlex graft replacement. What codes are assigned?

ICD-9-CM Diagnosis Code(s) with POA Indicator:

_____

ICD-9-CM Procedure Code(s): _____

ICD-10-CM Code(s): _____

ICD-10-PCS Code(s): _____

4.71. This is a 71-year-old female admitted with a complaint of right-sided weakness. She denies any fever, shortness of breath, cough, headaches, or chest pain. Patient has NIDDM, controlled by diet. Patient currently smokes. Mild right-sided paralysis was found on physical examination. Patient is right-handed. Gadolinium-enhanced brain MRI demonstrated subacute middle cerebral artery infarct in the left basal ganglia. Discharge diagnosis was CVA—subacute infarct. Physical therapy and speech therapy for her hemiparalysis and dysphasia started and will continue at the rehabilitation facility where she was transferred.

Which of the following answers would be correct?

ICD-9-CM Code(s):

a. 434.91, 438.21, 438.12, 250.00, 305.1, 88.91, 93.39, 93.72
b. 434.91, 342.91, 784.59, 250.00, 305.1, 88.91, 93.39, 93.74
c. 436, 250.00, 305.1, 88.91, 93.39, 93.74
d. 434.91, 342.91, 784.59, 250.00, 305.1, 88.91, 93.39, 93.72

ICD-10-CM Code(s): _____

ICD-10-PCS Code(s): _____

Newborn/Congenital Disorders

4.72. A 6-month-old baby with a left-sided, incomplete upper cleft lip and cleft soft palate is admitted and undergoes surgical repair of both deformities.

Which of the following codes would be correct?

ICD-9-CM Code(s):

a. 749.02, 749.12, 27.62, 27.54
b. 749.22, 27.54, 27.63
c. 749.02, 749.12, 27.69
d. 749.22, 27.62, 27.54

ICD-10-CM Code(s): _____

ICD-10-PCS Code(s): _____

4.73. The patient is an 18-day-old baby girl admitted after it was noticed she was developing drainage from the umbilical cord. Upon admission she was placed on intravenous Cefotaxime and Ampicillin, later changed to Cefotaxime and Clindamycin. A culture taken from the umbilical stump grew Staphylococcus aureus and Group H streptococcus. After the first day, there was great improvement, and the baby continued to improve. She remained afebrile, has continued to eat very well, and she shows no sign of abdominal tenderness or peritonitis. The mother was instructed to watch the child closely and to notify the office if there is any redevelopment of the redness, swelling, or discharge. Recheck in 2 weeks for 1 month check-up. Discharge diagnosis: *Staphylococcus aureus* and Group H streptococcus omphalitis of the newborn. What codes are assigned?

ICD-9-CM Diagnosis Code(s) with POA Indicator:

_____

ICD-10-CM Code(s): _____

4.74. An infant is born by cesarean section at 27 weeks' gestation. The baby weighs 945 g. The baby's lungs are immature, and the baby develops respiratory distress syndrome, requiring a 25-day hospital stay in the NICU. Discharge diagnosis: Extreme immaturity, with 27-week gestation, with respiratory distress syndrome, delivered by cesarean section.

Which of the following diagnosis codes would be correct?

ICD-9-CM Code(s):

a. V30.01, 765.03, 765.24
b. 765.03, 769
c. V30.01, 765.03, 765.24, 769
d. V30.01, 769

ICD-10-CM Code(s): _____

4.75. **Hospital Summary:** A male newborn, born at this hospital with pre-axial polydactyly of the thumbs and cleft deformities of both hands and feet, had a harsh murmur heard posteriorly and faint femoral pulses on initial newborn exam. The newborn was 39 weeks gestation and was born vaginally. Cardiology was consulted and determined a diagnosis of coarctation of the aorta and a very small conoventricular ventricular septal defect. The newborn had surgical repair of the coarctation but the VSD could not be repaired at this young age due to closeness to the aortic valve. Cardiology will follow to manage the VSD. Orthopedics was consulted for the hand and feet deformities and will schedule serial repairs after the age of about 1 year. The family will be seen by Medical Genetics as an outpatient for possible determination of a syndrome that encompasses this combination of defects. Assign the correct diagnostic code(s).

ICD-9-CM Diagnosis Code(s) with POA Indicator:

_____

ICD-10-CM Code(s): _____

4.76. This full-term female infant was born in this hospital by vaginal delivery. Her mother has been an alcoholic for many years and would not stop drinking during her pregnancy. The baby was born with fetal alcohol syndrome and was placed in the NICU. What codes are assigned?

ICD-9-CM Diagnosis Code(s) with POA Indicator:

_____

ICD-10-CM Code(s): _____

Pediatric Conditions

4.77. A child has second- and third-degree burns of the left lower leg and second- and third-degree burns of the lower back with a total of 16% total body surface area (TBSA), 9% third-degree. What is the correct code assignment?

ICD-9-CM Diagnosis Code(s) with POA Indicator and MS-DRG:

_____

ICD-10-CM Code(s): _____

4.78. Patient admitted with cervical lymphadenopathy. Left lymph node excisional biopsy confirmed Hodgkin's sarcoma disease. Megavoltage radiotherapy begun.

Which of the following is the correct code set?

ICD-9-CM Code(s):

a. 201.21, 40.40, 92.29
b. 201.91, 40.40, 92.29
c. 201.21, 40.11, 92.24
d. 201.91, 40.11, 92.24

ICD-10-CM Code(s): _____

ICD-10-PCS Code(s): _____ .

4.79. This 7-year-old child was brought to the hospital with congenital heart problems. During her stay a cardiac catheterization with a non-drug-eluting stent implantation to the left lower pulmonary vein is performed. The stent is implanted via the catheter. What is the correct code assignment for the percutaneous dilation of left pulmonary vein with insertion of stent?

ICD-9-CM Procedure Code(s): _____

ICD-10-PCS Code(s): _____

4.80. The 2-year-old female was admitted to the hospital after being seen in the ER because of vomiting and diarrhea. She received Phenergan suppositories but the vomiting and diarrhea persisted. She was given an intravenous bolus of normal saline followed by intravenous D5 one-quarter, with potassium added, to correct the 5% dehydration. At the time of admission, mucous membranes were tacky. The abdominal examination revealed markedly increased bowel sounds; abdomen was mildly distended, but nontender. There were no masses and no organomegaly. Laboratory evaluation at the time of admission included a Chem-7 profile, which was remarkable for a BUN of 22 and a CO_2 of 19.5. On repeat the following day, the Chem-7 revealed values that were essentially within normal limits. The CBC on admission revealed a white blood cell count of 13,500 with hemoglobin increased at 54.1%, and there was a left shift. On repeat evaluation, the white cell count was down to 5,100, and the indices were within normal limits. Throat culture revealed normal flora; Rotavirus antigen was positive and found to be the cause of the gastroenteritis.

Which of the following answers would be correct?

ICD-9-CM Code(s):

a. 008.61, 276.51
b. 276.51, 558.9
c. 276.51, 008.61
d. 008.8

ICD-10-CM Code(s): _____

ICD-10-PCS Code(s): _____

4.81. This 3-month-old infant was brought to the ER by the babysitter after she did not wake up from a nap. The babysitter admits to shaking the baby because she would not stop crying earlier in the day. She was admitted to ICU and was unconscious for 8 hours. Diagnosis at discharge: Shaken infant syndrome, subdural hematoma, loss of consciousness for 8 hours, and total retinal detachment, right eye. What codes are assigned?

ICD-9-CM Diagnosis Code(s) with POA Indicator and MS-DRG:

_____

ICD-10-CM Code(s): _____

Conditions of Pregnancy, Childbirth, and the Puerperium

4.82. The patient presented through the ED with severe abdominal pain, amenorrhea. Serum human chorionic gonadotropin (hCG) was lower than normal. There were also endometrial and uterine changes. Patient diagnosed with right tubal pregnancy. A laparoscopic salpingectomy with removal of tubal pregnancy was performed. Which of the following is the correct code assignment?

ICD-9-CM Code(s):

a. 633.80, 66.62
b. 633.10, 66.62
c. 633.10, 66.4
d. 633.10, 66.02

ICD-10-CM Code(s): _____

ICD-10-PCS Code(s): _____

4.83. From the health record of a patient experiencing a spontaneous abortion:

Diagnosis: Incomplete spontaneous abortion

Postoperative Diagnosis: Same

Operation: Dilatation and curettage

History: This 22-year-old female, gravida IV, para II, AB I, comes in today because of crampy abdominal pain and passing fetal tissue at home. Apparently her last menstrual period was 9 weeks ago, and she had been doing well, and this problem just started today.

Procedure: The patient was placed on the operating table in the lithotomy position, prepped, and draped in the usual manner. Under satisfactory intravenous sedation, the cervix was visualized by means of weighted speculum, grasped in the anterior lip with a sponge forceps. Cord was prolapsed through the cervix and vagina, and a considerable amount of placental tissue was in the vagina and cervix. This was removed. A sharp curet was used to explore the endometrial cavity, and a minimal amount of curettings was obtained. The patient tolerated the procedure well. What codes are assigned?

ICD-9-CM Code(s):

a. 635.91, 69.09
b. 634.91, 69.09
c. 634.91, 69.02
d. 635.91, 69.02

ICD-10-CM Code(s): _____

ICD-10-PCS Code(s): _____

4.84. This 25-year-old female was admitted at 38 weeks gestation for induction of labor due to mild pre-eclampsia. The patient failed to dilate during medical induction. The decision was made to perform a cesarean section due to the failed induction. What is the principal diagnosis?

ICD-9-CM Code(s):

a. 642.41
b. 659.11
c. 659.01
d. 652.51

ICD-10-CM Code(s): _____

4.85. This is a 26-year-old patient who had previous cesarean section for delivery for fetal distress. She had normal antepartum care and has had no complications. We are going to attempt a VBAC for this delivery. She is admitted in her 39th week in labor. The fetus is in cephalic position and no rotation is necessary. The labor continues to progress and 5 hours later she is taken to delivery. During the delivery she was fatigued, so low outlet forceps were required over a midline episiotomy which was subsequently repaired by an episiorrhaphy. A single liveborn infant was delivered. What codes are reported?

ICD-9-CM Diagnosis Code(s) with POA Indicator and MS-DRG:

_____

ICD-9-CM Procedure Code(s): _____

ICD-10-CM Code(s): _____

ICD-10-PCS Code(s): _____

4.86. The following documentation is from the OB record of a 33-year-old female patient.

Admit Note: 2/27

This is a 33-year-old G2 P0, with an estimated delivery date of 2/28, and estimated gestational age of 40 weeks. She presents for induction secondary to gestational diabetes mellitus. The diabetes has been managed by diet throughout the pregnancy. The patient also has diastasis recti that occurred three weeks ago, which has kept her at bedrest since that time. PNL: 0 positive, rubella immune. PE: AVSS, Abdomen FH 40 cm, EFW 3800-4000 grams. Cervix is closed/50%/-3/post/ceph. Plan is for Pitocin induction with epidural at the beginning of active labor.

Progress Note: 2/28 09:15

Patient is having uterine contractions every 3–8 minutes. Cervix is 1 cm/100%/ floating. Patient desires not to start Pitocin yet. Feels that she is in labor. FHR reactive, baseline 120's with accelerations.

Progress Note: 2/28 19:25

Patient's uterine contractions have resolved. Cervix unchanged. Discussed options, would like to go home to sleep and return in a.m. for Pitocin induction. Discharged home for tonight to sleep. Admit in a.m., start IV Pitocin as per protocol and clear liquid diet. Assign the correct diagnostic code(s).

ICD-9-CM Diagnosis Code(s) with POA Indicator:

_____

ICD-10-CM Code(s): _____

Disorders of the Respiratory System

4.87. The patient was admitted with increasing shortness of breath, weakness, and nonproductive cough. Treatment included oxygen therapy. Final diagnoses listed as acute respiratory insufficiency and acute exacerbation of chronic obstructive pulmonary disease (COPD). Which of the following is the correct diagnostic code assignment?

ICD-9-CM Code(s):

a. 491.21
b. 491.21, 518.82
c. 518.81, 491.21
d. 518.82, 491.21

ICD-10-CM Code(s): _____

4.88. A ventilator-dependent patient (due to emphysema) is admitted to the hospital at 10 a.m. on January 1. He is admitted for dehydration and is placed on the hospital's ventilator upon admission. The patient is discharged January 6 at 1 p.m. What is the appropriate code assignment?

ICD-9-CM Code(s):

a. 492.8, 276.51, 96.72
b. 276.51, 492.8, V46.11, 96.72
c. 276.51, 496, V46.11, 96.71
d. 492.8, 276.51, V46.11, 96.72

ICD-10-CM Code(s): _____

ICD-10-PCS Code(s): _____

4.89.   The patient is a 59-year-old female who is quadriplegic after C5–6 fracture and C5–6 spinal cord injury from motor vehicle accident 1 year ago. Admitted because of a 2-day history of shortness of breath, fevers, and productive cough of green yellow sputum. She has not had much of an appetite and has not been eating or drinking much for the past 2 days. The patient is allergic to Penicillin. An x-ray revealed left-sided pneumonia. She was admitted to the hospital and given intravenous antibiotics for her pneumonia, IV fluids for dehydration, and oxygen. Her pO_2 in the Emergency Room was 50 on room air. She was started on hand-held nebulizer treatment, and her hypoxemia rapidly improved. Serum electrolytes were normal except for potassium of 3.3. This was corrected with additional potassium. At the time of discharge, she was breathing easy on room air and was discharged home. What codes are assigned?

ICD-9-CM Diagnosis Code(s) with POA Indicator and MS-DRG:

_____

ICD-10-CM Code(s): _____

4.90.   **Discharge diagnosis:**

Moderate persistent asthma with status asthmaticus
Acute exacerbation of chronic obstructive pulmonary disease

Hospital Course: The patient presented with gradual increase in shortness of breath, which was unresponsive to home nebulizer treatments. In the emergency room, he received more respiratory treatments; however, he failed to improve. Therefore, the patient was admitted to the hospital. At the time of admission, the theophylline level was 5.9. Chest x-ray showed no evidence of active infiltrates. The patient was bolused with intravenous steroids and started on frequent respiratory therapy treatments. IV aminophylline boluses and drip were used to increase his theophylline level to therapeutic range. The patient gradually cleared and by the next day was much better. His IV aminophylline was changed to p.o. The Ventolin treatments were decreased to q 4 hr. and his steroids were rapidly tapered back to 10 mg. of Prednisone. What diagnosis codes are assigned?

ICD-9-CM Diagnosis Code(s) with POA Indicator:

_____

ICD-10-CM Code(s): _____

4.91.   A 75-year-old male was admitted to the hospital in acute respiratory failure. He has emphysema due to his continuous cigarette smoking for over 50 years. Sputum cultures showed streptococcus A pneumonia. He was intubated in the ER and started on mechanical ventilation. Thirty-six hours later he was extubated and was able to breathe on his own. He was started on Chantix™ to treat his dependence on nicotine. Diagnosis: Acute respiratory failure, pneumonia due to streptococcus A, and emphysema. What codes are assigned?

ICD-9-CM Diagnosis Code(s) with POA Indicator and MS-DRG:

_____

ICD-9-CM Procedure Code(s): _____

ICD-10-CM Code(s): _____

ICD-10-PCS Code(s): _____

Trauma and Poisoning

4.92. From the health record of a high-school athlete:

Discharge Summary: The patient is a 16-year-old male who received a hard tackle while playing football. He was unconscious at the playing field and was brought by ambulance to the emergency department. MRI brain showed a right subdural hematoma. Repeat MRI brain 1 hour later showed the hematoma to be growing. The patient remained unconscious. Vital signs were continuously monitored and remained within normal limits. The patient was taken to the OR, where the hematoma was evacuated via craniotomy. Postoperative course has been uneventful. The patient awakened and stated he was hungry. He has no memory of the event or the period of the football game. The patient is now discharged on the seventh postoperative day.

Which of the following code sets would be correct for this scenario?

ICD-9-CM Code(s):

a. 852.23, E886.0, E849.4, E007.0, E000.8, 01.31, 88.91, 88.91
b. 852.26, E886.0, E849.4, E007.0, E000.8, 01.31, 88.91, 88.91
c. 852.33, E886.0, E849.4, E007.0, E000.8, 01.39, 88.91, 88.91
d. 852.26, E886.0, E849.4, E007.0, E000.8, 01.39, 88.91, 88.91

ICD-10-CM Code(s): _____

ICD-10-PCS Code(s): _____

4.93. The patient is being seen due to right knee pain and decreased mobility. Previously the patient had a right total knee replacement for osteoarthritis. The patient also has extensive medical problems which were all monitored and treated while he was in the hospital: Parkinson's disease, hypertensive heart disease, congestive heart failure, bilateral capsular glaucoma, old MI six months ago, and recent abnormal cardiac stress test. Evaluation of the right knee indicated that patient had aseptic loosening of the tibial component of the knee. The orthopedic consultant indicated that the patient would need to be scheduled for a revision arthroplasty once he was cleared by cardiology for surgery. The cardiac clearance will be done as an outpatient and the procedure will then be scheduled. Assign the correct diagnostic code(s).

ICD-9-CM Diagnosis Code(s) with POA Indicator:

_____

ICD-10-CM Code(s): _____

4.94. This 35-year-old female patient was a driver involved in an automobile accident when she was rear-ended by another driver in a car. She was seen in the emergency room complaining of pain in the arm and neck. She was brought into the hospital by the EMTs on a backboard and after proper splinting to the right arm. It was evident that compound fractures were present. After a CT scan of the head and neck, the patient was removed from the backboard.

She was admitted to the hospital for an open reduction, internal fixation of the type II fractures of the radius and ulna. The surgery was completed without problems. Postoperative x-rays show the radial and ulnar shafts in good alignment. Patient was advised to wear a collar for her cervical strain.

Final Diagnoses, in Order of Significance:
   Compound radius and ulna shaft fractures
   Whiplash injury, cervical spine

What are the correct codes to report for this service?

ICD-9-CM Diagnosis Code(s) with POA Indicator and MS-DRG:

_____

ICD-9-CM Procedure Code(s): _____

ICD-10-CM Code(s): _____

ICD-10-PCS Code(s): _____

4.95. This 32-year-old patient was brought to the emergency department after a gas leak caused an explosion at his home. He was admitted with third-degree burns of the upper back involving 9 percent of the body surface. What codes are assigned?

ICD-9-CM Diagnosis Code(s) with POA Indicator and MS-DRG:

_____

ICD-10-CM Code(s): _____

4.96. This nursing home patient is admitted with extensive cellulitis of the abdominal wall. The examination performed reveals that his existing gastrostomy site is infected. He had a feeding tube inserted 4 months ago because of carcinoma of the middle esophagus. The physician confirms that the responsible organism is *Staphylococcus aureus*.

ICD-9-CM Diagnosis Code(s) with POA Indicator and MS-DRG:

_____

ICD-10-CM Code(s): _____

4.97. This patient was walking along the railroad tracks when a train hit him. He was taken to the Medical Center by ambulance. Surprisingly, there were no internal injuries, and the only injury sustained was significant trauma to both lower legs. Discharge diagnosis was bilateral traumatic amputation. A revision by further amputation of the traumatic amputations of the mid tibia and fibula to the high tibia and fibula was performed on both legs.

ICD-9-CM Diagnosis Code(s) with POA Indicator and MS-DRG:

_____

ICD-9-CM Procedure Code(s): _____

ICD-10-CM Code(s): _____

ICD-10-PCS Code(s): _____

4.98. From the health record of a patient who is status post joint replacement:

Discharge Summary: The patient is an active 61-year-old male, who underwent right total hip arthroplasty approximately 3 years ago. The patient is very active and walks several miles every day and enjoys playing golf. He has recently experienced several instances of failure of the right hip prosthesis. This is well documented in several ED visits for dislocation of the prosthetic hip. The patient was now admitted for scheduled replacement of the right hip arthroplasty. The patient was taken to surgery, where the old prosthesis was found to be eroded and bent, causing the repeated dislocations. The prosthesis was removed and replaced with a titanium/polyethylene prosthesis without incident. The patient was begun on physical therapy for gait training while in the hospital to help regain mobility. The patient was discharged on the fifth day postop to continue the physical therapy as an outpatient.

Which of the following codes would be used to report the above scenario?

ICD-9-CM Diagnosis Code(s) with POA Indicator:

_____

ICD-9-CM Procedure Code(s): _____

ICD-10-CM Code(s): _____

ICD-10-PCS Code(s): _____

4.99. **Discharge Summary:** The patient is a 45-year-old female who fell while walking her dog. She was walking on the sidewalk in her neighborhood and accidently tripped and subsequently fell. She sustained a comminuted fracture of the shaft of her right tibia confirmed by x-ray done in the emergency room. She also hit her head on a fire hydrant and suffered a slight concussion but no loss of consciousness. The patient was admitted and taken to surgery, where an open reduction with internal fixation was accomplished with good alignment of fracture fragments. Postop course was uneventful and the patient was discharged home with daily physical therapy.

ICD-9-CM Diagnosis Code(s) with POA Indicator:

_____

ICD-9-CM Procedure Code(s): _____

ICD-10-CM Code(s): _____

ICD-10-PCS Code(s): _____

Chapter 5

Case Studies from Ambulatory Health Records

Note: Even though the specific cases are divided by setting, most of the information pertaining to the diagnosis is applicable to most settings. Even the CPT codes in the ambulatory and physician sections may be reported in the same manner. The differences in coding in these two settings may involve modifier reporting, evaluation and management CPT code reporting, and other health plan reporting guidelines unique to settings. If you practice or apply codes in a particular type of setting, you may find additional information in other sections of this publication that may be pertinent to you.

Every effort has been made to follow current recognized coding guidelines and principles, as well as nationally recognized reporting guidelines. The material presented may differ from some health plan requirements for reporting. The ICD-9-CM codes used are effective October 1, 2011, through September 30, 2012, and the HCPCS (CPT and HCPCS Level II) codes are in effect January 1, 2011, through December 31, 2011. The current standard transactions and code sets named in HIPAA have been utilized. The 2011 draft edition of ICD-10-CM was utilized.

Instructions: Assign all applicable ICD-9-CM diagnosis codes including V codes and E codes. Assign all applicable ICD-10-CM diagnosis codes including Z codes and external cause codes. Assign all CPT Level I procedure codes and HCPCS Level II codes. Assign Level I (CPT) and Level II (HCPCS) modifiers as appropriate. Outpatient healthcare settings represented in the case examples include emergency room (ER), urgent care, outpatient surgery, observation, ancillary outpatient, wound care, interventional radiology, radiation therapy, or other outpatient department. Final codes for billing occur after codes are passed through payer edits. Medicare utilizes the National Correct Coding Initiative (NCCI) edits. CMS developed the NCCI edit list to promote national correct coding methodologies and to control improper coding leading to improper payments for Medicare Part B. The purpose of the NCCI edits is to ensure the most comprehensive code is assigned and billed rather than the component codes. In addition, NCCI edits check for mutually exclusive pairs.

Cases are presented as either multiple choice or fill in the blank.

- For multiple-choice cases:
  —Select the letter of the appropriate code set.

- For the fill-in-the-blank cases:
  —Assign up to three reasons for visit ICD-9-CM codes to describe the reason for unscheduled visits such as emergency room. Reason for visit coding is required on the claim submission for all "unscheduled" outpatient visits.
  —ICD-9-CM and ICD-10-CM: Sequence the first-listed diagnosis first followed by the secondary diagnoses including any appropriate Classification of Factors Influencing Health Status and Contact with Health Service codes, External Causes of Injury and Poisoning (ICD-9-CM) codes, and External Causes of Morbidity (ICD-10-CM) codes.
  —Sequence the CPT procedure code first followed by additional procedure codes including modifiers as appropriate (both CPT Level I and HCPCS Level II modifiers).
  —Assign HCPCS Level II codes only if instructed (case specific).
  —Assign evaluation and management (E/M) codes only if instructed (case specific).
    - Medicare Type A Emergency Department visits are reported with CPT Level I codes 99281–99285 and critical care codes 99291 and 99292.
    - Medicare Type B Emergency Department visits are reported with Level II HCPCS codes G0380–G0384.

The scenarios are based on selected excerpts from health records. In practice, the coding professional should have access to and refer to the entire health record. Health records are analyzed and codes assigned based on physician documentation. Documentation for coding purposes must be assigned based on medical record documentation. A physician may be queried when documentation is ambiguous, incomplete, or conflicting. The queried documentation must be a permanent part of the medical record.

The objective of the cases and scenarios reproduced in this publication is to provide practice in assigning correct codes, not necessarily to emulate complete coding that can be achieved only with the complete medical record. For example, the reader may be asked to assign codes based on only an operative report; in real practice, a coder has access to documentation in the entire medical record.

The *ICD-9-CM Official Guidelines for Coding and Reporting of Outpatient Services,* published by the National Center for Health Statistics (NCHS), supplements the official conventions and instructions provided within ICD-9-CM. Adherence to these guidelines when assigning ICD-9-CM diagnosis codes is required under the Health Insurance Portability and Accountability Act (HIPAA) of 1996. Additional official coding guidance can be found in the American Hospital Association (AHA)'s *Coding Clinic* publication.

Disorders of the Blood and Blood-Forming Organs

5.1.   This 35-year-old patient was brought to the ER for GI bleeding. He was given 3 units of packed red cells. He was taken to the same-day surgery suite, and the colonoscopy showed angiodysplasia of the transverse colon, which was controlled with laser. What codes are assigned for this case?

ICD-9-CM and CPT Code(s):

a. 569.85, 45382, 36430-59
b. 578.9, 569.84, 45382, 36430, 36430, 36430
c. 578.9, 45382, 36430-59
d. 569.84, 578.9, 45382

ICD-10-CM Code(s): _____

5.2. This 20-year-old female came to the outpatient procedure area with a diagnosis of anemia. A bone marrow aspiration was performed in the following manner.

Manubrial area was prepped with Betadine. Skin and periosteum anesthetized with 2 percent Xylocaine. Skin incision was made with #11 Bard Parker blade, and marrow aspirations performed with U of IL sternal needle. Patient tolerated the procedure with no complaints or complications. Advised to resume normal activity.

Diagnosis: Iron deficiency anemia

Pathology Report

Specimen Received: Bone marrow aspiration and biopsy

Pathologic Diagnosis: Slightly hypercellular marrow with diminished iron consistent with iron deficiency anemia

Microscopic Description: The bone marrow specimen is adequate. The marrow appears to be slightly hypercellular with a cell-to-fat ratio of 60/40. Megakaryocytes are easily found. Most of them are of normal morphology. There is nothing to suggest a primary or metastatic neoplastic proliferation. Granuloma is not found. The maturation of myeloid cells is complete. A Prussian blue stain obtained on both specimens shows diminished stainable iron. The specimen appears to be marrow aspiration. Bone trabecula are not seen in any of it. A reticulin stain was obtained. There is no evidence of significant increase in reticulin in the marrow stroma.

The marrow smears show adequate number of spicules. The complete maturation of myeloid cells is confirmed. Hemoglobinization of erythroid cells is slightly deficient. There is no evidence of excessive number of blasts. The myeloid/erythroid ratio is within normal limits. Plasma cells amount to less than 1 percent of the cells counted.

A review of the peripheral blood smear received shows no abnormal morphological changes in any of the cell lines.

What would be the correct codes assigned in this case?

ICD-9-CM and CPT Code(s):

a. 285.9, 38220
b. 280.9, 38220
c. 285.9, 38220, 38221-59
d. 280.8, 38230

ICD-10-CM Code(s): _____

5.3. This 18-year-old patient with an abnormal blood test underwent bone marrow aspiration from the sternum. The area was cleaned with antiseptic solution, and a local anesthetic was injected. The needle was inserted beneath the skin and rotated into the cortex and the sample taken. The needle was repositioned slightly, and a new syringe attached, and a second sample was obtained. These were sent to the laboratory for analysis. The results show acute lymphocytic leukemia. How is this coded?

ICD-9-CM and CPT Code(s): _____

ICD-10-CM Code(s): _____

5.4. A 40-year-old female had recent surgery for melanoma of the left arm, documented as Clark level IV. She has no obvious signs of metastasis or adenopathy, but staging needs to be done. Under general anesthesia, a sentinel node biopsy of the deep axillary nodes is performed with a gamma counter probe. An injection of isosulfan blue dye was performed, and the nodes followed carefully to the single bright blue node. This node was excised and sent for frozen section, which proved to be positive for melanoma. Before the procedure, lymphoscintigraphy was performed.

Assign the correct codes and modifier for this encounter.

ICD-9-CM and CPT Code(s): _____

ICD-10-CM Code(s): _____

5.5. This 12-year-old male African-American patient is admitted to the ER with chest pain and pulmonary infiltrates. He has sickle cell disease. Treatment was aimed at reducing the chest pain to improve breathing. He was transferred to a larger children's hospital for admission for his sickle cell crisis and acute chest syndrome. What code(s) would be assigned for the diagnosis in this case?

ICD-9-CM Reason for Visit Code(s): _____

ICD-9-CM and CPT Code(s): _____

ICD-10-CM Reason for Visit Code(s): _____

ICD-10-CM Code(s): _____

Disorders of the Cardiovascular System

5.6. The following documentation is from the health record of a 67-year-old male.

Procedure: Placement of a dual chamber implantable pacing cardioverter-defibrillator

Indications: Patient has moderate ischemic cardiomyopathy, prior infarct and stent

Description of Procedure: After informed consent was obtained, the patient was brought to the cardiac lab. The procedure was done under conscious sedation with fluoroscopic guidance. 1% Lidocaine was used to anesthetize the skin under the left clavicle, and a skin incision was made. A pocket was made for the ICD generator and leads, securing good hemostasis. The left subclavian vein was easily cannulated twice using a pediatric set, which was upsized to regular 037 wires, the position of which was checked under fluoro.

I then dilated the access volts with 9-French dilators and used 7-French access sheaths through which a 7-French ventricular lead was advanced and placed under fluoroscopic guidance. It was an active fixation lead. The numbers looked good, and the lead was sutured down. There was no diaphragmatic stimulation.

A 7-French lead was then advanced under fluoroscopic guidance and placed in the right atrial appendage. The numbers looked good. There was no diaphragmatic stimulation and the lead was sutured down. The leads were then attached to the generator, which was tested and sutured down in the pocket. The wound was irrigated several times with antibiotics during and at the end of the case. Wound was closed in layers. The patient tolerated the procedure well without any complications.

The ICD is Model Virtuoso DRD 154AWG. Atrial and ventricular leads are Medtronic. Battery voltage is 3.17 volts. Sensed P waves of 2.5 millivolts through the PSA, slew rate of 0.6 volts per second, impedance of 539 ohms, threshold of 17 volts at 0.5 milliseconds, current of 3.9 milliamperes, sensed R waves of 21 millivolts, slew rate of greater than 4 volts per second, impedance of 965 ohms, threshold of 0.8 volts at 0.5 milliseconds, and current of 0.8 milliamperes.

Through the device, sensed P waves of 2.3 millivolts, impedance of 472 ohms, threshold of 1 volt at 0.5 milliseconds, sensed R waves of 12.1 millivolts, impedance of 752 ohms, threshold of 1 volt at 0.1 milliseconds, HVB impedance of 38 ohms, HVA impedance of 44 ohms.

Defibrillator threshold testing was done. Battery was B2AX, rhythm induced was ventricular fibrillation with T shock, impedance of 43 ohms, energy delivered was 20 joules, charge time was 3.8 seconds, sensitivity was 1.2, and it was successful.

Tachy parameters are VF zone of 300 milliseconds at 200 beats. Therapies are 30 joules and then 35 times 5 with 80 P during charging for VT. Monitor zone is between 150 and 200 beats per minute. Brady parameters are AAI with backup DDD. Managed ventricular pacing at 50 to 120. PAV of 180. SAV of 150. Mode switch at 171.

Impression: Successful dual chamber ICD implantation as noted above. ESP testing of leads and generator. The patient will be monitored in observation, will get further doses of antibiotics, and be sent home when stable.

What CPT code(s) describe(s) this cardiac lab service?

a. 33240
b. 33225, 33240
c. 33249, 93641
d. 33249, 93640, 93641

5.7.   A pediatric patient requires a transesophageal echocardiogram to evaluate an atrioventricular canal defect present since birth. Which codes are reported for this outpatient service?

ICD-9-CM and CPT Code(s):

a. 745.4, 93315
b. 745.69, 93315
c. 745.69, 93312
d. 429.71, 93312

ICD-10-CM Code(s): _____

5.8. This 45-year-old patient is scheduled for the ambulatory surgical center to have an INFUSAID pump installed. He has primary liver cancer, and the pump is being inserted for continuous administration of 5-FU.

The right subclavian vein was cannulated without difficulty and the guidewire passed centrally. The subcutaneous tunnel and pocket were then created and the catheter passed through the tunnel. The central venous catheter was placed and connected to the secured pump. The pump was filled with the chemotherapy agent provided by the hospital, and the patient is observed for adverse reaction and then is discharged home.

What codes are assigned for this episode?

ICD-9-CM and CPT Code(s): _____

ICD-10-CM Code(s): _____

5.9. This 55-year-old patient has a history of unstable angina, hypertension, and chronic systolic heart failure. He is seen in the ER after prolonged chest pain that was not relieved by medication. Cardiac enzymes are elevated, and EKG shows anterior infarct. A decision was made to admit patient to observation and perform a cardiac catheterization and coronary angiography. Left heart catheterization was performed in order to perform a left ventriculogram. He tolerated the procedure well and will be discharged. Diagnosis: Acute anterior myocardial infarction (STEMI), chronic systolic heart failure, hypertension. What are the correct codes?

ICD-9-CM Reason for Visit Code(s): _____

ICD-9-CM and CPT Code(s): _____

ICD-10-CM Reason for Visit Code(s): _____

ICD-10-CM Code(s): _____

5.10. This 82-year-old male patient was shoveling snow and collapsed in his driveway. He arrived in the emergency department unresponsive and in asystole. A "code blue" was called, and CPR was administered without a return to consciousness. The final diagnosis on the ER record was "Cardiopulmonary arrest, probably secondary to an acute myocardial infarction induced by exertion." Which diagnosis codes are reported?

ICD-9-CM Reason for Visit Code(s): _____

ICD-9-CM Code(s): _____

ICD-10-CM Reason for Visit Code(s): _____

ICD-10-CM Code(s): _____

5.11. Under local anesthesia and ultrasound guidance, a patient underwent radiofrequency ablation of an incompetent greater saphenous vein in the right lower extremity. Assign the appropriate CPT code(s).

a. 36475-RT
b. 36475-RT, 36000
c. 36478-RT
d. 36475-RT, 76942

5.12. The elderly patient was seen in the same-day surgery unit for insertion of a subclavian venous catheter for treatment of his prostate carcinoma.

Operative Report: The patient's right upper chest was prepped and draped in the usual manner. Local anesthesia was obtained using Xylocaine. A percutaneous subclavian venous catheter was inserted and secured at the skin level with 4-0 nylon. A sterile dressing was applied. The catheter was irrigated with Heparin and the patient was sent to recovery.

What codes are assigned for this ambulatory surgery?

ICD-9-CM and CPT Code(s): _____

ICD-10-CM Code(s): _____

Disorders of the Digestive System

5.13. The following documentation is from the health record of a female patient.

Outpatient Operative Report

This patient with hiatal hernia is admitted to same-day surgery for repair.

Description of Procedure: The patient was placed under satisfactory general endotracheal anesthesia. She was then placed in the lithotomy position. Foley was placed. Orogastric tube was inserted. The abdomen was prepped and draped in normal sterile fashion. A supraumbilical incision was made to the midline, and the fascia was incised to enter the abdomen. Under direct visualization, a 0 VICRYL stitch was placed on each side of the fascia, and a blunt Hasson trocar was inserted. The abdomen was insufflated with CO_2. Under direct visualization, two 11-mm ports were placed in the left subcostal region, and 11-mm and 12-mm ports were placed in the right subcostal region.

The liver bed was then lifted up off the gastrohepatic ligament. The gastrohepatic ligament was taken down with harmonic scalpel. The right crus of the diaphragm was identified and dissected out with harmonic scalpel and blunt dissection. I dissected out the phrenicoesophageal ligament anteriorly and came around identifying the left crus. I then took down the short gastrics from the midportion of the greater curvature of the stomach up to the GE junction, using harmonic scalpel and taking care to not damage the spleen. Once we had adequately taken down the short gastrics, the posterior ligament was then mobilized behind the esophagus, and the stomach easily pulled through with no tension and no twist on the esophagus and easily laid in place.

The hiatal hernia was then repaired with a posterior cruropexy stitch of 0 ETHIBOND. The wrap was then brought around and was placed approximately 2 cm into the esophagus with a horizontal mattress pledgeted 0 ETHIBOND stitch. A second interrupted stitch was placed just through-and-through on the stomach below this. At the end of the procedure, there was no tension or twist on the esophagus and no bleeding apparent. All ports were removed under direct visualization and there appeared to be hemostasis. The fascia at the supraumbilical incision was closed with 0 VICRYL.

The skin was anesthetized with local anesthetic and then closed with 4-0 subcuticular MONOCRYL.

Which codes are reported for this case?

ICD-9-CM and CPT Code(s):

a. 553.3, 43327
b. 553.3, 43280
c. 551.3, 43280
d. 553.3, 43328

ICD-10-CM Code(s): _____

5.14.   This 59-year-old female patient came into the emergency room because of passing melanic stools. The emergency room physician initially saw her. The gastroenterologist was called into consultation. Because of the massive amounts of bleeding, it was decided to proceed with endoscopy. The endoscope was passed into the esophagus, stomach, and duodenum. Blood and clots were noted. This patient could possibly have a duodenal ulcer, but because of the amount of blood, it was difficult to delineate an ulcer crater. Diagnosis: Melenic stools, and possibly duodenal ulcer. What codes are assigned in this case?

ICD-9-CM Reason for Visit Code(s): _____

ICD-9-CM and CPT Code(s): _____

ICD-10-CM Reason for Visit Code(s): _____

ICD-10-CM Code(s): _____

5.15.   This 77-year-old patient admitted to the special procedures room is having an endoscopic-directed percutaneous endoscopic gastrostomy tube placed because of moderate malnutrition. The patient has had a stroke, with residual right dominant-sided hemiparesis. Assign the codes that the hospital would use to bill this service.

ICD-9-CM and CPT Code(s): _____

ICD-10-CM Code(s): _____

5.16.   A 39-year-old male has been treated for symptomatic cholelithiasis without improvement. Patient comes to outpatient surgery for a laparoscopic cholecystectomy. Due to previous abdominal surgery, adhesions were encountered. During the course of the laparoscopic cholecystectomy procedure, the adhesions were lysed, but this did not prolong the procedure.

What codes are assigned?

ICD-9-CM and CPT Code(s): _____

ICD-10-CM Code(s): _____

5.17. The following documentation is from the health record of an outpatient surgical patient.

Preoperative Diagnosis:	Rectal mass
	Change in bowel habits
Postoperative Diagnosis:	Rectal prolapse
	Colonic polyps. Biopsies × 2
	Significant sigmoid diverticulosis with nonspecific colitis
Procedure:	Colonoscopy performed to the level of the cecum, 110 cm

Procedure: The 62-year-old male patient was prepped in the usual fashion, followed by placement in the left lateral decubitus position. I administered 3 mg of Versed. Monitoring of sedation was assisted by a trained registered nurse. Next, the Pentax Video Endoscope was passed through the rectal verge after a negative digital examination and advanced to the level of the cecum. The scope was then slowly retracted with a circular tip motion. There was mild nonspecific colitis noted. She did have significant sigmoid diverticulosis and several small polyps just inside the rectum, as well as a large prolapsing mass of mucosa approximately 5 cm inside the rectum. This appears to have prolapsed previously. Two of the small polyps were biopsied using the cold biopsy forceps and sent to pathology for examination. The remainder of the examination was unremarkable. The patient tolerated the procedure well.

Pathology Report

Clinical Information: Change in bowel habits. Colonoscopy performed.

Gross Examination: The specimen is labeled polyps × 2 at 3 cm. Submitted are 2 fragments of tan tissue measuring up to 0.3 cm in greatest dimension.

Microscopic Examination: Sections examined at multiple levels show 2 fragments of rectal mucosa in which the surfaces and subjacent crypts show no evidence of adenomatous or neoplastic changes.

Diagnosis: Rectum, biopsies at 3 cm: rectal polyps

What codes are assigned in this case?

ICD-9-CM and CPT Code(s): _____

ICD-10-CM Code(s): _____

5.18. The following documentation is from the health record of an outpatient surgical patient.

Preoperative Diagnosis:	Right inguinal hernia
Postoperative Diagnosis:	Right inguinal hernia, direct and indirect
Procedures:	Repair of right inguinal hernia with mesh

Procedure: This 45-year-old male was prepped in the usual manner for an initial hernia repair. After satisfactory spinal anesthesia, the inguinal area was draped in the usual sterile manner. A transverse incision was made above the inguinal ligament and carried down to the fascia of the external oblique, which was then opened, and the cord was mobilized. The ilioinguinal nerve was identified and protected. A relatively large indirect hernia was found. However, there was an extension of the hernia, such that one could definitely tell there had been a long-standing hernia here that probably had enlarged fairly recently. The posterior wall, however, was quite dilated and without a great deal of tone and bulging, and probably fit the criteria for a hernia by itself. Nonetheless, the hernia sac was separated from the cord structures, and a high ligation was done with a purse-string suture of 2-0 silk and a suture ligature of the same material prior to amputating the sac. The posterior wall was repaired with Marlex mesh, which was sewn in place in the usual manner, anchoring two sutures at the pubic tubercle tissue, taking one lateral up the rectus sheath and one lateral along the shelving border of Poupart's ligament past the internal ring. The mesh had been incised laterally to accommodate the internal ring. Several sutures were used to tack the mesh down superiorly and laterally to the transversalis fascia. Then the two limbs of the mesh were brought together lateral to the internal ring and secured to the shelving border of Poupart's ligament. The mesh was irrigated with gentamicin solution. The subcutaneous tissue was closed with fine VICRYL, as was the internal oblique. Marcaine was infiltrated in the subcutaneous tissue and skin. The wound was closed with fine nylon. The patient tolerated the procedure well.

Pathology Report

Gross Description

Specimen: Right inguinal hernia sac

The specimen consists of a pink to blue-gray membranous piece of tissue measuring 5.5 cm in maximum dimension. Blocks are made.

Clinical: Right inguinal hernia

Assign the correct codes and modifier for this encounter.

ICD-9-CM and CPT Code(s): _____

ICD-10-CM Code(s): _____

5.19.   The following documentation is from the health record of an outpatient surgical patient.

Preoperative Diagnosis:	Chronic cholelithiasis
Postoperative Diagnosis:	Chronic cholelithiasis Subacute cholecystitis
Operation:	Laparoscopic cholecystectomy Intraoperative cholangiogram

Procedure: The patient is a 44-year-old female brought to the operating room, placed in supine position, and who underwent general endotracheal anesthesia. After adequate induction of anesthesia, the abdomen was prepped and draped in the usual fashion. The patient had several previous lower midline incisions and right flank incision; therefore, the pneumoperitoneum was created via epigastric incision to the left of the midline with a Verres needle. After adequate pneumoperitoneum was created, the 11-mm trocar was placed through the extended incision in the left epigastrium just to the left of the midline. The trocar was placed, and the laparoscope and camera were in place. Inspection of the peritoneal cavity revealed it to be free of adhesions, and an 11-mm trocar was then placed under direct vision through a small infraumbilical incision. The scope and camera were then moved to this position, and the gallbladder was easily visualized. The gallbladder was elevated, and Hartmann's pouch was grasped. Using a combination of sharp and blunt dissection, the cystic artery was identified. The gallbladder was somewhat tense and subacutely inflamed. Therefore, a needle was passed through the abdominal wall into the gallbladder, and the gallbladder was aspirated free until it collapsed. One of the graspers was held over this region to prevent any further leakage of bile. Again, direction was turned to the area of the triangle of Calot. The cystic duct was dissected free with sharp and blunt dissection. A small opening was made in the duct, and the cholangiogram catheter was passed. The cholangiogram revealed no stones or filling defects in the bile duct system. The biliary tree was normal. There was good flow into the duodenum, and the catheter was definitely in the cystic duct. The catheter was removed, and the cystic duct was ligated between clips, as was the cystic artery. The gallbladder was then dissected free from the hepatic bed using electrocautery dissection, and it was removed from the abdomen through the umbilical port. Inspection of the hepatic bed noted that hemostasis was meticulous. The region of dissection was irrigated and aspirated dry. The trocars were removed, and the pneumoperitoneum was released. The incisions were closed with Steri-Strips, and the umbilical fascial incision was closed with 2-0 Maxon. The patient tolerated the procedure well; there were no complications. She was returned to the recovery room awake and alert.

What codes would be assigned?

ICD-9-CM and CPT Code(s): _____

ICD-10-CM Code(s): _____

5.20. A 61-year-old male patient is being assessed for possible colon cancer and treated in the special procedure unit of the hospital. He undergoes a colonoscopy into the ascending colon with biopsy of a suspicious area in the transverse colon using the cold biopsy forceps. In addition, a colonic ultrasound of the area is performed, with transmural biopsy of an area of the mesentery adjacent to the transverse colon. Assign the appropriate CPT codes.

a. 45384, 45342
b. 45380, 45391
c. 45384, 45392
d. 45380, 45392

5.21. The following documentation is from the health record of an outpatient.

Preoperative Diagnosis: Aspiration pneumonitis

Postoperative Diagnosis: Aspiration pneumonitis

Operative Procedure: NJ Tube Placement

Description of Procedure: The identity of the patient was confirmed. The planned procedure was confirmed with staff. Consent was verified. The patient was prepared with IV sedation.

An 8 Fr CorPak tube was lubricated and inserted into stomach. Fluoroscopic guidance was provided by radiology. This allowed passage of the tube through the pylorus, through the duodenum, and into the jejunum. Position of the tube was confirmed by contrast instillation. Water flushed well through the tube. The tube was taped securely to the face. The patient was sent to the recovery room in good condition.

Impression: 1. Successful NJ tube placement

ICD-9-CM Reason for Visit Code(s): _____

ICD-9-CM and CPT Code(s): _____

ICD-10-CM Code(s): _____

5.22. The patient was seen in the ER after accidentally swallowing a crown from a tooth. A rigid esophagoscopy for foreign body removal was ordered.

Procedure: The 33-year-old was taken to OP surgery where conscious sedation was induced. An esophageal speculum was introduced and a small crown was grasped and removed using the speculum. Compression on the trachea was released. The esophagus was evaluated using a 6 × 30 esophagoscope and there appeared to be no remaining fragments or injuries to the esophagus. The esophagoscope was removed and the patient was sent to the PACU in good condition.

What code(s) are assigned for this outpatient encounter?

ICD-9-CM and CPT Code(s): _____

ICD-10-CM Code(s): _____

5.23. The patient was seen in the endoscopy suite for evaluation of previously diagnosed guaiac-positive stools. The EGD revealed no abnormalities except for a suspicious area in the duodenum which was biopsied. The scope was removed and a colonoscope introduced. The rectum, sigmoid colon, and descending colon were examined. After some difficulty, the scope was passed through the splenic flexure; the transverse colon had multiple polyps. Two large adenomatous polyps were removed by snare technique and two additional polyps were biopsied.

What code(s) are used to report this encounter?

ICD-9-CM and CPT Code(s): _____

ICD-10-CM Code(s): _____

5.24. The following documentation is from a health record from an OP surgery.

Preoperative Diagnosis:	Ventral hernia.
Postoperative Diagnosis:	Ventral hernia.
Operation Performed:	Ventral hernia repair via laparoscopy.

Description of Procedure: The patient was prepped and draped in the usual fashion after being placed in a supine position. A 1-cm incision was made and a Veress needle was introduced into the abdominal cavity. A ten mm trocar was inserted and the laparoscope introduced. Additional trocars were inserted. Direct observation of the abdomen revealed a 2- to 3-cm hernia defect just below the umbilicus. Following plication of the rectus abdominal muscle, mesh Marlex was fashioned to an appropriate size, applied around the area, and sutured using 2.0 Prolene suture. Two Jackson-Pratt drains were placed in the subcutaneous area and attached using 2-0 thread.

The scope and trocars were removed and incisions sutured. The patient tolerated the procedure well and left the OR in good condition.

What code(s) are assigned in this case?

ICD-9-CM and CPT Code(s): _____

ICD-10-CM Code(s): _____

Endocrine, Nutritional, and Metabolic Diseases and Immunity Disorders

5.25. This 17-year-old patient presents to the emergency room with a chief complaint of severe right lower quadrant abdominal pain. The patient describes the pain as tightness and an intense cramping feeling. She has had increased bowel movements that provide some relief from the cramping. The pain seems much more intense after milk or ice cream. The patient is also currently menstruating but describes these cramps as different and worse. She is on no medication, no birth control, and is not sexually active.

Emergency Department diagnoses: Lactose intolerance, menstrual cramps

ICD-9-CM Reason for Visit Code(s): _____

ICD-9-CM and CPT Code(s): _____

ICD-10-CM Reason for Visit Code(s): _____

ICD-10-CM Code(s): _____

5.26. The patient is diagnosed with a thyroglossal duct cyst. The surgeon locates the cyst using palpation, and an incision is created. The cyst is then excised. What is the correct CPT code assignment for this service?

a. 60200
b. 60210
c. 60280
d. 60281

5.27.   A 45-year-old female presents to the outpatient surgery unit of the hospital with a complaint of neck swelling. The physician noted diffuse swelling of the neck with enlargement of the thyroid gland. The patient exhibits no clinical signs of hyperthyroidism. The physician suspects lymphoma, and a biopsy is performed. A large, hollow core needle is passed through the skin into the thyroid. Tissue is sent for histopathology. A diagnosis of thyroid gland follicular lymphoma is confirmed and chemotherapy is planned.

What is the correct code assignment?

ICD-9-CM and CPT Code(s): _____

ICD-10-CM Code(s): _____

Disorders of the Genitourinary System

5.28.   A 55-year-old female patient presents to the same-day surgical unit with stress incontinence and requires repair for midline cystocele and incomplete vaginal prolapse. The physician elects to perform a paravaginal defect repair on both sides. An abdominal incision is made and entry into the space of Retzius is gained. Six sutures are placed through the anterior lateral edge of the vaginal wall and then through the fascia condensation over the obturator internus muscle from the inferior aspect of the pubic bone along the arcus tendinous to the ischial spine. Additional anchors were placed at the level of the urethrovesical junction on both sides to correct the cystocele.

Which of the following code sets is reported for this service?

ICD-9-CM and CPT Code(s):

a. 625.6, 618.01, 618.2, 57284, 51840
b. 625.6, 57284-50
c. 618.02, 57240
d. 618.01, 625.6, 57284

ICD-10-CM Code(s): _____

5.29.   This 77-year-old male patient is a nursing home patient who is admitted to the special procedure unit at the hospital. Patient is stress incontinent and continually leaks urine. To treat this, the urologist introduces a mechanical obstruction in the urethra that prevents leakage. Using an endoscope, the physician injects a solution of polytetrafluoroethylene into the region of the distal sphincter of the urethra, then inserts an inflatable bladder neck sphincter with pump, reservoir, and cuff. Which of the following code sets is reported for this surgery?

ICD-9-CM and CPT Code(s):

a. 788.37, 788.32, 53445, 51715
b. 788.39, 51715
c. 788.37, 53440
d. 788.37, 788.32, 53445

ICD-10-CM Code(s): _____

5.30. This 68-year-old male patient presents to the clinic with a chief complaint of inability to void. He has a history of several urinary tract infections in the past. The physician orders a urinalysis with a diagnosis of acute urinary retention. Urine is obtained by the nursing staff using a straight catheter. What codes would be submitted by the facility for the nursing services provided that day?

ICD-9-CM and CPT Code(s):

a. 788.20, V13.02, 51701
b. 788.20, 51702, P9612
c. 788.20, V13.02, P9612
d. 599.0, 51701

ICD-10-CM Code(s): _____

5.31. This patient, a 47-year-old male with adenoma of the prostate, is being treated in the outpatient surgery suite. The urologist inserts an endoscope in the penile urethra and dilates the structure to allow instrument passage. After endoscope placement, a radiofrequency stylet is inserted, and the diseased prostate is excised with radiant energy. Bleeding is controlled with electrocoagulation. Following instrument removal, a catheter is inserted and left in place. Which of the following code sets will be reported for this service?

ICD-9-CM and CPT Code(s):

a. 600.20, 53852
b. 600.20, 52601
c. 600.00, 53852
d. 222.2, 53850

ICD-10-CM Code(s): _____

5.32. The patient is a 22-year-old male with left testicular pain and scrotal swelling over the past 3 hours. No dysuria, no penile discharge, no fever and is able to void well. No trauma to groin. Pain 5/10. The physician orders an ultrasound which demonstrates a testicle that is free-floating in the scrotum with the spermatic cord looped once around the middle of the testicle. The patient was against surgical intervention and opted to try manual detorsion. The patient was warmed with hot packs to loosen the scrotal skin, and the physician manipulated the testicle until the spermatic cord felt loosened. Re-ultrasound confirmed proper position, and the patient's pain was substantially relieved. The patient was sent home with a list of precautions and instructions to return with any increase in pain.

What codes are reported by the facility? Do not include an E/M code for this case.

ICD-9-CM Reason for Visit Code(s): _____

ICD-9-CM and CPT Code(s): _____

ICD-10-CM Reason for Visit Code(s): _____

ICD-10-CM Code(s): _____

5.33.   A 90-year-old female nursing home patient with a long history of chronic urinary tract infections is brought to the emergency room after developing a fever of 102°F with generalized abdominal pain. The patient has senile dementia with delirium and is unable to communicate. The history was obtained from nursing home transfer records. Nonautomated urinalysis with microscopy was performed but was not remarkable. The physician's assessment stated "fever of unknown origin." The patient was treated with Tylenol and started on a broad-spectrum antibiotic and referred to her primary care physician for follow-up first thing in the morning.

What codes are reported by the ER facility coding? Do not include E/M codes in this example, but do include laboratory codes, even though they would be reported by the chargemaster.

ICD-9-CM Reason for Visit Code(s): _____

ICD-9-CM and CPT Code(s): _____

ICD-10-CM Reason for Visit Code(s): _____

ICD-10-CM Code(s): _____

5.34.   Patient is a 59-year-old admitted to the same-day surgery suite. Patient is a type I diabetic with diabetic nephropathy and end-stage renal disease now requiring dialysis. A Cimino-type direct arteriovenous anastomosis is performed by incising the skin of the left antecubital fossa. Vessel clamps are placed on the vein and adjacent artery. The vein is dissected free and the downstream portion of the vein is sutured to an opening in the artery using an end-to-side technique. The skin incision is closed in layers.

What codes are reported for this service?

ICD-9-CM and CPT Code(s): _____

ICD-10-CM Code(s): _____

5.35.   A 28-year-old patient admitted for same-day surgery with a history of abdominal surgery and is experiencing sharp pain in the pelvic area. Diagnostic workup has presented no etiology. An exploratory laparoscopy was performed and revealed adhesions around the fallopian tubes and ovaries. The adhesions were taken down during the procedure. What codes will be reported?

ICD-9-CM and CPT Code(s): _____

ICD-10-CM Code(s): _____

5.36.   A 59-year-old male is admitted to the special procedure unit of the hospital. He has been having increasing difficulty in urinating. A transurethral resection of the bladder neck is performed to treat urinary obstruction and retention due to vesicourethral obstruction with benign prostatic hypertrophy. What codes are reported?

ICD-9-CM and CPT Code(s): _____

ICD-10-CM Code(s): _____

5.37. A patient with advanced renal cell carcinoma is admitted to the interventional radiology department to undergo percutaneous radiofrequency ablation of four tumors of the right kidney. Assign the appropriate CPT code for this procedure.

Code(s): _____

Infectious Diseases

5.38. A 22-year-old male patient presents to the emergency room with symptoms of right upper quadrant pain, fever, profound malaise, and bloody diarrhea. An infectious consultation was obtained and diagnosis was made of acute *Entamoeba histolytica* dysentery. What code(s) are assigned?

ICD-9-CM Reason for Visit Code(s): _____

ICD-9-CM Code(s): _____

ICD-10-CM Reason for Visit Code(s): _____

ICD-10-CM Code(s): _____

5.39. A 29-year-old male patient presents to the hospital emergency room with a vesicular eruption and severe itching on the penis, scrotum, buttocks, and groin. Itching is severe at night. Assessment: Infestation with *Sarcoptes scabiei*. Plan: Permethrin 5% cream is applied to the affected area and a prescription provided for whole-body treatment of the entire household. What diagnosis code is reported for this encounter?

ICD-9-CM Reason for Visit Code(s): _____

ICD-9-CM Code(s): _____

ICD-10-CM Reason for Visit Code(s): _____

ICD-10-CM Code(s): _____

5.40. This 3-year-old patient presents to the emergency department with history of sudden bloody diarrhea. The stool culture demonstrated *Escherichia coli*. The patient went swimming with his child-care-center class the previous day at a nearby water park. The physician documented: acute enteritis, due to enterotoxigenic *E. coli*. What is the correct ICD-9-CM diagnostic code for this encounter?

ICD-9-CM Reason for Visit Code(s): _____

ICD-9-CM Code(s): _____

ICD-10-CM Reason for Visit Code(s): _____

ICD-10-CM Code(s): _____

5.41. The patient is seen for latent TB infection. He had a positive TB skin test last week and presents today for counseling on the start of INH 300 mg/day, orally. The patient also has moderate Bipolar I disorder and is currently depressed. Because of this, the physician spends considerable time discussing the need to take the INH daily, along with all other prescribed medication.

What diagnosis code(s) describe this case?

ICD-9-CM Reason for Visit Code(s): _____

ICD-9-CM Code(s): _____

ICD-10-CM Reason for Visit Code(s): _____

ICD-10-CM Code(s): _____

Disorders of the Skin and Subcutaneous Tissue

5.42. This is a record from a same-day surgery.

Preoperative Diagnosis:	Basal cell carcinoma of right nasal tip; lesion on right cheek.
Postoperative Diagnosis:	Pathology pending. Probable sebaceous hyperplasia.
Procedures:	Excision of lesion of the right nasal tip; placement of full thickness skin graft; excision of cheek lesion.

Description of Procedure: Under satisfactory premedication, the patient was brought to the Operating Room and using a loupe magnification, the area of excision was mapped out. 1% Xylocaine with Epinephrine was then utilized to anesthetize the nasal tip and also the keratosis on the right cheek. The 1.0-cm lesion in the right cheek was excised. The 0.9-cm nasal specimen was then excised after prepping and draping. The excision went down to the alar cartilage. Specimen was sent for frozen section. The specimen showed no basal cell cancer. The pathologist commented that it might be sebaceous hyperplasia. It appeared to be completely excised. Full thickness skin graft was then harvested from the right post auricular region. The area here was then closed after some cauterization of small bleeders with the battery-operated cautery. Closure was with interrupted 4-0 Vicryl and then a running 4-0 Prolene mattress suture. The graft was defatted and then sewn into position. The length of the graft was 1.1 × 1 cm. 5-0 Nylon was utilized to secure the graft. Xeroform and 2 × 2 gauze were then placed over the operative area. A Band-Aid was placed over the keratosis site. The patient tolerated the procedure quite well and was sent to the ASU.

Pathology Report

Tissue(s) Submitted:	Specimen A: Lesion - right nasal tip.
	Specimen B: Lesion - right cheek.

Gross Description:

A. Specimen is received in fixative and consists of a 1.3 × 0.7 cm ellipse of skin with a longitudinal cut. There is a suture along one long axis. This axis is marked with black ink and a central section through the ellipse is made. Frozen section diagnosis: sebaceous lobules, and a small follicular cyst.

B. Specimen is received in fixative and consists of an oval, gray, friable 0.6-cm piece of skin.

Microscopic Description:

Five microscopic slide(s) examined.

Diagnosis:

A. Basal cell carcinoma, skin of right nasal tip.

Comment: Surgical resection margins are free of neoplastic cells. Although initial frozen section did not reveal basal cell carcinoma, deeper sections of the frozen piece reveal basal cell carcinoma.

B. Seborrheic keratosis, skin of right cheek.

Assign the correct codes for this same-day surgery encounter.

ICD-9-CM and CPT Code(s): _____

ICD-10-CM Code(s): _____

5.43. **Preoperative Diagnosis:** Lipoma of the left posterior thigh.

Postoperative Diagnosis: Same.

Procedures: Excision of the above.

Description of Procedure: The patient was taken to the Operating Room where good anesthesia was obtained with 40 cc of 1% Carbocaine. The transverse incision was made centered over the visible and palpable mass, carried down through the skin and subcutaneous layer. The mass was noted and shelled out. It had no major neurovascular attachments. This was removed in its entirety. Copiously irrigated and aspirated. The fat layer was closed using 0 plain catgut. The skin was closed with 2-0 dermalon.

Estimated Blood Loss: Minimal. Dressings were applied and the leg wrapped with an ACE wrap for compression. She tolerated the procedure well and left the Operating Room in good condition.

Pathology Report

Clinical Diagnosis and History:

Operation: Excision soft tissue mass left thigh.

Tissue(s) Submitted: Specimen: soft tissue mass left lateral posterior thigh.

Gross Description: The specimen consists of several lobular portions of fatty tissue which together measure 4.5 × 3 × 2 cm in greatest dimension. Multiple sections through the specimen reveal no areas of softening or of unusual consistency.

Microscopic Description: Sections show mature fat with a scant amount of intervening fibrous stroma.

Diagnosis: "Soft tissue mass left lateral posterior thigh": The appearance is compatible with a lipoma.

What code(s) are used to report this encounter?

ICD-9-CM and CPT Code(s): _____

ICD-10-CM Code(s): _____

5.44.   A 55-year-old female patient who had a lesion removal 2 weeks ago returns now for a wide excision of a malignant melanoma on the back. The area excised consists of a 3-cm-diameter area. A layer closure is required to close the defect. The pathology report shows clear margins.

What are the correct codes to report? The procedure is performed in the outpatient surgery suite at the hospital.

ICD-9-CM and CPT Code(s):

a. 172.5, 11603
b. 709.9, 11603
c. 172.5, 11603, 12032
d. V76.43, 11603, 13121

ICD-10-CM Code(s): _____

5.45.   An ambulatory surgery operative report for a 75-year-old male patient states that the patient received a full-thickness graft of the cheek following lesion removal of a basal carcinoma. The lesion plus margins are documented to be 3.2 cm in diameter. A 10-sq-cm graft is applied with donor skin from his thigh, closed by suture.

Which of the following code sets is correct for this surgery?

ICD-9-CM and CPT Code(s):

a. 173.31, 15240, 11646
b. 173.31, 15240, 15004
c. 173.31, 15320, 15004, 11644
d. 173.31, 15240, 11644

ICD-10-CM Code(s): _____

5.46.   From the health record of a patient undergoing foot surgery in the outpatient surgical unit:

Indication for Procedure: The patient is a 60-year-old female who has a persistently ingrowing great toenail on the right foot that has had two past infections. The infection is now clear and the patient presents for wedge resection of the toenail. She also has pernicious anemia, Friedreich's ataxia, and heart disease. Because of these conditions, a digital block will be used for the procedure.

Procedure: Wedge resection of toenail

Procedure Description: The patient is placed in the supine position, with the knees flexed, and the right foot is flat on the table. The toe is prepped and cleansed. A standard digit block is performed with 1% lidocaine using a 10-ml syringe and a 30 gauge needle. Approximately 3 ml is instilled on each side of the toe.

After waiting 10 minutes, a sterilized rubber band is placed around the base of the toe. The toe is resterilized and draped with the toe protruding. A nail elevator is slid under the cuticle to separate the nail plate from the overlying proximal nail fold. The lateral one fourth of the nail plate is identified as the site for the partial lateral nail removal. A bandage scissors is used to cut from the distal end of the nail straight back beneath the proximal nail fold. A straight, smooth, new lateral edge to the nail plate is created. The lateral piece of nail is grasped with a hemostat and removed in one piece, pulling straight out.

Electrocautery ablation is used to destroy the nail matrix where the nail was removed. The matrix is treated twice. Antibiotic ointment is applied and a bulky gauze dressing is placed. The foot is placed in a surgical boot. Post-op instructions are given for daily cleansing with warm water, and strenuous exercise is to be avoided completely for at least 1 week. The patient tolerated the procedure well and understands the discharge instructions.

What codes would be assigned for reporting the facility services?

ICD-9-CM Reason for Visit Code(s): _____

ICD-9-CM and CPT Code(s): _____

ICD-10-CM Reason for Visit Code(s): _____

ICD-10-CM Code(s): _____

5.47. A 17-year-old male patient presents to the hospital outpatient surgery center for surgery. Destruction was performed on 8 viral warts on the left arm. Destruction was done using cryosurgery and curettage. What codes are reported?

ICD-9-CM and CPT Code(s): _____

ICD-10-CM Code(s): _____

5.48. This 4-year-old boy is seen in the emergency room today. He was helping his father outside, who was installing a new bedroom window, and the window fell. The glass broke, cutting the boy on his hand, forearm, and leg. He received a 2-cm laceration on his left hand, a 3-cm laceration on his left forearm, and a 2.5-cm laceration on his lower right leg. The lacerations on the hand and forearm were repaired with a simple repair. The laceration on the leg was deeper and required a layered repair. Assign the correct codes for this encounter.

ICD-9-CM Reason for Visit Code(s): _____

ICD-9-CM and CPT Code(s): _____

ICD-10-CM Reason for Visit Code(s): _____

ICD-10-CM Code(s): _____

5.49.   **Preoperative Diagnosis:**   Burn scar contracture with hypertrophic and keloid scarring anterior neck.

Postoperative Diagnosis: Burn scar contracture with hypertrophic and keloid scarring anterior neck.

Procedure Performed: Excision of keloid and release of anterior neck (20 × 8 cm).

Anesthesia: General.

Estimated Blood Loss: Minimal.

Indications for Procedure: This 18-year-old male had very severe hypertrophic burn scar to his anterior neck region. He is a keloid former by his previous history. He has been successfully treated with an acellular dermal replacement in the past. Our plan today after release of his neck and excision of the keloid is application of Integra to the defect on the anterior neck.

Description of Procedure: The patient was brought to the operating room and placed in the supine position on the OR table where general anesthesia and endotracheal intubation were accomplished without difficulty. After this was done, the patient was placed in a slightly hyper-extended position on the neck with a roll behind his shoulders and with sterile towels in the usual manner. A line was then drawn across the site of maximal contracture on the anterior neck and this was incised, carried down to scar into the platysma muscle. A large amount of hypertrophic and keloid scar was excised from the upper part of the flap. After this was released, the face was not distorted any longer and the contracture had been alleviated. The size of the defect with this was 20 × 8 cm. After bleeding was controlled with electrocautery, Integra was prepared, and one sheet was meshed 1:1 and applied on to the wound and secured with staples. Following this, stretched burn netting was applied over the Integra for support by Reston foam wet, irrigation catheters, and wet burn dressings. Spandex was used to complete the dressing.

The patient was then awakened, extubated, and transferred to the recovery room in good condition.

Assign the correct codes for this encounter.

ICD-9-CM and CPT Code(s): _____

ICD-10-CM Code(s): _____

5.50.   A 38-year-old female patient underwent a left lumpectomy and placement of an afterloading balloon catheter into the left breast in the special procedure room. Assign the appropriate CPT code(s).

   a. 19297-LT
   b. 19301-LT, 19297-LT
   c. 19301-RT
   d. 19120-LT

5.51.   A 75-year-old female patient is treated in the wound care clinic. She presents with a large sacral decubitus and a small decubitus on her buttock. The large sacral ulcer was a Stage II. Procedure performed by the surgeon: Full-thickness excisional debridement to the sacral decubitus. Scalpel was used to remove devitalized tissue down to bleeding. Patient tolerated the procedure well. Assign the diagnosis code(s).

ICD-9-CM Code(s):

a. 707.0, 707.22
b. 707.03, 707.05, 707.20
c. 707.03, 707.22
d. 707.03, 707.05, 707.22, 707.20

ICD-10-CM Code(s): _____

Behavioral Health Conditions

5.52.   A 35-year-old female patient presents to the Community Mental Health Center for group therapy with the diagnosis of obsessive-compulsive disorder. A psychiatrist provides group therapy for obsessive-compulsive disorder. Which of the following code sets would be reported for the facility code?

ICD-9-CM and CPT Code(s):

a. 301.4, 90853
b. 300.3, 90857
c. 300.3, 90853
d. 300.3, 90847

ICD-10-CM Code(s): _____

5.53.   A 66-year-old patient is seen as an outpatient in the community mental health center and participates in multiple-family group psychotherapy for 45 minutes. Diagnosis: Agoraphobia with panic attacks. List the diagnosis and CPT procedure codes for facility reporting.

ICD-9-CM and CPT Code(s): _____

ICD-10-CM Code(s): _____

5.54.   A 15-year-old depressed male is seen in the emergency department after a failed suicide attempt. Right wrist with a 3-cm laceration with no injury to the tendon. Left wrist with a 2.0-cm laceration with no injury to the tendon. Both wrists required simple suture repair. Patient used a razor to cut himself in a suicide attempt while at home in the bathroom today. He stated he has become increasingly depressed and has not experienced these types of symptoms before. He denies psychotic symptoms. Assessment: Laceration to both wrists, repaired. Major depression, severe. Plan: A 24-hour hold was instituted and the patient was transferred for psychiatric care. Stitches removed in 10 days. List the diagnosis and CPT procedure codes for facility reporting.

ICD-9-CM Reason for Visit Code(s): _____

ICD-9-CM and CPT Code(s): _____

ICD-10-CM Reason for Visit Code(s): _____

ICD-10-CM Code(s): _____

5.55.   This 25-year-old female was brought to the ER because of an overdose of prescription drugs. Her roommate found her and called 911. She has been treated recently for depression, and her bottle of amitriptyline was empty. The roommate also reports that her bottle of diazepam was empty. Roommate estimates that there may have been about 20 pills in each bottle. According to the evidence, it appears as if she used alcohol to take the pills, and this was confirmed during drug screening. She left a suicide note stating that she could not go on living. Aggressive measures included stomach pumping to remove pill fragments and cardiopulmonary resuscitation. She could not be revived and was pronounced dead at 2305. List the diagnosis and procedure codes for facility reporting.

ICD-9-CM Reason for Visit Code(s): _____

ICD-9-CM and CPT Code(s): _____

ICD-10-CM Reason for Visit Code(s): _____

ICD-10-CM Code(s): _____

Disorders of the Musculoskeletal System and Connective Tissue

5.56.   This 3-year-old male fell from a park bench at the playground and was unable to bear weight on the left leg. X-rays today determined that he sustained a midshaft fracture of the femur, which was reduced and placed in a spica cast under conscious sedation in the outpatient surgical suite. Total conscious sedation time was 1 hour and 40 minutes.

Which CPT codes are appropriate for reporting?

a. 27500, 99148, 99150
b. 27502
c. 27506, 99148 x4
d. 27506

5.57.   From the health record of a 16-year-old male patient requiring fracture care in the outpatient surgical unit:

Operative Report

Preoperative Diagnosis: Displaced comminuted fracture of the lateral condyle, right elbow

Postoperative Diagnosis: Same

Procedure: Open reduction, internal fixation

Description: The patient was anesthetized and prepped with Betadine. Sterile drapes were applied, and the pneumatic tourniquet was inflated around the arm. An incision was made in the area of the lateral epicondyle through a Steri-Drape, and this was carried through subcutaneous tissue, and the fracture site was easily exposed. Inspection revealed the fragment to be rotated in two planes about 90 degrees. It was possible to manually reduce this quite easily, and the judicious manipulation resulted in an almost anatomic reduction. This was fixed with two pins driven across the humerus. These pins were cut off below skin level. The wound was closed with some plain catgut suture subcutaneously and 5-0 nylon in the skin. Dressings were applied to the patient and tourniquet released. A long arm cast was applied.

Which of the following is the correct code assignment?

ICD-9-CM and CPT Code(s):

a. 812.52, 24577, 29065
b. 812.42, 24579, 29065
c. 812.42, 24579-RT
d. 812.52, 24579-RT

ICD-10-CM Code(s): _____

5.58. The patient was hit in the face by a soccer ball on the neighborhood soccer field, sustaining a 2.3-cm superficial laceration to the right medial cheek. X-rays revealed a nasal fracture that required stabilization. The emergency room physician stabilizes the fracture with a splint and tape and repairs the laceration.

ICD-9-CM Reason for Visit Code(s): _____

ICD-9-CM and CPT Code(s): _____

ICD-10-CM Reason for Visit Code(s): _____

ICD-10-CM Code(s): _____

5.59. This 52-year-old male was brought to the same-day surgery area for treatment of an open fracture of the distal phalanx of his index finger on the right hand. Patient is right-handed and this injury occurred when the food-processing machine at work tipped over and his hand got caught. He works in the local food factory here in town. The patient had open treatment performed to remove the fracture fragments without any internal or external fixation hardware used. What diagnosis and procedure codes are reported?

ICD-9-CM and CPT Code(s): _____

ICD-10-CM Code(s): _____

5.60. This 32-year-old male had an ORIF of a fractured metacarpal bone done 3 months ago. The fracture has completely healed, and he is scheduled for removal of deep internal fixation hardware involving the metacarpals of this left wrist. The plate and pins were removed without incident.

Assign the correct codes and modifier for this encounter.

ICD-9-CM and CPT Code(s): _____

ICD-10-CM Code(s): _____

5.61. The procedure that involves transplantation of a piece of articular cartilage and attached subchondral bone from a cadaver donor to a damaged region of the articular surface of the knee joint is called a(n):

a. Osteochondral autograft
b. Osteochondral allograft
c. Autologous chondrocyte implantation
d. Anterior cruciate ligament repair

5.62. From the health record of a 47-year-old patient admitted for outpatient surgery on his knee:

Operative Report

Preoperative Diagnosis: Severe chondromalacia patellar, right knee.

Postoperative Diagnosis: Severe chondromalacia patella and medial femoral condylar, right knee.

Procedure Performed:
1. Arthroscopy.
2. Chondroplasty/debridement of patella and medial femoral condyle.
3. Lateral retinacular release, right knee.

Anesthesia: General.

Indications: This 47-year-old man has a history of severe patellofemoral and anteromedial joint line pain. This has been treated with anti-inflammatory medications and physical therapy with persistent symptoms. He has tightness of his lateral retinaculum associated with lateral patellar compression syndrome and patellofemoral pain. He presents now for surgical treatment after failed conservative management.

Details of Operation: Patient was brought to the operating room and placed on the operating table in a supine position. After instillation of successful general anesthesia, the right knee was examined. Range of motion was full; no laxity to stress testing was noted. Marked patellofemoral crepitus was noted. The leg was then placed in the arthroscopic leg holder and the knee sterilely prepped and draped. The knee was injected with a total of 30 cc of 0.25 percent Marcaine with epinephrine. Standard arthroscopic portals were established. There were grade III changes over the superior aspect and medial aspect of the patella. The trochlear groove of the femur was softened and minimally fissured. The medial compartment was entered and showed grade III chondromalacia over the majority of the weight-bearing surface of the medial femoral condyle. The tibial plateau was mildly softened, as was the medial meniscus. Intercondylar notch revealed a normal anterior cruciate ligament. The lateral compartment also revealed mild degeneration of the posterior horn of the lateral meniscus and minimal chondromalacia of the tibial plateau. At that point, a full radius resector was placed, and a chondroplasty debridement was carried out of the patella and medial femoral condyle. An internal lateral retinacular release was then carried out using arthroscopic electrocautery to help decompress the patellofemoral area. The patient returned to the recovery room without complications.

What are the correct code assignments for this outpatient surgical case?

ICD-9-CM and CPT Code(s):

a. 719.46, 717.7, 29873-RT, 29877-RT-59
b. 719.46, 717.7, 27425-RT
c. 717.7, 29877-RT
d. 719.46, 717.7, 29999-RT, 29877-RT

ICD-10-CM Code(s): _____

5.63. **Operative Report:** Palmar Fasciectomy

Indications: This is a 93-year-old lady who presents with a Dupuytren contracture of the left palm, which has progressively involved the base of the middle and ring fingers with inability to straighten the fingers.

Preoperative Diagnosis:	Dupuytren contracture, left palm, involving the middle and ring fingers.
Postoperative Diagnosis:	Dupuytren contracture, left palm, involving the middle and ring fingers.
Procedure:	Palmar fasciectomy. Release of the contracture around the left middle and ring fingers.
Anesthesia:	IV Bier block.

Description of Procedure: With the patient under IV Bier block and in the supine position, the left hand was prepped and draped in a sterile fashion. A Z-shaped incision was made in the left hand and carried down to the median crease. The skin flap was dissected free from the palmar fascia. The thickened palmar ligament into the metocarpophalangeal joint of the ring and middle fingers was resected. The tourniquet was let down after about ½ hour and hemostasis was maintained in the operative field. There was good capillary refill to the fingers. The wound was copiously irrigated with saline. A Penrose drain was inserted and the wound was closed with interrupted 4-0 nylon. Pressure dressing was applied to the hand and a volar splint was applied.

The patient tolerated the procedure well. Blood loss during the procedure was less than 50 cc. The patient was sent home in good condition.

What CPT code(s) are assigned to this case?

Code(s): _____

5.64.

Preoperative Diagnosis:	Status post trauma with tri-malleolar fracture dislocation, left ankle.
Postoperative Diagnosis:	Same.
Procedure:	Removal of deep internal fixation devices from specified bone.

Description of Procedure: With the patient under general anesthesia, the right lower extremity was prepped and draped in the usual sterile manner. Pneumatic tourniquet was in place and inflated. There was a palpable lateral screw in the distal third of the fibula. An incision was made over the screw head through a previous area of incision, carried down through the skin and subcutaneous tissue and superficial fascia. The screw was identified and was removed. The tip of the medial malleolus and screw heads were identified and the incision carried down though the previous incision and carried down through the skin and a small split in the fascia and deltoid. The screw heads were each identified and removed. There was no evidence of infection. Irrigation was carried out throughout. The wounds were closed using 3-0 nylon.

The patient had a dry bulky dressing applied. There was good circulation in the foot. She tolerated the procedure well and went to the recovery room in good condition.

Pathology Report

Gross Description: The specimen is received fresh, labeled with the patient's name and consists of two metallic, partially threaded screws each measuring 5 cm in length and each measuring 0.2 cm in diameter. Additional material consists of a metallic, entirely threaded screw which is 6 cm in length and 0.3 cm in diameter. Gross only. No sections submitted.

Microscopic Description: None.

Assign the correct code(s) and modifier for this encounter.

ICD-9-CM and CPT Code(s): _____

ICD-10-CM Code(s): _____

Neoplasms

5.65.   A patient has squamous cell carcinoma of the posterior pharyngeal wall and metastasis to the cervical lymph nodes. Following consultation with the oncology team, the patient refused surgical intervention and elected to begin radiation therapy daily on a 6-MV linear accelerator. The radiation was delivered by hyperfractionation technique. Each field was treated twice each day, through a pair of large opposing lateral head and neck fields covering the primary cancer, the suspected areas of extension, and the lymph nodes in the neck. (Three separate treatment areas are involved, and customized shielding blocks are employed to shield normal tissue and shape the field to follow the anatomic boundaries.) Prior to the encounter under consideration, the clinical treatment parameters and dosimetry calculations have been completed, and the simulation-aided field settings have been accomplished.

Which of the following codes will be reported by the hospital for the encounters for radiation therapy, keeping in mind the number of treatments that will be reported in the unit's field on the UB-04?

ICD-9-CM and CPT Code(s):

a. V58.0, 77413
b. 149.0, 77408
c. V58.0, 149.0, 196.0, 77413
d. 149.0, 196.0, 77412

ICD-10-CM Code(s): _____

5.66. A patient with a lung mass discovered on prior x-ray presents to the outpatient surgery area for a diagnostic bronchoscopy. Following anesthetic to the airway, a fiberoptic bronchoscope is introduced into the bronchial tree. A needle is advanced through a channel in the scope, and tissue is aspirated from the lung mass for pathologic evaluation under fluoroscopic guidance. Pathology report confirmed parenchymal tissue of the lung was obtained and reported a diagnosis of oat cell carcinoma.

Which of the following is the correct code assignment?

ICD-9-CM and CPT Code(s):

a. 162.9, 31629
b. 162.9, 31629, 77002
c. 162.9, 31625
d. 235.7, 31629, 77002

ICD-10-CM Code(s): _____

5.67. A Medicare patient is scheduled for breast biopsy of a palpable lump in the right breast. A much smaller lesion in the left breast is identified by a radiological marker shown on mammography. An excisional biopsy is performed on both sides. The specimen on the right is diagnostic for breast malignancy with clear margins, whereas the small lesion in the left breast is found to be only fibrocystic disease, without evidence of malignancy. Which of the following is reported?

ICD-9-CM and CPT Code(s):

a. 174.9, 610.1, 19120-RT, 19125-LT, 19290-LT
b. 611.72, 610.1, 19120-50
c. 174.9, 610.1, 19120-50, 19125-50, 19290-50
d. 174.9, 610.2, 19120, 19125-59, 19290

ICD-10-CM Code(s): _____

5.68. A 50-year-old male patient with a personal history of colonic polyps presents to the outpatient surgery department for a colonoscopy to rule out colon cancer. The patient has been experiencing rectal bleeding for approximately 6 weeks and has lost a significant amount of weight. A colonoscopy to the terminal ileum is performed. Just beyond the rectal vault, two polyps are found and excised by hot biopsy forceps. Further up into the sigmoid colon, a lesion was biopsied. The pathology report confirms a diagnosis of colon cancer in the lesion found, and the polyps were found to be villous adenoma.

What codes are assigned in this case?

ICD-9-CM and CPT Code(s): _____

ICD-10-CM Code(s): _____

5.69.   A patient presents to the hospital outpatient department for chemotherapy treatment. She is a 15-year-old female with acute lymphocytic leukemia. The chemotherapy agent is listed as an injection of lyophilized cyclophosphamide, 200 mg IV push. What codes, including the medication, would be reported?

ICD-9-CM, CPT, and HCPCS Code(s): _____

ICD-10-CM Code(s): _____

Disorders of the Nervous System and Sense Organs

5.70.   A 36-year-old female patient presents to the ED with a severe headache, listlessness, light sensitivity, nausea, and vomiting. The headache has been growing in intensity over the last 3 days. The patient does not have a fever. The patient has a programmable cerebrospinal fluid shunt in place and after MRI of both the head and the abdomen, it is determined that there is fluid accumulation in the intracranial portion of the shunt, indicating malfunction. The neurosurgeon takes the patient to the outpatient surgical suite and performs a magnetic adjustment of the valve pressure. The diagnoses are documented as headache and idiopathic normal pressure hydrocephalus.

Excluding the E/M code and the MRI codes assigned by the chargemaster, what codes would be assigned for the facility in this case?

ICD-9-CM and CPT Code(s): _____

ICD-10-CM Code(s): _____

5.71.   A patient with Lou Gehrig's disease presents to the hospital-based outpatient neurology department for EMG testing. A needle electromyography of the legs and both of the eyes was conducted. Which of the following code set combinations would be reported?

ICD-9-CM and CPT Code(s):

a. 335.20, 92265-50, 95861
b. 335.24, 95868, 95861
c. 335.20, 95861, 92265
d. 335.29, 95861

ICD-10-CM Code(s): _____

5.72.   From the health record of a patient requiring outpatient eye surgery:

Operative Report

Preoperative Diagnosis:	Type I diabetes patient with severe retinal microaneurysmal diabetic retinopathy, OU
Postoperative Diagnosis:	Same
Operation:	Vitrectomy followed by laser photocoagulation, OU

Description of Procedure: An Ocutome is used to go behind the iris and cut and suction the vitreous mechanically. After vitreous removal, a laser is used to treat the remaining retinal disorders in all four retinal quadrants and prevent further retinal hemorrhage. Procedure repeated.

Which of the following code sets is reported for this service?

ICD-9-CM and CPT Code(s):

a. 250.51, 362.01, 67040-50
b. 362.01, 362.81, 67040-50
c. 250.50, 362.02, 67039-LT-RT
d. 250.51, 362.02, 67105, 67145

ICD-10-CM Code(s): _____

5.73.   From the health record of a patient with cataracts treated in outpatient surgery at the Eye Center:

Operative Report

Procedure: Extracapsular cataract extraction with intraocular lens implantation, left eye

Diagnosis: Bilateral cataracts

Technique: The patient was given a retrobulbar injection of 2.5 to 3.0 cc of a mixture of equal parts of 2 percent lidocaine with epinephrine and 0.75 percent Marcaine with Wydase. The area about the left eye was infiltrated with an additional 6 to 7 cc of this mixture in a modified Van Lint technique. A self-maintaining pressure device was applied to the eye, and a short time later, the patient was taken to the OR.

The patient was properly positioned on the operating table, and the area around the left eye was prepped and draped in the usual fashion. A self-retaining eyelid speculum was positioned and 4-0 silk suture passed through the tendon of the superior rectus muscle, thereby deviating the eye inferiorly. A 160° fornix-based conjunctival flap was created, followed by a 150° corneoscleral groove with a #64 Beaver blade. Hemostasis was maintained throughout with gentle cautery. A 6-0 silk suture was introduced to cross this groove at the 12 o'clock position and looped out of the operative field. The anterior chamber was then entered superiorly temporally, and after injecting Occucoat, an anterior capsulotomy was performed without difficulty. The nucleus was easily brought forward into the anterior chamber. The corneoscleral section was opened with scissors to the left and the nucleus delivered with irrigation and gentle lens loop manipulation. Interrupted 10-0 nylon sutures were placed at both the nasal and lateral extent of the incision. A manual irrigating-aspirating setup then was used to remove remaining cortical material from both the anterior and posterior chambers.

At this point, a modified C-loop posterior chamber lens was removed from its package and irrigated and inspected. It then was positioned into the inferior capsular bag without difficulty, and the superior haptic was placed behind the iris at the 12 o'clock location. The lens was rotated to a horizontal orientation in an attempt to better enhance capsular fixation. Miochol was used to constrict the pupil, and a peripheral iridectomy was performed in the superior nasal quadrant. In addition, three or four interrupted 10-0 nylon sutures were used to close the corneal scleral section. The silk sutures were removed, and the conjunctiva was advanced back into its normal location and secured with cautery burns at the 3 o'clock and 9 o'clock positions. Approximately 20 to 30 mg of both gentamicin and Kenalog were injected into the inferior cul-de-sac in a subconjunctival and sub-Tenon fashion. After instillation of 2 percent pilocarpine and Maxitrol ophthalmic solution, the eyelid speculum was removed and the eye dressed in a sterile fashion. The patient was discharged to the recovery room in good condition.

Assign the correct codes and modifier for this encounter.

ICD-9-CM and CPT Code(s): _____

ICD-10-CM Code(s): _____

5.74.   The following documentation is from the health record of a 10-year-old female.

Indication for Procedure: The patient is a 10-year-old girl who has a history of refractory seizure disorder, now in almost a continual seizing state.

Description of Procedure: This is a digital electroencephalogram recorded using the 10-20 Electrode Placement System. The recording was performed after sleep deprivation. The patient was both awake and asleep during the recording.

During the EEG hookup the patient began having a seizure. At the beginning of the recording, well into the seizure, there were generalized polyspikes overlying 1–2 hertz diffuse delta waves that evolved in frequency. The patient was given diastat to stop the seizure. Post-ictally, there was diffusely increased beta range activity and intermittent vertex waves. The patient fell asleep and there was a buildup of diffuse delta activity with overlying beta activity. This appeared to be a buildup to another seizure. The recording was stopped before another seizure began.

Impression: Very abnormal EEG with a generalized idiopathic epileptic seizure. Refractory seizure disorder, per history.

Assign the correct codes and modifier for this encounter.

ICD-9-CM Reason for Visit Code(s): _____

ICD-9-CM and CPT Code(s): _____

ICD-10-CM Reason for Visit Code(s): _____

ICD-10-CM Code(s): _____

5.75.   The patient has known chronic glaucoma, more severe in the left eye. She is brought to the outpatient procedure suite and anesthetized with a periocular anesthetic. The left eye is prepared and sterilely draped, followed by insertion of a lid speculum. A clear corneal incision is made temporally with the diamond blade approximately 3.4 mm in width. Viscoelastic material is injected into the anterior chamber over the pupil and lens to increase and maintain anterior chamber depth. Viscoelastic is then injected under the iris for 180° to visualize the ciliary body processes with the endoscope. The endoscope is inserted through the temporal incision, viewing the nasal ciliary processes. The ciliary processes are coagulated through the endoscope with the endpoint of shrinkage and whitening.

Assign the appropriate CPT code for the described procedure.

a. 66710-LT
b. 66711-LT
c. 66720-LT
d. 66700-LT

5.76.   From the health record of a patient scheduled for eye surgery:

Surgery Date: 04/10/XX

Preoperative Diagnosis: Endophthalmitis, left eye.

Postoperative Diagnosis: Endophthalmitis, left eye.

Operative Procedure: 1. Pars plana vitrectomy, left eye.
                              2. Intravitreal vancomycin (1 mg left eye).
                              3. Intravitreal ceftazidime (2 mg left eye).
                              4. Intravitreal triamcinolone (4 mg left eye).

Anesthesia: Retrobulbar anesthesia with 5 cc of a 50/50 mixture of 2 percent lidocaine and 0.75 percent Marcaine.

Indications: This patient is status post tap and injection on April 1, 20XX. She presents with vitreous debris, poor vision, and a history of endophthalmitis.

Description of Procedure: After informed written consent was obtained, the patient was brought to the operating room and was prepped and draped in the usual sterile fashion. Retrobulbar anesthesia was performed with 5 cc of a 50/50 mixture of 2 percent lidocaine and 0.75 percent Marcaine in the retrobulbar space of the left eye without any complications. She was then prepped and draped in the usual sterile fashion. A speculum was placed in the left eye.

A standard 20-gauge pars plana vitrectomy was carried out with the pars placed 3 mm posterior to the limbus. A full vitrectomy was performed. Posterior vitreous detachment was induced and then further vitrectomy was carried out. The sclerotomy was closed with 7-0 VICRYL, as was the conjunctiva. Then, 0.1 mL of vancomycin (1 mg), 0.1 mL of ceftazidime (2 mg), and 0.1 mL of triamcinolone (4 mg) were injected into the vitreous cavity at the end of the case.

The patient was patched after atropine and Maxitrol were applied to the eye. The patient will follow up tomorrow at 8 a.m.

No qualified resident was available for the case.

What are the correct codes for this ambulatory surgery?

ICD-9-CM and CPT Code(s):

a. 360.00, 67036-LT, 66030-LT
b. 360.03, 67036-LT, 66030-LT
c. 360.00, 67036-RT
d. 998.59, 360.00, 67036-LT, 66030-LT

ICD-10-CM Code(s): _____

Newborn/Congenital Disorders

5.77.   A baby was born in the hospital to a woman who lacked prenatal care and contracted rubella during pregnancy, passing it on to her fetus. The baby was born with multiple deformities, including a congenital cortical and zonular cataract of the left eye. The baby is now 7 months old and ready for extracapsular phacoemulsification with intraocular lens replacement.

Which of the following code sets and modifier, if needed, would be reported for the surgery?

ICD-9-CM and CPT Code(s):

a. 743.30, 760.2, 66984-50
b. 366.03, 66984-LT
c. V30.00, 771.0, 743.32
d. 743.32, 66984-LT

ICD-10-CM Code(s): _____

5.78.   A newborn female is born with polydactyly of the right foot with a total of 5 normal toes and 2 extra digits that do not contain bony structures. Which of the following code sets would be reported by the ASC facility tying off and removing these digits at the age of 2 weeks?

ICD-9-CM and CPT Code(s):

a. 755.02, 11200
b. 755.02, 11200-RT, 11200-59
c. 755.00, 28899
d. 755.02, 26587

ICD-10-CM Code(s): _____

5.79.   A baby boy is born with hypospadias. At 7 months of age, the first stage of surgical correction is undertaken, which requires transplantation of the prepuce, but no skin flaps. What are the correct codes for this ambulatory surgery, as reported by the hospital?

ICD-9-CM and CPT Code(s): _____

ICD-10-CM Code(s): _____

5.80.   This child was born with a bilateral hydrocele. He also has reducible inguinal hernias on both sides. The condition has become troublesome, and the parents and pediatrician have decided that surgical correction is warranted for this 3-year-old. Surgeon performed a bilateral hernia repair with hydrocelectomy.

Postoperative Diagnosis: Bilateral hernia repair with hydrocelectomy

Report diagnosis and CPT procedure codes.

ICD-9-CM and CPT Code(s): _____

ICD-10-CM Code(s): _____

Pediatric Conditions

5.81. The following documentation is from the health record of a 6-year-old female patient.

Preoperative Diagnosis:	Unilateral incomplete cleft of lip
Postoperative Diagnosis:	Unilateral incomplete cleft of lip
Operation:	Secondary correction with complete take-down of unilateral cleft lip

Description of Procedure: After the proper operative consent was obtained from the parents, the patient was brought to the operating room. She was comfortably placed on the operating room table and induced with general endotracheal anesthesia. The patient's oral facial region was then prepped with Betadine and draped sterilely. Normal anatomical landmarks were then carefully marked out on the patient's lip. This was tattooed with methylene blue. 2% Xyocaine with 1:100,000 epinephrine was infiltrated into the lip. A revision rotation advancement flap was carefully marked out. This included cutting out an area at the nasal base where there was a significant depression. The rotation flap was cut first. This was done with a 15-blade. The dissection was carried down through skin. There was significant scar on the lip, and it was completely cut through. The advancement flap was then cut. Tissue was left on the advancement flap to be rotated up when the flap was thin at the nasal base. Hemostasis was again secured. The orbicularis muscle was dissected from the skin and from the mucosa. Hemostasis was again verified. Muscle was then brought together. This was done with interrupted 4-0 Vicryl suture. Vermillion was closed with 5-0 Chromic. The lip itself was closed with 5-0 Rapid Catgut. The patient tolerated the procedure well. Sponge, instrument, and needle count were correct.

ICD-9-CM Reason for Visit Code(s): _____

ICD-9-CM and CPT Code(s): _____

ICD-10-CM Reason for Visit Code(s): _____

ICD-10-CM Code(s): _____

5.82. Tonsillectomy and Adenoidectomy: Chronic Adenoiditis and Tonsillitis

Preoperative Diagnosis:	Chronic adenoiditis and tonsillitis.
Postoperative Diagnosis:	Chronic adenoiditis and tonsillitis.
Anesthesia:	General.
Complications:	None.

Descriptions: The 6-year-old female was brought to the operating room where general anesthesia was induced and maintained through an endotracheal tube. A Crowe-Davis mouthgag was inserted and red rubber Robinson placed through the nose and retrieved through the oropharynx for retraction of the palate. An adenoid curette was used to remove the adenoid tissue from the nasopharynx.

Hemostasis was obtained with electrocautery. The left tonsil was grasped, and using electrocautery it was dissected from the fossa and transected at the base. The right tonsil was removed in a similar manner. The patient was awakened, extubated, and then taken to the recovery room in satisfactory condition.

Which CPT codes would be used to report this encounter?

a. 42825, 42830
b. 42820, 42820
c. 42821
d. 42820

5.83. Emergency Room Service

Chief Complaint: Coughing, history of asthma, on Albuterol MDI, no allergies.

S: Patient is an 11-year-old male, who is seen today with cough that started 3 days ago, growing progressively worse. He states that he coughs when walking short distances. Peak flows have been around 200 at home but hard to measure due to coughing. Personal best is 300. Has been using Albuterol MDI with little success today. He had some loose stools yesterday, and Mom says that his activity level is severely reduced. Appetite moderate to minimal, totally unlike him. Some nasal allergy symptoms due to tree season. No chest pain. No nausea or vomiting.

O: Young white male in moderate respiratory distress. W: 81 lbs P: 64 RR: 24 T: 100.4 HEENT: PERRLA. TMs bilaterally are clear. Nose: congested with rhinorrhea. Oropharynx: mild erythema. Neck: supple. Full ROM. Thyroid normal. Lungs have bilateral wheeze in the left lower lobe. Heart RRR w/o gallop or murmur. Abdomen: positive bowel sounds, soft, nontender. No organomegaly is noted.

Data: Peak flows here are 200, 210, 200 with coughing. Pulse Ox is 97. Albuterol 0.5 cc aerosol via nebulizer is given with resulting peak flows of 230, 240, and 220 and repeat nebulizer at .05 cc in 15 minutes with improvement to 250.

A: Cough, acute asthma exacerbation due to seasonal allergies.

P: Albuterol 2 puffs QID. Prednisone 40 mg qd x 3 days, rest at least today, until appetite and energy improve. Follow up with PMD in 3 days for adjustment in asthma care plan or sooner if symptoms don't improve.

Excluding the E/M code, assign the correct codes for this encounter.

ICD-9-CM, CPT, and HCPCS Level II Code(s): _____

ICD-10-CM Code(s): _____

5.84. The child has a syndactyly of 1 web space without bone or tendon involvement and has undergone previous surgery to insert a tissue expander. After multiple expansions, there is sufficient tissue present to proceed with repair today. The tissue expander is removed and the fingers are now separated, carefully placing the incisions to form flaps to be used for closure. The defect is 4.5 cm in length along both fingers. The flaps are now approximated to cover the defects on the 2 individual fingers. The skin and subcutaneous tissue are closed in layers.

Which of the following CPT code sets is correct for reporting this surgery?

a. 14040, 11971
b. 26560, 11971
c. 26561
d. 26562

5.85. This 4-year-old child was brought to the ER because of cough and fever. The mother was worried about pneumonia, and the physician's office was closed for the weekend. X-ray was negative. Diagnosis: upper respiratory infection with bilateral acute conjunctivitis. What diagnosis code(s) are assigned?

ICD-9-CM Reason for Visit Code(s): _____

ICD-9-CM Code(s): _____

ICD-10-CM Reason for Visit Code(s): _____

ICD-10-CM Code(s): _____

Conditions of Pregnancy, Childbirth, and the Puerperium

5.86. A patient in the 26th week of pregnancy had a 1-hour glucose screening test. Results of this test showed a blood sugar level of 160 mg/dL. Subsequently, the patient presents to the outpatient laboratory department with a physician order for a 3-hour glucose tolerance test. The reason for the test as documented on the order is: abnormal glucose on screening, rule out gestational diabetes. What is the correct code set for this outpatient ancillary services encounter?

ICD-9-CM and CPT Code(s):

a. 790.22, V22.2, 82951
b. 648.83, 82951
c. 648.83, 82950
d. 648.80, 82951, 82952

ICD-10-CM Code(s): _____

5.87. This 26-year-old gravida 1, para 0 female has been having spotting and has been on bedrest. She awoke this morning with severe cramping and bleeding. Her husband brought her to the hospital. After examination it was determined that she has had an incomplete early spontaneous abortion. She is in the 10th week of her pregnancy. She was taken to outpatient surgery, and a dilatation and curettage was performed. There were no complications from the procedure. She is discharged home with instructions to follow up with the physician in the office.

Which of the following is the correct code set?

ICD-9-CM and CPT Code(s):

a. 637.91, 58120
b. 634.91, 59812
c. 634.91, 58120
d. 634.92, 59812

ICD-10-CM Code(s): _____

5.88. This 23-year-old female is expecting her first child. She comes into the radiology department for an outpatient antenatal ultrasound to confirm the gestational age of the fetus and rule out fetal growth retardation. A real-time image was taken of the fetus estimated to be at 16 weeks. What diagnosis codes and associated codes (even though they may be chargemaster-assigned codes) are assigned?

ICD-9-CM and CPT Code(s): _____

ICD-10-CM Code(s): _____

5.89. This patient has a history of infertility and has been seeing her OB/GYN physician for more than 2 years. It was elected to perform a hysterosalpingogram at the outpatient surgery center to assess the patency of the fallopian tubes.

Procedure Report

The patient was prepped and draped in the usual manner. The cervical os was cannulated and Sinografin injected in retrograde fashion under fluoroscopic control. The body of the uterus appears normal. No filling defects are seen. There is no evidence of synechiae. The right fallopian tube is occluded approximately 1 cm from the body of the uterus. The left fallopian tube is patent and demonstrates free spill of contrast into the peritoneal cavity.

Assign the codes for this encounter.

ICD-9-CM and CPT Code(s): _____

ICD-10-CM Code(s): _____

Disorders of the Genitourinary System

5.90. Operative Report

Preoperative Diagnosis:	A 5-mm stone in the right lower pole.
Postoperative Diagnosis:	A 5-mm stone in the right lower pole.
Operation Performed:	Right extracorporeal shockwave lithotripsy.
Anesthesia:	Intravenous sedation.

Indications for Procedure: This is a 32-year-old young man who recently presented with right renal colic. An x-ray showed a stone in the proximal ureter. On June 1, 20XX, he underwent cystourethroscopy, the stone was successfully flushed into the kidney, and a double-J stent was placed in the ureter. Today, he presents for ESWL. An x-ray confirmed location of the stone in the right lower pole.

Description of Procedure: The patient was placed onto the treatment table and sedated. He was positioned over the shockwave electrode. Biaxial Fluoroscopy was utilized to position the stone at the focal point of the shockwave generator. The stone was treated with a total of 3,000 shocks. At the conclusion of the procedure, the stone appeared to have fragmented nicely, and the patient was discharged to the PACU.

Which of the following CPT code(s) are reported for this service?

a. 52332, 50590
b. 50590
c. 52353
d. 50590, 52353

5.91. Operative Report

Indications: The patient is a 50-year-old gentleman with 4 children. He desires a permanent form of birth control via vasectomy.

Preoperative Diagnosis:	Elective vasectomy.
Postoperative Diagnosis:	Elective vasectomy.
Procedure:	Bilateral trans-scrotal segmental vasectomy.
Anesthesia:	Local with 1% Xylocaine infiltration.
Estimated Blood Loss:	Minimal.
Drains:	None.
Complications:	None.
Findings:	Normal testes and normal vas deferens.

Description of Procedure: The patient was taken to the procedure room where, in the supine position, he was prepped and draped in routine fashion. The left vas deferens was identified and isolated. Local anesthesia was obtained using infiltration of 1% Xylocaine without epinephrine. An incision was made overlying the vas deferens. The vas deferens was identified and delivered to the operative field. A 2.5-cm segment of vas deferens was then excised between hemostats. The ends of the vasa were then cauterized with electrocautery. The distal end was sutured and folded back upon itself with 3-0 chromic. The proximal end was sutured and folded back upon itself. Hemostasis was obtained. Next, attention was directed to the right side where the procedure was performed in mirror-image fashion. After confirming adequate hemostasis, the vasa were returned to the normal location within the scrotum. The skin was closed using interrupted sutures of 3-0 chromic. The patient was returned to the recovery room in good condition.

What code(s) are assigned for this encounter?

ICD-9-CM and CPT Code(s): _____

ICD-10-CM Code(s): _____

5.92.   This is a record of an emergency room visit:

Admission Date:	1/1/20XX
Discharge Date:	1/1/20XX
Discharge Diagnosis:	Torsion, right appendix testis.
Operation:	Right scrotal exploration; excision appendix testis
Surgeon:	
Complications:	None.
Allergies:	None.
Disposition/Medications:	Follow-up in 2 weeks. No medications.
Special Instructions:	Parents instructed to keep incision clean.

Summary: HPI - patient is a 4-year-old white male patient who is known mentally retarded with obesity; otherwise he gets along reasonably well. However, the patient presented to his pediatrician this morning with a 1 hour history of sudden onset of testicular pain. Physical exam at that time was suggestive for testicular torsion, and he was admitted for surgical repair. Physical exam showed an obese white male, who was crying. Lungs clear. Heart regular, without murmur or gallop. Abdomen obese; no masses appreciated; bowel sounds normal active. Genital exam showed a small penis which was engulfed in the suprapubic fat; testes down bilaterally; the right side was exquisitely tender.

Laboratory values on admission: WBC 8.7, with 33 segs, 58 lymphs; hgb 14.3.

Patient was admitted and taken to the Operating Room immediately, and right scrotal exploration was undertaken. The appendix testis was found to be hemorrhagic and cyanotic. It was excised. The testicle otherwise appeared fine. The right testicle was fixed in the scrotum. It was not felt necessary to explore the left side for fixation. Postoperatively the patient did well. He was discharged later that evening in good condition.

Pathology Report

Gross Description: The specimen consists of a dark reddish-brown polyp-like tissue fragment, 8 × 4 × 4 mm. The entire specimen is submitted.

Microscopic Description: The specimen consists of histologic sections of a papillomatous tissue fragment lined by what appears to be mesothelium. The core of the specimen is composed of extremely loose connective tissue showing vascular congestion and hemorrhage.

Diagnosis: Appendix – testis: Edema and hemorrhage.

What code(s) are assigned to this case?

ICD-9-CM and CPT Code(s): _____

ICD-10-CM Code(s): _____

Disorders of the Respiratory System

5.93.   A patient with chronic obstructive asthma and an acute exacerbation of chronic bronchitis presents to the ED in respiratory distress.

   Which answer represents the correct diagnosis coding for this case?

   ICD-9-CM Code(s):

   a. 493.22
   b. 493.21, 491.21
   c. 493.20
   d. 491.21

   ICD-10-CM Code(s): _____

5.94.   This 65-year-old smoker with hemoptysis and chronic cough is scheduled for an outpatient bronchoscopy with an endobronchial biopsy of the lesion in the bronchus. The pathology report states "well-differentiated oat cell carcinoma of the upper bronchus." What codes would be reported?

   ICD-9-CM and CPT Code(s): _____

   ICD-10-CM Code(s): _____

5.95.   This 59-year-old male patient has recovered from an extended period of time on a ventilator with a tracheostomy and is now ready for closure. The physician repairs the tracheal defect with good result, not requiring plastic repair. What codes are reported?

   ICD-9-CM Reason for Visit Code(s): _____

   ICD-9-CM and CPT Code(s): _____

   ICD-10-CM Reason for Visit Code(s): _____

   ICD-10-CM Code(s): _____

Trauma and Poisoning

5.96. While running, a 10-year-old boy began choking on a small latex balloon and was rushed from the amusement park to the emergency department. The balloon is lodged in the trachea just past the larynx and threatening to obstruct her breathing. The piece of latex balloon is carefully removed from the trachea by use of biopsy forceps through flexible fiberoptic laryngoscope following administration of topical anesthesia.

Which codes are reported for this service in addition to the ED visit code?

ICD-9-CM Code(s):

a. 934.0, E912, E000.8, E849.4, 31577
b. 934.0, E912, E849.4, 31511
c. 784.99, E912, E000.8, E849.4, 31530
d. 933.1, 31577

ICD-10-CM Code(s): _____

5.97. This 23-year-old female is brought to the emergency department after being found by her college roommate. Sometime within the last hour and a half after the roommate left, the patient ingested her entire bottle of verapamil (estimated at over 20 pills) as a suicide attempt, evidenced by a note. The physician ordered a high-dose glucagon HCl administration as an antidote, consisting of 10 mg/100 ml of D5W in an IV over 2 minutes, followed by a 5 mg/100 ml of D5W per hour for 2 more hours. A gastric lavage and aspiration were also performed. The patient's vital signs stabilized and lab work returned to normal over the next several hours. The patient was transferred to an inpatient psychiatric facility for follow-up treatment on her suicide attempt.

Assign the correct codes for this encounter.

ICD-9-CM, CPT, and HCPCS Level II Code(s): _____

ICD-10-CM Code(s): _____

5.98. This 32-year-old female was burned by hot grease in her kitchen 1 week ago. She is seen in the hospital-based wound clinic for large dressing changes on both upper extremities following second-degree burns to both arms. This is accomplished without requiring anesthesia.

What codes are assigned for this service?

ICD-9-CM and CPT Code(s): _____

ICD-10-CM Code(s): _____

5.99. A physician performed an aspiration via thoracentesis on a patient in observation status in the hospital. The patient has advanced lung cancer with malignant pleural effusion. Later the same day, due to continued accumulation of fluid, the patient was returned to the procedure room and the same physician performed a repeat thoracentesis.

Report diagnosis and procedure codes. Do not report observation codes.

Assign the correct codes and modifier for this encounter.

ICD-9-CM and CPT Code(s): _____

ICD-10-CM Code(s): _____

5.100. A 12-year-old boy presents with his father to the ER due to open wounds to his arm, hand, and upper leg. The injury occurred when the boy fell on a barbed-wire fence at the farm while running. Diagnosis: Multiple open wounds to the right forearm, right hand, and left thigh. Procedure: Suture repair of the following: single-layer closure, 4.0 cm, forearm; layered closure, 3.0 cm, hand; 6.0 simple repair, thigh.

ICD-9-CM Reason for Visit Code(s): _____

ICD-9-CM and CPT Code(s): _____

ICD-10-CM Reason for Visit Code(s): _____

ICD-10-CM Code(s): _____

5.101. From the health record of a patient seen in the emergency room/observation area for an allergic reaction:

Discharge Summary

Date of Discharge: 01/08/XX

Chief Complaint: Allergic reaction to Bactrim, resulting in angioedema and mild respiratory distress.

Hospital Course: Fifty-six-year-old male admitted for angioedema after taking Bactrim for an ear infection. The patient had mild respiratory distress and marked swelling of his hands, face, and his oropharynx. The patient was given IV steroids in the Emergency Room and was admitted overnight for observation. The patient's swelling rapidly improved and by the morning after his admission he was back to baseline. He had no complaints of shortness of breath and desired to go home.

Condition on Discharge: Good. Activity: As tolerated. Diet: As tolerated.

Medications: Home medications only including:

1. Celebrex 200 mg one b.i.d.

2. Isosorbide 30 mg once a day.

3. Atenolol 25 mg per day.

4. Lipitor 10 mg per day.

Follow-Up: Will be as needed with primary care physician if ear problem returns and/or if he has any evidence of recurrent swelling and/or respiratory distress.

Emergency Assessment

Chief Complaint: Swelling, itching, and change in voice.

Present Illness: This is a 56-year-old white male with a history of allergic reaction to an antibiotic in the past, who presents today after taking his second dose of Bactrim this morning at home. He then had acute onset of swelling, redness, itching, and change in voice; also states that he was slightly short of breath but no wheezing. He denies any nausea, vomiting, fevers, chills.

Past Medical History: Coronary artery disease, MI 2 years ago, is currently taking Celebrex, Isosorbide, Atenolol, Lipitor, and Bactrim that he just started on this morning.

Physical Examination: Appears very red, swollen diffusely with erythematous rash, macular type rash. Blood pressure is 146/77, heart rate of 120, respiration rate 18 and 02; saturation is 96%. On room air. HEENT: He does have swollen eyelids, both upper and lower eyelids, with also some facial swelling and some uvular swelling as well as some lateral pharyngeal and uvular swelling, which appears to be allergic in nature. His tongue appears also slightly swollen, does not have any neck swelling, also has an erythematous rash. Lungs: Clear to auscultation with no wheezing noted. Abdomen: Soft, nontender.

Ed Course: Received Benadryl 25 mg IV, Pepcid 20 mg IV, Solu-Medrol 125 mg IV. At this point, his voice was still changing, and decision was made to admit the patient to the hospital for observation and then to observe and given a second dose of Solu-Medrol and Benadryl. Consultation between patient's private physician.

Select the correct codes for this observation patient.

ICD-9-CM Code(s):

a. 961.0, 786.09, 995.1, 693.0, E857, E849.0
b. 995.20, E931.0, E849.0
c. 995.1, 786.09, E931.0, E849.0
d. 995.1, 786.09, 693.0, E930.9, E849.0

ICD-10-CM Code(s): _____

5.102. Operative Report

Preoperative Diagnosis: Circular saw injury with complex laceration of left index finger with laceration of extensor tendon and joint capsule; laceration collateral ligament, radial side; displaced fracture at base of the middle phalanx, articular involvement.

Postoperative Diagnosis: Circular saw injury with complex laceration of left index finger with laceration of extensor tendon and joint capsule; laceration collateral ligament, radial side; compound fracture, base of the middle phalanx, articular involvement.

Operation Performed

Debridement and repair extensor tendon and joint capsule. Repair radial collateral ligament and wound closure.

Anesthesia: Digital block

This is a 42-year-old white male who accidentally injured his left index finger on a circular saw while working on broken shutters at home in his garage. The patient sustained a jagged laceration over the dorsal radial aspect of the index finger at the proximal interphalangeal joint. The wound was deep, involving the joint capsule, extensor tendon, and collateral ligament. The bone was also involved, especially at the base of the middle phalanx into the apical surface. The sensation to the tip of the finger was intact, especially all of the radial side. The wound measured about 3 cm in length.

Procedure: 0.5 percent Marcaine was used as local anesthetic digital block. After anesthesia had been obtained, the hand was prepped and draped in the usual manner. Tourniquet then was placed at the base of the fingers. The wound was then debrided. The minute loose bone and articular surface had to be removed. Some skin debrided also was removed. After satisfactory debridement, the joint capsule and extensor tendon then were repaired with 5-0 PDS suture material. The radial collateral ligament also was repaired with the same suture material. The skin then was carefully approximated with 5-0 nylon. After completion, a dressing was applied. The tourniquet was released and there was good perfusion throughout the fingers. An aluminum splint was placed.

The patient received 1 g of Ancef in the emergency room. He will continue to take Keftab 500 mg twice daily for 4 days and Vicodin 1 tablet q.4h. p.r.n. for pain. The postoperative instructions were given. Also the patient was informed about his injury and complications, especially wound infection and some stiffness of the finger. The patient will be followed up in my office.

Assign the correct codes and modifier for this encounter.

ICD-9-CM and CPT Code(s): _____

ICD-10-CM Code(s): _____

Chapter 6

Case Studies from Physician-based Health Records

Note: Although the specific cases are divided by setting, much of the information pertaining to the diagnosis is applicable in most settings. Even the CPT codes in the ambulatory and physician sections may be reported in the same manner. The differences in coding in these two settings may involve modifier reporting, evaluation and management CPT code reporting, and other health plan reporting guidelines unique to settings. If you practice or apply codes in a particular type of setting, you may find additional information in other sections of this publication that may be pertinent to you.

Every effort has been made to follow current recognized coding guidelines and principles, as well as nationally recognized reporting guidelines. The material presented may differ from some health plan requirements for reporting. The ICD-9-CM codes used are effective October 1, 2011, through September 30, 2012, and the HCPCS (CPT and HCPCS Level II) codes are in effect January 1, 2011, through December 31, 2011. The current standard transactions and code sets named in HIPAA have been utilized. The 2011 draft edition of ICD-10-CM was utilized.

Instructions: Assign all applicable ICD-9-CM diagnosis codes including V codes and E codes. Assign all CPT Level I procedure codes and HCPCS Level II codes. Assign Level I (CPT) and Level II (HCPCS) modifiers as appropriate. Final codes for billing occur after codes are passed through payer edits. Medicare utilizes the National Correct Coding Initiative (NCCI) edits. CMS developed the NCCI edit list to promote national correct coding methodologies and to control improper coding leading to improper payments for Medicare Part B. The purpose of the NCCI edits is to ensure the most comprehensive code is assigned and billed rather than the component codes. In addition, NCCI edits check for mutually exclusive pairs.

Cases in this workbook are presented as either multiple choice or fill in the blank.

- For multiple-choice cases:
  —Select the letter of the appropriate code set.
- For fill-in-the-blank cases:
  —Sequence the primary diagnosis first followed by the secondary diagnoses including appropriate V codes and E codes (both cause of injury and place of occurrence).

—Sequence the primary CPT procedure code first followed by additional procedure codes including modifiers as appropriate (both CPT Level I and HCPCS Level II modifiers).

—Assign HCPCS Level II codes only if instructed (case specific).

—Assign evaluation and management (E/M) codes only if instructed (case specific).

The scenarios are based on selected excerpts from health records. In practice, the coding professional should have access to and refer to the entire health record. Health records are analyzed and codes assigned based on physician documentation. In physician practice, valuable information for coding purposes is available on the superbill; however, documentation for coding purposes must be assigned based on medical record documentation. A physician may be queried when documentation is ambiguous, incomplete, or conflicting. The queried documentation must be a permanent part of the medical record.

The objective of the cases and scenarios reproduced in this publication is to provide practice in assigning correct codes, not necessarily to emulate complete coding, which can only be achieved with the complete medical record. For example, the reader may be asked to assign codes based on only an operative report; in real practice, a coder has access to documentation in the entire medical record.

The *ICD-9-CM Official Guidelines for Coding and Reporting of Outpatient Services,* published by the National Center for Health Statistics (NCHS), supplements the official conventions and instructions provided within ICD-9-CM. Adherence to these guidelines when assigning ICD-9-CM diagnosis codes is required under the Health Insurance Portability and Accountability Act (HIPAA) of 1996. Additional official coding guidance can be found in the American Hospital Association (AHA)'s *Coding Clinic* publication.

Anesthesia Services

Note: The reporting of the anesthesia section code versus the CPT code is a payer-specific policy. For these exercises, the anesthesia section code is to be reported for practice in assigning these codes. The exercises in this section are not based on payer-specific requirements.

6.1.   Correctly apply the anesthesia code for 19367, a breast reconstruction with TRAM flap. Do not assign modifiers in this example.

CPT Code(s):

a. 00404
b. 00406
c. 00402
d. 00400

6.2. An epidural was given during labor. Subsequently, it was determined that the patient would require a C-section for cephalopelvic disproportion because of obstructed labor. Assign the correct codes. Modifiers are not used in this example.

ICD-9-CM and CPT Code(s):

a. 660.11, 653.41, 64493
b. 660.11, 653.01, 01961
c. 660.11, 653.41, 01967, 01968
d. 660.11, 653.91, 01996

ICD-10-CM Code(s): _____

6.3. A 3-year-old child came to the outpatient surgery center to have dental caries filled and caps placed on his teeth due to nursing bottle decay syndrome. Anesthesia was provided by an anesthesiologist. Assign the correct codes for the anesthesia services. Modifiers are included in this example.

ICD-9-CM and CPT Code(s):

a. 521.00, 00170-AA-23
b. 521.00, 00170-AA
c. 520.7, 00170-P1-23-AA
d. 521.30, 00170

ICD-10-CM Code(s): _____

6.4. A 5-year-old patient was brought into the emergency room with a deep 2-cm laceration of his scalp. The child was combative and would not allow staff to cleanse the wound. The mother held the child in her lap while the ED physician administered 10 mg of Versed intranasally. When the child was sufficiently sedated, one of the ED nurses monitored the patient's vital signs, and the physician performed a layered repair of the laceration. The intra-service time for the procedure did not exceed 30 minutes.

Assign the correct CPT code(s) for the procedure and sedation for this case:

a. 12031, 99143
b. 12031, 99144
c. 12031-47
d. 12031-QS

6.5. A 2-month-old infant is brought to the operating room for repair of coarctation of the aorta with a pump oxygenator. Anesthesia is provided by an anesthesiologist. The infant is in critical condition and may not survive. Assign the correct codes, including physical status, Level I and II modifiers, and qualifying conditions for this procedure.

ICD-9-CM and CPT Code(s): _____

ICD-10-CM Code(s): _____

Disorders of the Blood and Blood-Forming Organs

6.6. The physician diagnoses acquired coagulopathy due to vitamin K deficiency. How is this coded?

ICD-9-CM Code(s): _____

ICD-10-CM Code(s): _____

6.7. A patient is admitted with cervical lymphadenopathy. A needle biopsy of a cervical lymph node is performed, and Hodgkin's sarcoma disease is confirmed. Which of the following is the correct code assignment?

ICD-9-CM and CPT Code(s):

a. 201.21, 38505
b. 201.91, 38505
c. 201.21, 38500
d. 785.6, 38510

ICD-10-CM Code(s): _____

6.8. From the physician services documentation of a 39-year-old male:

History of Present Illness: The patient is a 39-year-old African-American male who has a known history of sickle cell anemia. He was admitted to the hospital with diffuse extremity pains with minor complaints of pain along the right inguinal area. They started on Friday, became a little bit better on Saturday, then improved, and started again in the past 24 hours. He denies any problems with cough or sputum or production. He denies any problems with fever.

Past Medical History: See recent medical records in charts. He does have a new onset of diabetes, probably related to his hemochromatosis. He does have evidence of iron overload with high ferritins.

Review of Systems: Otherwise unremarkable except for those related to his pain. He denies any problems with fever or night sweats. No cough or sputum production. Denies any changes in gastrointestinal or genitourinary habits. No blood from the rectum or urine.

Physical Examination: This is a 39-year-old, African-American male who is conscious and cooperative. He is oriented x 3 and appears in no acute distress. Vital signs are stable. HEENT is remarkable for icterus present in oral mucosa and conjunctivae, which is a chronic event for him. The neck is supple. No evidence of any gross lymphadenopathy of the cervical, supraclavicular, or axillary areas. The heart is abnormally irregular in rate without any murmurs heard. Lungs are clear to auscultation and percussion. The abdomen is soft and benign without any gross organomegaly. Extremities reveal no edema. No palpable cords. He does have some tenderness along the inner aspects of his right lower extremity near the inguinal area; however, no masses were palpable and no point tenderness is noted.

The patient was treated for his painful sickle cell crisis with IV fluids and pain medications. He had a problem with his right inguinal area. He had evidence of pain. There was some pain on abduction of his right lower extremity. The examination really was unremarkable. There was no evidence of any Holman; no palpable cords, no masses were palpable.

Because of his sickle cell anemia, rule out the possibility of osteonecrosis of the femur. Complete x-rays of his femur and hip were carried out. However, these were both negative. Patient is being discharged after improvement. To follow up with me in 1 week.

Diagnoses:
1. Painful sickle cell crisis
2. Type II diabetes mellitus
3. Chronic atrial fibrillation

Condition on Discharge: Stable

What diagnosis code(s) would the physician report on this case?

ICD-9-CM Code(s):

a. 282.61, 789.09, 427.31, 250.00
b. 282.62, 733.42, 427.31, 250.00
c. 282.62
d. 282.62, 427.31, 250.00

ICD-10-CM Code(s): _____

6.9.   This established patient comes to the physician's office and after evaluation requires a glucose tolerance test. The physician drew the three specimens and performed the test at the office. List the correct CPT procedure code(s).

Code(s): _____

6.10.   The physician documents that the patient has blood-loss anemia. Which diagnosis code is supported by this documentation?

ICD-9-CM Code(s):

a. 280.0
b. 285.1
c. 285.8
d. 285.9

ICD-10-CM Code(s): _____

Disorders of the Cardiovascular System

6.11.   **Chief Complaint:** Left knee pain

Reason for Admission: Hypotension, bradycardia, and possible GI bleed

This 83-year-old patient presented to my office this morning complaining of knee pain and wanting to see an orthopedic surgeon for a knee replacement. My first impression of the patient was that he appeared lethargic and extremely tired-looking. Upon questioning, he stated that he was far more tired than normal and "just didn't feel good," attributing this to the chronic pain in the knee. I reviewed his meds and completed a 10-point review of systems, which revealed increasing bouts of periodic diarrhea with dark stool. He has overall poor health with multiple previous surgeries and hypertension that has been difficult to control. Other systems are negative for new complaints today. At the completion of our office visit, I arranged for a direct admission to the hospital. I saw him again at the hospital and continued the diagnostic workup.

No known allergies. Takes Lisinopril 40 mg daily, Coreg, half of a 25 mg pill twice per day, and Protonix daily. He is married and lives with his second wife. The first wife died in 1996. His mother lived to 93 and father lived to 96. He reports that they died of "old age."

Vital Signs: Blood pressure is 96/62. RR 18, P 54, T 97.3, Wt 197, down 6 pounds from last month with BMI of 28.67. General: Elderly male in no acute distress. Skin: Laminectomy scar on his lower back. No clubbing or cyanosis of his fingers and no suspicious lesions. Neurologic: He is alert and oriented but his timeline is unclear, especially relating to the diarrhea. Is far more concerned about his knee than anything else. Cranial nerves grossly intact and motor strength is 5/5. HEENT: Atraumatic, normocephalic. Anicteric sclera. No sinus tenderness. Posterior oropharynx is very irritated. Lips without cyanosis. NECK: Supple without adenopathy. No thyromegaly, nodules, or carotid bruits. CHEST: Normal symmetry. CARDIOVASCULAR: Rate is somewhat bradycardiac and very difficult tones to auscultate. Regular rhythm. LUNGS: Clear. ABDOMEN: Soft, nontender, nondistended, decreased bowel sounds, no hepatosplenomegaly, rebound, or rigidity. No inguinal adenopathy, 2+ inguinal pulses bilaterally. MUSCULOSKELETAL: Left leg shows some atrophy in the muscles and left knee looks larger than the right knee. No real swelling appreciated. Not warm. GU: Normal scrotal exam. No hernia. RECTAL: Perianal area is somewhat irritated. There is a large external hemorrhoid. Prostate is slightly enlarged. Stool is dark brown but heme negative.

Labs are pending. EKG shows a significant sinus bradycardia around 50–55 beats per minute. This does not appear to be atrial fibrillation. He has a somewhat widened QRS complex or intraventricular conduction delay. He does not peak T waves or have any other significant issues regarding arrhythmia.

Assessment:

1. Hypotension, potentially due to antihypertensive medication or based on decreased volume due to diarrhea and potential GI bleed.
2. Sinus bradycardia. Cause unclear but could also be due to volume depletion.
3. Diarrhea. Has had problems with anemia in the past but not currently. Potentially upper GI source since stool is dark.
4. Localized osteoarthrosis of left knee.

Plan: IV fluids, 2L over 8 hours and then will switch to 100 ml/hour of D5 normal saline. Blood was drawn in the office. Recheck comprehensive metabolic panel after IV hydration. Hold Lisinopril and Coreg until blood pressure stabilizes. Cardiology consult requested. GI consult requested. Will hold on evaluating any orthopedic issues until seen in follow-up in the office.

Assign the correct codes for this encounter.

ICD-9-CM and CPT Code(s): _____

ICD-10-CM Code(s): _____

6.12. The following documentation is from the health record of a 63-year-old female patient.

Admission Date:	11/19/XX
Discharge Date:	11/24/XX
Final Diagnoses:	1. Coronary artery disease
	2. Sick sinus syndrome
Procedures:	1. Permanent AV sequential pacemaker insertion
	2. Percutaneous transluminal coronary angioplasty

History of Present Illness: The patient is a 63-year-old female who was admitted to another hospital on 11/19 after experiencing tachycardia. At that hospital, she underwent a cardiac catheterization, showing the presence of severe single-vessel coronary artery disease. The patient has a history of sick sinus syndrome. She was transferred to our hospital to undergo a percutaneous transluminal angioplasty.

Physical Examination: No physical abnormalities were found on the cardiovascular examination. Pulse 50, blood pressure 100/66. HEENT: PERRLA, faint carotid bruits. Lungs: Clear to percussion and auscultation. Heart: Normal sinus rhythm with a 2.6 systolic ejection murmur. Extremities and abdomen were negative. Laboratory data: Unremarkable.

Hospital Course: To manage the patient's sick sinus syndrome, a permanent AV sequential pacemaker was implanted by transvenous technique on 11/19. On 11/20, the patient underwent a PTCA without complications and good results were obtained. Postoperatively, the patient was stable and was subsequently discharged. Patient was discharged on the following medications: Cardizem, 30 mg p.o. q. 6 hours; ASA, 5 grains q. a.m.; Metamucil and Colace p.r.n; Nitro paste 1/2 inch q. 6 hours.

Which of the following is the correct code assignment for the procedures performed?

ICD-9-CM and CPT Code(s):

a. 427.0, 414.01, 92982, 33206
b. 414.01, 427.81, 92995, 33208
c. 414.01, 427.81, 92982, 33208
d. 427.81, 414.01, 92982, 33206

ICD-10-CM Code(s): _____

6.13. A patient is seen in the hospital with a diagnosis of congestive heart failure due to hypertensive heart disease. The patient responds positively to Lasix therapy. The patient also has chronic kidney disease stage V and is a type I diabetic. Assign the correct diagnostic codes.

ICD-9-CM Code(s): _____

ICD-10-CM Code(s): _____

6.14. This 55-year-old male was brought to the ER with chest pain. The final diagnostic statement on the patient's record stated "preinfarction syndrome." What is the correct diagnostic code?

ICD-9-CM Code(s): _____

ICD-10-CM Code(s): _____

6.15. A patient had an implantable vascular access device placed 7 weeks ago for chemotherapy administered each week in the ambulatory surgery department of the hospital. The full cycle is now complete and it is no longer needed. The physician surgically removed the centrally tunneled central venous catheter. No services for the carcinoma of the sigmoid colon are provided. The cancer has not been resected yet because the chemotherapy was utilized in an attempt to shrink the tumor before surgery was initiated. The correct codes for reporting by the physician will be:

ICD-9-CM and CPT Code(s): _____

ICD-10-CM Code(s): _____

Disorders of the Digestive System

6.16. This 30-year-old male patient has exhausted all types of conservative treatment for his morbid obesity due to his excess calories intake. He has been treated by me in this clinic for 3 years. He has also been treated for hypertension and hypercholesterolemia. With these risk factors and with careful review of his condition and symptoms and with multiple consultations with him regarding the risks and benefits of the surgery, it is decided to perform a vertical-banded gastroplasty.

What diagnosis and CPT procedure codes are used in this surgical case?

ICD-9-CM and CPT Code(s):

a. 278.00, 43842, 43846–51
b. 278.01, 401.9, 272.0, 43842
c. 278.01, 401.1, 272.0, 43842, 43843–59
d. 278.01, 43848

ICD-10-CM Code(s): _____

6.17. This 25-year-old woman has been treated for Crohn's disease of the small intestine since 18 years of age. She has had several exacerbations but has been maintained on drug therapy. She is being seen now for extreme pain, which on x-ray shows small bowel obstruction. Patient is taken to surgery immediately. During the surgery, a partial excision of the terminal ileum is performed to release the obstruction. There is also a section of the jejunum that is very inflamed. This section is also resected. An end-to-end anastomosis is completed on all segments. The patient tolerates the procedure well. Which of the following is the correct code assignment?

ICD-9-CM and CPT Code(s):

a. 560.89, 555.0, 44120, 44121-51
b. 555.0, 560.89, 44120, 44121-51
c. 555.0, 560.89, 44120, 44121
d. 555.2, 560.89, 44020

ICD-10-CM Code(s): _____

6.18. During a colonoscopy, the surgeon biopsies an inflamed area in the ascending colon and removes a polyp in the descending colon with use of hot biopsy forceps. What is the correct CPT and modifier code assignment?

CPT Code(s): _____

6.19. The patient has a history of abdominal pain and blood in the stool. A colonoscopy was done earlier today and did not identify a bleed. As a further evaluation, the patient is undergoing a capsule endoscopy of the entire GI tract. The physician documentation states:

The patient was able to swallow the capsule orally without difficulty. Images were downloaded. The capsule was seen traversing the small bowel all of the way down to the cecum. Gastric images demonstrated no ulceration. Gastric passage time was 1 hour and 37 minutes. Careful review of small bowel images, which were of good quality, did not demonstrate any significant mucosal lesion. There was one single site suggestive of possible erosion seen in the ileum. The capsule was seen entering the ileocecal valve into the cecum.

Assign the correct codes for this encounter.

ICD-9-CM and CPT Code(s): _____

ICD-10-CM Code(s): _____

6.20. This 50-year-old male patient had a cholecystectomy done with exploration of the common duct for stones. During the procedure an incidental appendectomy was performed. How are the CPT procedure codes reported if the third-party payer requires that both procedures be reported?

CPT Code(s): _____

6.21. The patient has both internal and external thrombosed hemorrhoids in a single group, excised in the outpatient surgical suite. What codes would be assigned by the surgeon?

ICD-9-CM and CPT Code(s):

a. 455.4, 455.1, 46255
b. 455.5, 455.2, 46260
c. 455.4, 455.1, 46945, 46320
d. 455.7, 46083, 46320

ICD-10-CM Code(s): _____

6.22. A laparoscopic cholecystectomy with cholangiography was performed on a 35-year-old female patient due to symptomatic cholelithiasis. The pathology report showed acute and chronic cholecystitis with lithiasis and was documented by the physician. What codes would be assigned?

Assign the correct codes for this encounter.

ICD-9-CM and CPT Code(s): _____

ICD-10-CM Code(s): _____

6.23. The patient's gastric band has been adjusted so many times that it is losing its elasticity and starting to slip on her stomach and migrate up around her esophagus. She enters to undergo removal of her current gastric band and placement of a new adjustable band. Her weight loss has been steady and appropriate. Assign the CPT code(s) for the procedure of laparoscopic removal and replacement of an adjustable gastric band.

a. 43773
b. 43771, 43770
c. 43774, 43770
d. 43888

6.24. This is the health record of a patient treated in the ambulatory surgery center.

Preoperative Diagnosis:	Ankyloglossia
Postoperative Diagnosis:	Same as above
Procedure:	Lingual frenoplasty
Anesthesia:	General

Technique: The 4-year-old was brought to the operating room and was placed in the supine position. The patient was prepped and draped in the normal fashion and induced under general anesthesia. The patient was intubated with a pediatric tube with no problem. The ventral surface of the tongue with injected with 2% lidocaine with epinenphrine and retracted superiorly using a retraction suture placed through the tip of the tongue. A Bovie cautery was used to incise the lingual fenulum from the ventral surface of the tongue approximately 1 cm posteriorly. Using 3-0 chromic sutures, the ventral surface of the tongue was sutured in an interrupted fashion to obtain hemostasis and to prevent reattachment of the frenulum. The wound was covered with moist dressings and the patient was sent to recovery in good condition.

Assign the correct codes for this outpatient surgery.

ICD-9-CM and CPT Code(s): _____

ICD-10-CM Code(s): _____

6.25. **Pre-Procedure Diagnosis:**

Post-Procedure Diagnosis: Diverticulosis; diminuitive sigmoid polyp at 20 cm (removed); internal hemorrhoids

Procedure: Colonoscopy

Anesthesia: Conscious Sedation

Procedure: After informed consent was obtained and history and physical examination performed, the patient was placed in the left lateral decubitus position. While being continuously monitored for heart rate, blood pressure, cardiac rhythm, and oxygen saturation, conscious intravenous sedation was established using intravenous Fentanyl and Versed. A digital rectal examination was unremarkable.

The Olympus video colonoscope was inserted into the rectum which revealed internal hemorrhoids. The colonoscope was then advanced through a sigmoid and left colons which revealed scattered diverticulosis. A diminutive 6- to 8-mm polyp was noted 20 cm from the anal verge and was removed using standard hot biopsy technique. The colonoscope was then advanced to the cecum, identified by the ileocecal valve and appendiceal opening. The colonoscope was advanced through the appendiceal opening and into the small bowel which was unremarkable.

The colonoscope was then withdrawn carefully inspecting the walls for mucosal abnormalities. Once back in the rectum retroflexion revealed internal hemorrhoids. The colonoscope was straightened and withdrawn. The patient tolerated the procedure well. There were no complications. She was sent to the Recovery Room in stable condition.

Plan:
1. The patient will remain on a high fiber diet.
2. Will await histology of the benign appearing sigmoid polyp.
3. Schedule the patient for surveillance colonoscopy in 36 months.

Assign the correct codes for this outpatient encounter.

ICD-9-CM and CPT Code(s): _____

ICD-10-CM Code(s): _____

Evaluation and Management (E/M) Services

6.26. A 45-year-old patient was found unconscious in a park and was brought to the emergency department by ambulance. A comprehensive physical examination was performed, and the medical decision making was of high complexity. The ED physician documents that he was unable to obtain a history due to the condition of the patient.

What is the correct E/M code assignment for the physician's services for this encounter?

a. 99284
b. 99285
c. 99285-52
d. 99291

6.27. Dr. Jones saw Mr. Stone at the VA domiciliary after the patient had an episode of severe choking at the noon meal. He did not aspirate any food, but had a slight sore throat after the episode. The patient stubbornly refused to go to the clinic but agreed to be seen if the doctor came over. Mr. Stone has had several episodes of choking in the past few days, which he attributed completely to his sinus medication causing a very dry mouth. Dr. Jones documented a problem-focused interval history and an expanded problem-focused examination on this established patient. Medical decision making was of low complexity. Another medication was substituted. He was advised to drink liquids with his meals and take smaller bites. Give the correct codes for this visit.

ICD-9-CM and CPT Code(s):

a. 784.99, 783.3, 99335
b. 933.1, 99334
c. 933.1, 99335
d. 783.3, 99334

ICD-10-CM Code(s): _____

6.28. A 59-year-old male established patient is scheduled for his routine physical examination; however, the physician finds a mass in the abdomen, schedules an abdominal CT scan, and orders laboratory for blood work and a UA. The physician performs a detailed history and an expanded problem-focused examination with medical decision making of moderate complexity. The patient has been a patient of this physician for several years. What E/M code(s) are assigned?

Code(s): _____

6.29. An elderly patient is brought to the emergency department by an ambulance due to a cardiac arrest suffered at home. The ED physician provides and documents critical care services to the patient for a total duration of 2 hours before the attending physician admits the patient to the cardiac care unit.

What codes are assigned for the ED physician? (Include E/M code(s).)

ICD-9-CM and CPT Code(s): _____

ICD-10-CM Code(s): _____

6.30. Summary of the clinic record of a family practice physician:

The patient is a 3-year-old male with Down's Syndrome who was seen in the office yesterday for bilateral otitis media. He was given a prescription for Septra liquid suspension. On repeat visit today, the mother reports that the patient complained of a "tummy ache" after the first dose and has vomited six times since being seen yesterday. PO intake is decreased but still sufficiently hydrated. Has not been able to keep down any antibiotic. A detailed history is documented.

Documentation states that the ears have increased redness with the right TM bulging more than yesterday. Considerable wheezing is noted on lung exam. No other significant findings are documented on the detailed exam.

The patient is treated with 500 mg of Ceftriaxone sodium, IM, and given a prescription for an albuterol metered dose inhaler with spacer. The patient and mother are taught the proper use of the inhaler.

The physician documents the diagnoses as:

1. Acute otitis media
2. First-time wheezer
3. Vomiting
4. Down's Syndrome

What codes would be reported for this visit (include E/M code)?

ICD-9-CM and CPT Code(s):

a. 381.4, 493.90, 787.03, 758.0, 99214, 96372, J0696
b. 382.9, 758.0, 99214, 94640, 96372, J0696 × 2 units
c. 382.9, 786.07, 787.03, 758.0, 99214-25, 94664, 96372, J0696 × 2 units
d. 382.9, 786.07, 787.03, 758.0, 99214-25, 96372, J0696

ICD-10-CM Code(s): _____

6.31. Dr. Smith sees his patient, Bob Jones, in the nursing home where he has resided for 11 months. Bob is pretty stable and happy, and Dr. Smith performs an annual physical examination and completes the minimum data set instrument. He performs and documents a detailed interval history, comprehensive examination, and performs medical decision making of and low complexity. Assign the appropriate CPT code.

a. 99304
b. 99308
c. 99318
d. 99306

6.32. An established patient sees his doctor in the office with complaints of chest pain. The physician admits the patient on December 1 under observation status at the local community hospital. The physician completes a comprehensive history that includes a complete review of all body systems and a complete past, family, and social history. The physician performs a comprehensive examination but finds no significant issues. The patient does admit to a great deal of stress at work. Medical decision making is of moderate complexity. On the second day of care, the physician continues to observe the patient when he conducts a detailed examination and medical decision making of moderate complexity. The patient is subsequently discharged home the next day with a diagnosis of mild depression. The patient was in observation status for three days.

What E&M codes would the physician report for the second day of care?

Code(s): _____

6.33. The patient was brought by ambulance to the ER after being shot in the head in a random drive-by shooting. Critical care services are provided by the physician for 125 minutes. During this time the physician performed CPR, reviewed ECG and blood gas results on the EHR, and intubated the young man. However, the patient died from his extensive injuries. What E/M codes are used to report the services supplied by the physician?

   a. 99292, 92950
   b. 99291, 99292, 92950
   c. 99291, 99292, 99090, 92950, 43752
   d. 99291, 99292, 92950

Endocrine, Nutritional, and Metabolic Diseases and Immunity Disorders

6.34. A repeat thyroidectomy is performed after a previous right partial thyroidectomy was completed several years ago. All thyroid tissue is removed from the right side, and a total left thyroidectomy is performed. The parathyroid glands are separated from the thyroid tissue and replanted. What is the correct CPT code assignment for the services of the surgeon?

   a. 60220-50
   b. 60240
   c. 60260-50, 60512
   d. 60260-RT, 60220-LT, 60512

6.35. A 6-year-old child, an established patient, is seen in the pediatrician's office for routine immunization. The physician speaks with the child's father about national immunization recommendations, and the risks and benefits of vaccine provided, and gives follow-up instructions for possible side-effect treatment. The patient receives a DtaP immunization IM. Assign the appropriate CPT procedure code(s).

   a. 90461, 90700
   b. 99213, 90460, 90700
   c. 90460, 90461, 90700
   d. 90460

6.36. A 35-year-old man was referred to the endocrinology clinic for symptoms that involved headaches, deepening voice, and enlargement and coarsening of facial features, hands, and feet. This has been gradual over the past 3 years. The patient was referred by his dentist, who noticed increased spacing between his teeth over the same time period. Growth hormone levels tested by the endocrinology clinic were elevated for an adult male. Follow-up IGF-1 tests confirmed the diagnosis. The patient was scheduled for a CT scan of the brain to rule out pituitary tumor. Diagnosis after the second clinic visit was acromegaly and ruled out pituitary adenoma. Give the correct code(s) for the second clinic visit.

ICD-9-CM Code(s):

a. 253.0, 225.0
b. 253.0
c. 227.3
d. 253.0, 227.3

ICD-10-CM Code(s): _____

6.37. The following documentation is from the health record of a 54-year-old female patient:

CC: Refill of estrogen patch and follow-up.

HPI: Severe hot flashes have been controlled. Energy level is back to a reasonable level.

ROS: All other systems are reviewed and are negative.

She is able to meet her work commitments as a community college instructor.

Exam: Unremarkable.

Assessment: Menopausal symptoms controlled by estrogen patch. Refill for 6 months given. Return PRN.

Which of the following lists the correct codes for this clinic visit?

ICD-9-CM and CPT Code(s):

a. 627.2, V07.4, 99213
b. V07.4, V49.81, 99212
c. 627.2, 99213
d. V07.4, 99212

ICD-10-CM Code(s): _____

6.38. This 45-year-old female diabetic patient comes in for her quarterly evaluation of her condition. She has type I diabetes, which has been in good control now. She has diabetic nephropathy and retinopathy. What diagnosis codes are assigned?

ICD-9-CM Code(s): _____

ICD-10-CM Code(s): _____

6.39. From the hospital record of a patient requiring diabetic management:

Hospital Course: This 49-year-old female patient has a history of type I diabetes mellitus and is on 15 units of NPH and 10 of Regular in the morning, and 10 units of NPH and 5 of Regular in the evening. The patient started having symptoms of nausea and vomiting. The patient at the same time had increased frequency of urination and polydipsia. The patient was severely dehydrated on admission. There was no evidence of thrombophlebitis, varicosities, or edema on examination of the extremities. The patient was hydrated and, as a result, her blood sugar decreased from more than 600 to normal levels. The patient was discharged with the diagnosis of diabetic ketoacidosis, dehydration, polydipsia, and increased frequency of urination.

What diagnosis codes would be assigned for this admission for the physician's services?

ICD-9-CM Code(s): _____

ICD-10-CM Code(s): _____

6.40.   Assign the code(s) for a patient with type II diabetic gastroparesis who is presently on insulin.

ICD-9-CM Code(s):

a. 250.60, 536.3, V58.67
b. 250.60, 586.3, 337.1, V58.67
c. 250.61, 536.3
d. 250.62, 536.3, V58.67

ICD-10-CM Code(s): _____

6.41.   A 65-year-old female patient has a long history of type II diabetes mellitus with diabetic retinopathy. She is being seen today for her retinal ischemia and diabetic macular edema. What codes are assigned for this proliferative retinopathy?

ICD-9-CM Code(s):

a. 250.50, 362.07
b. 250.50, 362.06, 362.07
c. 250.50, 362.02, 362.07
d. 362.02, 363.07

ICD-10-CM Code(s): _____

Disorders of the Genitourinary System

6.42.   **Procedure:** Transrectal prostatic biopsy under ultrasound guidance

Preoperative Diagnosis: Nocturia and hesitancy

Postoperative Diagnosis: Prostatic calcifications, BPH

History: Elevated PSA of 11.8. Digital rectal examination revealed a nodular prostate gland. Patient complains of frequent need to urinate during the night and hesitancy when urinating.

Procedure: The patient was placed in the left lateral position and endorectal scanning of the prostate gland was carried out utilizing the Toshiba Just Vision 400 ultrasound. Both axial and sagittal scanning probes were utilized.

The prostate gland was enlarged in size and shape with a gland volume of 112.5 cc. The seminal vesicles appeared symmetrical. The capsule was smooth and intact. There were no hypoechoic areas noted but nodules were seen throughout the entire left peripheral zone.

The Bard biopsy guide was then attached to the sagittal scanning probe. Biopsies were obtained utilizing a prostatic block through the left and right sides of the prostate gland including the apical, mid, and basilar portion of the peripheral as well as the lateral base and lateral apex for a total of 10 biopsies.

What codes are used to report this ambulatory surgery?

ICD-9-CM and CPT Code(s): _____

ICD-10-CM Code(s): _____

6.43. A patient in end-stage renal failure requires outpatient hemodialysis 3 times a week while he is awaiting kidney transplant. He has an A-V fistula in his left arm for vascular access. Which of the following code set combinations is appropriate for reporting physician services for this 55-year-old male for the month of August?

ICD-9-CM and CPT Code(s):

a. 585.6, 90970
b. V56.0, 90960
c. 585.6, V56.8, 90999
d. 585.6, 90960

ICD-10-CM Code(s): _____

6.44. From the health record of a patient receiving endoscopy services:

The patient presents to the hospital outpatient department for follow-up cystoscopy for a history of high-grade bladder cancer. This was resected 7 years ago and was found to be grade III with superficial muscle invasion. A cycle of chemotherapy was provided, but no radiation. No recurrence has been noted since then. CT scan of the pelvis 6 months ago was negative for masses. Sometimes the patient experiences painful ejaculation, but no hematospermia has been found. Cytology to date has been negative, so a biopsy will not be performed because there has been 7 years without recurrence.

Cystoscopy examination today shows a normal anterior urethra and prostatic urethra. There is some lateral lobe prostatic hypertrophy, just barely touching in the midline. The bladder is nontrabeculated. There are no tumors, stones, or carcinoma in situ evident on examination. There is clear efflux from each orifice. The area of resection was around the right ureteral orifice, which appears a little atrophic, but patent.

Impression: Stable transitional cell of the bladder without recurrence with mild benign prostatic hypertrophy.

Which of the following code sets is appropriate for this case?

ICD-9-CM and CPT Code(s):

a. V67.6, V10.51, 600.00, 52000
b. 188.9, 600.0, 52000
c. 600.00, V10.51, 52010
d. V67.00, 188.9, 52000

ICD-10-CM Code(s): _____

6.45. The following documentation is from the health record of a 42-year-old female patient:

Preoperative Diagnosis:	Menometrorrhagia and endometrial polyp
Postoperative Diagnosis:	Same
Operation:	Diagnostic hysteroscopy Endometrial ablation Fractional dilatation and curettage
Specimens:	Endometrial curettings

Operative Findings: The uterus sounded to a depth of 8.5 cm. The cervical length was 4 cm and the cavity depth was 4.5 cm. Cavity width was 4 cm and the treatment cycle was 80 seconds. The power setting was 99.

Description of Procedure: The patient was brought to the operating room suite and general anesthesia was administered. The patient is placed in the dorsal-lithotomy position and her vagina and perineum were sterilely prepped and draped in the usual fashion.

The bladder was decompressed with an in-and-out catheter. The weighted speculum was placed into the vagina after bimanual pelvic examination had been performed revealing a midline positioned uterus. The anterior lip of the cervix was grasped with a single-tooth tenaculum. The uterus was sounded to a depth of 8.5 cm; however the internal cervical os could not be palpated with the uterine sound. Sure sound was therefore used to find a cervical length of 4 cm and a cavity length of 4.5 cm. This being accomplished, the diagnostic hysteroscopy was performed. Both tubal ostia were visualized. There was no evidence of intracavitary defect. Endometrial tissue was visible including polyps. Glycine was used as the distending media. The hysteroscope was withdrawn. The cervix was dilated to allow the admission of a #4 sharp curette. Uterine curettage was performed until a good uterine cry was noted. The polyp forceps was used to extract remaining fragments of tissue. The tissue was sent to Pathology for evaluation. Now the NovaSure instrument was placed and the settings accomplished giving a power setting of 99. After cavity assessment was passed, the ablation procedure was initiated. The ablation procedure treatment cycle lasted 80 seconds.

The array was closed, the instrument withdrawn, and then general anesthesia was reversed. The patient was taken to the recovery room in stable and satisfactory condition having tolerated the procedure well. All sponge, instrument, and needle counts were correct. The estimated blood loss was 3 cc.

What CPT code(s) would be assigned in this case?

Code(s): _____

6.46. This 35-year-old female has had 4 cesarean births in the past 6 years and has decided to proceed with sterilization.

Operative Report

Procedure: Laparoscopic tubal ligation with application of Falope-Rings

Diagnosis: Multiparity; desired sterilization

Anesthesia: General

Under general anesthesia and in the supine lithotomy position, the patient was prepped and draped in the usual sterile fashion. A two-puncture laparoscopy was performed in the usual manner with insufflation through a Verres needle inserted infraumbilically. Through the first puncture, a trocar was inserted infraumbilically, followed by the laparoscope. A second trocar was inserted suprapubically in the midline, followed initially by a probe and then a Falope-Ring applicator. Both tubes were ligated in their midsegment. On the left side, two rings were applied because of the round position of the Falope-Ring director. The right tube was singly ligated. The operation was completed, and the trocar sites were closed with subcuticular sutures of 2-0 VICRYL. The patient was transferred to the recovery room in good condition.

What are the correct codes to assign for this service?

ICD-9-CM and CPT Code(s): _____

ICD-10-CM Code(s): _____

6.47. This 35-year-old man has had an eruption of molluscum contagiosum on the penis for several months. He finally sought medical attention. He was advised to have these lesions removed. He is here now for the procedure. The patient had destruction of a penile molluscum contagiosum performed by cryosurgery and laser surgery. What are the correct code(s)?

ICD-9-CM and CPT Code(s): _____

ICD-10-CM Code(s): _____

Infectious Diseases

6.48. The patient is a 10-year-old girl who presents with a sore throat, fever of 101.4, swollen glands in the neck, and a red blotchy rash over the neck, face, chest, and back. She has significant nausea and has vomited 3 times since this morning and is complaining of severe pain when swallowing. A detailed history and examination are documented, with medical decision making of moderate complexity. The physician ordered a rapid strep test, which was performed in the office and was positive. Because of the significant nausea and questionable antibiotic compliance in the past, the physician administers 1.2 million units of Bicillin L-A (long-acting Penicillin G) via a deep intramuscular injection. The patient will be seen again in 5 days. Diagnoses were documented as strep throat with scarlatina.

Assign the codes, including E/M codes and laboratory codes, for this case.

ICD-9-CM, CPT, and HCPCS Code(s): _____

ICD-10-CM Code(s): _____

6.49.   The employees of this clinic who work in the patient care areas are receiving the vaccination for hepatitis B in the employee health clinic. What codes would be reported for this service given as an IM injection?

ICD-9-CM and CPT Code(s): _____

ICD-10-CM Code(s): _____

6.50.   This 5-year-old patient of ours is here in the office for her routine annual child exam. She has been healthy, but reports that she is challenged in K-4 to concentrate and pay attention. Mother would like to schedule an evaluation for possible attention deficit disorder. Active immunization with live measles, mumps, and rubella virus vaccine was given during her annual preventive medicine visit for this established patient. The physician requests a consultation with a psychologist for concentration deficit; they rule out attention deficit disorder.

What are the correct codes?

ICD-9-CM and CPT Code(s): _____

ICD-10-CM Code(s): _____

Disorders of the Skin and Subcutaneous Tissue

6.51.   An elderly patient has an abscess formation around a pacemaker pocket on his chest wall that requires that the device be removed and the pocket reformed in another location. Which of the following code sets is appropriate for this outpatient surgical service? Do not assign E codes in this case.

ICD-9-CM and CPT Code(s):

   a. 996.61, 682.2, 33222
   b. 682.2, 33222
   c. 996.61, 33233
   d. 996.72, 682.2, 33999

ICD-10-CM Code(s): _____

6.52.   This 18-year-old male patient has pustular acne that requires periodic opening and/or removal of milia and comedones from his face in the dermatology clinic on a recurring basis. These visits do not include medical history or examination by the physician—only the procedure.

Assign the correct codes for this encounter.

ICD-9-CM and CPT Code(s): _____

ICD-10-CM Code(s): _____

6.53. This 54-year-old female has noticed areas of raised skin on her face, mostly on her forehead. She states that they have grown quickly with the size almost doubling in 3 weeks. She has concerns that this may be skin cancer and wants an evaluation. She is scheduled for surgery, and the physician abraded 6 areas on the patient's face. They were determined to be keratoses. What codes would be assigned for the surgery episode of care?

ICD-9-CM and CPT Code(s): _____

ICD-10-CM Code(s): _____

6.54. A patient with significant second- and third-degree burns over his back and buttocks underwent debridement of approximately 175 sq cm of necrotic eschar tissue and application of 325 sq cm of Mediskin as a temporary wound closure. Assign the appropriate CPT code(s).

Code(s): _____

6.55. This patient received 45 sq cm of TranCyte to an ulcer of the lateral left foot. Assign the appropriate CPT procedure code(s).

Code(s): _____

6.56. This is the record from an outpatient encounter.

Chief Complaint: Warts on the sole of the left foot

The 12-year-old patient is seen with complaints of painful warts on the sole of the left foot. He states that the warts first appeared about 3 weeks ago but have become progressively painful. The patient was seen in the office 2 months ago with chronic otitis media and he had no problems at that time with warts.

The physical examination of the bottom of the left foot reveals four separate lesions of the following sizes and locations: 4-mm verruca on the heel of the foot, two 3-mm verruca on the ball of the foot, and a 6-mm verrucous papule near the base of the big toe.

Initial impression is that of plantar warts.

After consent from the mother, cryocautery was used to destroy each of the lesions. The patient experienced minor discomfort which abated soon after. The wounds were dressed and the patient was advised to make an appointment for 1 week.

Which codes are used to report this office visit?

ICD-9-CM and CPT Code(s): _____

ICD-10-CM Code(s): _____

Behavioral Health Conditions

6.57.   A patient in a clinic received individual insight-oriented psychotherapy for more than 25 minutes. The physician also provided E/M services that included a problem-focused history, problem-focused examination, and straightforward level of medical decision making. What CPT code(s) would this physician report?

   a. 90805
   b. 90804, 99212
   c. 90811
   d. 90810, 99212

6.58.   A young adult who is self-referred presents as a new patient in the clinic with complaints of an increasing inability to concentrate and complete tasks. He states that he has always been easily distracted and often leaves tasks uncompleted, but in recent years his restlessness has increased. He is perceived as unreliable at work and is concerned about future job advancements. The physician takes a comprehensive history and exam and performs medical decision making of moderate complexity. The physician's diagnosis is attention deficit disorder, DSM-IV 314.9, and the plan of treatment is to begin Ritalin and to follow up to assess dosage and efficacy. The physician documents that he spent 45 minutes in counseling with the patient.

   What are the correct codes to report this encounter?

   ICD-9-CM and CPT Code(s):

   a. 314.00, 99214
   b. 314.00, 99204
   c. 314.01, 99204
   d. 314.9, 99214

   ICD-10-CM Code(s): _____

6.59.   This 25-year-old man is seen by the psychiatrist for repeated attempts to stop smoking. An hour-long hypnotherapy session is completed to help eliminate the need for smoking. What CPT code(s) are assigned in this case?

   Code(s): _____

6.60.   Physician progress note states: This patient is a 75-year-old female who has severe Alzheimer's disease. The patient shows no acute change in mental status from her last visit. She requires continuous care because of her dementia, but the family is insistent on keeping her at home. She has made repeated attempts to leave and has wandered off in the past, hence the need for continuous care. She at times recognizes her daughter, the primary caregiver, but most of the time she is unaware of her identity. What diagnosis codes are reported for this visit?

   ICD-9-CM Code(s): _____

   ICD-10-CM Code(s): _____

Disorders of the Musculoskeletal System and Connective Tissue

6.61. A patient had an osteopathic physician as a primary care provider. The patient suffered from sternoclavicular somatic dysfunction. An evaluation was done using a detailed history and an expanded problem-focused examination with low medical decision making. The physician performed osteopathic manipulation to the affected body region. What codes should be assigned to this office visit?

ICD-9-CM and CPT Code(s):

a. 739.7, 99213-25, 98925
b. 739.2, 98925
c. 786.59, 99212-25, 98925
d. 739.8, 99213

ICD-10-CM Code(s): _____

6.62. From the health record of a young athlete:

Preoperative Diagnosis: Fracture of fibula, left

Postoperative Diagnosis: Left distal fracture of fibula

Procedure: Reduction of fibular fracture

Indications and Description: This 14-year-old girl who is a gymnast felt pain in her leg after hitting the vault at practice. She is unable to bear any weight on her left leg.

Physical examination revealed foot and ankle to be normal. The neurovascular status of the foot is normal. The ankle is nontender and not swollen. Findings are confined to the distal fibula, 2 inches proximal to the lateral malleolus. There is point tenderness in this area. An x-ray of the tibia and fibula shows a displaced comminuted fracture of the distal fibula.

The fracture was reduced, and the patient was put in a short leg splint molded for her from fiberglass, with extensive padding placed over the fracture site. Crutches were provided, and she is instructed not to place any weight on the foot. She was given a supply of Tylenol 3 for pain and will follow up at the clinic in 10 days.

Which of the following is the correct code combination assignment?

ICD-9-CM and CPT Code(s):

a. 824.8, E917.0, 27788, Q4046
b. 824.2, E917.0, 27788, 29515–51
c. 823.81, E917.0, 27786, L4350
d. 824.4, E917.0, 27810, 29515–51, L4396

ICD-10-CM Code(s): _____

6.63. This 16-year-old was tackled during a football game 3 weeks ago and received fracture care with a cast for a displaced, comminuted fracture of the right fibula. He is coming in today for a walking cast, which was applied after a 2-view x-ray in the clinic. This converted an existing cast to one that did not require crutches. What are the codes that will appear on the CMS-1500 form that is sent to the insurance company?

ICD-9-CM and CPT Code(s): _____

ICD-10-CM Code(s): _____

6.64. The physician treats a patient who has osteomyelitis of the scapula following an injury. A piece of dead bone is removed from the body of the scapula.

What CPT code is assigned by the surgeon?

a. 23140
b. 23172
c. 23182
d. 23190

6.65. From the health record of a patient having hand surgery:

Operative Report

Preoperative Diagnosis: Foreign body on the left little finger at the metacarpophalangeal joint is a broken piece of glass.

Postoperative Diagnosis: Same.

Operation: Exploration of the MP joint of the left little finger with excision and removal of foreign body.

Indication of Surgery: The patient was a passenger in a vehicle that was struck by a large rock. The rock from a hillside hit the windshield, breaking the glass. She tried to brace herself with her left hand and sustained a laceration on the dorsum of the metacarpal phalangeal joint of the left little finger. The injury didn't seem significant at the time and she did not even see a physician. The wound subsequently healed, but she started noticing some pain in that region. Over three months later, she accidentally hit the metacarpal phalangeal joint of the left little finger against something and since then she has been complaining of severe pain and numbness. She had an x-ray of her left hand which revealed a foreign body in the metacarpal phalangeal joint of the left little finger. The patient was referred to me. I explained to the patient I need to open up the wound, explore the area, and remove the foreign body. The possible risks, benefits, and possible complications of the procedure were explained.

Technique: The patient was placed on the OR bed assuming the supine position. Blood pressure monitoring and pulse oximetry monitoring were in progress. The left hand and forearm were then prepped and draped. Initially, I tried to palpate the metacarpophalangeal joint until I found the area that had the most tenderness. This area is located at the dorsum of the MP joint of the left little finger proximal to the previously healed scar. This area was then marked out and infiltrated with 1% Carbocaine solution. An oblique incision was then made over the area parallel to the old scar. Incision was deepened and bleeders were fulgurated with high temperature. By careful sharp and blunt dissection, the foreign body was searched for. For a while, I could not find the foreign body. Therefore, the incision was extended distally towards the previous area of the laceration. After searching for some time, it was found that the dorsal digital nerve in this area was intact. It was retracted out of harm's way and the area near the extensor tendon towards the foot of the extensor tendon. The foreign body was wedged in the soft tissue of the joint capsule. It was a piece of broken glass and measures about $2 \times 3 \times 1$ mm. It was completely extracted and removed. The wound was irrigated with a large amount of saline solution. Wound closure was accomplished with 5-0 nylon interrupted mattress sutures. Compression dressing was applied. The patient withstood the procedure well. She was advised to keep the hand elevated and keep it dry and clean. She was advised to use an ice compress and change dressing in 48 hours. The patient was placed on Vicodin 1 tablet q.4h p.r.n. for pain. She was cautioned not to take pain medicine if she was driving. She was instructed to return to my office in six days.

Assign the correct codes for this encounter.

ICD-9-CM and CPT Code(s): _____

ICD-10-CM Code(s): _____

6.66. When back pain is due to a psychological condition, how is this diagnosis coded?

ICD-9-CM Code(s):

a. 724.5
b. 724.5, 307.89
c. 307.89
d. 307.89, 724.5

ICD-10-CM Code(s): _____

Neoplasms

6.67. A non-Medicare patient with carcinoma of the oral cavity and lower lip is receiving daily intramuscular injections of interferon alfa-2a (3 million units) in the outpatient cancer center. Which of the following will be reported for this service? The payer does accept HCPCS Level II codes for drugs.

ICD-9-CM Code(s):

a. V58.12, 149.8, 96401, J9213
b. 149.8, 96372, J9213
c. 145.9, 140.9, 96372
d. V58.12, 96549

ICD-10-CM Code(s): _____

6.68. This 32-year-old female with asthma and known cervical dysplasia is admitted for an endoscopic cervical biopsy with endocervical curettage. The procedure was performed without incident. The pathology report shows carcinoma in situ of the cervix. What diagnosis and CPT procedure codes are assigned?

ICD-9-CM and CPT Code(s): _____

ICD-10-CM Code(s): _____

6.69.   This patient had a history of carcinoma of the colon 5 years ago without reoccurrence or metastasis. After several tests he is admitted now for probable renal cell carcinoma, thought to be a new primary. Laparoscopic partial nephrectomy of the kidney was performed without incident. Frozen-section pathology report reveals a lipoma. What diagnosis and CPT procedure codes are assigned for the procedure performed in the hospital?

ICD-9-CM and CPT Code(s): _____

ICD-10-CM Code(s): _____

6.70.   The patient had a 2.0-cm lesion removed from the neck, including 0.2-cm margins. The frozen section returned with a diagnosis of Merkel Cell tumor and clear margins.

What are the appropriate diagnosis and CPT procedure codes for this service?

ICD-9-CM and CPT Code(s):

a.   173.49, 11622
b.   209.32, 11623
c.   209.36, 11422
d.   216.4, 11423

ICD-10-CM Code(s): _____

6.71.   This 42-year-old female patient has known ovarian carcinoma, and she is being admitted for right oophorectomy. Patient has type I diabetes mellitus, and during her stay we had a hard time controlling her blood sugar level. Right oophorosalpingectomy with lymph node samplings and peritoneal biopsies was completed to stage the cancer. Diagnosis: Ovarian carcinoma, without metastasis, and diabetes out of control. What are the correct diagnosis and CPT procedure codes for this admission?

ICD-9-CM and CPT Code(s): _____

ICD-10-CM Code(s): _____

Disorders of the Nervous System and Sense Organs

6.72.   A patient has right trigeminal neuralgia, and it is decided that gamma knife stereotactic radiosurgery will be performed. A Leksell stereotactic head frame was placed prior to the procedure, which consisted of a single shot to a total dose of 7,500 cGy delivered to the 50 percent isodose line.

What is the correct CPT code assignment for this service?

a.   61796, 20660
b.   61796, 61800
c.   64600
d.   61796

6.73. The following documentation is from the health record of a surgical patient.

A Medicare beneficiary has a procedure to promote nerve regeneration at a pain management center. The patient is placed in a prone position, and a midline incision overlying the affected vertebrae is made. The fascia is divided and the paravertebral muscles are retracted. The physician places the inductive electrode pads in the epidural space proximal to the damaged spinal segment. The pulse generator is sutured over the muscles, just below the skin, and closed with a layer closure.

What CPT procedure code is reported by the physician?

a. 63655
b. 63685
c. 63650
d. 63688

6.74. From the health record of a patient having eye surgery:

Operative Report

Preoperative Diagnosis: Mild stage open-angle glaucoma, right eye; diabetes mellitus, type I

Postoperative Diagnosis: Same

Operation: Initial trabeculectomy, right eye

Anesthesia: Local

Procedure: Full-thickness lid speculums were placed. A fornix-based, conjunctival flap was performed in the superior temporal quadrant. An angulated blade breaker was used to make grooves at the site of the future scleral flap at approximately the 10 o'clock position. Next, a three-sided, partial-thickness, scleral flap was created using a #64 Beaver blade. A trabeculectomy was performed using a sharp blade. A peripheral iridectomy was performed. The scleral flap was irrigated and found to be free flowing. The conjunctiva was closed using two 8-0 collagen sutures at the 12 o'clock position and one 8-0 collagen at the nine o'clock position. Decadron 10 mg was injected subconjunctivally in the inferior fornix. Maxitrol ointment, patch, and shield were applied.

What are the correct codes for this procedure performed in the hospital surgery center?

ICD-9-CM and CPT Code(s):

a. 365.9, 365.70, 250.00, 66172–RT
b. 365.11, 250.01, 65850
c. 250.51, 365.44, 365.71, 66170–52
d. 365.10, 250.01, 66170–RT

ICD-10-CM Code(s): _____

6.75.   From the health record of a patient having office-based surgery:

Operative Report

Preoperative Diagnosis: Bilateral entropion

Postoperative Diagnosis: Bilateral entropion

Operation: Repair of entropion of right eye

Anesthesia: Local

Procedure: The patient was sterilely prepped and draped for ocular solution of 2 percent lidocaine, mixed in equal proportions with 0.75 percent Marcaine with the addition of Wydase, and a modified Van Lint technique was performed on the right eye. Incision was made in the inferior lid margin extended inferiorly. This consisted of a diamond shape, with 6-mm lengthwise incisions interconducted. Hemostasis was obtained using wet-field cautery. The incision was then sutured using a tapered needle. The first suture was placed through the approximate lash line, in addition to one suture through the area of the meibomian gland. Using the tapered needle, the tarsal plate was approximated and reapproximated. The incision was then reapproximated with subcuticular sutures. This was followed by implantation of approximately four interrupted skin sutures using 6-0 nylon.

What are the correct codes for this procedure performed in the hospital surgery center?

ICD-9-CM and CPT Code(s):

a. 374.00, 67921–RT
b. 374.00, 67921–50
c. 374.10, 67921–RT
d. 374.00, 67923

ICD-10-CM Code(s): _____

6.76.   This 71-year-old male had a stroke 6 months ago. He is being followed during his therapy for the residuals of his stroke with evaluation of progress. He has right-sided hemiplegia and aphasia (right side is dominant). He also has hypertension and diabetes mellitus, type II. What diagnosis codes are assigned?

ICD-9-CM Code(s): _____

ICD-10-CM Code(s): _____

6.77.   The patient presents to the ophthalmologist with a foreign body in the anterior segment of the right eye. The patient is a metalworker in a factory and had just taken off his protective eyewear when his co-worker's grinder malfunctioned. The metal fragment penetrated his eye. The eye was anesthetized and the metal shaving was removed with a magnet. How would this injury be coded (diagnosis codes?) What are the correct external cause and procedure codes?

ICD-9-CM and CPT Code(s): _____

ICD-10-CM Code(s): _____

6.78. **Preoperative Diagnosis:**   Chronic otitis media

Postoperative Diagnosis: Same as above

Anesthesia: General

Procedure: Myringotomy, bilateral with insertion of tubes

Technique: The 10-month-old was brought to the operating room where general anesthesia was induced. An operating microscope was used to incise the anterior tympanic membrane of the right ear and suction any purulent effusion. None was noted. A ventilating tube was inserted into the eardrum. The procedure was repeated on the left ear in a mirror fashion. Ear drops were inserted into the auditory canal and the patient was sent to recovery.

Which codes were reported by the physician for this outpatient encounter?

ICD-9-CM and CPT Code(s):

a. 382.9, 69436-50
b. 381.00, 69421-50
c. 382.9, 69433-50
d. 382.9, 69436

ICD-10-CM Code(s): _____

Newborn/Congenital Disorders

6.79. A neonatologist is treating a spontaneously delivered newborn with respiratory failure and erythroblastosis fetalis due to Rh antibodies. An exchange transfusion is required to stabilize this critically ill baby receiving services in the neonatal intensive care unit. The baby remains on CPAP to assist breathing and prevent further respiratory failure.

Which of the following code sets is reported by the neonatologist for this second day of care following birth?

ICD-9-CM and CPT Code(s):

a. 773.0, 770.84, 99469
b. V30.00, 99468, 36450, 94660
c. V30.00, 773.0, 770.84, 99469, 36450
d. 773.0, 770.84, 99469

ICD-10-CM Code(s): _____

6.80. A 22-year-old patient presents for a closure of a patent ductus arteriosus. The patient's thorax is opened posteriorly and the vagus nerve is isolated away. The PDA is divided and sutured individually in the aorta and pulmonary artery.

What is the CPT code for this procedure?

a. 33813
b. 33820
c. 33822
d. 33824

6.81. A newborn is born with a large gastroschisis and is transferred to a specialty hospital. The surgeon repairs the defect on the newborn's first day of life, without the use of a prosthesis.

Which of the following code set combinations is used to report the surgical service?

ICD-9-CM and CPT Code(s):

a. 569.89, 49580
b. 756.73, 49605
c. 569.89, 49600
d. 756.73, 49600

ICD-10-CM Code(s): _____

6.82. A hospital-based pediatric clinic is treating a newborn with talipes equinovarus by manipulation and short leg casting. Which of the following code sets is reported for a visit where the condition is evaluated with a problem-focused history and examination and parents' questions are answered, followed by foot and ankle manipulation and replacement of the plaster cast?

ICD-9-CM and CPT Code(s):

a. 754.69, 29450
b. 736.71, 29405
c. 754.51, 29405
d. 754.51, 99212–25, 29450

ICD-10-CM Code(s): _____

6.83. From the health record of a newborn delivered in a birthing room setting:

This infant was born in the New Beginnings Birthing Center adjacent to Children's Hospital at 10:58 a.m. on September 1. He weighed 8 lb, 5 oz and was 21 inches long with Apgar scores of 9 and 9. Dr. Smith performed a history and examination immediately following the vaginal delivery with no abnormal findings. Parents declined circumcision or administration of hepatitis B. The patient was discharged at 6:30 p.m. with his mother.

Which of the following code sets is appropriate for Dr. Smith's services on September 1?

ICD-9-CM and CPT Code(s):

a. V30.2, 99460, 99238
b. V30.00, 99463
c. V30.2, 99460
d. V30.2, 99463

ICD-10-CM Code(s): _____

Pediatric Conditions

6.84. A 6-month-old infant, born prematurely, presents for his monthly injection for RSV. The nurse documents Synagis 40 mg, IM.

Which of the following code sets is correct for reporting this office visit?

a. 99212, 90378, 96372
b. 90378, 90471
c. 99212, J1459
d. 90378, 96372

6.85. This 5-year-old female patient presents to the office for bilateral ear drainage, fever, and ear pain. The patient is in foster care and brought in by the new foster mother. There is a large perforation in the left eardrum visible. She was given Augmentin twice a day for 7 days and will be seen in follow-up.

Diagnosis: Acute suppurative otitis media. An expanded problem-focused history and examination were performed, with medical decision making of moderate complexity.

What are the correct diagnosis and CPT procedure codes (including E/M) for this case?

ICD-9-CM and CPT Code(s): _____

ICD-10-CM Code(s): _____

6.86. The same patient in item 6.85 is scheduled for tubes now after the acute otitis media has resolved.

Surgery Center Report

Preoperative Diagnosis: Chronic recurrent suppurative otitis media

Postoperative Diagnosis: Same

Operation: Bilateral myringotomy, placement of permanent ventilating tube

Anesthesia: General

Procedure: A standard myringotomy incision was made and a copious amount of serous fluid suctioned from the middle ear cleft. A Goode T-tube was placed without problems. The procedure was then repeated on the left side in the same manner.

What are the diagnosis and procedure codes (including E/M) reported by the surgeon for this procedure? The procedure was performed in the hospital same-day surgery center.

ICD-9-CM and CPT Code(s): _____

ICD-10-CM Code(s): _____

6.87. This 7-year-old child with an acute attack of his childhood asthma is taken to ER. Spirometry, both pre- and post-bronchodilator, reveal continued bronchospasm with intractable wheezing. An expanded problem-focused history and examination were performed with moderate medical decision making. He is subsequently admitted to the hospital. What diagnosis and procedure codes (including E/M) are assigned by the ER physician?

ICD-9-CM Code(s): _____

ICD-10-CM Code(s): _____

CPT Code(s): _____

Conditions of Pregnancy, Childbirth, and the Puerperium

6.88. This 29-year-old female has had 2 spontaneous abortions because of incompetent cervix. Because of this, she had a cervical cerclage placed in the third month of this pregnancy. She is coming in now to have the cerclage removed under general anesthesia. She was taken to surgery, and the cerclage was removed without complication. She was discharged that evening. There are no signs of labor, and the membranes are intact. She was instructed on the signs of labor and will see me in the office in 2 days. Estimated due date is in 2 weeks, but labor could begin at any time.

What are the correct code assignments for this case?

ICD-9-CM and CPT Code(s):

a. 654.53, 59871
b. 654.53 (The cerclage removal is part of the global package.)
c. 622.5, with appropriate E/M procedure
d. 622.5, 59871

ICD-10-CM Code(s): _____

6.89. The following documentation is from the health record of a 24-year-old female patient.

Preoperative Diagnoses:	1. Term intrauterine pregnancy at 39-weeks plus three-days gestational age
	2. Polyhydramnios
	3. Failure to progress
Postoperative Diagnoses:	1. Term intrauterine pregnancy at 39-weeks plus three-days gestational age
	2. Viable male infant. Apgars 8 at one minute and 9 at five minutes. Birth weight 7 lbs, 10 oz.

Operation: Primary cesarean section with low-transverse uterine incision

Anesthesia: Spinal

Estimated Blood Loss: 500 cc.

Complications: None

Description of Procedure: The patient was brought to the surgical delivery room suite and anesthesia was administered. The patient was placed in a supine position with left lateral uterine displacement. The abdomen was sterilely prepped and draped in the normal fashion for cesarean section.

After ascertaining the adequacy of the anesthetic level with an Allis test, a Pfannenstiel incision was made approximately three finger breaths above the pubic symphysis and carried down to the level of the fascia. The fascia was dissected off in the midline, and the peritoneum was carefully entered. The bladder was retracted inferiorly with a DeLee retractor and then a bladder flap was created. The DeLee retractor was repositioned to further retract the bladder inferiorly.

A transverse curvilinear incision was made in the lower uterine segment and extended upward and laterally using blunt dissection. Fetal membranes were ruptured and a viable male infant was delivered from a vertex presentation in an atraumatic fashion. The oropharynx and nares were suctioned on the operative field. The umbilical cord was doubly clamped and cut. The infant was handed off to the awaiting pediatric personnel.

Cord blood was obtained after a segment of cord was clamped and saved for cord blood gases pending Apgars. The placenta was delivered by manual extraction. The uterus was explored to remove any remaining fragments of membranes. The uterus was exteriorized. The uterine incision was reapproximated using No. 1 chromic suture in a running and locking fashion. A second layer of No.1 chromic suture was placed in a Lembert fashion to imbricate the first layer, creating a double layer closure. The uterine incision was inspected and hemostasis confirmed.

The uterus was returned to the abdominal cavity. The uterine incision was inspected once again for hemostasis. All blood and clots were cleared from the lateral gutters and then a final inspection confirmed hemostasis of the uterine incision. The rectus muscles were brought together with three simple interrupted 2-0 Vicryl sutures. Hemostasis was confirmed at the level of the rectus muscles and then the fasciad was reapproximated using two separate 0-Vicryl sutures in a running fashion. The subcutaneous tissues were irrigated and the skin was reapproximated with surgical steel staples. A sterile dressing was applied. The patient was taken to the recovery room in stable and satisfactory condition having tolerated the procedure well.

What is the correct CPT code assignment for this service?

Code(s): _____

6.90. This 26-year-old gravida 1 para 1 female has been spotting and has been on bed rest. She awoke this morning with severe cramping and bleeding. Her husband brought her to the hospital. After examination, it was determined that she has had an incomplete early spontaneous abortion. She is in the 12th week of her pregnancy. She was taken to surgery, and a dilation and curettage was performed. There were no complications from the procedure. She is to follow up with me in the office. She has had 4 antepartum visits during her pregnancy.

What are the correct codes to assign?

ICD-9-CM and CPT Code(s):

a. 637.91, 59812
b. 634.91, 59812, 59425
c. 634.91, 58120
d. 634.92, 58120, 59425

ICD-10-CM Code(s): _____

6.91. This 30-year-old female comes to the clinic because of excessive vomiting. She has been vomiting for 3 days. She has had no problems with vomiting in her early pregnancy. She is now estimated to be in her 24th week. What is the correct diagnostic code assignment for this case?

ICD-9-CM Code(s): _____

ICD-10-CM Code(s): _____

6.92. This 29-year-old female is admitted to the hospital with pneumonia due to *Pneumocystis carinii*. She is in her 30th week of pregnancy and has AIDS. What diagnosis codes are assigned?

ICD-9-CM Code(s): _____

ICD-10-CM Code(s): _____

6.93. **Procedure:**   McDonald's cerclage placement

Postoperative Diagnosis: Intrauterine pregnancy at 14 weeks; patient has a history of cervical incompetence

Anesthesia: Epidural

History: The patient is a 31-year-old gravida 4, para 2. A positive HCG was noted approximately six weeks ago. Ultrasound reveals an intrauterine pregnancy in the second semester. Her previous pregnancies were brought to term using cerclage.

Findings: Preoperatively the internal os was approximately 1.2 cm dilated. The posterior cervix was approximately 2 cm long and the interior cervix was approximately 1.1 cm long.

The patient was placed in the dorsal lithotomy position and prepped and draped for cerclage. A Mersilene band was used with one needle placed in at the 6 o'clock position and brought out at the 3 o'clock position and replaced at the same position and brought out at the 12 o'clock position. A second needle was taken in at 3 o'clock and brought out at 9 o'clock and then replaced and brought out in the 12 o'clock position.

The Mersilene band was then tied at the 12 o'clock position and the internal os was closed. At the end of the procedure the knot could be felt at the appropriate position and the internal os was closed to digital examination.

The procedure was without complications, and the patient was taken to the PACU in good condition.

What codes are used to report this outpatient encounter?

ICD-9-CM and CPT Code(s): _____

ICD-10-CM Code(s): _____

6.94. **History of Present Illness:** This is a 31-year-old, gravida IV, para 0 who presents today for follow-up of a suspected spontaneous abortion. She had a history of having had elective abortions at ages 17 and 19. At age 27 she became pregnant and experienced a spontaneous abortion and became pregnant again approximately 9 weeks ago. She presents today after experiencing blood loss, cramping, and pain during the early hours of the morning.

Physical Examination: Abdomen is soft and non-tender but vaginal vault does show remnants of bloody discharge. Ultrasound showed no fetal heart tones or movement. A dilation and curettage is performed to treat this incomplete spontaneous abortion. The diagnosis and procedure codes for this encounter would include:

ICD-9-CM and CPT Code(s):

a. 634.91, 59820
b. 634.92, 59820
c. 634.81, 59812
d. 634.91, 59812

ICD-10-CM Code(s): _____

Disorders of the Respiratory System

6.95. A patient is respirator-dependent and has a tracheostomy in need of revision due to redundant scar tissue formation surrounding the site. Under general anesthesia and after establishing the airway to maintain ventilation, the scar tissue is resected and then repair is accomplished using skin flap rotation from the adjacent tissue of the neck. What codes will be used to report this procedure performed in the hospital short-stay surgery area?

ICD-9-CM and CPT Code(s):

a. 519.00, V46.11, 31614
b. V55.0, V46.11, 31614
c. V55.0, 31610
d. 519.00, 31613

ICD-10-CM Code(s): _____

6.96. This 60-year-old patient was admitted with emphysematous nodules. A thoracoscopic wedge resection was performed in the left lung to remove the lung nodules. A resection was done in the upper and lower lobes. Which of the following answers is correct?

ICD-9-CM and CPT Code(s):

a. 518.89, 32657
b. 492.8, 32657, 32657-51
c. 518.89, 32500
d. 492.8, 32657

ICD-10-CM Code(s): _____

6.97. From the health record of a patient newly diagnosed with a malignancy:

Preoperative Diagnosis: Suspicious lesions, main bronchus

Postoperative Diagnosis: Carcinoma, in situ, main bronchus

Indications: Previous bronchoscopy showed two suspicious lesions in the main bronchus. Laser photoresection is planned for destruction of these lesions because bronchial washings obtained previously showed carcinoma in situ.

Procedure: Following general anesthesia in the hospital same-day surgery area, with a high-frequency jet ventilator, a rigid bronchoscope is inserted and advanced through the larynx to the main bronchus. The areas were treated with laser photoresection.

Which codes are reported for this service?

ICD-9-CM and CPT Code(s):

a. 231.2, 31641
b. 162.2, 31641, 31623–59
c. 231.2, 31641, 31623–59
d. 162.2, 31641

ICD-10-CM Code(s): _____

6.98. This 80-year-old male presented to the ER with acute pulmonary edema after experiencing a 3-day history of increasing shortness of breath and cough. He was admitted to the critical care unit with a diagnosis of congestive heart failure and treated with Procardia, Nitro Paste, and Lasix with resolution of his respiratory distress.

The patient responded to treatment with increasing nitroglycerin and Lasix. The patient was also given intravenous fluids and low-dose dopamine to maintain an adequate wedge pressure and cardiac output.

Final Diagnosis: Acute pulmonary edema with congestive heart failure.

What diagnosis code(s) are reported?

ICD-9-CM Code(s): _____

ICD-10-CM Code(s): _____

6.99. This 82-year-old nursing home patient presents with aspiration pneumonia. The patient aspirated food particles. Treatment included clindamycin 600 mg IV q 6 hours. He also has superimposed staphylococcal pneumonia. The condition resolved with treatment, and patient transferred back to the nursing home. What is the correct diagnosis code assignment?

ICD-9-CM Code(s): _____

ICD-10-CM Code(s): _____

6.100. Under conscious sedation, administered by the endoscopist, a patient underwent a bronchoscopy with biopsy of the walls of the left upper lobe bronchus and left mainstem bronchus, dilation of the left mainstem bronchus, and placement of a bronchial stent in the left mainstem bronchus. Assign the appropriate CPT codes.

a. 31622, 31625, 31636, 99144
b. 31628, 31632, 31636
c. 31625, 31636
d. 31625, 31636, 99144

6.101. Procedure: Direct microlaryngoscopy using general anethesia

Diagnosis: Dysphonia

Technique: This 22-year-old patient was taken to the outpatient surgical suite where general anesthesia was administered. A Jako laryngoscope was inserted with an operating microscope to perform a laryngoscopy. The vocal cords were examined and no evidence of abnormality was discovered. They were within normal limits. The entire endolarynx was also well visualized and showed no evidence of subglottic stenosis. No other abnormalities were noted. The procedure was terminated and the patient sent to PACU in good condition.

What codes are used to report this outpatient encounter?

ICD-9-CM and CPT Code(s): _____

ICD-10-CM Code(s): _____

Trauma and Poisoning

6.102. Assign the correct diagnosis codes for a 29-year-old patient with deep third-degree burns of the chest and right leg. He was the victim of a house fire. He has third-degree burns over 25 percent of his body.

ICD-9-CM Code(s): _____

ICD-10-CM Code(s): _____

6.103. The patient in question 6.102 was treated with skin grafting over a period of time until his burns healed. Six months later, he is being seen with severe scarring due to third-degree burns of his right leg and chest received in a house fire. What diagnosis codes are assigned for this case?

ICD-9-CM Code(s): _____

ICD-10-CM Code(s): _____

6.104. This 79-year-old patient had a gastrostomy performed because of dysphagia due to a stroke. He has been doing fairly well but is now admitted with extensive cellulitis of the abdominal wall. Examination reveals that the existing gastrostomy site is infected. The physician confirms that the responsible organism is *Staphylococcus aureus*. What diagnosis codes are assigned?

ICD-9-CM Code(s): _____

ICD-10-CM Code(s): _____

6.105. What is the correct CPT code assignment for a 36-square-centimeter adjacent tissue transfer performed on the hip to cover a large open wound?

CPT Code(s): _____

6.106. What diagnosis codes are reported for an encounter where the patient is seen for a crushing injury of the left toes, foot, and ankle? He was crushed in a metal rolling mill machine at work.

ICD-9-CM Code(s): _____

ICD-10-CM Code(s): _____

Part III
Advanced Coding Exercises

Chapter 7

Case Studies from Inpatient Health Records

Note: Even though the specific cases are divided by setting, most of the information pertaining to the diagnosis is applicable to most settings. If you practice or apply codes in a particular type of setting, you may find additional information in other sections of this publication that may be pertinent to you.

Every effort has been made to follow current recognized coding guidelines and principles, as well as nationally recognized reporting guidelines. The material presented may differ from some health plan requirements for reporting. The ICD-9-CM codes used are effective October 1, 2011, through September 30, 2012. The current standard transactions and code sets named in HIPAA have been utilized, which require ICD-9-CM Volume III procedure codes for inpatients. The 2011 draft editions of ICD-10-CM and ICD-10-PCS are utilized in this chapter.

Instructions: Cases are presented as either multiple choice or fill in the blank.

- For multiple-choice cases:
  —Select the letter of the appropriate code set.
- For the fill-in-the-blank cases:
  —Assign the MS-DRG, where indicated.
  —Assign present on admission (POA) indicator for each ICD-9-CM diagnosis code.
  - Y: Yes (POA)
  - N: No (Not POA)
  - U: Unknown (Documentation is insufficient to determine if condition is POA.)
  - W: Clinically undetermined (Provider is unable to clinically determine whether or not the condition was POA.)
  - Leave blank for the exercises in this book all codes that are exempt from POA reportirng. See the Exempt List as published in the *ICD-9-CM Official Guidelines for Coding and Reporting.* These codes are exempt because they represent circumstances regarding healthcare encounters or factors influencing health status that do not represent a current disease or injury, or are always present on admission.

ICD-9-CM Coding Instructions:

- Sequence the ICD-9-CM principal diagnosis in the first diagnosis position.
- Assign all reportable secondary diagnosis codes including V codes and E codes (both cause of injury and place of occurrence).
- Sequence the ICD-9-CM principal procedure code in the first procedure position.
- Assign all reportable secondary ICD-9-CM procedure codes.

ICD-10-CM and ICD-10-PCS Coding Instructions:

- Sequence the ICD-10-CM principal diagnosis code in the first diagnosis position.
- Assign all reportable secondary ICD-10-CM codes.
- Sequence the principal ICD-10-PCS code in the first procedure position.
- Assign all reportable secondary ICD-10-PCS codes.

The scenarios are based on selected excerpts from health records. In practice, the coding professional should have access to and refer to the entire health record. Health records are analyzed and codes assigned based on physician documentation. Documentation for coding purposes must be assigned based on medical record documentation. A physician may be queried when documentation is ambiguous, incomplete, or conflicting. The queried documentation must be a permanent part of the medical record.

The objective of the cases and scenarios reproduced in this publication is to provide practice in assigning correct codes, not necessarily to emulate complete coding, which can be achieved only with the complete medical record. For example, the reader may be asked to assign codes based on only an operative report when in real practice, a coder has access to the entire medical record.

The *ICD-9-CM Official Guidelines for Coding and Reporting*, published by the National Center for Health Statistics (NCHS), includes Present on Admission (POA) Reporting Guidelines in Appendix I. These guidelines supplement the official conventions and instructions provided within ICD-9-CM. Adherence to these guidelines when assigning ICD-9-CM diagnosis codes is required under the Health Insurance Portability and Accountability Act (HIPAA) of 1996. Additional official coding guidance can be found in the American Hospital Association (AHA)'s *Coding Clinic for ICD-9-CM* publication.

Disorders of the Blood and Blood-Forming Organs

7.1.   The following documentation is from the health record of an 87-year-old female patient.

Discharge Summary

History of Present Illness: The patient is an 87-year-old female who was admitted from a nursing home with dehydration and pleural effusion, as well as urinary tract infection and thrombocytopenia with petechial hemorrhage. On admission, she was found to have a platelet count of 77,000 and a hematology consultation was done. The patient denied any bleeding diathesis in the past. She stated that she had recent bruising of the hands related to needle sticks but otherwise has not had any past history of any bleeding disorder. She stated she was taking aspirin on a regular basis. No specific history of hematuria, hematemesis, gross rectal bleeding, or black stools.

Past Medical History: Significant for congestive heart failure, diabetes

Medications: Coreg, isosorbide, aspirin, Actos, digoxin, glyburide, hydralazine, furosemide, Ditropan, and potassium

Family History: No family history of any bleeding disorder

Physical Examination: She is an elderly-appearing white female, somewhat short of breath, using supplemental oxygen. Examination of the head and neck revealed no scleral icterus. Throat was clear. Tongue was papillated. There was no thyromegaly or JVD. There was no cervical supraclavicular, axillary, or inguinal adenopathy. Chest examination revealed rales, bilaterally. There were decreased breath sounds at the right base. There were coarse rales heard in the right midlung field. Heart examination showed rhythm was irregularly irregular. Abdomen examination was difficult to perform. I was unable to palpate the liver or spleen. Bowel sounds were active. Extremities revealed no clubbing, cyanosis, or edema. There were diffuse ecchymoses, especially in the dorsum of the right hand.

Laboratory Studies: Hematocrit was 43, white blood cell count 9,000 with 82 percent neutrophils, and the platelet count 77,000. The MCCV was 102. Creatinine was 1.7. Bilirubin was 1.7. The alkaline phosphatase was 122. AST 498, ALT 493, and albumin 3.6. The prothrombin time was 18 seconds and the PTT was 25 seconds. The chest x-ray showed a right pleural effusion.

Course in Hospital: The patient was admitted and started on IV fluids. Her diuretics were increased, and she showed a good response with a resolution of her pleural effusion and better control of her congestive heart failure. Hematology consult recommended holding platelet transfusion unless there was evidence of active bleeding. No platelets were given during this admission.

The patient was discharged back to the nursing home on day 6 in improved condition to continue with the same medication regimen as previous to hospitalization.

Final Diagnoses: 1. Pleural effusion from congestive heart failure
2. Dehydration
3. Primary thrombocytopenia with petechial hemorrhage and hematoma of the eyelids and arms and hands
4. Urinary tract infection
5. Type II diabetes mellitus

Which of the following code sets would be correct for this hospitalization?

a. 428.0, 276.51, 287.30, 599.0, 250.00
b. 428.0, 276.51, 287.5, 599.0, 250.00
c. 428.0, 511.9, 276.51, 287.30, 599.0, 250.00
d. 276.51, 511.9, 428.0, 287.30, 782.7, 599.0, 250.00

ICD-10-CM Code(s): _____

Optional MS-DRG Exercise (for users with access to MS-DRG software or tables)

What is the correct MS-DRG for this case? _____

Which of the following is an incorrect statement regarding the MS-DRG assignment on this case?

a. MS-DRG assignment in this case is based on the principal diagnosis; the secondary codes do not impact the DRG.
b. A principal diagnosis of CHF results in a higher-paying DRG than a principal diagnosis of dehydration.
c. This patient's LOS exceeded the average length of stay for the assigned DRG.
d. All of the above are true.

7.2.   The following documentation is from the health record of a 34-year-old male patient.

Admission Diagnosis: Sickle cell pain crisis.

Discharge Diagnosis: Sickle cell pain crisis/Staph (Staphylococcus) aureus bacteremia.

Secondary Diagnosis: Sickle cell disease, priapism, chronic lower back pain secondary to sickle cell diagnosis, asthma, gastroesophageal reflux disease (GERD), and hemorrhoids.

Consults: None.

Procedures: PICC line placement, bone scan, and transesophageal echocardiogram (heart and aorta).

Hospital Course: The patient is a 34-year-old African-American male with a history of sickle cell disease who presented with back pain and whole body pain, a remote history of some diarrhea and nausea, and some fevers and chills. Blood cultures taken on admission and during his first night as an inpatient grew four out of four bottles of Staph. aureus. The patient received 1 gm of ceftriaxone in the Emergency Department and received approximately six days of vancomycin IV as an inpatient. Thereafter he was switched to Ancef 1 gm IV g.8 hours.

In order to find a source for the patient's Staph. bacteremia, a transesophageal echocardiogram was done which did not show evidence of any cardiac vegetations. A bone scan was also done which did not show any deep-seated abscesses or any evidence of osteomyelitis. In light of the fact that the patient had Staph. bacteremia of unknown source, Infectious Disease was consulted. As per their recommendation, the patient is to be on five weeks of IV Ancef.

At the time of admission, the patient was placed on a PCA pump. He was rapidly weaned off of this and he was also placed on some oxygen and was bolused with fluids and kept on maintenance fluids. The patient's clinical status improved rapidly. He was soon weaned off the oxygen, fluids, and pain medications.

At the time of discharge, the patient is afebrile and stable. A PICC line was placed in order to ensure access for the next five weeks, during which he will receive his IV antibiotics. Home care and home IV teaching was arranged for the patient and his family.

Follow-Up: Hematology was contacted and follow-up will be arranged within the next two weeks. Follow-up will also be arranged with Infectious Disease in five weeks. Home medications include folate 1 mg p.o. q.d.; Flexeril 10 mg p.o. b.i.d.; Ancef 2 gm q.12 IV times five weeks; Phenergan 12.5 mg p.o. q.4 p.r.n. nausea; and Zantac 150 mg p.o. b.i.d. The patient was told to return for fevers, chills, sweats, nausea, vomiting, or bone or muscle pain.

Disposition is to home with home care.

Code Assignment Including POA Indicator

ICD-9-CM Principal Diagnosis: _____

ICD-9-CM Additional Diagnoses: _____

ICD-9-CM Procedure Code(s): _____

Issues To Clarify: _____

ICD-10-CM Code(s): _____

ICD-10-PCS Code(s): _____

7.3. The following documentation is from the inpatient record of a patient with anemia.

Discharge Summary

Date of Admission: 11/19/XX

Date of Discharge: 11/21/XX

Discharge Diagnoses:
1. Anemia of chronic disease.
2. Chronic renal insufficiency.
3. Diabetes mellitus, insulin-dependent.
4. Hypertension.
5. Coronary artery disease.
6. Congestive heart failure.
7. Hypokalemia.

Attending Physician for Service: Family Practice Service.

Consultations: None.

Procedures: None.

Hospital Course: The patient is a 66-year-old gentleman with multiple medical problems including coronary artery disease, insulin-dependent diabetes mellitus, and chronic renal insufficiency, who presented to the Emergency Department at Anytown Hospital on 11/19/XX complaining of shortness of breath. He had been seen in the office earlier that week and seemed to be doing reasonably well at that point in time.

On admission he said that over the last two to three days his shortness of breath had been increasing, and he had orthopnea and a nonproductive cough. He denied chest pain at that point in time. He denied other symptomatology.

In the Emergency Department he was noted to have significant anemia with hemoglobin of 7.0 and a hematocrit of 21.2 with an MCV of 78.3. He was given two units of packed red blood cells via peripheral vein and admitted to the Transitional Care Unit to rule out myocardial infarction and to receive blood.

Problems

1. **Anemia.** Initial H&H of 7.0 and 21.2. He received two units of packed red blood cells and at discharge his H&H was 9.1 and 27.0, respectively. His reticulocyte count was pending at discharge. Iron level was 51, total iron binding capacity was 371, and ferritin level was 14. He had been on iron as an outpatient. This was stopped secondary to diarrhea, which he felt was probably from the iron. We will restart this at this time consisting of Niferex one p.o. q day. Follow his H&H as an outpatient. I would consider him for erythropoietin therapy at some point in time.

2. **Cardiac.** History of coronary artery disease and congestive heart failure. He had one elevated troponin on day 1 of hospitalization. He had had two normal troponins previous to this and two post this. I am uncertain of the significance of this one elevation of his troponin to 1.6. He had no chest pain throughout. Electrocardiogram

showed no changes. He was briefly started on heparin. This was subsequently discontinued the following day. We will send him home on his regular cardiac regimen consisting of Digoxin, an ACE inhibitor, diuretics consisting of Lasix and Carbatolol. He will also be given p.r.n. nitrates. From a congestive heart failure perspective on admission he was felt to have mild congestive heart failure. He diuresed well, and once he was transfused, his shortness of breath, and orthopnea improved significantly.

3. **Hypokalemia.** The day after admission revealed this and his potassium was replaced. Being we were restarting his Lasix therapy, we will send him home on potassium supplementation as well.

4. **Diabetes mellitus.** Well-controlled. Continue Glucotrol at 5 mg p.o. b.i.d.

5. **Hypertension.** Controlled. Continue Lotensin, Coreg, and will add Lasix as above.

6. **Gastrointestinal.** He had weakly heme-positive stools on admission. He has had this recently and has actually undergone upper and lower endoscopy twice this year already. He has had no complaints of melena or bright red blood. I am wondering if this was not secondary to trauma during the rectal examination. We will continue to follow for now.

Code Assignment Including POA Indicator

ICD-9-CM Principal Diagnosis: _____

ICD-9-CM Additional Diagnoses: _____

ICD-9-CM Principal Procedure: _____

ICD-9-CM Additional Procedures: _____

ICD-10-CM Code(s): _____

ICD-10-PCS Code(s): _____

Disorders of the Cardiovascular System

7.4.   The following documentation is from the health record of a 66-year-old male patient.

Discharge Summary

Admission Date: 6/19/XX

Discharge Date: 6/28/XX

History of Present Illness: This patient is a 66-year-old man admitted on 6/19 because of unstable postinfarct angina. He underwent cardiac bypass surgery here 15 years ago. He did well until 1989, when he developed angina and underwent angioplasty here. On 6/9, he was awakened with severe chest pain and was taken to a nearby community hospital where he was found to have a small anterior wall ST elevation myocardial infarction, with the CPK only slightly elevated.

Because of this small infarction, he was referred here for consideration for further coronary arteriography. He was discharged from the hospital on 6/16. On 6/19, as the patient was walking from the car to the office, he developed quite significant chest pain and was therefore admitted to rule out further infarction.

Hospital Course: He was taken to the cardiac catheterization laboratory the day after admission. At that time, complete left heart catheterization, left ventricular cineangiography, coronary arteriography, and bypass visualization were performed. We found that his left ventricle showed severe anterior hypokinesis, although it did still move. The left main coronary artery was narrowed by about 70 percent.

The bypass to the circumflex looked good, but the bypass to the left anterior descending had a very severe stenosis in the body of the graft. There was a very large, marginal circumflex artery that had an orificial 80 percent stenosis. I felt that he was not a candidate for angioplasty but should have bypass surgery. He was seen in consultation by Dr. Reed, who agreed with this, so he was taken to the operating room on 6/21 for that procedure.

Using extracorporeal circulation, the left internal mammary artery was anastomosed to the left anterior descending coronary artery and a venous graft was placed from the aorta to the marginal circumflex. It was found that the old venous graft to the main circumflex was in excellent condition with very soft, pliable walls, so that vessel was left intact. There were no complications of this surgery.

His postoperative course was singularly uncomplicated. He never had any arrhythmia problems; his wounds healed nicely. He had a tiny left pleural effusion that never needed to be tapped. He was walking about the ward participating in the cardiac rehab program at the time of discharge.

Discharge Instructions: Discharge medications will simply be aspirin grains 5 q. d., Tylenol with Codeine 1 or 2 p.r.n. for pain, Lopressor 50 mg a day, and Colace, as necessary. He was instructed to contact his private physician upon return home for resumption of his medical care. He is to call me here at the medical center if there are any questions or problems that he wishes to discuss.

Discharge Diagnoses: 1. Unstable angina (intermediate coronary syndrome)
2. Recent incomplete anterior wall myocardial infarction
3. Coronary atherosclerosis, three vessel
4. Successful double-bypass surgery

What are the correct codes for this admission?

a. 414.01, 414.05, 410.12, 411.1, V45.82, 36.11, 36.15, 39.61, 37.22, 88.53, 88.57
b. 414.01, 414.05, 410.12, 411.1, V45.81, 36.12, 39.61, 37.22, 88.53, 88.57
c. 414.00, 414.05, 410.11, 411.1, 36.11, 36.15, 39.61, 37.22, 88.53, 88.57
d. 414.01, 414.05, 410.12, 411.1, 412, V45.81, 36.11, 36.15, 39.61, 37.22, 88.53, 88.57

ICD-10-CM Code(s): _____

ICD-10-PCS Code(s): _____

Optional MS-DRG Exercise (for users with access to MS-DRG software or tables)

Indicate the principal diagnosis. _____

Which of the codes affects the MS-DRG assignment on this case?

_____

True or False: For this MS-DRG, the presence of a complication/comorbid condition affects the MS-DRG assignment?

7.5.   Discharge Summary

Date of Admission: 4/19

Date of Discharge: 4/24

Discharge Diagnosis: Acute myocardial infarction
Hyperlipidemia
Complete heart block
Upper gastrointestinal hemorrhage
Arteriosclerotic heart disease

Admission History: This is a 45-year-old white male with a history of hyperlipidemia and tobacco use. He presented to the hospital with an acute myocardial infarction. He was treated with intravenous TPA and had a reperfusion. The patient continued to have chest pain with an inferior ST elevation on EKG.

Course in Hospital: The patient sustained an acute myocardial infarction. The patient presented with an acute myocardial infarction and underwent catheterization. The patient was found to have stenosis of the mid right coronary artery and right distal coronary artery. The left coronary branches have minimal noncritical disease. The left ventricular ejection fraction was approximately 45% with inferior wall hypokinesis.

The patient had a successful stent PTCA to the mid-RCA with a stent. I initially attempted to dilate with a balloon, but the results were inadequate and we proceeded to place a 4.0-mm J&J stent. The patient continued to have anginal symptomatology and for this reason was taken to the OR for CABG × 2. He did well after the CABG × 2 without any anginal symptoms.

The patient also had gastrointestinal bleeding following the PTCA. The patient developed retching and hematemesis and anemia for which he required blood transfusion. The probable cause of the nausea and vomiting was a reaction to anesthesia. Upper endoscopy revealed no evidence of peptic ulcer disease.

At the present time the patient has been treated with aspirin and Ticlid and has been doing very well. The plan is to discharge him home with follow-up in my office next week.

Instructions on Discharge: Follow up in 1 week in my office. Medications include: aspirin 1 tablet per day, Ticlid 250 mg twice per day, Tagamet 400 mg twice per day, and sublingual nitroglycerin as needed for chest pain. Condition upon discharge is stable. Activity is restricted until cardiac rehabilitation.

History and Physical

Admitted: 4/19

Acute myocardial infarction

Complete heart block

Ventricular ectopy

Possible ASHD

Reason for Admission: Pain in chest

History of Present Illness: This is a pleasant 45-year-old male with a history of hyperlipidemia and previous tobacco use. He also has a family history of coronary artery disease. He denies any prior history of coronary artery disease, myocardial infarction, or CVAs. The patient has been essentially very healthy, except for occasional skipped heartbeat in the past for which he has never taken any medications. The patient is presently on no medications.

Two days ago, he started complaining of a dull chest ache that appeared to radiate to his left arm and lasted for a few minutes. He was brought to the emergency department and was noted to have an acute inferior myocardial infarction with complete heart block. I was consulted to evaluate the patient and proceeded with administration of TPA therapy and IV Atropine for complete heart block. At the present time the patient is in sinus rhythm and is presently receiving IV TPA. He denies any melena, hematochezia. Denies any shortness of breath, PND, orthopnea.

Past Medical History: He denies any history of hypertension or diabetes. He has a history of high cholesterol. He states that he had his cholesterol checked approximately 3 months ago and it was around 310. He used to smoke tobacco, one pack a day for 20 years. He quit smoking 6 months ago. He denies any history of coronary artery disease, myocardial infarction, or cerebrovascular accident.

He has a history of heart palpitations that he describes as skipped heartbeat in the past for which he is not taking any medications. He has never had an evaluation.

He has a history of kidney stones two years ago. He denies any history of peptic ulcer disease. He has a history of hemorrhoidal bleeding in the past. The last episode of bleeding was 6 or 7 months ago.

The patient denies any trauma or recent surgery.

Allergies: Patient has no known drug allergies

Chronic Medications: None

Social History: He quit tobacco 6 months ago and denies alcohol abuse. He is a construction worker.

Review of Systems: Denies melena, hematochezia, hematemesis, and he denies change in weight

Physical Examination: This is a pleasant gentleman who appears slightly diaphoretic and is expressing having mild chest pain which is better from admission. He is presently receiving IV TPA. Vital signs are as follows: Blood pressure is 100/70; heart rate in the 80s. The neck shows no JVD, no carotid bruits. The lungs are clear and heart is regular rate with S4 gallop rhythm and no murmurs. The abdomen is soft and nontender. Extremities show no edema. The pulses of his femoral and dorsalis pedis are 2+ bilaterally. Neurological examination reveals an alert and oriented male × 3.

Laboratory Data: SMA-7, sodium 138, potassium 3.7, BUN 7, creatinine 0.9. CBC showed a white blood cell count of 12. Hematocrit 37, hemoglobin 13. Platelet count is 312. His EKG showed complete heart block with significant ST elevation in the inferior leads with reciprocal changes in the anteroseptal leads, consistent with an acute inferior wall myocardial infarction. His chest x-ray is pending.

Impression and Plan: Acute myocardial infarction that appears to have started around 10:30 in the morning. He presented very early to the emergency department and was treated aggressively with intravenous TPA, intravenous aspirin, intravenous nitroglycerin.

We will continue the TPA and begin lidocaine. We will obtain cardiac enzymes and admit to CCU. The patient will need cardiac catheterization evaluated within 48 hours. If symptoms recur or patient does not have evidence of reperfusion, will need urgent cardiac catheterization. If heart block occurs, will treat with intravenous Atropine on a p.r.n. basis. We will check a cholesterol and lipid profile in the hospital.

Consultation

Date: 4/20

Chief Complaint: Vomiting blood

Review of Systems: This 45-year-old white male was seen in consultation because of GI bleeding. The patient was admitted 1 day ago with acute myocardial infarction. He was treated with TPA and later went to cardiac catheterization where he was found to have a lesion of the mid RCA and distal RCA. Today the patient exhibited hematemesis with retching. He has no past history of ulcer disease or GI bleeding.

Physical Examination: Physical examination reveals an adult male lying in bed. Blood pressure is 120/80, pulse 60. HEENT: Pale. Lungs: Clear. Heart: Regular rate and rhythm. Abdomen: Benign.

Laboratory: WBC is 12, hemoglobin 12, and hematocrit 37

Impression: Upper GI bleeding; rule out ulcer disease

Recommendation: We will perform an upper endoscopy to be performed today after informed consent is obtained. Further recommendations are to follow.

Progress Notes

4/19   This is a 45-year-old white male with a history of increased cholesterol, no prior coronary artery disease, MI, or CVA. He presented with acute ischemia and heart block. He was given IV TPA; 1–1 1/2 hours after TPA he had severe chest pain with elevated ST inferior leads. He was treated emergently for urgent catheter and PTCA.

Post Catheter/Stent

Procedure: Left heart catheter, coronary angio, left ventricular angiography

Results: Normal LCA, 99% mid-RCA and 70 stenosis distal RCA, successful stent PTCA to mid RCA with excellent results

4/20   **Cardiac:** Patient continues to have pain. Will prepare for CABG when patient stable from GI perspective.

       GI: The patient experienced vomiting with flecks of blood after the cardiac catheterization. In light of apparent acute blood loss anemia, will check for peptic ulcer. Probable reaction to anesthetics.

       Endoscopy Note:

       Preop: Gastrointestinal bleeding

       Postop: Gastrointestinal bleeding, etiology unknown

       Procedure: EGD

       Complications: None

4/21   Patient is scheduled for the OR today. Bleeding stable.

       OP Note:

       Preop: Critical stenosis of the mid-RCA and distal RCA

       Postop: Same

       Operation: CABG × 2

       Complications: None

4/22   Patient recovering well. No chest pain or shortness of breath. The wound looks good. Will monitor blood loss anemia. The patient declines blood transfusion.

4/23   Chest clear, no chest pain, abdomen is soft with bowel sounds. Will transfer to the floor.

4/24   Wound healing well, patient OOB ambulating, no chest pain, lungs clear.

4/25   Will discharge today. Patient to follow up in 1 week.

Operative Report

Date: 4/21

Preoperative Diagnosis: Critical stenosis of mid right coronary artery and distal right coronary artery

Postoperative Diagnosis: Same

Operation: Coronary bypass × 2 using saphenous vein from aorta to right mid coronary artery and distal right coronary artery

Anesthesia: General

Under general anesthesia with arterial and pulmonary artery monitoring with sterile prep and drape, a sterile midline sternotomy was performed. The pericardium was opened. Purse-string sutures were placed in the ascending aorta and the right atrium. Extracorporeal circulation was undertaken at this point. The greater saphenous vein was harvested from the right leg endoscopically. The patient was then placed on cardiopulmonary bypass. Cardioplegia was affected. The right coronary artery was dissected. Using a 6-0 Prolene suture an end-to-side anastomosis was created between the right mid coronary artery and the aorta. A second opening for end-to-side anastomosis was performed from the aorta to the distal right coronary artery. Following spontaneous contraction of the heart, the patient was removed from cardiopulmonary bypass. Approximating the pericardium then began closure. Hemostasis was obtained. The sternum was approximated with a parasternal wire and fascia and skin with vicryl. The patient tolerated the procedure well and was transferred to the recovery room in stable condition.

Endoscopy Report

Date: 4/20

Pre-gastrointestinal bleeding; rule out ulcers

Post-upper gastrointestinal bleeding; stomach and duodenum appear unremarkable

Meds: Demerol 50 mg IV
Versed 3 mg IV

Procedure: Esophagogastroduodenoscopy

The patient was sedated and the scope inserted into the hypopharynx. There was fresh blood oozing from an area in the hiatal hernia pouch just below the gastroesophageal junction. The scope was passed further down to visualize the remainder of the stomach and the duodenum. All areas appeared unremarkable with no other ulcers or lesions identified. The patient tolerated the procedure well. He did have some retching and vomiting after the scope was removed.

Cardiac Catheterization Report

Date: 4/19

Procedure: Left heart catheterization

Left ventricular angiography

Coronary angiography

Stent to mid right coronary artery

After obtaining informed consent the patient was taken to the cardiac catheterization laboratory. He was prepped and draped in the usual fashion and 2% Xylocaine was used to anesthetize the right groin. 6-French sheaths were introduced into the right femoral artery and vein, and a 6-French multipurpose catheter was used for left heart catheterization, coronary angiography, and left ventricular angiography. I then proceeded to perform a stent/PTCA to the mid RCA. An HTF wire was used to cross the RCA stenosis and a 4.0-mm J&J stent was placed in the mid right coronary artery with excellent results. The final angiogram was obtained and the guiding catheterization was removed. The sheaths were securely sutured and the patient tolerated the procedure well without complications.

Findings

1. Left heart catheterization revealed an elevated resting left ventricular end-diastolic pressure of 18 mm Hg.
2. Left ventricular angiography revealed mild to moderate inferior wall hypokinesis with overall mildly depressed left ventricular systolic function and an estimated global ejection fraction of 45%.
3. Coronary angiography (using single catheter): The left coronary artery arises normally from the left sinus of Valsalva. The left main artery, left anterior descending coronary artery and its branches, and the circumflex artery and its branches have minimal irregularities.

   The right coronary artery arises normally from the right sinus of Valsalva. There is a 99% very eccentric stenosis in the large mid right coronary artery and a 70% stenosis of the distal right coronary artery.

Impression: Arteriosclerotic coronary artery disease was found. There was a successful implantation of 4.0-mm J&J stent in the mid right coronary artery. This site was predilated with a 4.0-mm balloon, and then followed by the insertion of a stent.

The mid right coronary artery shows excellent results. Pending the patient's progress we may have to proceed with CABG. The patient will remain on aspirin, Coumadin, and nitrates in the hospital. He will remain on intravenous heparin while his PT levels are adjusted.

Radiology Reports

Date: 4/19

Chest, Supine: There is no gross evidence of acute inflammatory disease or congestive heart failure.

Impression: No acute disease

Date: 4/21

Diagnosis: The patient appears to have undergone sternotomy. The heart appears normal. The endotracheal tube is in place as is the Swan-Ganz catheter.

Impression: Stable postoperative chest

EKG Reports

Date: 4/19

Impression: Elevated ST changes. Cannot eliminate the possibility of ischemia. Complete heart block is also noted.

Date: 4/20

Impression: Acute inferior myocardial infarction. Complete heart block has resolved.

Code Assignment Including POA Indicator

ICD-9-CM Principal Diagnosis: _____

ICD-9-CM Additional Diagnoses: _____

ICD-9-CM Procedure Code(s): _____

ICD-10-CM Code(s): _____

ICD-10-PCS Code(s): _____

7.6. A patient is admitted with severe atherosclerosis of the left common carotid artery. He undergoes a percutaneous atherectomy of the artery, along with infusion of streptokinase to assist with clot resolution. A carotid artery stent was also inserted to ensure that the artery would remain open. Assign the appropriate procedure code(s) to report this procedure.

ICD-9-CM Code(s):

a. 00.61, 99.10, 00.63
b. 00.61, 99.10, 00.64
c. 00.61, 00.63
d. 00.61

ICD-10-PCS Code(s): _____

7.7. Joe Jones was admitted to the hospital with severe angina. At cardiac catheterization he was found to have major atheromatous involvement of the left anterior descending coronary artery, with near-total occlusion, but well-preserved flow in the remainder of the coronary arteries. Because only one vessel was involved, the attending physician decided on a percutaneous treatment and stent placement. Mr. Jones underwent percutaneous atherectomy of the LAD with placement of two sirolimus-eluting stents. Intracoronary Urokinase administered to assist with clot dissolution. Assign the appropriate procedure codes for the hospital to report this inpatient procedure. Do not assign codes for the cardiac catheterization for this exercise.

ICD-9-CM Code(s):

a. 00.66, 00.40, 36.07, 36.07, 99.10
b. 00.66, 36.07
c. 00.66, 00.40, 00.46, 36.07, 99.10
d. 36.09, 00.40, 00.46, 36.06, 99.10

ICD-10-PCS Code(s): _____

7.8. A patient with severe arterial disease involving the lower abdominal aorta and the iliac bifurcation is admitted to the hospital as an inpatient for endovascular repair. Incisions are made over each femoral artery, and a catheter with modular attachments is inserted via the right femoral artery. The catheter carries a self-deploying endovascular prosthesis, which consists of an aortic component with a modular bifurcated prosthesis to extend into each of the iliac arteries. Via the femoral incisions, the components are aligned and are noted to be secure. The small incisions are closed, and the patient is taken to the recovery area for further observation. Assign the appropriate procedure code(s) to describe this procedure.

ICD-9-CM Code(s):

a. 38.44
b. 39.79
c. 39.71
d. 39.7

ICD-10-PCS Code(s): _____

7.9. **History and Physical:** The patient is a 67-year-old male who was transferred from Down-the-Street Hospital, where he was admitted six days ago with chest pain, shortness of breath, elevated cardiac enzymes, and EKG changes indicating an anterolateral ST elevation myocardial infarction. He subsequently underwent a cardiac catheterization, which revealed significant four-vessel disease. He was transferred here for a coronary artery bypass procedure.

Past History:	Type 2 diabetes (on insulin), hypercholesterolemia, and status post appendectomy
Medications:	See transfer list
Allergies:	None known

Physical Exam

General: Normal appearing male in no acute distress

Cardio: Rate and rhythm regular

Lungs: Normal

Tests: Chest x-ray normal; EKG nonspecific T-wave changes

Impression and Plan: Anterolateral myocardial infarction, coronary artery disease, diabetes mellitus, and hypercholesterolemia; patient will undergo CABG tomorrow

Operative Report

Preoperative Diagnosis: CAD

Postoperative Diagnosis: Same

Procedure: CABG × 4; saphenous vein graft of obtuse marginal diagonal artery and posterior descending artery; left internal mammary artery to the left anterior descending artery. Cardiopulmonary bypass.

Description of Procedure: After obtaining adequate anesthesia, the patient was prepped and draped in the usual fashion. A primary median sternotomy incision was made, and the pericardium was opened. The left internal mammary artery was dissected as a pedicle using electrocautery and small hemoclips at the same time that the greater saphenous vein was harvested endoscopically from the left lower extremity. Cardiopulmonary bypass was instituted, and the patient was taken to a mild degree of hypothermia.

The aorta was cross-clamped, and electrical arrest effect was administered via cold blood cardioplegia. The saphenous vein graft was placed end-to-side with the posterior descending artery, and then a separate graft was placed to the obtuse marginal artery and finally a separate graft was placed to the diagonal artery. Each anastomosis was done with running 7-0 Prolene suture and verified no bleeders were present. The left internal mammary artery was subsequently brought through a subthalamic tunnel and placed end-to-side with the left anterior descending coronary artery.

Following completion of the grafts, warm blood cardioplegia was administered. During this time, two atrial and ventricular pacing wires were attached to the heart's surface; in addition, mediastinal tubes also were placed. The cross clamps were released following this, and sinus rhythm returned spontaneously. The patient was weaned from cardiobypass without incident.

After all grafts were checked for diastolic flow, which revealed no problems, the incisions were closed. The patient was taken to the recovery room in good condition and will be monitored in the intensive care unit for complications.

Progress Notes

Day 1: Patient progressing well; all vital signs are stable. Will transfer to step-down unit today.

Day 2: Heart rate stable and incision healing nicely. If patient continues to progress will be ready for discharge in a few days.

Day 3: Stable; patient ambulating in hallway without difficulty.

Day 4: Continues to progress in ambulation; ready for discharge tomorrow.

Day 5: Discharge patient today to follow up with myself next week.

What is the correct code assignment for this admission?

ICD-9-CM Code(s):

a. 411.1, 414.01, 250.00, 272.0, 36.12, 36.15, 39.61
b. 414.01, 411.1, 250.00, 272.0, 36.12, 36.15, 39.61
c. 414.00, 413.9, 995.89, 250.00, 36.12, 36.15, 39.61
d. 414.01, 411.1, 272.0, 250.00, 36.13, 39.61

ICD-10-CM Code(s): _____

ICD-10-PCS Code(s): _____

7.10. The following documentation is from the health record of a patient admitted with angina.

Coronary Artery Bypass Graft

Surgery Date: 03/14/XX

Preoperative Diagnosis: Unstable postinfarct angina, mitral insufficiency, and severe left ventricular dysfunction.

Postoperative Diagnosis: Unstable postinfarct angina, mitral insufficiency, and severe left ventricular dysfunction.

Operative Procedure: On-pump coronary artery bypass surgery × 3: Saphenous vein to the right, saphenous vein to the marginal, internal mammary to the left anterior descending, and mitral valve reconstruction with a #26 Future ring and posteromedial papillary muscle repositioning.

Anesthesia: General endotracheal, Dr. Anesthesiologist.

Operative Findings: The patient had marked RV and LV dysfunction, ejection fraction of left ventricle about 20 percent. There was moderately severe mitral insufficiency related to tethering of the posteromedial papillary muscle. Vein and mammary were adequate.

Description of Procedure: Patient brought to the OR and placed on the OR table in supine position. Arterial line and Swan-Ganz catheter were placed, general endotracheal anesthesia induced, and the patient prepped and draped in usual fashion. Midline sternotomy performed. Left greater saphenous vein endoscopically harvested, left mammary harvested. Cooled the patient to 32 degrees, gave 1,200 cc of antegrade cardioplegia, and performed a distal anastomosis to the right with 7-0 Prolene. 500 cc of cardioplegia given. Distal anastomosis to the OM completed with 7-0 Prolene. Another 1,000 cc of cardioplegia given antegrade and retrograde as well as down the graft. The extended transseptal approach to the mitral valve was utilized, the mitral valve exposed, and the papillary muscle repositioned using pledgeted two Gore-Tex sutures sutured to the annulus. Complete partially flexible, partially rigid ring #26 Future was then implanted with 2-0 Ethibond sutures, the left atrial appendage oversewn in two layers, and left and right atria closed with running 4-0 Prolene, the mammary anastomosis with 8-0 Prolene, and the proximal anastomosis with 6-0 Prolene. Cardioplegia given every 15 to 20 minutes at 500- to 1,000-cc boluses. Warm blood potassium cardioplegia given prior to removal of crossclamp. Left atrium, left ventricle, and ascending aorta were deaired. Pericardial wall flooded with CO_2 to minimize air emboli. The aortic crossclamp was removed and the patient discontinued from cardiopulmonary bypass on epinephrine, Levophed, Neo-Synephrine, vasopressin, and milrinone, as well as inhaled Flolan. Cannulae were removed, heparin reversed with protamine, and the wound closed in layers with antibiotic irrigation of soft tissue. Sterile dressing applied.

Which of the following is the correct code set for this inpatient procedure?

ICD-9-CM Code(s):

a. 411.1, 424.0, 429.81, 36.12, 36.15, 39.61, 35.12, 35.31
b. 411.1, 424.0, 36.12, 36.15, 39.61, 35.12, 35.31
c. 411.1, 424.0, 429.81, 36.13, 39.61, 35.12, 35.31
d. 411.0, 424.0, 429.81, 36.12, 36.15, 39.61, 35.12, 35.31

ICD-10-CM Code(s): _____

ICD-10-PCS Code(s): _____

Disorders of the Digestive System

7.11. The following documentation is from the health record of an 81-year-old female patient.

Operative Report

Diagnoses: Acute cholecystitis with gallstone, bile duct obstruction, acute gallstone pancreatitis.

Operation: Cholecystectomy; exploration of common bile duct; insertion of feeding tube; intraoperative colangiogram performed under fluoroscopy

History: The patient is an 81-year-old female admitted 48 hours ago with evidence of acute gallstone pancreatitis. The patient had some thickening of her gallbladder wall and pericholecystic fluid. The patient had marked elevation of amylase and was given 48 hours of medical therapy with chemical clearance of her pancreatitis. The patient was thought to be a candidate for open exploration of her biliary tract, with concomitant cholecystectomy and possible common duct exploration.

Description of Procedure: After discussion with the patient and her family and obtaining informed consent, she was taken to the operating room where, after induction of general anesthesia, the abdomen was prepped and draped in a standard fashion. Following this, a right upper quadrant incision was used to gain access to the abdominal cavity. Manual exploration revealed no abnormalities of the uterus, ovaries, colon, or stomach. The pancreas was enlarged and edematous in the area of the head. Attention was then turned to the right upper quadrant, where the gallbladder was noted to be somewhat distended. This decompressed with a 2-0 VICRYL purse string stitch using the trocar. The cystic artery was dissected free and double clipped proximally, singly distally, and divided. The duct was then dissected free and subsequently clipped proximally.

Low osmolar cholangiogram with fluoroscopy was then obtained by opening the cystic duct and placing a cholangiogram catheter. The common bile duct measured roughly 1.5 cm in size. The duct tapered out in the area of the intraduodenal portion of the common duct to near-occlusion. The gallbladder was removed by transecting the cystic duct and removing it in a retrograde fashion. The gallbladder contained several stones.

Following removal of the gallbladder, attention was turned to the common bile duct, which was opened. No stones were retrieved initially from the bile duct. A biliary Fogarty was passed distally and, with some difficulty, was negotiated into the duodenum. On return, no calculus material was obtained. Palpation of the distal duct revealed thickening because of the pancreatic inflammation, which was noted to improve somewhat over the inside portion of the C-loop to the duodenum. The patient was felt to have bile duct obstruction from some other primary duct process other than a stone or inflammation.

Following this, cholangiography revealed some mild emptying of the distal common duct into the duodenum. With the overall picture, it was thought that the patient might benefit from a feeding jejunostomy, because she might well sustain postoperative or perioperative complications of respiratory insufficiency or perhaps other imponderables. As such, jejunum was identified roughly one foot beyond the ligament of Treitz, and 2-0 VICRYL purse-string stitches × 2 were placed. The jejunotomy was performed, and a 16 French T-tube was then placed and brought out through a stab wound in the left upper quadrant. The tube was anchored anteriorly with interrupted 2-0 silk stitches and externally with 2-0 stitches. Jackson-Pratt drain was placed through a lateral stab wound in the right upper quadrant and used to drain the duodenotomy and choledochotomy. This was anchored with several 3-0 silk stitches.

Following this, the wound was irrigated with Kantrex irrigation, 1 g/L, and the wound was closed by closing the posterior rectus sheath with running #1 VICRYL suture. The sub-q was irrigated and the skin was closed with staples. The wound was then dressed, and the patient was taken to the recovery room postop in stable condition. Estimated blood loss was 400 cc. Sponge and needle counts were correct × 2.

Code Assignment

ICD-9-CM Principal Diagnosis: _____

ICD-9-CM Additional Diagnoses: _____

ICD-9-CM Principal Procedure: _____

ICD-9-CM Additional Procedures: _____

ICD-10-CM Code(s): _____

ICD-10-PCS Code(s): _____

7.12.   The patient is a 56-year-old male who was admitted with a history of hematemesis for the past 36 hours. He also had some tarry black stools and was noted to have a giant gastric ulcer which was actively bleeding. Patient was subsequently referred for surgical intervention.

Final Diagnosis: 1. Acute gastric ulcer
                            2. Chronic pancreatitis
                            3. Liver cirrhosis due to alcoholism
                            4. Cirrhosis due to chronic hepatitis C

Procedure Performed: Subtotal gastrectomy with Billroth II anastomosis

Operative Procedure: The patient was brought to the operating room and placed on the table in a supine position, at which time general anesthesia was administered without difficulty. His abdomen was then prepped and draped in the usual sterile fashion. An upper midline incision was made. The peritoneum was then entered using the Metzenbaum scissors and hemostats. A retractor was placed, and he was noted to have a cirrhotic liver with micronodular cirrhosis. The left lobe of the liver was mobilized at that point, and the retractors were placed. On palpation of the stomach along the lesser curvature at approximately the mid portion, there was a large gastric ulcer located just above the pyloric antrum in the body of the stomach. At this point, the gastrocolic omentum was taken off the greater curvature of the stomach to the level of the pylorus. Additionally, the lesser omentum was taken down off the lesser curvature of the stomach to the level of the pylorus. The stomach was then transected approximately 3 cm above the ulcer. At that point, the stomach was reconstructed in a Billroth II fashion by bringing the jejunum through the transverse colon mesentery. Two stay sutures were placed to align the jejunum along the posterior wall of the stomach, and a GIA stapler was used to create the anastomosis without difficulty. The stomach and jejunum were then pulled below the transverse colon mesentery, and this was tacked in several places using 3-0 silk sutures. A feeding jejunostomy tube was then placed distal to this using the feeding jejunostomy kit without difficulty. The abdomen was then irrigated thoroughly using normal saline solution. Hemostasis was achieved using Bovie electrocautery. The midline incision was then closed using #1 PDS in a running fashion. The skin was closed using skin staples. A sterile dressing was applied. The patient was extubated in the operating room and returned to the Intensive Care Unit in guarded condition.

Code Assignment Including POA Indicator

ICD-9-CM Principal Diagnosis Code(s): _____

ICD-9-CM Additional Diagnoses Code(s): _____

ICD-9-CM Principal Procedure Code(s): _____

ICD-9-CM Additional Procedures Code(s): _____

ICD-10-CM Code(s): _____

ICD-10-PCS Code(s): _____

Optional MS-DRG Exercise (for users with access to MS-DRG software or tables)

What are the results when you group this case? _____

Which MS-DRG is appropriate for this case? _____

Excluding the principal diagnosis, what other code affects the MS-DRG assignment for this admission? _____

7.13. Discharge Summary

Principal Diagnosis: Morbid obesity

Principal Procedure: Open Roux-en-Y gastric bypass, removal of gastroplasty ring, gastric (G) tube prior placement

History of Present Illness: The patient is a 55-year-old white female with a history of gastroplasty ring placement in 1979 who comes to Dr. Smart for revision by doing a Roux-en-Y gastric bypass because of recurrence of her morbid obesity. Her morbid obesity is complicated by gastroesophageal reflux disease (GERD) and obstructive sleep apnea (OSA).

Past Medical History: (1) Morbid obesity. (2) OSA. (3) GERD.

Past Surgical History: (1) Gastroplasty in 1979. (2) Laminectomy.

Allergies: Keflex

Medications: Pepcid q. d.

Physical Examination: Vital signs: Afebrile, vital signs stable. General: No acute distress. CV RRR. PULMONARY CTAB. Abdomen: Soft, nontender, nondistended.

Impression: A 55-year-old white female with a history of gastroplasty, needing a revision into a Roux-en-Y gastric bypass after morbid obesity not secured.

Hospital Admission: The patient was admitted through same-day surgery and taken to the operating room for open Roux-en-Y gastric bypass with removal of a gastroplasty ring, liver biopsy, and G tube placement. Afterward, she was taken to the ICU because of her obstructive sleep apnea. She was monitored closely, did very well, and afterward, she was transferred to the floor. She was full advanced to activities of daily living through our gastric bypass protocol. She advanced to gastric bypass soft diet by postoperative day four. She did well with this. On postoperative day five, she was deemed ready to go home. She understands her discharge instructions and will be given pain medications as well as continue prescription for Zantac for her GERD and for marginal ulcer prophylaxis.

Condition on Discharge: Stable on postoperative day five from open Roux-en-Y gastric bypass

Disposition: The patient was discharged home with family.

Medications: Resume previous home medications. The patient can resume her Pepcid, or she can continue taking Zantac 150 b.i.d.

Follow-up: The patient will follow up with Dr. Smart.

Diet on Discharge: Gastric bypass soft diet. She has been instructed by a dietician two times already.

Operative Report

Preoperative Diagnosis: Morbid obesity with gastroplasty dysfunction

Postoperative Diagnosis: The same

Operation: Revision gastroplasty to Roux-en-Y gastric bypass and liver biopsy.

Indications: This 55-year-old lady had undergone a Silastic ring gastroplasty by another surgeon in 1979 at a weight of more than 250 lb. She had done well for a long time and then had started regaining her weight and also developed significant gastroesophageal reflux disease. A gastric endoscopy done preoperatively showed that the Silastic ring of her gastroplasty had eroded into the gastric lumen with a wide outlet from the pouch and also with a separate dehiscence of the staple line. In the interim, she had developed sleep apnea but did not have hypertension or diabetes. Following the endoscopy and because of being on disability related to a laminectomy and to spinal problems, the excess weight seemed to aggravate her disability and seemed a justifiable reason for a surgical intervention.

Description of Procedure: With the patient supine on the operating table and under satisfactory general anesthesia, we attempted a right and then left subclavian line but had difficulties with the wire guide. Subsequently, a neck central line was placed and the abdomen was prepped and draped in a sterile manner. An upper midline incision was made and carried through the fat by tearing and through the fascia with the cautery. There were adhesions immediately of omentum to the anterior abdominal wall and also to the lower abdominal wall where a paramedian incision had been. These were all lysed, which was not difficult. A Tru-Cut needle was used to obtain a biopsy from the left lobe, which was moderately fatty by examination. The gallbladder was emptied sufficiently to know that there were no stones. The uterus and ovaries were surgically absent. We began by lysing adhesions on the undersurface of the left lobe of the liver to the stomach until we were able to uncover the old gastric pouch and appreciate the location of the staple line. I could also appreciate where the Silastic ring was, separate from the nasogastric tube, which was brought inside. We dissected around the distal esophagus and brought a long Penrose drain around it for retraction purposes. I held up the portion of the stomach near the lesser curve where the Silastic ring was palpable, and we used the cautery to enter into the lumen to find the ring. Its suture was cut and the ring was removed and sent to pathology. The opening made for the gastrotomy was closed with interrupted 2-0 silk sutures. We then dissected a little more proximal to this location along the lesser curve to go around the serosa of the stomach to its backside. A 12 French Robinson catheter was put along this tract and turned around to come to hold the lesser omentum on traction. We also divided some of the gastrocolic omentum to gain access from the lateral side to the posterior lesser sac. We then used a 45-mm blue load endoscopic autosuture stapler to staple and transect the stomach at the lesser curve transversely to create the posterior part of our pouch. When this was done, there was still a small hole into the distal stomach and perhaps into the proximal pouch where the staples had found the tissue too thick to seal completely. On the gastric pouch side, this was managed by an over-and-over suture of 2-0 Prolene from one edge to the other. On the gastric side, this was managed with interrupted 2-0 silk sutures. We then dissected behind the stomach up to the angle of His and eventually were able to pass the 12 French Robinson catheter through the angle of His and around the stomach to represent the pathway for the stapler to go at a later time. We lifted the omentum upward and identified the ligament of Treitz. The jejunum was divided a measured 7.5 inches beyond that ligament, and the mesentery at that level was divided using the endoscopic stapler. The small bowel was then measured from that point to the cecum, which proved to be 204 inches, and we selected a 72-inch Roux limb length. The side-to-side jejunojejunostomy was created with the biliopancreatic limb and the Roux limb using an outer running 3-0 Prolene seromuscular layer and an inside GIA stapled anastomosis. The Prolene was continued over the holes made for the stapler and also used to invert the stapled edge of the biliopancreatic limb. The aperture between the two mesenteric leaves was closed with a couple of 3-0 silk sutures. We then made a channel through the omentum up to the transverse colon and then across the gastrocolic omentum to allow the Roux limb to lie easily antecolic up near the pouch. When this placement was assured, the Roux limb was fixed to the end of our pouch with three interrupted 3-0 silk seromuscular sutures. The cautery was used to make an opening in the jejunum in the gastric wall and the posterior part of the anastomosis was done with interrupted 3-0 VICRYL suture. An opening was made in the Roux limb through which a 10-mm Hegar dilator was passed through the jejunal and gastric sides of the anastomosis. That anastomosis was then sutured with the VICRYL over the dilator and then further reinforced with interrupted 3-0 silk seromuscular sutures. When this was done, we removed the dilator and passed the nasogastric tube through the anastomosis to lie in the Roux limb. The end of the Roux limb was then oversewn with a running 3-0 Prolene suture. After this, we used the 60-mm blue load endoscopic stapler to begin to transect the gastric pouch from the remainder of the stomach, going vertically towards the angle of His. It ultimately took three 45-mm cartridges after the first 60-mm cartridge in order to complete this, but it was done satisfactorily. We used 2-0 Prolene to oversew that vertical staple line throughout its length. We also used the 2-0 Prolene to oversew the gastric staple line throughout its length. The anastomosis in the pouch looked fine, and we made sure that the nasogastric tube was movable within the pouch. We then created a gastrostomy to the distal stomach, with a 2-0 silk purse-string suture near the greater curve. A 22 French Foley catheter was brought through a left upper quadrant stab wound and on into the stomach, and the balloon was filled. A purse-string suture was tied, and a couple of

2-0 silk sutures between stomach and abdominal wall were placed. After this, we irrigated the abdomen with an antibiotic solution containing Kantrex and bacitracin. All of the bowel and omentum was laid back in its normal position, and there was no tension on the Roux limb. The fascia was then closed with a running #1 loop PDS suture. The subcutaneous fat was cleaned with antibiotic solution and the skin was closed with 3-0 VICRYL dermal sutures and 3-0 VICRYL subcuticular sutures. The patient tolerated the procedure well and was taken to the SICU. Estimated blood loss was 350 mL, and the sponge count was correct.

Code Assignment

ICD-9-CM Principal Diagnosis: _____

ICD-9-CM Additional Diagnoses: _____

ICD-9-CM Principal Procedure: _____

ICD-9-CM Additional Procedures: _____

ICD-10-CM Code(s): _____

ICD-10-PCS Code(s): _____

Optional MS-DRG Exercise (for users with access to MS-DRG software or tables)

What is the MS-DRG assignment for this admission? _____

Which of the following would change the MS-DRG assignment of this admission?

a. Secondary diagnosis of a complication/comorbid condition or a major complication/comorbid condition
b. Additional procedure codes
c. If one of the current diagnoses was not present on admission
d. All of the above

Endocrine, Nutritional, and Metabolic Diseases and Immunity Disorders

7.14.   This 56-year-old female was admitted for resection of an adrenal mass. The patient has had hypertension and palpitations of several years' duration treated with Toprol under good control. Ultrasound was done in consideration of the possibility of a mass, and catecholamine studies have been normal. A 4- to 5-cm right adrenal mass was identified. Dr. White had obtained a 24-hour urinary free cortisol, ACTH, and short suppression tests, all of which confirmed the presence of Cushing's syndrome. The patient was not diabetic. She did report weight gain, some shift in body configuration, and easy bruising of several years' duration. The easy bruising was identified on examination in the hospital.

Surgery: A 5-cm, well-circumscribed round cortical tumor was resected from the adrenal gland via an open approach. Pathology report confirmed that the tumor was benign.

Allergies: No known drug allergies

Medications on Discharge: Hydrocortisone, rapidly tapering dose, currently on 40 mg daily; Toprol 50 mg q. a.m.; Prevacid 30 mg q. d.; Lipitor 10 mg q. a.m.; Prempro 0.625/2.5

Physical Exam: Vital signs stable. HEENT: Sclerae and conjunctivae clear. Neck: Supple. No palpable thyroid. Lungs: Somewhat decreased breath sounds currently. There is mild splinting with deep breathing. Abdomen: Tenderness in the incision area. She has active bowel sounds at this time. Extremities: No definite bruises currently. No edema noted.

Discharge Diagnosis: Right adrenal tumor with Cushing's syndrome secondary to tumor

Plan: The patient appears to have tolerated the surgery well. She will require steroid replacement. Excess cortisol output is presumed entirely due to her tumor, and her ACTH was suppressed previously. As with exogenous steroid therapy, there will be contralateral adrenal suppression. The patient will be tapered rapidly to replacement hydrocortisone levels. We will try the remaining hydrocortisone withdrawal over the next 6 months or so, depending on her ACTH and cortisol responses. She is discharged to home with follow-up in my office in 1 week.

Which of the following is the correct code set for this hospitalization?

ICD-9-CM Code(s):

a. 239.7, 255.0, 401.9, 785.1, 07.21
b. 194.0, 401.9, 785.1, 07.22
c. 227.0, 255.0, 401.9, 785.1, 07.21
d. 227.0, 255.0, 07.29

ICD-10-CM Code(s): _____

ICD-10-PCS Code(s): _____

Optional MS-DRG Exercise (for users with access to MS-DRG software or tables)

Which of the following MS-DRGs is correct for this admission?

a. 644, Endocrine Disorders with CC
b. 615, Adrenal and Pituitary Procedures without CC/MCC
c. 614, Adrenal and Pituitary Procedures with CC/MCC
d. 628, Other Endocrine, Nutritional and Metabolic OR Procedures with MCC

7.15.   The following documentation is from the health record of a 57-year-old male patient.

Discharge Diagnoses: 1. Lung cancer currently undergoing chemotherapy with Taxol and carboplatin with dexamethasone
2. Type II diabetes, with neuropathy and nephropathy, not controlled
3. Hyperlipidemia
4. Hepatomegaly

History: This patient is a 57-year-old man who presented for outpatient chemotherapy. He had surgery for lung cancer in September and is now undergoing chemotherapy with Taxol and carboplatin, including dexamethasone as part of his chemo and prophylaxis for nausea. He has done very well with the chemotherapy. When he presented for outpatient treatment on the day of admission, he was found to be hypoglycemic. He is a known type II diabetic. His diabetes is complicated by neuropathy and nephropathy. Due to his blood glucose levels, it was decided to postpone this chemo session, and he was admitted for control of his diabetes. Dr. Johnson consulted with the patient to manage his diabetes regimen. He has been on 70/30 insulin, 25 units in the morning and 15 units in the evening. He had problems in the hospital with hypoglycemia several times the first day, with blood sugar levels ranging from 30 to greater than 450. An IV insulin drip was started, and he also had q. 1 hour Accu-Cheks. His hepatomegaly has enlarged from the last time that I saw him. Question whether this is fatty infiltration due to poor diabetes control, or whether there is now some involvement with metastatic carcinoma.

Laboratory Data: Sodium 128, potassium 5.5, chloride 89, CO_2 34, BUN 13, creatinine 0.8, glucose range 30–460, with final glucose of 210. Calcium 9.4, WBC 9.8, hemoglobin 11.6, hematocrit 34.3, platelets 277,000

Plan: One difficulty here is the cyclic nature of his chemo treatment regimen, likely to produce major shifts in his glucose, which is already difficult to control. The patient will need to monitor his glucose levels closely. He is discharged on 70/30 insulin, 35 units in the morning and 20 units in the evening. Dr. Johnson will be managing his diabetes, and the patient has instructions to call his nurse on a daily basis for the next week. He is to follow up with me for further chemotherapy in the oncology clinic next week.

Code Assignment Including POA Indicator

ICD-9-CM Principal Diagnosis: _____

ICD-9-CM Additional Diagnoses: _____

ICD-9-CM Procedure Code(s): _____

Issues To Clarify:_____

ICD-10-CM Code(s): _____

ICD-10-PCS Code(s): _____

7.16.   The following documentation is from the health record of a 52-year-old patient.

Discharge Summary

Admission Date: 11/14/XX

Discharge Date: 11/17/XX

Discharge Diagnosis: 1. Diabetic ketoacidosis
2. Dehydration
3. Congestive heart failure
4. Aortic valve disorder
5. Urinary tract infection
6. Hyperkalemia
7. Peripheral vascular disease

8. Hypertension
9. *Escherichia coli* infection
10. Hyperlipidemia
11. Renal ureteral disease
12. Old myocardial infarction
13. Tobacco use
14. Coronary atherosclerosis with native coronaries

Admitting Diagnosis:
1. Diabetic ketoacidosis
2. Diabetes mellitus Type I
3. Dehydration
4. Congestive heart failure
5. Hyperkalemia
6. Hyperlipidemia
7. Hypertension
8. Tobacco abuse
9. Severe peripheral vascular disease
10. Atherosclerotic coronary artery disease
11. Urinary tract infection
12. Renal insufficiency

Present Illness: A 52-year-old white female with known diabetes mellitus Type I, CVAs, cellulitis, hypertension, chronic hypertension, hyperlipidemia, poorly compliant diabetic. Most recently in hospital from September 3 to September 8 with cellulitis, congestive heart failure, poorly controlled diabetes. Most recently in the hospital with diabetic ketoacidosis. Discharged home. She was supposed to be following up with her primary care physician doing b.i.d. Accu-Cheks. She was nauseated for the previous two weeks. As soon as she got nauseated, she quit checking her blood sugar level. She cancelled her doctor's appointment because she was "too sick to go." She had decreased appetite and was feeling poorly overall. She came to the emergency room with a blood sugar of 737. She had ketones 200 to 250. Her blood urea nitrogen was 75, creatinine 1.8. Her potassium is 6.1, chloride 5, bicarb at 13. Patient is a poor historian, although she is awake and alert at the time of evaluation, on an insulin drip. Overnight her nausea had resolved. The nausea probably occurred because she was in the beginning stages of diabetic ketoacidosis.

Hospital Course: The patient was put on insulin drip. Blood sugars got down. She was put on q.i.d. Accu-Cheks. Once her blood sugar level came down to the 100s, potassium was lowered. I had a very lengthy discussion with patient about the need for keeping doctor's visits and checking blood sugars. The patient was placed on Cipro. Her electrocardiogram showed a prolonged Q T. The patient went to ultrasound and had sludge and possible small stones in her gallbladder, and it was felt that she was able to be discharged home improved.

Discharged Medications/Instructions: Insulin 70/30, 20 units in the a.m., 20 in the p.m., Rezulin 400 mg q. a.m., Tenormin 50 q.d., Plavix 75 q.d., Monoket 10 mg b.i.d., Lasix 20 mg b.i.d., aspirin 325 q. a.m., Zocor 20 once a day, Oxycotin 20 b.i.d., Prozac 20 q. a.m., Vasotec 5 mg q. a.m., Propulsid 10 mg at Ac and HS, Bactrim DS one tablet every 12 hours. She is to see her primary care physician in one week. She is to call if she has any difficulties.

Disposition: Discharged home

History and Physical

Past Medical History: The patient has history of renal insufficiency with a blood urea nitrogen of 30 to 40 with a creatinine of 1.2 to 1.4. She has had a CVA, severe peripheral arterial disease. Echocardiogram done shows aortic sclerosis, mitral leaflet thickening, normal left ventricular size, normal diabetes. Smokes three to four packs of cigarettes a day. She has hypertension. She has hyperlipidemia. She is dehydrated. She has a history of atherosclerotic coronary artery disease.

Medications: At the time of admission included Rezulin 40 mg q.d., Prozac 20 q.d., Propulsid 10 a.c. and h.s., Vasotec 2.5 two every morning, Atenolol 50 q. a.m., Plavix 75 q. a.m., Lasix 20 milligrams b.i.d., Novolin 70/30 20 units every a.m., aspirin 325 q. a day, vitamin E, iron, Oxycotin 20 a.m. and h.s., Zocor 20 mg at dinner. The patient has no known drug allergies.

Social History: She is married but her husband lives out of state and works there. She has one daughter. She does not drink and has smoked about 3 to 4 packs a day since a teenager.

Physical Exam: At the present time, the patient is afebrile, vital signs are stable. She is awake and alert, oriented × 3.

HEENT: Pupils equal, round, reactive to light and accommodation, extraocular muscles intact, oropharynx benign

Neck: Supple without adenopathy or jugular venous distention

Lungs: Clear to auscultation

Heart: Reveals a regular rate and rhythm without murmurs, gallops, or rubs

Abdomen: Soft, nontender, positive bowel sounds, no masses noted

GU: Deferred

Extremities: No edema. She has a baseline edema currently. Pulses are absent, pedal pulses.

Laboratory: At the time of admission, her glucose was 737, blood urea nitrogen 75, creatinine 1.8, acetone greater than 200, less than 250, sodium 136, potassium 6.1, chloride 95, bicarb of 13. Her hemoglobin was 13.9 and hematocrit of 44.1, white blood cell count of 9.2 with a left shift showing 80.2 percent neutrophils, 16.2 percent lymphocytes. Platelets were 241,000. Urinalysis shows positive nitrites, greater than 1,000 glucose, 30 protein, 15 ketones, trace hemoglobin. She had 13 white blood count per high power field. Rare red per high power field, 2+ bacteria. Gram stain on her u/a showed no organisms seen.

Impression(s):
1. Diabetic ketoacidosis
2. Diabetes mellitus type I
3. Dehydration
4. Congestive heart failure
5. Hyperkalemia
6. Hyperlipidemia
7. Hypertension
8. Tobacco abuse
9. Severe peripheral vascular disease, arterial in nature
10. Atherosclerotic coronary artery disease
11. Urinary tract infection
12. Renal insufficiency

Plan: Admit, hydrate. She has been on insulin drip, we will d/c this now and change to q. 4 Accu-cheks and continue sliding scale. Hopefully on 16th be able to reinstitute her routine meds. Her potassium has now come down to the mid 4's secondary to her hydration and her sugar being driven intracellular with the insulin drip. I have impressed upon the patient the need for checking blood sugars and keeping M.D. appointment versus death in the future. The patient is on Cipro for her urinary tract infection. Further workup as indicated during hospital stay.

Exam: 9005 EK EKG REG
    Compared with 9/25/07 no change

Impression: Normal EKG

Code Assignment Including POA Indicators

ICD-9-CM Principal Diagnosis: _____

ICD-9-CM Additional Diagnoses: _____

Issues To Clarify:_____

ICD-9-CM Diagnosis Code(s): _____

ICD-10-CM Code(s): _____

Disorders of the Genitourinary System

7.17.   The following documentation is from the health record of a 48-year-old female patient.

Discharge Summary

Discharge Diagnoses

1. Dysfunctional uterine bleeding

2. Anemia

Therapies

1. Transfusion of four units of packed red blood cells

2. Fractional D&C

3. ThermaChoice balloon endometrial ablation

Discharge Medications: Tylenol III and iron supplementation

Hospital Course: The patient presented to the emergency department with complaints of heavy vaginal bleeding which had progressively gotten worse over the previous three months. Prior to the patient's admission, she was using seven maxi pads in an hour. Assessment at that time showed that she was hemodynamically stable. However, she did have a hemoglobin of 8.5 and was continuing to bleed. She was admitted for IV premarin therapy and transfusion.

The patient has a mechanical heart valve and for this reason, she was on Coumadin. A PT with INR was obtained to make sure that the patient was not supra therapeutic. However, she was in the normal range. Despite the Premarin, the patient did continue to bleed. After the first two units of blood were transfused, her hemoglobin was only 8.8. She was given two additional units and scheduled for a D&C and a balloon ablation of her endometrium. This was performed. The procedure was uncomplicated. She was discharged home to follow up in the office.

History & Physical Exam

Admission: For surgery

Present Illness: This is a 48-year-old gravida 10, para 7 who had been seen in the office with complaints of some bleeding after being menopausal for approximately one year. On examination, her uterus was found to be slightly enlarged, six to eight weeks' sized, the adnexa were non palpable. An ultrasound was performed which showed the endometrial thickness was 25 rom and had a complex echogenicity to it. Uterus measured 10.5 × 8.2 × 6.1 cm, right ovary 3.7 × 3.8 × 3.5 cm, left ovary 3.1 × 2.1 × 3.2 cm. There is no evidence of fluid in the cul-de-sac. An endometrial biopsy was performed which showed a small amount of proliferative-type endometrium with breakdown consistent with dysfunctional uterine bleeding. She was scheduled to have a D&C later this month. However, the patient presented to the Emergency Department with complaints of very heavy vaginal bleeding requiring the use of seven maxi pads in an hour. The patient was found to be hemodynamically stable, blood pressure and pulse were in the normal range. However, hemoglobin was found to be 8.5. She was bleeding rather heavily; there was a large amount of clot in her vagina. She was admitted for a blood transfusion. She received two units of packed red cells and was also started on IV Premarin 25 mg every six hours. The patient has a history of having a mechanical heart valve for which she takes Coumadin; the fear was that perhaps she was overly anticoagulated. However, a PT with INR was found to be in the therapeutic range. Due to the patient's heavy bleeding, I felt that a D&C with some kind of therapeutic intervention was warranted. In this particular circumstance, an endometrial ablation would serve the patient very well. Plan is to perform a D&C with a balloon thermo-ablation.

Past Medical History: Significant for mechanical valve placement

Surgery: Valve replacement

Current Medications: Lasix, Lanoxin, Coumadin. Allergies: No drug allergies

Obstetrical History: Gravida 10, para 7

Social History: No tobacco, alcohol, or drugs

Family History: Significant for diabetes in her mother

Physical Exam: Blood pressure 120/80, weight 224

HEENT: Moist mucous membranes without thyromegaly or lymphadenopathy

Breasts: Symmetrical without additional mass, nipple discharge

Lungs: Clear to auscultation

Heart: Regular rate and rhythm

Abdomen: Soft, no mass. No lesions are seen on the vulva, vagina or the cervix. Uterus is approximately six to eight weeks' sized. The adnexa were not palpable.

Assessment and Plan: 48-year-old gravida 10, para 7 with dysfunctional uterine bleeding. Plan is to perform a D&C (dilation and curettage) with a ThermaChoice balloon ablation. The patient is currently in-house and this is scheduled for Thursday morning at 8 a.m.

Operative Report

Pre-Operative Diagnoses

1. Dysfunctional uterine bleeding
2. Anemia

Post-Operative Diagnoses: Same

Operations: Fractional D&C and Therma-Choice balloon endometrial ablation

Anesthesia: General with endotracheal tube intubation

Complications: None

Estimated Blood Loss: Less than 50 cc. Drains: None

Specimen(s) to Lab

1. Endocervical curettings
2. Endometrial curettings

Operative Procedure: The patient was taken to the Operating Room and under adequate general anesthesia. She was prepped and draped in the dorsolithotomy position for a vaginal procedure. The uterus was sounded to approximately 9–10 cm. Using Pratt cervical dilators, the cervix was dilated to the point that a Sims sharp curette could be inserted. A Kevorkian curette was first used to obtain endocervical curettings and the Sims sharp curette was passed to obtain endometrial curettings. After the curettings were obtained, the Therma-Choice system was assembled and primed. The catheter with the balloon was placed inside the endometrial cavity and slowly filled with fluid until it stabilized at a pressure of approximately 175 to 180 mmHg. The system was then preheated, and after preheating to 87 degrees C, eight minutes of therapeutic heat was applied to the lining of the endometrium. The fluid was allowed to drain from the balloon and the system was removed. The procedure was then discontinued.

All sponge, instrument, and needle counts were correct. The patient tolerated the procedure well and was taken to the Recovery Room. She will be discharged home when stable.

Pathology Report

Endocervical mucosa with squamous metaplasia, negative for dysplasia

Inactive endometrium with features of non-cycling endometrium

No evidence of hyperplasia or malignancy

Code Assignment Including POA Indicator

ICD-9-CM Principal Diagnosis: _____

ICD-9-CM Additional Diagnoses: _____

ICD-9-CM Procedure Code(s): _____

Issues To Clarify:_____

ICD-10-CM Code(s): _____

ICD-10-PCS Code(s): _____

Optional MS-DRG Exercise (for users with access to MS-DRG software or tables)

What are the results when you group this case with the code for acute blood loss anemia versus anemia due to blood loss?

MS-DRG assignment with the acute blood loss anemia code:

_____

MS-DRG assignment with the anemia due to blood loss code:

_____

Which MS-DRG is appropriate for this case? _____

7.18. The following documentation is from the health record of a 92-year-old female patient.

Admission Diagnoses

1. Fever

2. Delirium

Discharge Diagnoses

1. Left lower extremity cellulitis

2. Probable urosepsis with streptococcal bacteremia

3. Status post acute renal failure likely secondary to acute tubular necrosis

4. Insulin-requiring diabetes mellitus

5. Probable chronic obstructive pulmonary disease

6. Hypothyroidism

7. Hypertension

Consultations: Infectious Disease

Procedures Performed

1. Doppler ultrasound of the left lower extremity which showed no evidence of DVT

2. Transthoracic echocardiogram which showed normal left ventricular function

Hospital Course: The patient is a 92-year-old white female with past medical history significant for hypertension, hypothyroidism, and non-insulin-dependent diabetes mellitus who was brought to the Emergency Room for evaluation of fever and dyspnea. The patient at that time was a poor historian; however, family corroborated abrupt onset of symptoms with no clear source. Generally the patient has been healthy although she is minimally active and most of her activities of daily living consist of ambulating around her bedroom with the assistance of family.

In the Emergency Room the patient was febrile to 40:C. Urinalysis was significant for pyuria with evident bacteria. No focal infiltrate was seen on chest x-ray. The patient had marked leukocytosis with a white count of 25,000, 80 polys and 15 band forms. She was admitted for intravenous antibiotics. She was treated with Ceftriaxone and by the following morning was noticeably brighter and more alert. She remained afebrile for the duration of her hospital course. Also on the morning of first hospital day, blood cultures were reported as positive for gram positive cocci in chains. This was subsequently confirmed as group C streptococcus which was Penicillin sensitive. Urinalysis grew out mixed flora. It was somewhat unclear as to the specific source of the patient's bacteremia. It is somewhat unusual for a UTI to yield this organism. The patient had some mild erythema on her left lower extremity and had marked discomfort to touch over both of her ankles, which she attributed to her "diabetes." She remained on Rocephin and was actually tolerating near normal diet.

On the evening of the second hospital day, the patient complained of increased pain and was noted to be increasingly incoherent. She had been placed on nasal cannula overnight for have markedly increased erythema in her left lower extremity concerning for desaturation. On evaluation by cross covering physician, she was noted to have markedly increased erythema in her left lower extremity concerning for possible DVT. Doppler ultrasound showed no evidence of clot. She was started on Vancomycin for improved gram positive coverage. Respiratory status remained stable. However, the patient was minimally arousable later that morning. She had been administered a 1-mg dose of morphine for leg pain. Chest x-ray showed increased interstitial edema possibly consistent with heart failure. The patient received Narcan with some improvement in her mental status. Arterial blood gas showed evidence of significant CO_2 retention with pH of 7.19, pCO_2 70, p02 50, serum bicarbonate of 26. She was diuresed and administered nebulizer treatments. She was moved to the Medical Intensive Care Unit for possible ventilation with BiPAP. Echocardiogram showed no wall motion abnormalities and no left ventricular dysfunction. Chemstix remained greater than 100 mg/dL. The patient had prompt improvement in her respiratory status with diuresis and prevision of Narcan. No further invasive ventilation was necessary.

Of note during these events the patient's family was in close attendance including her three daughters and grandson. There was extensive consultation with them regarding any advanced directives that the patient might have specified previously. It was the consensus of the family that reasonable attempts at aggressive intervention were indicated as long as there was a possibility of a reversible etiology for her problems. Fortunately the patient's condition stabilized.

For the remainder of her hospital course, intervention focused on improving her pulmonary status as well as renal function. Her creatinine had increased from prior baseline of 1.2 up to 1.7 with noticeable drop-off in her urine output. The patient had received intravenous antibiotics during her hospital course but had not had any noticeable hypotensive episodes. She was receiving diuretics, which complicated calculation of her urine sodium; however, overall picture appeared consistent with acute tubular necrosis. Renal ultrasound was obtained and showed no evidence of hydronephrosis or obstruction. She was restarted on her oral Indapamide and continued to have steady improvement in her pulmonary status. She did not require any supplemental oxygen following resolution of her pulmonary edema.

Infectious Disease was consulted with regards to her cellulitis and was concerned that it was not resolving as would be expected with a streptococcal organism. Therefore she was continued on Vancomycin for an additional five days and by the time of this dictation erythema had completely resolved and the patient was consistently alert, sitting up in bed and actually ambulating around her room. Leukocytosis resolved and, as noted above, renal function normalized. The plan was to continue her on oral Dicloxacillin for an additional 10 days of oral antibiotic therapy. Only additional intervention was provision of a combined albuterol Atrovent inhaler given the patient's signs of chronic interstitial lung disease. This appeared to improve her ventilatory status as she had no further episodes of nocturnal desaturation. The patient at this time is stable for discharge.

I briefly discussed her hospital course with her primary physician, who will continue to follow her. Family is requesting the assistance of home health nurse for overall assessment over the next two weeks while the patient continues to recuperate at home. Other peripheral issues addressed during this hospitalization included the patient's probable iron deficiency anemia. Recent colonoscopy and endoscopy showed evidence of diverticular disease but no other pathology. The patient has had upper GI bleeding. She was guaiaced during this admission, had stable hematocrit. B-12 and folate were checked and were within normal limits. Other issue was the patient's diet and she was evaluated by a speech therapist who noted that she did fine without any aspiration as long as she was provided with somewhat *thickened* feeds and had her usual foods provided. It was particularly requested that she be given pills, tablets, and capsules with a spoonful of pudding, applesauce, or yogurt instead of fluid. It was also recommended that she continue to have thickener available. The family was aware of these recommendations and is extraordinarily attentive to the patient's needs.

Medications on Discharge: Insulin NPH 10 units qam; Synthroid .05 mg po qd; Aspirin 325 mg po qd; Lorazepam 0.5 mg po qhs; Iron 324 mg po tid; Colace 100 mg po qd; Dulcolax 10 mg prn constipation; Combivent MDI 2 puffs bid; Indapamide 2.5 mg po qd; Dicloxacillin 125 mg po qid × 10 days

Follow-up: The patient's family has been instructed to call for appointment.

Diet: Soft mechanical 1,800 calorie ADA

Activities: The patient may ambulate to a chair with assistance.

Special Instructions: The patient should seek prompt medical attention for any recurrent fever, increased erythema in her lower extremity, or mental status changes as reported by the family.

Code Assignment Including POA Indicator

ICD-9-CM Principal Diagnosis: _____

ICD-9-CM Additional Diagnoses: _____

ICD-9-CM Procedure Code(s): _____

Issues To Clarify:_____

ICD-10-CM Code(s): _____

ICD-10-PCS Code(s): _____

7.19. The following documentation is from the health record of a 14-year-old male patient.

Discharge Summary

The patient is a 14-year-old male with a history of renal failure and failed left kidney transplant. The patient was admitted for his second kidney transplant.

Prior to surgery, the patient underwent hemodialysis, through the existing AV fistula. The transplant was accomplished within 48 hours of the harvesting of the donor organ. Tissue samples confirmed adequate donor match. The previously transplanted, now failing, kidney was first removed; then the new kidney was placed.

One postoperative dialysis session was required before the transplanted kidney was functioning adequately. Postoperatively, the patient was watched carefully for signs of rejection. Patient's postoperative course was relatively uneventful.

The patient was discharged, to be followed weekly in the office.

Which of the following code sets will be reported for the above admission?

ICD-9-CM Code(s):

a. 996.81, 586, 55.53, 55.69, 39.95 × 2
b. 586, 996.81, 55.69, 39.95 × 2
c. 586, V42.0, 55.53, 55.69, 39.95
d. 584.9, V42.0, 55.69, 39.95

ICD-10-CM Code(s): _____

ICD-10-PCS Code(s): _____

7.20. The following is from the health record of a 77-year-old female.

Discharge Summary

Admission Date:	04/12/XX
Discharge Date:	04/15/XX
Discharge Diagnosis:	1. Acute renal failure
	2. Congestive heart failure
	3. Chronic obstructive pulmonary disease (COPD)
	4. Leg cellulitis, resolved
	5. Seizure disorder
	6 Venous insufficiency
	7. Osteoarthritis
	8. Morbid obesity
	9. Acute ankle arthritis, likely pseudogout
Discharge Medications:	Resume home medications
Procedures:	None
Consults:	None

Present Illness: This is a 77-year-old female transferred to the acute care ward from a subacute unit for treatment of renal insufficiency. She was originally admitted with a BUN of 32, creatinine 1.4. While on the subacute unit she was diuresed for congestive heart failure and developed acute renal failure. Her BUN rose to 78, creatinine to 2.3. She was transferred to the trauma care unit (TCU) for IV fluids and monitoring for her redevelopment of congestive heart failure. She was developing some rales with IV fluids on the subacute unit. She was monitored closely over the next 3 days. As her BUN and creatinine fell she seemed to tolerate it fairly well symptomatically, having some rales. She had a BUN of 60 and a creatinine of 1.3 on the day of discharge. She was released by the cardiologist that day when he felt she was in no significant congestive heart failure and her BUN and creatinine were improving. She should follow up with the cardiologist in the near future for follow-up electrolytes and reevaluation of her congestive heart failure.

While the patient was on the TCU, she also developed some ankle pain. It was somewhat swollen and was given a dose of steroids. She had quick resolution to the pain and swelling and likely this was an episode of pseudogout.

History and Physical Exam

Admission Date: 04/12/XX

Chief Complaint: Acute renal failure.

Present Illness: This is a 77-year-old white female who was transferred down from the subacute unit to the acute care unit for increasing renal insufficiency. The patient was originally admitted on 03/28 with a BUN, creatinine of 32 and 1.4. The patient has been treated with I.V. Ancef and I.V. Lasix for cellulitis and pulmonary edema. Yesterday, her BUN and creatinine were found to be 78 and 2.3. She was transferred to the acute care unit for I.V. fluids and to monitor her renal function. This a.m., she complains of right ankle pain. She denies any trauma to the right ankle, but she does give a history of generalized osteoarthritis. She reports that there is excruciating pain with weight bearing and with any movement. In addition, she reports that the right ankle is very tender to touch.

Past Medical History:		
	1.	Obesity
	2.	Renal failure
	3.	Bilateral lower extremity cellulitis
	4.	Hypertension
	5.	Anemia
	6.	COPD
	7.	Seizure disorder
	8.	Intertrigo

Current Medications:		
	1.	Lotrisone, b.i.d. topical to breast and groin
	2.	Prinivil, 40 mg po q.day
	3.	Dilantin — mg po b.i.d.
	4.	Benadryl, 25 mg q. 4 hours prn
	5.	Catapres, 0.1 mg prn
	6.	Hydrocortisone cream, 1% topical b.i.d. prn
	7.	Tylox, 1–2 tabs po q.i.d. prn
	8.	Norvasc, 5 mg po q.day

Allergies: No known drug allergies

Review of Systems: The patient reports that she does have arthritis in her back and multiple joints. She denies a history of gout. She denies sporadic fevers, chills, cough, abdominal pain, GI or GU complaints.

Social History: The patient is a smoker; she has smoked two packs per day for the previous 20 years.

Physical Exam: BP 140/70, pulse 100, respirations 24, temperature 97.5. In general, this is an obese white female in no acute distress. HEENT: Atraumatic, normocephalic. Pupils equal, round, and reactive. Oropharynx is clear. Neck: Supple; no lymphadenopathy; trachea midline. Lungs: Lungs reveal few crackles, right base. Heart: Regular rate and rhythm; SI, S2, no murmur, click, gallop, or rub. Abdomen: Protuberant, positive bowel sounds, and nontender. Extremities: Chronic venous changes bilaterally with trace edema. Right lateral malleolus is very tender to palpation, range of motion is limited by pain. There is no calf or thigh tenderness.

Laboratory Data/Clinical Tests: Glucose 98, BUN 76, creatinine 2.1, calcium 8.2, sodium 134, potassium 4.4, chloride 94, total CO2 30

Assessment/Plan

1. Renal failure. This is most likely prerenal secondary to overdiuresis. We will hold her diuretics and continue with general I.V. fluids. Her BUN, creatinine is slightly improved today since yesterday with this therapy. Urine electrolytes and eosinophils are currently pending.

2. Right ankle pain. Etiology not completely certain. There is no history of trauma. I question if this could possibly be an inflammatory arthritis monoarticular such as gout or pseudogout. We will check a sed rate and a rheumatoid factor. We will hold off on giving the patient any nonsteroidal anti-inflammatories, in light of her renal failure. We'll continue with the Tylox and give her a trial of SoluMedrol. We'll also check a foot x-ray.

3. Cellulitis. This is stable, off of her antibiotics.

4. Hypertension. We will continue her current treatment.

Which of the following is the correct code assignment?

ICD-9-CM Code(s):

a. 584.9, 428.0, 496, 345.90, 459.81, 721.90, 715.89, 278.01, 275.49, 712.37, 401.9
b. 403.90, 584.9, 428.0, 496, 345.90, 459.81, 721.90, 715.89, 278.01, 275.49, 712.37
c. 586, 428.0, 496, 345.90, 459.81, 721.90, 715.89, 278.01, 275.49, 712.37
d. 404.90, 584.9, 428.0, 496, 345.90, 459.81, 721.90, 715.89, 278.01, 275.49, 712.37

ICD-10-CM Code(s): _____

Optional MS-DRG Exercise (for users with access to MS-DRG software or tables)

True or False: The assigned MS-DRG for this admission contains a CC or MCC.

Infectious Diseases

7.21. The following documentation is from the health record of a 71-year-old male patient.

Discharge Summary

History and Physical Findings: This 71-year-old male is a nursing home resident as a result of a cerebrovascular accident 2 years ago. He has had numerous hospital admissions for pneumonia and other infectious complications. On the day of admission (4/21), the patient was noted to be clammy, with tachypnea, to have decreased level of responsiveness, and to show increased fever. He was seen in the ER, where evaluation revealed the presence of probable urosepsis. The patient was also found to have renal insufficiency with BUN and creatinine elevated. His WBC count was 23,000 with decreased hemoglobin and hematocrit. He was admitted for treatment of *Escherichia coli* septicemia. Physical examination revealed an elderly male who was aphasic and with a right hemiplegia from a previous CVA. The heart had a regular rhythm. The lungs were clear. The abdomen was soft.

Significant Lab, X-Ray, and Consult Findings: Follow-up chemistry showed progressive decline in the BUN and creatinine to near-normal levels. Initial white blood cell count was 23,700. Final blood count was 9,000. The urinalysis showed white cells too numerous to count. The urine culture had greater than 100,000 colonies of *E. coli* and group D strep, which revealed the cause of the UTI. Repeated blood cultures grew *E. coli* with the same sensitivities as that of the urine. There were no acute abnormalities noted. EKG showed sinus tachycardia and low lead voltage, otherwise was normal and unchanged.

Course in Hospital: The patient was initially started empirically on Primaxin. He underwent fluid rehydration and his electrolytes were followed closely. Electrolytes improved through his hospital stay. He was continued on IV Primaxin until the date of discharge, when he was changed to Cipro by tube. All of the bacteria grown in the urine and in the blood were sensitive to the Cipro. The chest x-ray showed no change from previous admissions, and he was followed closely with additional oxygen as needed. The patient does have a history of chronic obstructive lung disease and has required intermittent oxygen therapy at the nursing home. At this time, the patient had reached maximal hospital benefit. He was switched to oral antibiotics. He was to continue on tube feedings, which he was tolerating quite well. The patient was discharged back to the nursing home on 5/4.

Discharge Diagnoses: *E. coli* septicemia
UTI
Renal insufficiency
Chronic obstructive lung disease
CVA with right hemiplegia

Code Assignment Including POA Indicator

ICD-9-CM Principal Diagnosis: _____

ICD-9-CM Additional Diagnoses: _____

Issues To Clarify: _____

ICD-10-CM Code(s): _____

Optional MS-DRG Exercise (for users with access to MS-DRG software or tables)

What is the correct MS-DRG for this case?

_____

7.22.   The following documentation is from the health record of a 34-year-old male.

Discharge Summary

History of Present Illness: The patient is a 34-year-old male who was transferred to the hospital with the diagnosis of rule out AIDS. The patient dates the onset of his current illness to two months prior to admission when he had a tooth extraction. The patient doesn't know whether he was treated with antibiotics at that time; however, he does note that the socket was packed. The patient states that after the above tooth extraction, he developed a fever with shaking chills, night sweats, and anorexia. He lost about 12 pounds. He also notes the onset of mild right flank pain associated with foam in urine and urinary frequency. There was no hematuria, dysuria, incontinence, urinary retention, hesitancy, or slow stream. The patient also complains of occasional diarrhea but no melena or bright red blood per rectum. Medications on transfer are Codeine, Lasix, Amphojel, Mylanta, Penicillin, Ranitidine, Halcion. Social history is remarkable for continuous IV drug abuse, both heroin and cocaine. There's no history of homosexual activity. He doesn't drink alcohol but smokes a half-pack of cigarettes a day.

Pertinent Lab, X-Ray, and Consult Findings: This patient is a 34-year-old, well-developed, well-nourished male in no acute distress. Mucous membranes are moist. There is a questionable white area at the outer aspect of the right lower gingiva near second tricuspid. There are small mobile submandibular and posterior cervical nodes. The patient also has bilateral inguinal adenopathy and two left epitrochlear nodes. Chest x-ray showed minimal blunting of both costophrenic angles, no definite effusions are noted. There are confluent patches of infiltration in the left midlung field spanning from the hilum to the periphery as well as in the right lower lung. These findings are nonspecific, but could very well fit in with the diagnosis of Pneumocystis carinii pneumonia. Urinalysis negative. CBC: Hemoglobin 9.0, hematocrit 27.2, MCV 87, WBC 5.1, 11 lymphs, S monos, platelets 206,000. Sodium 130, potassium 3.98, chloride 112, C02 10, BUN 50, creatinine 4.7, glucose 82, calcium 7.0, albumin 0.80. Sputum culture showed normal respiratory flora with normal Enterobacter aerogens. Urine culture showed no growth.

Hospital Course by Problem List

Problem #1. Acquired immunodeficiency syndrome: The patient's history was significant for weight loss. Social history significant for IV drug abuse. Physical examination revealed diffuse lymphadenopathy. Laboratory data revealed neutropenia with lymphopenia. Serological test was positive for HIV.

Problem #2. Pneumocystic carinii pneumonia: The patient underwent bronchoscopy and brushings from the left and right lower lobes revealed changes consistent with pneumocystic carinii and reactive bronchial cells and pneumocytes. The patient was treated with two weeks of intravenous Septra therapy. However, there was no improvement in his clinical status. After two weeks of therapy, the patient was still afebrile. His chest x-ray did not improve and WBC count progressively declined to a low of 2.5. The infectious disease service recommended Pentamidine therapy at that point. The patient became afebrile.

Problem #3. Chronic renal failure: The patient's renal failure deteriorated during his hospitalization prior to transfer. Workup was negative and the etiology remains unclear. The patient's renal function remained stable throughout this hospitalization. At the time of transfer, his BUN and creatinine were 50 and 5.0, respectively. He was started on Bicitra therapy to correct the metabolic acidosis felt secondary to his renal failure.

Problem #4. Nephrotic syndrome secondary to renal failure: The patient was found to have edema, hypoalbuminemia, proteinuria, and high triglyceride levels, all consistent with the diagnosis of nephrotic syndrome. The patient did have a renal biopsy done prior to transfer to this hospital and the results per phone report are as follows: Interstitial nephritis, no deposits over capillary loops, no immunofluorescence of CMV. The patient was treated with bed rest, a low-sodium, high-protein fluid restriction diet. In spite of this therapy, the patient's albumin level had not improved at the time of transfer.

Problem #5. Chronic normocytic normochromic anemia secondary to external hemorrhoid bleeding. The patient required transfusion of two units of packed red blood cells. Otherwise, his hematocrit remained relatively stable throughout the admission. Physical examination revealed swollen hemorrhoids with stool heme negative.

The patient was transferred in stable condition to the local hospital. Medications at the time of transfer were Bicitra, Pentamidine, Restoril, Lorazepam.

Which of the following is the correct code assignment for this admission?

ICD-9-CM Code(s):

a. 042, 136.3, 276.2, 581.89, 585.9, 280.0, 305.61, 305.51, 455.5, 305.1, 33.24, 99.04
b. 042, 136.3, 276.2, 581.89, 585.9, 280.0, 455.5, 33.24, 99.04
c. 042, 136.3, 581.89, 585.9, 280.0, 305.61, 305.51, 305.1, 33.24, 99.04
d. 136.3, 042, 581.89, 585.9, 280.0, 305.61, 305.51, 305.1, 33.24, 99.04

ICD-10-CM Code(s): _____

ICD-10-PCS Code(s): _____

7.23.   The following documentation is from the health record of a two-year-old boy.

Discharge Summary

Admission Date: 7/18/20XX

Discharge Date: 7/20/20XX

Admitting Diagnosis: Fever of unknown origin

Discharge Diagnosis: 1. Primary herpetic gingivostomatitis
                          2. Kawasaki's disease
                          3. Strep pharyngitis

History: The patient is a 2-year-old male who presented to the ER this evening from his primary medical doctor's office with 4 days of fever, rash, cracked lips, and drooling. Mom states that he has had a decreased activity level, decreased p.o. intake, and increased irritability. He has received Tylenol and Motrin at home. Mom denies vomiting or diarrhea. He has had a sick contact at day care. He also has dysphagia and rhinorrhea.

Past Medical History: Significant for a VSD that has not been repaired. He is followed by a cardiologist and the abnormality is currently stable.

Physical Exam: This young male is quite irritable. He has bulbar conjunctival injection without discharge. His tympanic membranes are dull bilaterally. His tonsils are enlarged. He also has an exudate in his oropharynx. Heart shows regular rate and rhythm with a IV–VI systolic murmur at the left lower sternal border. He has a diffuse maculopapular rash on his lower extremities, trunk, back, and diaper area. He also has perineal desquamation.

Hospital Course: Patient presented to the ER with a 4- to 5-day history of fever, rash, cracked lips, drooling, and sore throat. Due to lymphadenopathy, perineal desquamation, bilateral bulbar conjunctivitis, and rash found on physical exam, he was treated for Kawasaki's disease with IVIG 2 g/kg and aspirin 80 mg per day. He was also tested for herpes due to the perioral, paranasal, and oral lesions. His test came back positive for herpes I virus and he was treated with Kefzol. Cardiologist performed an echocardiogram to evaluate his VSD. His lesions slowly improved and are largely healed at this time. He remained afebrile for the past 4 nights. His medications were changed to oral form. He is no longer taking antibiotics, and he will be continued on oral acyclovir. Follow-up with cardiologist is in 4 weeks.

Which of the following is the correct code set for this hospitalization?

ICD-9-CM Code(s):

a. 523.10, 054.9, 745.4, 446.1, 034.0
b. 054.2, 745.4, 034.0, 446.1, 785.6, 372.30, 782.1
c. 054.2, 745.4, 446.1, 034.0
d. 054.2, 446.1, 034.0

ICD-10-CM Code(s): _____

7.24.   History

The patient is a 78-year-old female who was initially admitted to the intensive care unit for sepsis and urinary tract infection and decreased level of consciousness. After admission to the intensive care unit, the patient was found to have a massive right-sided cerebrovascular accident, which was felt to be secondary to an embolic phenomenon. The patient also had severe mitral regurgitation, moderate tricuspid regurgitation, and aortic insufficiency. CT of the head revealed an acute left middle cerebral arterial infarction involving the temporal and parietal lobes with localized mass effect and mild midline shift. No hemorrhage was seen.

The patient's sepsis was treated with IV antibiotics as was her urinary tract infection. Discussion was undertaken with the patient's next of kin as to the patient's resuscitation status. The patient was made a Do Not Resuscitate. Decision was made to keep the patient comfortable, and she was transferred to a medical bed. The patient's antibiotics were adjusted by an infectious disease group. Her renal failure which was determined to be due to her sepsis was followed by nephrology. Neurology was consulted for the patient's cerebrovascular accident. They did an EEG, which showed marked slowing; however, there was no total absence of brain activity. Cardiology consultation was obtained because of new onset atrial fibrillation. Cardiology felt that no aggressive intervention was needed; however, she would be given medicine to control her ventricular rate. The patient remained unresponsive. She was started on tube feeding and her antibiotics were continued. The patient was noted to have some thrombocytopenia as well as her continued renal failure and anemia. Diuresis was attempted with IV diuretics by nephrology in an attempt to help the patient's congestive heart failure. The patient was retaining copious amounts of fluid despite the diuretics. Her prothrombin time eventually normalized. Her blood sugar was elevated, and she was placed on insulin once per day at bedtime to cover her tube feedings. The patient was found without audible or visible respirations and no heart tones. She was pronounced dead at 12:40, and her body was released to the funeral home.

Which of the following code sets would be assigned by the hospital for this admission?

ICD-9-CM Code(s):

a. 038.9, 995.91, 599.0, 434.11, 394.1, 397.0, 398.91, 427.31, 287.5, 285.9
b. 995.91, 599.0, 586, 434.11, 424.0, 397.0, 428.0, 427.31, 287.5, 285.9
c. 038.9, 995.92, 599.0, 586, 434.11, 396.3, 397.0, 398.91, 427.31, 287.5, 285.9
d. 434.11, 038.9, 995.92, 586, 428.0, 424.0, 397.0, 427.31, 287.5, 285.9

ICD-10-CM Code(s): _____

Optional MS-DRG Exercise (for users with access to MS-DRG software or tables)

What is the correct MS-DRG for this case?

a. 064, Intracranial Hemorrhage or Cerebral Infarction with MCC
b. 871, Septicemia without mechanical ventilation 96+ hours with MCC
c. 872, Septicemia without mechanical ventilation 96+ hours without MCC
d. 868, Other Infectious and Parasitic Disease Diagnoses with CC

7.25. Discharge Diagnosis

1. *Escherichia coli* and *Staphylococcus aureus* urinary tract infection with sepsis
2. Sepsis syndrome
3. Advanced dementia
4. Hypothroidism
5. Hypertension
6. Protein calorie malnutrition
7. Dysphagia

Discharge Medications: Levoxyl 88mcg p.o. q. a.m., Paxil 20mg p.o. q. a.m., Namenda 10mg p.o. q. a.m., Ativan 0.5 q. 8 hours agitation, Augmentin 500 mg p.o. b.i.d. for 15 days, and Megace 400 mg p.o. b.i.d.

Discharge Disposition: Improved and home with home healthcare.

History of Present Illness: The patient is an 85-year-old female who was apparently brought into the emergency room by her family this evening for multiple problems. According to the family, she has not been eating recently and has been getting extremely weak. She has been unable to stand without assistance for quite some time now. The patient, although awake and alert, will not answer any questions. All history is obtained from the computer records, as well as the ER staff and ER physician. Initial workup reveals significant urinary tract infection. She is also most likely septic secondary to her presentation given her hypotension and acute encephalopathy.

Laboratory/Radiology: Admission labs significant for a white blood cell count of 9.8, hemoglobin 14.9, platelets of 328,000 with a BUN of 29 and creatinine of 1.4. Urinalysis was small bilirubin, 15 mg ketones, large blood, 100 mg protein, positive nitrates, large leukocytes, and too many WBCs to count, with many bacteria and many red cells. CT of the head was normal. Portable chest x-ray showed hyperexpanded lung fields but no mass.

Hospital Course: The patient was admitted to the general medical floor with the diagnosis of sepsis. After discussion with family, she was made DNR III and was hydrated and started on IV ciprofloxacin. She has a significant advanced dementia and does not speak but was somewhat more encephalopathic secondary to her sepsis, and this improved to her baseline. Her BUN and creatinine normalized, and she was continued on her usual medications for dementia. Her hydrochlorothiazide was held, but she was continued on her Toprol. Levoxyl was held and a TSH was within normal limits. She was continued on her Paxil. Subsequently, her urine culture grew out *E. coli,* pan sensitive, and *S. aureus,* pan sensitive, and she was changed from ciprofloxacin to Augmentin 500mg p.o. b.i.d., which she tolerated well. Speech therapy was consulted, and an MBS was performed. Diet with thin liquids was recommended. She does have protein calorie malnutrition.

Disposition: The daughter has been contacted because the patient is stable for discharge. She is discharged to her daughter's care with physical and occupational therapy.

Code Assignment Including POA Indicator

ICD-9-CM Principal Diagnosis: _____

ICD-9-CM Secondary Diagnosis: _____

ICD-10-CM Code(s): _____

Behavioral Health Conditions

7.26.   In the following case scenario, a 26-year-old white male was admitted after being transferred from the outpatient evaluation service with severe homicidal and suicidal ideation. Admitting diagnosis was severe major depressive disorder with psychotic features. Pharmacologic treatment was initiated and suicide precautions were instituted. After a thorough neuropsychological, personality, and behavioral psychologic evaluation, the risks and benefits of ECT were reviewed. Due to the severity of the psychotic episode and the patient's delusional state, it was determined that ECT was warranted. Extensive efforts were made to secure informed consent from the patient, and a course of single seizure unilateral ECT was begun.

ECT was administered three times per week, and the course of therapy was completed in a three-week period. On the fourth treatment of ECT, postictal observation was notable for cardiac arrhythmia, which subsided without sequelae. Otherwise, the patient tolerated the therapy well and responded quickly with resolution of the psychotic features and overall improvement in the acute phase of his depressive disorder. Suicide precautions could be lifted after the fifth treatment with ECT. After establishing adequate therapeutic levels of lithium, the patient was discharged to be managed as an outpatient.

Discharge Diagnosis: Severe major depressive disorder with suicidal ideation, stabilized after a course of ECT.

Which is the correct code set for reporting this case scenario?

ICD-9-CM Code(s):

a. 296.24, V62.84, 94.27, 94.22, 94.08
b. 296.23, V62.84, 94.27, 94.22, 94.08
c. 296.24, V62.84, 427.9, 94.26, 94.22, 94.08
d. 296.23, V62.84, 997.1, 427.9, 94.27, 94.22, 94.08

ICD-10-CM Code(s): _____

ICD-10-PCS Code(s): _____

7.27.   The following documentation is from the health record of a 56-year-old male patient.

Final Diagnosis

Axis I: Chronic schizophrenia, paranoid type with acute exacerbation, improved
Axis II: None
Axis III: Cardiomyopathy secondary to hypertension
          COPD
          Type II diabetes mellitus
Axis IV: Psychosocial and environmental stressors are severe
Axis V: Admission GAF 25 to 30
          Discharge GAF 55

Physical Examination: For pertinent findings on medical examination, see the medical doctor's dictation.

Pertinent Laboratory Results: Electrolyte panel within normal limits. Digoxin level was 0.6, hemoglobin A1C 6.5, triglycerides 138, CBC unremarkable. TSH 1.3, urinalysis negative. EKG showed normal sinus rhythm.

Hospital Course: This is a 56-year-old male who was admitted due to decompensating at his apartment where he thought people were trying to get into his apartment, and he continued to decompensate with his paranoia and persecutory-type delusions, so that it was felt he needed longer hospitalization. During this time he also switched his medications from Zyprexa to Seroquel to Risperdal, and then he was admitted on Prolixin. We reviewed his records, and it appears he did quite well on Risperdal so he went back to taking that, and he was titrated up to 30 mg q. h.s. of Risperdal and 100 mg of trazodone. These two medications helped significantly to eliminate his delusions and paranoid ideation. He slept better. Patient started going on therapeutic passes that went well. His sister reports that he is doing the best that she has seen him in quite some time. During his stay here his mother passed away from a long medical illness, and he was able to go to the funeral and dealt with that loss in an appropriate way. He continued to show improvement and was placed on Level E. He continued to go to psychosocial programming. A discharge meeting was held, and it was agreed that he could get most of his services through the outpatient program. It was felt by everyone that the patient was stable enough to be discharged, and discharge was scheduled.

Pertinent Findings on Mental Status at Discharge: 45 minutes spent in the final examination with the patient. Appearance: Pleasant, white male who looks his stated age. Behavior is cooperative, fair eye contact. Speech is of normal rate and volume. Not rapid or pressured. Mood euthymic, affect appropriate. Thought process is goal directed, decreased paranoid ideation. Negative for racing thoughts and flight of ideas. Thought content: He denies signs of active psychosis, denies current suicidal or homicidal intent. Insight and judgment improved. Impulse control is fair.

Prognosis: Fair. The main problem is that the patient is on so many medications for his medical problems. He did do well with the pill organizer and self-medications, but his mental illness may be exacerbated if his medical conditions are not well controlled.

Discharge Medications: Digoxin 0.25 mg q. d, Glucotrol 2.5 mg a.m. and 7.5 mg q. 5:00 p.m., potassium 10 mEq q. a.m., Spironolactone 25 mg q. a.m., an aspirin 325 mg q. a.m., Lasix 10 mg q. d., lisopril 2.5 mg q. d., Atrovent inhaler two puffs q. i.d., isosorbide dinitrate 10 mg t.i.d., beclomethasone inhaler four puffs b.i.d., Risperdal 3 mg q. h.s., Colace 100 mg b.i.d., and trazodone 100 mg q. h.s.

Aftercare Recommendations: The patient will be discharged to his apartment. Social services will follow the patient. He will follow up with a psychiatrist and medical care through the outpatient program. Also, a home health nurse will come to see the patient.

Which of the following code sets is correct for reporting this inpatient hospitalization?

ICD-9-CM Code(s):

a. 295.34, 425.4, 401.9, 496, 250.01, 94.25
b. 295.32, 402.90, 496, 250.01, 94.25
c. 295.34, 402.90, 496, 250.00, 94.25
d. 295.84, 402.90, 496, 250.00, 94.25

ICD-10-CM Code(s): _____

ICD-10-PCS Code(s): _____

7.28. The following documentation is from the health record of a 17-year-old male patient.

History of Present Illness: The patient is a 17-year-old white male who was brought to the ED after being found passed out in the town park. The patient was in restraints and accompanied by two police officers. The patient was combative and aggressive, threatening physical harm to himself as well as the physician and hospital staff. The patient has a long history of alcohol and drug abuse, was in the local treatment center, and walked off campus two days ago.

Allergies: NKDA

PMH: Attention deficit hyperactivity disorder (ADHD), drug and alcohol dependence, aggressive behavior

Family History: Noncontributory

ROS: As above

Physical Examination: Vital signs: Temp. 100.1 degrees; BP 144/88 mm Hg; General: Alternating between lethargy and combativeness; HEENT: Pupils pinpoint, 1 mm bilaterally; Skin: Cool, clammy to touch, feet and hands cold, slightly diaphoretic; Heart: Rate tachy, no murmurs; Lungs: Clear, respiratory rate 28 and shallow; Abdomen: Benign; Neurological: Mental status as above; follows commands inconsistently, responds to voice; Cranial nerves: Pupils as noted, gag intact; Motor: Moving all four extremities with equal power; Sensory: Responds to touch in all four extremities; deep tendon reflexes +3 throughout, but plantar reflexes down going bilaterally.

Laboratory: U/A shows 2+ blood, done after Foley catheter was placed; drug screen positive for amphetamines; ETOH 0.30; ABG within normal limits; EKG sinus tachycardia

Hospital Course: Family was contacted, IV fluids were initiated, and the patient was admitted to ICU with suicide protocol, Ativan 1 to 2 mg IV q. 2 hours p.r.n. He was maintained on soft restraints with checks every 15 minutes and monitored with telemetry and neuro checks through the night. By the morning he was no longer tachycardic. By hospital day three he was medically stable, but still saying he wants to "kill himself." Psychiatric consult requested; see dictated report.

Disposition: Discharge to psych. Psychiatric liaison service agreed to accept him in transfer to the inpatient adolescent psychiatric unit at children's hospital.

Discharge Diagnoses: Drug overdose with amphetamines and alcohol
                            Apparent suicide attempt
                            Continued verbalization of suicidal ideation

Which of the following code sets would be correct for this case?

ICD-9-CM Code(s):

a. 969.7, 785.0, 304.40, E950.3, 980.0, 303.00, E950.9, 314.01, 312.00
b. 785.0, E939.7, 305.90, 314.01, 312.00
c. 969.7, 785.0, 304.00, E980.3, 303.00, 314.01, 312.00
d. 785.0, 303.00, 304.40, 969.7, E950.3, 980.0, E950.9, 314.01, 312.00

ICD-10-CM Code(s): _____

Disorders of the Musculoskeletal System and Connective Tissue

7.29. **Preoperative Diagnosis:**   Bucket-handle tear left medial meniscus

Postoperative Diagnosis: Bucket-handle tear left medial meniscus

Procedure: Arthroscopic partial medial meniscectomy

Indications: The patient is a 16-year-old male who tore his left medial meniscus while playing football at the local high school football field. The patient is a wide receiver for the high school football team and was tackled resulting in the torn medial meniscus. I saw and treated the patient initially in the emergency room three weeks ago for this injury.

Technique: After induction with general anesthesia, a standard three-portal approach of the knee was evaluated. Mild synovitic changes were noted in the suprapatellar pouch. No chondromalacia changes were noted. The anterior portion of the medial meniscus had a flap tear, which was removed.

After all instruments were withdrawn, 4-0 nylon horizontal mattress stitches were used to close the wound, and pressure dressings were applied. The patient was awakened and taken to the recovery room in good condition.

Code Assignment Including POA Indicator

ICD-9-CM Principal Diagnosis: _____

ICD-9-CM Additional Diagnoses: _____

ICD-9-CM Procedure Code(s): _____

ICD-10-CM Code(s): _____

ICD-10-PCS Code(s): _____

7.30. **Preoperative Diagnosis:**   Primary osteoarthritis of right knee

Postoperative Diagnosis: Primary osteoarthritis of right knee

Procedure: Right posterior stabilized total knee arthroplasty

Implants: DePuy Sigma System size 4 right posterior stabilized femoral component, size 3 modular tibial tray with 8 mm noncrosslinked polyethylene spacer and 35 mm × 8.5 mm thick patella. Antibiotic cement was used.

Procedure Description: After obtaining informed consent, the patient was brought to the operating room whereupon the smooth induction of right femoral block and general anesthesia was performed. The patient was positioned in supine fashion on the operating room table, and all bony prominences were well-padded. A bump was placed under the right hip, and a tourniquet was placed on the right proximal thigh. A gram of Kefzol was given intravenously. The right lower extremity was prepped and draped in standard sterile fashion for arthroplasty including an alcohol pre-prep.

After exsanguinations of the extremity with an Ace wrap, the tourniquet was inflated to 300 mg Hg. An approximately 6-inch longitudinal incision was made about the anterior aspect of the knee centered on the inferior pole of the patella. The skin and subcutaneous tissue were dissected sharply down to the level of the fascia, and a medial parapatellar incision was made in the fascia with the medial most split proximally. The patella was everted, and the knee was flexed. Care was taken to protect the patellar tendon insertion. The osteophytes about the femoral notch were removed and a partial resection of the posterior patellar fat pad was carried out. The femoral canal was entered with a drill, and the sword with distal femoral cutting guide were attached set for a resection of 10 mm. The lateral femoral condyle was noted to be eroded distally and posteriorly; however, a 10-mm cut was sufficient for the distal cut.

Using anterior-referenced system, the femur was sized to a size 4. Rotation was set at 3 degrees external rotation. This was checked using the epicondylar axis. The four-in-one cutting guide was then applied, and the distal femoral anterior and posterior cuts as well as the chamfer cuts were completed. Care was taken to protect the collateral ligaments during these cuts. The femoral notch was then completed using the notch-cutting guide supplied with the system. Once that was done, attention was turned to the tibia. Using an external referenced guide, a tibial cut was made with a zero degree posterior slope with 2 mm off the low (lateral) side. This resection resulted in a similar amount of resection medially and laterally. The tibia was exposed using a Homan placed posteriorly and laterally. The osteophytes were removed laterally and posteriorly.

At this point the osteophytes about the posterior femoral condyles were removed using a curved osteotome under direct visualization. The tibia was then sized to a size 3. A thin cut was then made for the modular tibial tray system. An 8-mm posterior stabilized trial spacer, size 3 tibia tray, and size 4 femur were then applied. The knee was taken through a range of motion. Following this, stability was symmetric medially and laterally. The patella was then prepared. The osteophytes were removed with a rongeur, and the thickness was measured to be 25 mm. An 8.5-mm resection was made down to 16.5 mm and a 16.5 x 35 mm patellar trial was applied after the cut was completed. Stability of this component was then trialed, and it was found to be excellent.

The trial components were removed, and the knee was copiously irrigated with normal saline. The final components were then cemented into place in the sizes mentioned above. Order of cement was patella, tibia, femur. The tibial tray was placed and the knee brought out into full extension to compress the tibial and femoral components. Again, antibiotic gentamicin-containing cement was used. The wound was then cleared of excess cement and bony debris and irrigated one final time. It was then closed in layers over a ConstaVac drain. Number 1 Vicryl was used for the extensor fascia and Scarpa fascia in a simple interrupted fashion, 3-0 Monocryl was used for the subcutaneous tissue in a simple buried fashion, and staples were placed at the level of the skin.

A sterile dressing was placed. The ConstaVac drain extension and reservoir were attached and activated, and a compressive wrap was placed from the toes to the thigh. The tourniquet was released for a total tourniquet time of 112 minutes. EBL was minimal. Postoperatively the patient was taken to the recovery room in stable condition.

Which of the following is the correct code assignment?

ICD-9-CM Code(s):

a. 715.16, 81.54
b. 715.36, 81.47
c. 715.16, 81.55
d. 715.36, 81.54

ICD-10-CM Code(s): _____

ICD-10-PCS Code(s): _____

7.31.   The following documentation is from the health record of an ORIF patient.

Operative Report

Preoperative Diagnosis: Displaced comminuted fracture of the lateral condyle, right elbow

Postoperative Diagnosis: Same

Procedure: Open reduction, internal fixation

Description: The patient, with malignant hypertension and type I diabetes mellitus, was anesthetized and prepped with Betadine, sterile drapes were applied, and the pneumatic tourniquet was inflated around the arm. An incision was made in the area of the lateral epicondyle through a Steri-Drape, and this was carried through subcutaneous tissue, and the fracture site was easily exposed. Inspection revealed the fragment to be rotated in two planes about 90 degrees. It was possible to manually reduce this quite easily, and the judicious manipulation resulted in an almost anatomic reduction. This was fixed with two pins driven across the humerus. These pins were cut off below skin level. The wound was closed with some plain catgut subcutaneously and 5-0 nylon in the skin. Dressings were applied to the patient and tourniquet released. A long arm cast was applied.

Which of the following is the correct code assignment?

ICD-9-CM Code(s):

a. 812.52, 401.9, 250.01, 79.32
b. 812.42, 401.0, 250.01, 79.31
c. 812.42, 401.0, 250.01, 78.52
d. 812.52, 401.9, 250.00, 79.32

ICD-10-CM Code(s): _____

ICD-10-PCS Code(s): _____

7.32.   ## Discharge Summary

Admission Date: November 15, 20XX

Discharge Date: November 20, 20XX

Description: The patient is a 49-year-old male who was admitted on November 15. He underwent revision laminectomy and stabilization of his lumbar spine with a Dynesys system. The patient tolerated the procedure well and had an uneventful hospital course, except experienced acute pain after the surgery requiring additional physical therapy and pain control.

By postoperative day 5, he was tolerating a regular diet, had obtained pain control, and cleared physical therapy. He was subsequently discharged home with written instructions. He is to follow up in 3 weeks after discharge. He was given Percocet and Flexeril for pain and spasms, as needed.

History and Physical

Admit Diagnosis: Recurrent herniated disc

Procedure: Lumbar laminectomy, disc stabilization with Dynesys

History of Present Illness: 49-year-old male with left leg and back pain. Diagnosed with recurrent disc herniation

Past Medical History: Status post laminectomy and diskectomy 2 years ago

Physical Examination

Neck: Supple

Heart: Regular rate and rhythm

Lungs: Clear to auscultation

Neuro: Left leg weakness, numbness, and pain

Skin: No lesions, masses, or rashes

Assessment and Plan: Recurrent HNP L5 to S1

Operative Report

Preoperative Diagnosis: Radiculopathy and degenerative disc disease at L5–S1 with recurrent disc herniation at L5–S1

Postoperative Diagnosis: Same

Procedure Performed: Revision L5 laminectomy, revision S1 laminectomy and diskectomy, stabilization of L5 to S1 with flexible rod Dynesys system

Anesthesia: General

Blood Loss: Minimal

Complications: Intraoperative dural tear, which was repaired with watertight seal with interrupted 4-0 Nurolon sutures

Description of the Procedure: Under sterile conditions, the patient was brought to the operating room and was placed under general endotracheal anesthesia and placed in a prone position. Lumbar spine was then prepped and draped in the usual sterile manner with a Betadine prep. A lateral x-ray was obtained with an 18-gauge spinal needle placed for level localization. Based upon the x-ray, a direct posterior approach to the lumbar spine was performed. This was carried down to the transverse process of L5 and the sacral ala bilaterally. After adequate exposure, complete laminectomy was performed in a subperiosteal fashion with a combination Leksell and Kerrison rongeurs at the L5 and S1 levels. Mobilization of the left S1 and L5 nerve roots was performed, although there was a significant amount of scar tissue. There was a large free L5-S1 recurrent disc fragment, which was removed with a pituitary rongeur. There was a small dural tear within the axilla of the L5 nerve root repaired with watertight seal with interrupted 4-0 Nurolon sutures. After adequate decompression, attention was brought to stabilization. Using the usual internal and external landmarks, pedicle screws were placed in the L5 and S1 pedicles bilaterally. These were drilled, probed, dilated, and then a combination of 7.2 mm × 40 mm screws and 7.2 mm × 45 mm screws were placed in the L5 and S1 pedicles bilaterally. AP and lateral x-rays were obtained, noting appropriate placement of the screws. Measuring of the cord device was performed bilaterally. The cord was placed in the usual fashion, tensioned, and then finally tightened. The wound was copiously irrigated with bacitracin solution. No drain was utilized. The fascia was closed with interrupted 0 VICRYL suture. The subcutaneous tissue and skin were closed in three sequential layers. The patient was awakened in the operating room, extubated, and brought to the recovery room in satisfactory condition.

Code Assignment Including POA Indicator

ICD-9-CM Principal Diagnosis: _____

ICD-9-CM Additional Diagnoses: _____

ICD-9-CM Procedure Code(s): _____

ICD-10-CM Code(s): _____

ICD-10-PCS Code(s): _____

Neoplasms

7.33. Discharge Summary

Date of Admission: 2/3

Date of Discharge: 2/4

Discharge Diagnosis: Malignant ascites from metastatic adenocarcinoma of the colon

Course in Hospital: This 59-year-old white female patient was admitted for continuous infusion chemotherapy with 5-FU and Leucovoran. Patient had a central venous catheter placed in the superior vena cava which was used for the chemotherapy treatment. This was done under the care of Dr. ZXY. The patient tolerated her chemotherapy very well. She had no complications throughout her hospital course, and she was discharged to be followed further as an outpatient by her oncologist.

Instructions on Discharge: Follow up in the office

History and Physical

Admitted: 2/3/20XX

Reason for Admission: Chemotherapy

History of Present Illness: The patient is a 59-year-old white female with peritoneal carcinomatosis and malignant ascites from colon carcinoma. She is admitted for continuous chemotherapy. The patient has a sigmoid colostomy and has had multiple abdominal surgeries for carcinoma; the first one was an anterior and posterior repair in 1982. She had six weeks of radiation therapy completed two years ago and has been on weekly chemotherapy consisting of 5-FU and methotrexate recently. Because of increasing abdominal girth, she was admitted in June and diagnosed with malignant ascites and carcinomatosis. At that time, she had an extensive evaluation including an upper gastrointestinal series, barium enema, CT scan, and ultrasound of the abdomen. She was told she had adhesions causing a partial obstruction. No further surgery was pursued. For the past week, she has complained of frequent vomiting. Her weight has decreased another six pounds. She denies any abdominal pain. She has occasional diarrhea for which she takes Questran. She has had no blood in her colostomy drainage.

Past Medical History: No hypertension, myocardial infarction, diabetes, or peptic ulcer disease. Anterior and posterior repair in 1982, colectomy, cholecystectomy, appendectomy, hysterectomy with bilateral salpingo-oophorectomy for uterine fibroids in 1968.

Allergies: None

Chronic Medications: Pancrease three times a day; Questran as needed for diarrhea; Os-Cal 2× a day, 250 mg

Family History: Mother died at age 80. Father died of colon cancer at age 60.

Social History: Prior to that time, she smoked a pack a day for 20 years. She denies any alcohol intake. She works in the shipping department.

Review of Systems: Unremarkable

Physical Examination: An alert, white female in no acute distress

General Appearance

  Skin, Head, Eyes, Ears, Nose, Throat: Pupils are equal, reactive to light and accommodation. Extraocular movements are intact. Fundi are benign. Tympanic membranes are normal.

  Mouth: No oral lesions are seen.

  HEENT: Within normal limits

  Neck: Carotids are plus 2 with no bruits. Thyroid is normal. There is no adenopathy at present.

  Lungs: Clear

  Heart: Regular sinus rhythm. No murmur, rub, or gallop.

  Breasts: A small, approximately 3-mm, cystic lesion the medial aspect of her left breast at around eight o'clock. It is freely movable and nontender. There are no axillary nodes.

  Abdomen: Distended. Sigmoid colostomy present. Right lower quadrant induration is present. There is no abdominal tenderness. There is no hepatosplenomegaly. Bowel sounds are normal.

  Pulses: Femorals are plus 2 with no bruits. There are good pedal pulses bilaterally.

  Genitalia: Normal

  Rectal: Deferred

  Extremities: No edema

  Neurologic: Deep tendon reflexes are plus 2 throughout

Laboratory Data: Pending

Impression

  Peritoneal carcinomatosis from colon cancer

  Small left breast cyst

Plan: The patient will be admitted for continuous chemotherapy.

Progress Notes

2/3   Patient tolerating chemo well. No complaints offered.

2/4   Patient well hydrated, nausea and vomiting under control. Will discharge.

Code Assignment Including POA Indicator

ICD-9-CM Principal Diagnosis: _____

ICD-9-CM Additional Diagnoses: _____

ICD-9-CM Procedure Code(s): _____

ICD-10-CM Code(s): _____

ICD-10-PCS Code(s): _____

7.34   Discharge Summary

Date of Admission: 1/3

Date of Discharge: 1/7

Discharge Diagnosis: Recurrent carcinoma, left lung

This is a 63-year-old female who is two years status post left upper lobe resection for adenocarcinoma. Pathology at that time revealed a positive bronchial margin of resection. She was treated with postop radiation and has done extremely well. She has remained asymptomatic with no postoperative difficulty. Follow-up serial CT scans have revealed a new lesion in the apical portion of the left lung, which on needle biopsy was positive for adenocarcinoma. She was admitted specifically for a left thoracotomy and possible pneumonectomy.

Past Medical History: Positive for tobacco abuse 2 PPD × 30 years in the past. Significant for a right parotidectomy and also significant for hypertension, degenerative joint disease of lumbar spine, and chronic pulmonary disease. The patient also suffered a stroke in the left brain with resulting hemiparesis three years ago. Medications on discharge: Tenormin 25 mg once a day, Calan SR 240 mg twice a day, Moduretic one tablet q. day, K-Dur 10 meq q. day, Proventil MDI 2 puffs PO q.i.d. p.r.n., Azacort MDI 2 puffs PO t.i.d., Vioxx 25 mg PO daily.

Physical Examination: Revealed a well-healed right parotid incision. No supraclavicular adenopathy. She has a healed left posterior lateral thoracotomy scar. Impression is that of local recurrence, status post left upper lobectomy. She is to undergo a left pneumonectomy.

Operative Findings and Hospital Course: There was a large mass in the remaining lung, extensive mediastinal fibrosis, bronchial margin free by frozen section. Following surgery she was placed in the intensive care unit postoperatively. The chest tube was removed on postoperative day number two.

She experienced some EKG changes consistent with acute nontransmural MI. Cardiology was consulted, and she was started on nitroglycerin and IV heparin. She was eventually weaned from her oxygen therapy.

She was started on regular diet and was discharged in good condition. Her wound was clean and dry.

Instructions on Discharge: Discharged home with instructions to follow up with cardiology next week. Also follow up with me in the office.

History and Physical

Admitted: 1/3

History of Present Illness: Patient is a 63-year-old right-handed female with history of recurrent adenocarcinoma of apical segment of left upper lobe of lung. She has received radiation therapy to her chest. She weighs 123 pounds. She also has chronic obstructive pulmonary disease.

Review of Systems: She can climb two flights of steps with minimal difficulties. She has a significant underbite. She has stiffness in lower spine, worse in the a.m. She has hypertension and took her Tenormin 25 mg, Calan SR 240 mg this a.m.

Past Surgical History: She had a right parotidectomy seven years ago and was told they needed to use a "very small" ETT. Two years ago she underwent a left upper lobe resection at this facility. Previous medical records are being requested.

Allergies: She is allergic to sulfa. Postoperatively last time she received Demerol. She also had hallucinations in the ICU for several days. She blames the hallucinations on the Demerol. The only allergy sign was hallucinations.

Physical Examination: Revealed a well-healed right parotid incision. No supraclavicular adenopathy. She has a healed left posterior lateral thoracotomy scar. Impression is that of local recurrence, status post left upper lobectomy. She is to undergo a left completion pneumonectomy, muscle flap coverage of bronchial stump. The patient has hemiparesis in the right extremities which is her dominant side.

Impression: Recurrent carcinoma left lower lobe of lung

Plan: Pneumonectomy of left lung. The patient is agreeable to general endotracheal anesthesia or the use of epidural narcotic. She is agreeable to postoperative ventilation if necessary.

Progress Notes

1/3   **Attending Physician:** Admit for recurrent lung carcinoma, s/p radiation therapy. Consent signed for pneumonectomy. Epidural morphine usage postop explained to and discussed with the patient. She is agreeable.

         Anesthesia Preop: Patient evaluated and examined. General anesthesia chosen. Patient agrees. Will provide postop epidural morphine for pain management s/p thoracotomy.

         Procedure Note:

         Preop Dx: Local recurrence of carcinoma of the lung

         Postop Dx: Same

         Procedure: Pneumonectomy with muscle flap coverage of bronchial stump

Complications: R/O intraop MI

Anesthesia Postop: Patient in stable condition following GEA with possible intraoperative MI due to hypotension. CPK to be evaluated as available. Patient comfortable with epidural morphine. No adverse effects of anesthesia experienced.

1/4 **Attending Physician:** Path report confirms recurrent adenocarcinoma. Patient stable but with persistent hypotension resolving slowly—will consult cardiology. CPK MB positive. Incision clean and dry. COPD stable, arthritis stable.

Cardiology Consult: The patient has resolving intraoperative myocardial infarction. Will continue to monitor.

1/5 **Attending Physician:** Looks and feels well, weaning off morphine. Blood pressure stable. Left pleural space expanding and filling space. Chest tube removed, epidural cath removed.

Cardiology Consult: The patient looking and feeling better.

1/6 **Attending Physician:** Patient stable for discharge in a.m. Cardiology to follow.

Operative Report

Date: 1/3

Operation: Pneumonectomy

Preoperative Diagnosis: Recurrent carcinoma of left lung

Postoperative Diagnosis: Same

Anesthesia: General endotracheal anesthesia

Operative Findings: There was a large mass in the left lower lobe.

The patient was prepped and draped in the usual fashion. Following thoracotomy the left lung was completely removed. A muscle flap coverage was used for the bronchial stump. During the procedure the patient experienced an episode of hypotension, watch for resulting MI. The patient was fluid resuscitated and sent to the recovery room in good condition.

Pathology Report

Date: 1/3

Specimen: Left lung, resected

Clinical Data: This is a 63-year-old female with recurrent disease on CT scan

Diagnosis: Adenocarcinoma of the apical portion of the lung, bronchial margin is free of disease

Radiology Reports

Date: 1/3

Chest X-Ray: Reveals mass in the left lower lobe. There are surgical clips in the thorax from apparent previous surgery. The thoracic organs are midline and the vasculature is normal.

Impression: Carcinoma LLL, no congestive heart failure

Date: 1/4

Chest X-Ray: Reveals absence of left lung. Other architecture is normal other than post-operative changes. The thoracic organs are midline and the vasculature is normal.

Impression: Postop changes consistent with lobectomy, no congestive heart failure.

EKG Report

Date: 1/3

Normal sinus rhythm

Date: 1/4

There are nonspecific ST changes consistent with possible evolving myocardial infarction.

Date: 1/5

Possible acute myocardial infarction, please correlate with other clinical findings.

Code Assignment Including POA Indicator

ICD-9-CM Principal Diagnosis: _____

ICD-9-CM Additional Diagnoses: _____

ICD-9-CM Procedure Code(s): _____

ICD-10-CM Code(s): _____

7.35.   The following documentation is from the health record of a 50-year-old female patient.

Discharge Summary: The patient is a 50-year-old female with known carcinoma of the right breast with widespread pulmonary and bone metastases. She recently completed the third of six outpatient chemotherapy treatments for the metastases. The patient also has a history of a right mastectomy for the breast carcinoma two years ago and is no longer receiving any treatment for this carcinoma. The patient was now admitted for treatment of lumps of the lower-outer quadrant of the left breast. A left mastectomy with bilateral insertion of tissue expanders has been recommended as treatment for the lumps of the left breast due to the patient's history of right breast carcinoma with metastases. The patient has agreed to the recommended treatment.

The patient was taken to surgery, and a left simple mastectomy was performed. Via an open approach, tissue expanders were inserted under both pectoral muscles bilaterally, to start the reconstruction process.

Pathology report revealed benign fibroadenoma.

The patient was discharged in satisfactory condition to see me in the office in 10 days.

Code Assignment Including POA Indicator

ICD-9-CM Principal Diagnosis: _____

ICD-9-CM Additional Diagnoses: _____

ICD-9-CM Procedure Code(s): _____

ICD-10-CM Code(s): _____

ICD-10-PCS Code(s): _____

7.36. The following documentation is from the health record of a 72-year-old male patient.

Discharge Summary

History of Present Illness: The patient is a 72-year-old male with a history of abdominal perineal resection for colon cancer in 1985 and left hemicolectomy in 1995 for splenic flexure recurrence of cancer. Subsequent right nephrectomy, right adrenalectomy, right posterior hepatic wedge resection in February for metastatic colon carcinoma. The patient is admitted with complaints of lower back pain and bilateral thigh pain for 2 months, increasing in intensity.

Physical Examination: Examination on admission: Temperature 99°F, pulse 72, respirations 24, blood pressure 150/90. The examination was remarkable for left lower quadrant colostomy from previous operation, mildly tender lumbar spine, and the patient was barely able to stand. It was also noted that the patient had decreased sharp/dull discrimination on the neural examination of the lateral thighs.

Laboratory Data: On admission the laboratory values were: Urinalysis: Specific gravity 1.021, pH 5; chem. tests were negative; nitrite negative; blood negative, 12 white cells, moderate bacteria. The clinical chemistry results were: Serum sodium 141, BUN 42, potassium 4.9, chloride 104, CO_2 28, glucose 99, creatinine 1.8, SGOT 12, SGPT 16, alkaline phosphatase 68, total protein 6.6, albumin 3.8, total bilirubin 0.7, direct bilirubin 0.0, GGT 87, calcium 10.3, magnesium 2.0, phosphorus 3.2, uric acid 5.7, PT 12.9, PTT 28.4, white blood cell count 8.0, hemoglobin 15.0, hematocrit 43.8, platelets 223,000. The CEA level was noted to be 508 nanograms per mL on admission. Metastatic workup for the colon carcinoma revealed no evidence of metastatic disease to the head or the thoracic and cervical spine.

Radiologic Studies: CT and MRI revealed left celiac ganglion node plexus enlarged, diagnosed as metastasis. Multiple small lung nodules, bilaterally, suspicious for metastasis. Pathological fractures of L2 and L4, with compression of L2, effacement of the spinal canal space and apparent cord compression at the L2 level. Subsequent urine culture grew out greater than 10 to the 5th *Pseudomonas aeruginosa,* which was sensitive to ciprofloxacin. The patient was treated for this UTI with ciprofloxacin 500 mg p.o. q. 8 hours and subsequent urine culture showed no growth.

Hospital Course: The patient went to the operating room for L2 laminectomy with decompression and anterior allograft bone fusion. The patient fell 3 days after surgery while ambulating without significant injuries. Further physical therapy was marked by continued improvement in ambulation with walker and no further setbacks. Clinically, the patient is afebrile without signs and symptoms of infection, no CVA tenderness, and no dysuria. The patient will be discharged home today. Condition on discharge fairly good.

Treatment: The patient will go home on Vicodin p.o. q 4 to 6 hours for pain, and Capoten. He will resume Capoten b.i.d. dosing per his internist's recommendations for his hypertension, 25 p.o. b.i.d. Prognosis: The long-term prognosis is poor as the patient has extensive metastatic colon CA; short-term prognosis is fairly good with improvement in ambulation. Ambulation is with walker assistance. Follow-up: The patient will return to see me next Wednesday.

Final Diagnoses: Metastatic colon cancer to lung and bone
Pathologic fracture of L2 secondary to metastasis, with cord compression

Code Assignment Including POA Indicator

ICD-9-CM Principal Diagnosis: _____

ICD-9-CM Additional Diagnoses: _____

ICD-9-CM Procedure Code(s): _____

ICD-10-CM Code(s): _____

ICD-10-PCS Code(s): _____

7.37.   The following documentation is from the health record of a 59-year-old cancer patient.

History and Physical Examination

Present Illness: The patient is a 59-year-old female admitted with a diagnosis of seizure disorder and acute seizure. This patient's illness began last year when she was diagnosed with a metastatic lesion in her brain, which was a metastatic hypernephroma from her right kidney. She had the isolated metastasis removed surgically, had been on Tegretol since then, but she has only been taking her nighttime dosages. The dosages she felt kind of wiped her out a little bit. She then was scheduled for renal surgery but developed chest pain, and a coronary angiogram revealed severe three-vessel disease, inoperable and not a candidate for any kind of surgical procedure. Since then her treatment has been expectant with treatment of chemotherapy per usual protocols. She did not have any radiation to the brain previously. Her CT scan in the ER last night was showing some questionable areas.

Past Medical History: She has had the metastatic lesion to the head, renal carcinoma, and severe coronary artery disease. She had no prior surgeries or illnesses.

Review of Systems: Was doing well until yesterday, but she was taking the treatment and taking her Tegretol mainly at night. Her level was 5.9 where 8 or 9 is therapeutic.

Family History: She is adopted but has a brother. She is divorced with two children. She is living with her daughter. She is on disability from work. She was employed actively.

Physical Examination: She is a well-developed, well-nourished white female.

HEENT: Negative

Neck: No bruits

Chest: Clear

Heart: Regular sinus rhythm

Abdomen: Soft; no masses

Pelvic/Rectal: Deferred at this time

Extremities: Negative

Neurologic: Negative. At this time, the daughter states that her right leg and arm stiffened out during her seizure.

Impression(s): Seizure disorder secondary to metastatic renal to brain. She is to get an MRI done today, and we are going to increase dosage to the Tegretol. I think she can go home and if she does have metastatic lesion, she will probably need to have radiation done and will be set up through a radiation oncologist whom I think has been consulted previously on her condition.

Discharge Summary

Admission Date: 06/01/XX

Discharge Date: 06/03/XX

Consultants: 1. Oncologist
                                  2. Neurosurgeon

Discharge Diagnosis

1. Convulsion, secondary to malignant neoplasm of the brain secondary to a hypernephroma

Hospital Course: The patient was seen by the neurosurgeon, who felt conservative management was needed. She is going to begin radiation treatment to her head. This will be done as an outpatient in order to control the metastatic disease to the brain.

Discharge Medications/Instructions: She was discharged home on:

1. Lopressor 50 mg each morning

2. Decadron 4 mg twice a day

3. Tegretol 200 t.i.d. Her Tegretol level was a little low at the time of admission.

So, she will be followed then to begin radiation treatment on Monday for follow-up there.

Consultation

Physical Examination: She is a well-developed, well-nourished white female with partial baldness to the right side of her head. Her neck exam reveals turbulence transmitted from the thorax bilaterally to both carotids. On lung exam there were no crackles or wheezes and her respiratory effort is normal. Cardiac exam reveals S1 and

S2 to be physiologic with no S3 or S4 gallop. There is a murmur at the left ventricular apex most compatible with a flow murmur. The apex is not well palpated. She has no gallop or rub appreciated. Abdominal exam is supple without organomegaly. The back exam is normal. Her extremity exam reveals no clubbing, cyanosis, or edema. HEENT exam reveals partial baldness of the right side of the scalp. There is a well healed craniotomy scar. She has no xanthelasma nor is there any gum bleeding. Her musculature and gait are relatively normal without any obvious lateralizing signs.

Final Assessment: This is a lady who has incredibly severe coronary disease and a poor prognosis with regard to her heart. She tolerated a craniotomy 6 months ago before knowledge of her coronary artery disease. She could probably tolerate another craniotomy but would be at increased risk for a perioperative infarction during general anesthesia. This would be obviously magnified if she had hemodynamic instability. The anticipated surgery would not involve a vascular challenge as would the nephrectomy. Nonetheless, the general anesthetic would pose a cardiovascular risk that seems to be unpreventable. The plan is to proceed with radiation and reserve surgery for nonavoidable indication. I have discussed this with the radiation oncologist, and the patient is most agreeable with this sort of approach as well. I hope this information can be of some help to you. Thanks again.

History of Present Illness: This 59-year-old woman is well known to me, undergoing craniotomy for resection of a metastatic renal cell carcinoma in January of 20XX. At that time she presented with weakness of her left upper and lower extremity. She was continued on a daily Tegretol dose as she did not tolerate Dilantin. She was doing well until she presented with a generalized tonic clonic seizure yesterday and postictal Todd's paralysis which is now resolving. She was brought to the hospital, underwent a CT scan and subsequent MRI scan that does show a solitary lesion in the postoperative bed consistent with recurrence of her metastatic disease. She has never received whole brain radiation postoperatively. Currently she tells me her right kidney was never resected as she has significant cardiovascular disease and was thought by the cardiologist not to be able to tolerate a nephrectomy. Currently treatment options include:

1. Whole brain radiation
2. Surgical removal of the lesion followed by whole brain radiation if she can obtain surgical clearance
3. Possibility of doing stereotactic radiosurgery on the lesion, again followed by whole brain radiation

Recommendations: Currently, I have placed the patient on Decadron 400 mg twice daily and will ask the neurosurgeon and his associates to evaluate the possibility of a craniotomy on the patient.

Which of the following is the correct code assignment?

ICD-9-CM Code(s):

a. 198.3, 189.0, 780.39, 414.01
b. 780.39, 198.3, 189.0, 414.01
c. 189.0, 198.3, 780.39, 414.01
d. 198.3, 189.0, 414.01

ICD-10-CM Code(s): _____

Optional MS-DRG Exercise (for users with access to MS-DRG software or tables)

What is the correct MS-DRG for this case? _____

Which MDC does this MS-DRG belong to? _____

Disorders of the Nervous System and Sense Organs

7.38.   The following documentation is from the health record of a 62-year-old male patient.

Discharge Summary

Admission Diagnosis: Transient ischemic attack, possible stroke

Final Diagnoses

1. Transient vertigo versus posterior circulation transient ischemic attack

2. Non-insulin-dependent diabetes

3. Coronary artery disease status post coronary bypass grafting

4. Hyperlipidemia

Consultants: Neurology

History

This is a 62-year-old white male who was admitted through the Emergency Department with a variety of symptoms, somewhat vague, describing components of dizziness, double vision, slightly slurred speech, vague numbness and tingling of the upper extremities for two or possibly three days. He has had intermittent different episodes off and on over the last two to three months. The patient has several risk factors including coronary disease, hyperlipidemia, and he is a smoker. He was admitted with possible TIAs or CVA.

Hospital Course: After being admitted to the Intermediate Care Unit and Stepdown Unit for monitoring and being started on Heparin, his symptoms resolved very rapidly.

Diagnostics: A CT of the brain indicated a possible ischemic event in the right frontoparietal region and an old lacunar infarct to the basal ganglia on the right. The chest x-ray showed mild congestive heart failure, although this was not clinically apparent. Carotid studies showed minimal abnormalities with approximately 30% disease on the left internal carotid. The right side was normal.

An echocardiogram of the heart indicated minor valvular abnormalities of no significance and an ejection fraction of 35–40%, and no embolic clots were noted. A routine cardiogram showed some old findings of left anterior hemiblock.

As mentioned, the patient's symptoms rapidly resolved. He was seen in consultation by Dr. G. the following morning who felt that he did not need IV heparin for the current event and that aspirin should be sufficient. Some consideration was given that if he had future episodes, of starting either Plavix or possible long-term Coumadin. Arrangements were made for discharge, as the patient's basic clinical status has returned to baseline.

Discharge Medications

1. Glucophage 500 mg b.i.d.
2. Glyburide 5 mg b.i.d.
3. Lipitor 20 mg daily
4. Ecotrin 325 mg daily

Discharge Instructions

Diet—ADA diet, low fat. He was advised at length about smoking cessation. Activity—As tolerated, but no heavy exertion. It was suggested that at some point the patient have an MRI and an MRA as an outpatient and consideration be given to stronger anticoagulation if he has further episodes. Follow-up in the office in approximately one to two weeks.

Emergency Department

History of Present Illness: This is a 62-year-old male who complains of five days of dizziness and three days of weakness, decreasing ambulation, and unsteadiness. He complains of no pain or numbness of the lower extremities, chest pain, fever, or headache. He does complain of having mild vision blurring with turning when he turns his head. The patient has also had slurring of his speech. He was seen yesterday by his private physician who noticed his ataxia and has him scheduled for a magnetic resonance imaging today.

Past Medical History

1. Diabetes mellitus
2. Myocardial infarction times three in the past
3. Coronary artery bypass graft done in the last five years
4. Hypertension
5. Mild neuropathy secondary to his diabetes mellitus

Social History: The patient lives in a private home by himself. He smokes two packs of cigarettes a day. He denies any drinking.

Medications

1. Glucophage
2. Talacen

Allergies: No known allergies.

Review of Systems: Negative except for the pertinent positives and negatives noted in the history of present illness.

Physical Examination

Vital Signs: Temperature is 97. Pulse of 84. Respirations 20. Blood pressure 132/73. General: The patient is mildly sleepy but very alert and cooperative with the examination. HEENT: He is normocephalic. Atraumatic. He has some mild preauricular swelling on the right as compared to the left. His tympanic membranes were normal bilaterally. Extraocular muscles intact. Pupils equal, round, reactive to light and accommodation. Oral pharynx is normal. He did have some staining consistent with tobacco.

Neck: Supple. No adenopathy.

Heart: Regular rate and rhythm without any murmurs, thrills, or rubs. He has 2+ pulses radial and brachial bilaterally.

Lungs: Breath sounds are clear bilaterally with no tachypnea or retraction.

Abdomen: Mildly tender at the left upper quadrant over the rib area. Otherwise the abdomen was soft and nondistended.

Extremities: He had upper and lower extremity strength of +5.

Neurology: There is 212 and grossly intact. He had no pitting edema or other lesions noted. The patient was ataxic.

Laboratory and Diagnostics: Labs were obtained. Basic metabolic profile showed a sodium of 138, potassium 4.0, chloride of 107, bicarbonate of 22, glucose of 106, blood urea nitrogen of 21, and creatinine of 0.8. Calcium is 9.4. PT and partial prothrombin time were 13.2 and 29.8. White blood cell count was 11.4. H&H is 15.4 and 45.7. He had 222,000 platelets, 62 segs, 29 lymphs, 4 monocytes, 3 eosinopllils, and no basophils. CT scan of the head showed a new infarction of the brain and old lacunar infarct.

Emergency Room Course: We talked to the primary care doctor who agreed with the admission of this patient.

Plan: The patient was admitted to a monitored bed. Assisting physician helped coordinate the care, management, and treatment of this patient with myself. The patient is being admitted to the primary care doctor's service.

Neurologic Consultation

History: This is a 62-year-old white male whom we were asked to evaluate regarding dizziness and a possible new stroke.

The patient's neurologic history recently appears to date back to approximately one month ago when he developed what he described as some double vision. He was seeing things side by side. He did see his primary care physician who felt this may have been due to a diabetic extraocular movement palsy, and the patient was given a patch. After three weeks, his symptoms resolved. Around that same time, about a month ago, he noticed some numbness and tingling in his fingertips which at times is still bothersome. He was doing fine until this past Saturday when he had the onset of what sounds like dysequilibrium or vertigo where he had difficulty walking. This was transient and then seemed to resolve. This is not currently a problem for him now, and he is much better. The patient tells me that his son told him he may have had some slurred speech, but he is not aware of it. He reported no other specific symptoms. Specifically, he reported no headache. He denies any new change in his vision in the last week. He reported no other areas of focal numbness or tingling.

He reported no trouble with focal weakness. He felt like his balance was only off for a short period of time but then resolved. His bowel and bladder function had been fine. He has had no nausea or vomiting. He denies any chest pain, palpitations, or shortness of breath. He did see his primary care physician who told him that some of his problems may have been related to recent medication change and felt that otherwise he would be okay. However, when seeing the physician the day of admission, he was noted to be somewhat ataxic and was admitted to rule out a new stroke.

Laboratory Data: Current blood work on admission showed normal electrolytes. Digoxin level was less than 0.3. CPK levels have been normal. White count was 11.4 with the remainder of his CBC normal. INR was normal at 1.3. He has remained neurologically stable since admission.

Diagnostics: MRI and MRA are pending. Echocardiogram was grossly suboptimal with an ejection fraction of 35% to 40%. Carotid ultrasound preliminarily showed no stenosis. Heparin is on hold at this time pending our evaluation and the results of the MRI and MRA.

Current Medications

1. Glucophage
2. Insulin coverage
3. Lasix
4. DiaBeta
5. Lipitor

Neurologic Examination: On exam, the patient is awake and alert. He is fully oriented. He is able to name and repeat. Attention, concentration, and memory are okay. Cranial nerves II–XII are grossly intact. Neck is supple with no bruits. Motor exam appears symmetric with no significant focal weakness. He has fairly good bulk and tone. There is no tremor. Sensory exam is remarkable for stocking glove sensory loss. Reflexes are symmetric and somewhat diminished in the lower extremities. Gait is only minimally wide based and he is able to ambulate on his own without any clear ataxia noted at this time. Coordination testing is symmetric. Romberg is negative. He does have difficulty with heel-to-toe walk.

Impression: The patient presents now with transient vertigo along with some slurred speech. This combined with the recent history of double vision certainly warrants a workup for vertebrobasilar insufficiency.

Recommendations

Echocardiogram as done

Carotid ultrasound as done

MRI and MRA as done

IF MRI and MRA are negative, along with the other studies, then treatment with antiplatelet therapy is certainly reasonable.

Physical therapy

Blood pressure and blood sugar control while avoiding relative hypotension

We will likely need to stop heparin or discontinue its use even while being held, as long as studies appear normal. If all of this is okay, and the patient is stable on his feet, discharge then could be shortly.

Code Assignment Including POA Indicator

ICD-9-CM Principal Diagnosis: _____

ICD-9-CM Additional Diagnoses: _____

ICD-10-CM Code(s): _____

7.39.   The following documentation is from the health record of a 67-year-old female patient.

Discharge Summary

This is a 67-year-old lady with complaints of low back pain, with radiation down her right leg to her foot. This pain has been progressively worse over the past 6 months. She had an MRI scan that showed degenerative disc disease at L2–L3, L3–L4, and L4–L5; L3–L4 with mild central canal stenosis; and facet arthropathy at L3–L4 and L4–L5. She has a past medical history of coronary artery disease, hypertension, and lumbar osteoarthritis. Her current medications include Lipitor, Avapro, Ecotrin, Imdur, Lasix, K-Dur, calcium, and Vioxx. She had a CABG 2 years ago. She also had PTCA with cardiac stents placed 3 years ago. Patient is admitted for lumbar epidural steroid injections for her lumbar radiculopathy—as noted on MRI results.

Which of the following is the correct code assignment?

ICD-9-CM Code(s):

a. 722.52, 721.3, 724.02, 724.4, 414.00, 401.9, V45.81, V45.82, 03.92, 99.23, 88.93
b. 724.4, 414.00, 401.9, V45.81, V45.82, 03.92, 99.23, 88.93
c. 722.52, 721.3, 414.00, 401.9, V45.81, V45.82, 03.92, 99.23, 88.93
d. 722.52, 721.3, 414.00, 401.9, V45.81, V45.82, 03.91, 88.93

ICD-10-CM Code(s): _____

ICD-10-PCS Code(s): _____

Optional MS-DRG Exercise (for users with access to MS-DRG software or tables)

Which of the following statements is true regarding the MS-DRG assignment for this case?

a. This case is assigned to a medical MS-DRG.
b. This case is assigned to a surgical MS-DRG.
c. MS-DRG assignment is changed based on the procedure code (03.92).
d. The MS-DRG assigned to this case falls into MDC 1, diseases and disorders of the nervous system.

Newborn/Congenital Disorders

7.40. The following documentation is from the health record of an 18-day-old baby boy.

Discharge Summary

This is an 18-day-old male infant who was admitted after he was noticed to be developing omphalitis. He was immediately placed on intravenous cefotaxime and ampicillin, later changed to cefotaxime and clindamycin. A culture taken from the umbilical stump grew *Staphylococcus aureus* and group H *Streptococcus*.

After the first day, there was great improvement, and the patient continued to improve completely. Now there is no redness or swelling whatsoever. The child has remained afebrile and has continued to eat very well. He shows no sign of abdominal tenderness or peritonitis. I feel that we have treated this well. He has had 5 days of intravenous antibiotics. I will finish the treatment with Keflex by mouth seeing that both *Streptococcus pyogenes* and *Staphylococcus aureus* are sensitive. The mother will watch the child closely and let me know if any problems occur. I have instructed her to watch for any more redevelopment of the redness, swelling, or discharge. We will recheck this in 2 weeks at his 1-month checkup.

Which of the following answers contains the correct diagnostic code(s) for this admission?

ICD-9-CM Code(s):

a. 771.2, 041.09
b. 686.9, 041.11, 041.09
c. 771.4
d. 771.4, 041.11, 041.09

ICD-10-CM Code(s): _____

7.41. The following documentation is from the health record of a three-day-old baby boy.

Discharge Summary

The patient is a 3-day-old male infant. He was born at home after approximately 38 weeks' gestation and brought to the Emergency Room shortly thereafter with difficulty breathing. The baby's respirations were very quick and shallow. This was the mother's fourth child, all of whom have been born at home. This was the first child born with complications.

The newborn was resuscitated and placed in the NICU under continuous oxygen therapy.

Admission history and physical examination were otherwise unremarkable. Chest x-ray showed wet lungs. Repeat chest x-ray 24 hours later showed the lungs had cleared. PKU specimen was taken and sent to the state laboratory, as required.

By the second day of hospitalization, the patient was able to be weaned off the oxygen and discharged from the NICU to a bassinet.

The mother requested that the baby be circumcised. This was accomplished without incident.

The infant is discharged to be seen in the clinic at 1 month for a well-baby visit.

Which of the following answers is correct to code this admission?

ICD-9-CM Code(s):

a. 770.6, V30.10, V50.2, 96.04
b. V30.1, 770.6, V50.2, 64.0, 93.93, 93.96
c. V30.1, 769, V50.2, 64.0, 96.04
d. V30.10, 768.6, V50.2, 64.0, 96.05, 93.96

ICD-10-CM Code(s): _____

ICD-10-PCS Code(s): _____

Optional MS-DRG Exercise (for users with access to MS-DRG software or tables)

In addition to the principal diagnosis, the MS-DRG for this admission is based upon which of the following factors listed below?

a. Complication or comorbid condition
b. Major complication or comorbid condition
c. Procedure code
d. Other significant problems

7.42.   The patient is a 3-year-old child with congenital patent ductus arteriosus. The patient has had several open-heart surgeries attempting to correct the defect. The patient was born prematurely at 34 weeks' gestation. The patient continues to be below average on standard growth charts in size and weight, and the mother states the child is not very active.

Recent echocardiogram revealed an area of the aorta leaking blood into the pulmonary artery. The child is now admitted for further corrective surgery.

On the day after admission, the child was taken to the OR. Open-chest surgery was performed through the existing scar, and the ribs were spread to gain access to the operative field. Several areas of communication between the aorta and the left pulmonary artery were identified and closed. The chest was then closed. Throughout the procedure, the patient's vital signs were monitored and remained at satisfactory levels. The patient tolerated the procedure well.

The day after surgery, the patient was allowed to be up and walking. The child appeared to have increased energy and was a healthy pink color. The child was eating and asking for more.

The patient was discharged on the third postop day to be followed as an outpatient in the cardiac education center.

Final Diagnosis: Patent ductus arteriosus

Which of the following answers is correct to code this admission?

ICD-9-CM Code(s):

a. 747.0, 765.10, 765.27, 38.85
b. 745.9, 35.39
c. 747.0, 38.85
d. 745.0, 38.85

ICD-10-CM Code(s): _____

ICD-10-PCS Code(s): _____

7.43. The following documentation is from the health record of a five-year-old girl.

Discharge Summary

The patient is a 5-year-old female child born with myelomeningocele spina bifida. The patient has previously undergone several procedures to cover the defect at the bottom of her spine, including the insertion of a ventriculoperitoneal (VP) shunt to drain the cerebrospinal fluid (CSF) accumulation from her hydrocephalus.

The patient was admitted this morning through the emergency department with a plugged shunt. The child was rushed to the OR for emergent irrigation of the shunt. Irrigation was attempted several times but was unsuccessful. Therefore, the shunt was removed and replaced with another VP shunt.

The patient tolerated the procedure, although she was very anxious about having surgery and being in the hospital. Her parents were very caring and present to calm her at all times.

The patient was discharged on the second day postop to be followed in the office.

Final Diagnoses: Congenital myelomeningocele spina bifida
                                Plugged VP shunt

Which of the following answers is correct to code this admission?

ICD-9-CM Code(s):

a. 996.75, 741.03, 02.42
b. 996.2, 741.03, 02.41, 02.42
c. 741.03, V45.2, 02.42, 02.43
d. 996.75, 742.3, 741.00, 02.42

ICD-10-CM Code(s): _____

ICD-10-PCS Code(s): _____

Pediatric Conditions

7.44.   The following documentation is from the health record of a 13-year-old boy.

Preoperative Diagnosis:	Right inguinal hernia, hypospadias
Postoperative Diagnosis:	Same
Operation:	Right inguinal herniorrhaphy, repair of hypospadias

Indications: The patient is a 13-year-old male with reducible right inguinal hernia and hypospadias who now presents for definitive care.

Procedure: The patient was brought to the operating room and placed in the supine position. After the adequate general endotracheal anesthesia, a 4-cm incision was made in the right inguinal region. The subcutaneous tissues were divided, and hemostasis achieved with electrocautery. The external oblique fascia was identified and cleaned using Metzenbaum scissors. An incision was made in the external oblique and carried down to the external ring using Metzenbaum scissors. The external oblique was freed from the underlying cord using two pairs of forceps. The cremasteric fibers were divided and the hernia sac grasped. Pulling the hernia sac up on some tension, we were then able to tease off the cremasteric fibers, as well as the vas and vessels. At this point, we were able to control the hernia sac between the two hemostats. We then teased off the vas and vessels as we dissected proximally toward the internal ring. At this point, the sac was twisted, sutured ligated, × 2, amputated, and then the sac was allowed to fall back into the peritoneal cavity. We continued the dissection distally. The anterior wall was opened using electrocautery. At this point, we placed the cord back into the inguinal canal. The external oblique fascia was closed using interrupted 4-0 silk sutures. The external oblique fascia and the structures below it were infiltrated using .05 percent Marcaine. The Scarpa's fascia was closed using 5-0 VICRYL. The skin was closed using interrupted 5-0 subcuticular stitches. Steri-Strips were applied.

With this completed, attention was then turned to repairing the hypospadias. Procedure commenced by placing a 4-0 Prolene stay suture through the glans for traction and observing the distal shaft penile hypospadias without chordee and with a dorsal hooded foreskin.

The urethroplasty was begun by making parallel lines with a marking pen on either side of the urethral meatus, going out to the tip of the glans, connecting these proximally from the meatus for a distance of about 2.5 cm. With a tourniquet used intermittently, an incision was made in these lines to create two rectangular flaps connected at the urethral meatus. On the left side of the meatus there was a small nevus just lateral to the incision line, and the incision was extended around this to excise a small nevus, less than 0.6 cm in diameter, which will be sent for pathology. After mobilization of both skin flaps, the proximal one off of the shaft and the ventral one off of the underlying tissue of the glans, optical magnification was used to convert these two flaps into a neourethral tube using 6-0 PDS sutures. The neourethral tube came together quite well.

Next, an incision was made in the midline, out to the tip of the glans, through the incision point at the previous site of the distal flap, to accomplish mobilization of the urethra and advance this urethra out to the tip of the glans. Wedge-shaped areas of glandular tissue were excised to make a smooth passageway for the neourethra. Then the neourethra was sutured into position at the tip of the glans with 6-0 and 5-0 PDS sutures.

Next, a second layer was created by approximating the subcutaneous tissue, adventitial tissue, and elements of the corpus spongiosum over the neourethral reconstruction at the corona, and carrying this with a running 6-0 PDS suture proximally to provide a second layer of coverage.

When this was done, the glans itself was approximated with 4-0 PDS sutures, placing about three sutures into position to firmly reconnect the wings of the glans and to keep them from pulling apart. This left an aperture for the neourethra, which was then sutured into position with 4-0 and 5-0 PDS sutures. When this was done, a #11 French Silastic catheter was used, and a portion of its wall was cut out to turn it into a splint. It was positioned into the urethra and sutured into place at the meatus with a 4-0 Prolene suture to hold it into position. The next step was to close the skin defect on the ventral shaft with interrupted 3-0 chromic catgut suture.

The next part of the operation involved performing circumcision of the redundant dorsal and lateral preputial tissue. First, this was marked with a marking pen, and then an incision was made in the pen lines to allow excision of the redundant foreskin. Hemostasis was obtained with electrocautery, and 3-0 chromic catgut suture was used to complete the circumcision.

The next step was to consider the ability of this patient to void. Because of his hernial repair and this operation on the prepuce, I was afraid he would be in urinary retention. I therefore inserted a #8 French feeding tube through the #11 French Silastic catheter, passed it all the way into the bladder, and allowed it to drain urine freely. Then a light sterile dressing of 1-inch Adaptic roller gauze soaked in tincture of benzoin was loosely wrapped around the shaft for mild compression and hemostasis. The last few wraps of this incorporated the catheter.

The patient was taken to the recovery room in satisfactory condition.

Which of the following code sets is correct for reporting this operative episode?

ICD-9-CM Code(s):

a. 752.61, 550.91, 752.69, 58.49, 53.02, 64.0, 57.94
b. 752.61, 605, 550.90, 239.5, 58.47, 53.01, 64.2, 57.94
c. 752.61, 550.91, 752.69, 58.49, 53.00, 57.94
d. 752.61, 605, 550.90, 222.1, 58.45, 53.02, 64.0, 64.2, 57.94

ICD-10-CM Code(s): _____

ICD-10-PCS Code(s): _____

7.45. The following documentation is from the health record of an 11-year-old boy.

Preoperative Diagnoses: 1. Ewing sarcoma, left scapula
2. Down syndrome

Postoperative Diagnosis: Same

Findings: This is an 11-year-old boy with Down syndrome who presented 4 days ago with a large mass in the left scapular region. Outpatient x-ray and CT scan showed laminated new bone with a large, expansile, permeative lesion in the scapular body. It did not appear to involve the glenohumeral joint. Outpatient bone scan showed marked increased uptake and questionable area of uptake in the right seventh rib and left first vertebral body. CT of the lungs was reportedly normal. At the time of biopsy, there was obvious stretching of the posterior trapezius and deltoid musculature over the mass and a very soft calcific mass noted within the central area of the substance. Frozen pathology sections showed many small cells, but definitive diagnosis could not be made off the frozen section. Final pathologic diagnosis was malignant bone tumor consistent with Ewing sarcoma. He will be started on a chemotherapy program, and definitive surgery will be planned.

Procedure: Following an adequate level of general endotracheal anesthesia, the patient was turned to the right lateral decubitus position with the left side up. The left shoulder region was prepped and draped in routine sterile fashion. Before beginning the biopsy, a venous access device was inserted into the subcutaneous tissue of the abdominal wall on the right side using an open approach.

A 3-cm incision was then made over the spine of the scapula. Electrocautery was used for hemostasis and the incision deepened with electrocautery. When we were in the area of the soft-tissue mass noted on the CT scan, biopsies were taken. The initial biopsies showed primarily muscle fibers, so we deepened the incision at this point and obtained some of the obvious calcific soft-tissue mass. These cultures were more consistent with tumor, and, at this point, hemostasis was achieved with a combination of bone wax, packing, and electrocautery. Meticulous hemostasis was achieved prior to closure, and then a two-layer interrupted closure was performed, closing the skin with a running subcuticular suture of 4-0 VICRYL. Bulky dry sterile dressing was applied, and the patient was awakened and returned to the recovery room in good condition.

Which of the following is the correct code set to report this procedure?

ICD-9-CM Code(s):

a. 170.4, 758.0, 77.41
b. 170.4, 170.3, 170.2, 77.81
c. 170.4, 758.0, 77.61, 86.07
d. 170.4, 758.0, 77.41, 86.07

ICD-10-CM Code(s): _____

ICD-10-PCS Code(s): _____

Optional MS-DRG Exercise (for users with access to MS-DRG software or tables)

What is the correct MS-DRG assignment for this admission?

a. 517, Other musculoskeletal system and connective tissue OR procedure without CC/MCC

b. 497, Local excision and removal internal fixation devices except hip and femur without CC/MCC

c. 479, Biopsies of musculoskeletal system and connective tissue without CC/MCC

d. 477, Biopsies of musculoskeletal system and connective tissue with MCC

Conditions of Pregnancy, Childbirth, and the Puerperium

7.46. The following documentation is from the health record of a 19-year-old female patient.

Discharge Diagnosis:
1. Term pregnancy
2. Previous cesarean section
3. Failed attempt at vaginal birth after cesarean delivery
4. Arrest of descent, secondary to occiput posterior position

Procedures Performed: Repeat low transverse cesarean delivery

History of Present Illness: The patient is a 19-year-old, gravida 3, para 1 with an estimated date of delivery in two weeks. She is with a 37-week-plus pregnancy. She has prior beta strep culture, positive. She underwent spontaneous rupture of membranes. Upon admission, the patient's membranes were ruptured.

Hospital Course: The patient was started on intravenous Clindamycin for positive group B strep. Further, she was started on Pitocin for induction of labor because of the premature rupture of membranes. The patient had a slow labor course, eventually establishing a good labor curve. She dilated completely to a zero station but failed to descend with pushing. Then the decision was made to perform a low transverse cesarean delivery because of arrest of descent. She underwent a cesarean delivery without complications. Estimated blood loss was 600 cc. This resulted in delivery of a live male infant weighing 7 pounds 4 ounces having Apgars of 9 at one minute and 9 at five minutes.

Postoperatively, the patient did well. She was ambulating and tolerating her diet. She was afebrile and her incision looked clear so the patient was discharged home on the third postoperative day.

Medications/Aftercare Plan

1. The patient is to limit her activity around the home for a one-week period.

2. She will be followed up in the office in one to two weeks.

3. Birth control method was discussed and the patient is considering Depo-Provera. She will finalize her decision on this and let us know in the office.

The patient's discharge medications consist of:

1. Motrin 800 mg one every eight hours p.r.n.
2. Tylenol #3 1–2 every four hours p.r.n.
3. The patient should continue her prenatal vitamins and irons.
4. Colace 100 mg b.i.d.
5. There are no diet restrictions.

Assign the correct codes:

ICD-9-CM Principal Diagnosis: _____

ICD-9-CM Additional Diagnoses: _____

ICD-9-CM Procedure Code(s): _____

ICD-10-CM Code(s): _____

ICD-10-PCS Code(s): _____

7.47.   Discharge Summary

Date of Admission: 2/3

Date of Discharge: 2/5

Discharge Diagnosis: Full-term pregnancy—delivered male infant

Patient started labor spontaneously three days before her due date. She was brought to the hospital by automobile. Labor progressed for a while but then contractions became fewer and she delivered soon after. A midline episiotomy was done. Membranes and placenta were complete. There was some bleeding but not excessive. Patient made an uneventful recovery.

History and Physical

Admitted: 2/3

Reason for Admission: Full-term pregnancy

Past Medical History: Previous deliveries normal and mitral valve prolapse

Allergies: None known

Chronic Medications: None

Family History: Heart disease—father

Social History: The patient is married and has one other child living with her.

Review of Systems

  Skin: Normal

  Head/Scalp: Normal

  Eyes: Normal

  ENT: Normal

  Neck: Normal

  Breasts: Normal

  Thorax: Normal

  Lungs: Normal

Heart: Slight midsystolic click with late systolic murmur II/VI

Abdomen: Normal

Impression: Good health with term pregnancy. History of mitral valve prolapse—asymptomatic

Progress Notes

2/3: Admit to Labor and Delivery. MVP stable. Patient progressing well. Delivered at 1:15 p.m. one full-term male infant.

2/4: Patient doing well. MVP prolapse stable. The perineum is clean and dry, incision intact.

2/5: Will discharge to home.

Delivery Record

Date: 2/3

The patient was 3 cm dilated when admitted. The duration of the first stage of labor was 6 hours, second stage was 14 minutes, third stage was 5 minutes. She was given local anesthesia. An episiotomy was performed with episiorrhaphy repair. The cord was wrapped once around the baby's neck, but did not cause compression. The mother and liveborn baby were discharged from the delivery room in good condition.

Code Assignment Including POA Indicator

ICD-9-CM Principal Diagnosis: _____

ICD-9-CM Additional Diagnoses: _____

ICD-9-CM Procedure Code(s): _____

ICD-10-CM Code(s): _____

ICD-10-PCS Code(s): _____

7.48. The following documentation is from the health record of a 32-year-old female patient.

Inpatient admission: The patient, gravida II, para 1, was admitted at approximately 33 weeks gestation with mild contractions. She was contracting every 7-8 minutes. An ultrasound showed twins of approximately 4 pounds each. The patient was given magnesium sulfate to stop the contractions, but she contracted through the drug. After developing a fever with suspected chorioamnionitis, a low cervical cesarean section was performed. The umbilical cord was wrapped tightly around the neck of twin 1.

Discharge diagnoses: Cesarean delivery of liveborn twins prematurely at 33 weeks gestation; chorioamnionitis; umbilical cord compression.

Code Assignment Including POA Indicator

ICD-9-CM Principal Diagnosis: _____

ICD-9-CM Additional Diagnoses: _____

ICD-9-CM Procedure Code(s): _____

ICD-10-CM Code(s): _____

ICD-10-PCS Code(s): _____

7.49.   **Discharge Summary**

Admission Diagnosis: A 38-week intrauterine pregnancy with leaking amniotic fluid

Discharge Diagnosis: Postpartum female—status post classical cesarean section secondary to prolonged second stage of labor; endomyometritis, postoperative ileus, persistent fever—suspected septic pelvic thrombophlebitis; wound seroma

Operative Procedure: Classical cesarean section

Admission History: This is a 26-year-old gravida 1, para 0 female who presented at 38 weeks gestation complaining of leaking fluid in the morning. She had very mild leaking noted. She had positive nitrazine. She had no gush of fluid at that time and good fetal movement. She had some mild cramping and minimal contractions. No nausea, vomiting, headache, or shortness of breath. No chest pain. Her pregnancy had been uncomplicated. She has had mildly elevated blood pressures over the past couple of weeks, but otherwise nothing significant.

Past medical and social history is negative.

Ob-Gyn History: She is gravida 1

OB Laboratory Data: Blood type is O positive. Antibody screen negative. HIV negative. GBS negative. Rubella nonimmune. RPR nonreactive. Hepatitis B negative.

Objective

Vital Signs: Stable; BP: Elevated at 152/102; it did come down between the 130 to 140s/70 to 80

Lungs: Clear to auscultation

Heart: Regular rate and rhythm

Abdomen: Soft and nontender

Pelvic: Cervix is 1 cm, 70% effaced, and –2 station. The amniotic bag could still be palpated, but it was thought that the patient might be leaking fluid; therefore, artificial rupture of membranes was performed with clear fluid. Tocol showed irregular contractions.

Assessment and Plan: Term intrauterine pregnancy at 38 weeks with mild leaking of fluid. The patient is admitted, and she is given an IV Hep-lock with expectant management.

Hospital Course: The patient did require Pitocin augmentation, as after several hours, she was not contracting adequately. She progressed slowly but adequately over the next 24 hours. She was completely dilated at approximately 7:00 in the morning. She began pushing. She pushed for 3 hours. The baby progressed from a +1 to a +2–3 station. She had no further progression. She was counseled on the risks regarding cesarean section versus forceps delivery. The patient did elect for a cesarean section. She is, therefore, taken for a C-section; see operative report for details. The patient did undergo a classical cesarean section due to the fact that the fetal head could not be reduced from the vagina, and a classical was performed in order to grab the fetal feet and deliver in a breech fashion.

Postoperatively the patient did become febrile within a few hours, and this was felt to be caused by endomyometritis due to the prolonged rupture, prolonged labor, and the significant manipulation of the uterus with cesarean section. The patient was started on Ancef during the procedure and was started on gentamicin within 12 hours of the surgery. The patient continued on IV antibiotics. Her temperature continued to spike on a fairly regular basis over the next 2 postoperative days. She was tolerating a regular diet and ambulating, in addition to passing minimal flatus. On postoperative day 1 she did have a fever as high as 103°F with a tachycardic episode in the 160s. She was somewhat lightheaded when she was out of bed to go to the restroom, but improved with rest. Her heart rate did decrease at that point. An EKG was done and this showed sinus tachycardia. She denied any shortness of breath or chest pain. No nausea or vomiting. Her laboratory studies showed her hemoglobin to be 8.9, white count 12, with a morning repeat of 8.8 and a white count of 9. Blood cultures also were done at that time.

On postoperative day 2, the patient was beginning to feel distended. Her pain was getting worse secondary to the descent. She denied any shortness of breath or chest pain. She was still passing some flatus, but minimal. No nausea or vomiting. On examination her temperature was 103.3°F, which was the maximum. Her abdomen is soft; however, she did have moderate to severe distention at that time. She had good bowel sounds in all the quadrants. Her incision was intact. The extremities showed no calf tenderness. A chest x-ray was done because of the continued elevated temperature; there was bowel distension and suspected ileus. Abdominal x-rays were then done which did confirm an ileus, but no signs of bowel obstruction. Her hemoglobin was repeated and showed 7.4 with stable platelets. Blood cultures were negative, as well as her urine. BUN and creatinine were normal. The patient was made n.p.o. and given an NG tube for the postoperative ileus. She did note some relief to her abdominal discomfort and pain. She was afebrile throughout most of the day at that time. The NG tube had 250 cc out initially.

On postoperative day 3, the NG tube was continued, and her belly was somewhat less distended. She continued to pass flatus and her pain was otherwise controlled. Her temperature was 101.6°F, and clindamycin was added to the antibiotic regimen to treat the persistent fevers. On examination, her distention was improved. She was still having some bowel sounds, although hypoactive. The incision showed no significant erythema. Blood cultures remained negative, and the NG tube was continued with intermittent suction.

On postoperative day 4, the patient was feeling better and producing stools. No nausea or vomiting or shortness of breath, chest pain, dizziness, or lightheadedness. She was having normal lochia and pain was controlled. The NG tube had collected a minimal amount overnight, and her temperature was 101.6°F. She was then started on a clear diet and, if tolerated, the NG tube was to be discontinued. Her hemoglobin level was 6.9, with a decreased potassium level of 3.2. All other lab work was essentially normal. The NG tube was discontinued, and she was given KCl to replace her potassium.

On postoperative day 5, she continued to be febrile with a temperature of 101.5°F. The abdomen was soft and nondistended. She was appropriately tender, more on the left side than the right. The incision still appeared well. Laboratory studies showed the hemoglobin to be 6.8 and stable. Her potassium continued to decrease to 3.1. At that time a CT of the abdomen and pelvis was ordered to rule out a pelvic abscess. *C. difficile* was ordered due to continued diarrhea. Another physician was consulted. A suspicion of septic pelvic thrombophlebitis was then entertained as her fever continued despite adequate antibiotic therapy. The patient was started on Lovenox, and the CT scan showed normal postoperative changes, but no evidence of an abscess.

On postoperative day 6, she was feeling better and had no further diarrhea. *C. difficile* was negative and she was tolerating a regular diet. Her incision did show some erythema, and it was probed with some serosanguineous drainage from the left side, but no purulent drainage. Her laboratory studies were stable, and she was continued on Lovenox and antibiotics. The incision was to be cleaned twice daily.

Postoperative day 7, the patient continued to improve and was feeling well. She was tolerating a regular diet and remained afebrile in which she remained for 27 hours and therefore was discharged home.

Consultation Report: The patient is a 26-year-old female who is gravida 1, now para 1. The patient required a C-section because of prolonged labor and maternal exhaustion. The patient was ruptured for a little over 24 hours prior to delivery. The C-section was complicated by the inability to reduce the fetal head from the vaginal canal and was converted to a breech extraction; therefore, the patient had a primary low transverse C-section that had to be converted to a classical C-section. The patient had some tachycardia on the date of delivery. Ancef was continued and gentamicin was started. On postoperative day 1, she developed a temperature up to 103°F. Urinalysis was unremarkable, along with blood cultures. A chest x-ray revealed some atelectasis at the bases, which the radiologist ultimately felt was possibly consistent with bibasilar pneumonia. At that point the patient was switched from Ancef to ceftriaxone; clindamycin was added on postoperative day 2.

It was noted on the chest x-ray that she had a probable ileus, which was confirmed on the abdominal films. She was placed n.p.o. and an NG tube to intermittent suction wa° started. The fevers persisted with concomitant chills through today, postoperative day 5; however, now her temperature spikes are more in the 101°F range. The patient's ileus has resolved, and she is tolerating a normal diet. The patient clinically had endometritis after the delivery with a tender lower abdomen. However, this has gradually improved even though her fevers are persisting.

Review of systems performed in addition to physical examination.

Data Interpretation: Laboratory data reviewed; chest x-ray also reviewed by myself revealed some atelectatic changes in the lung bases with bibasilar patchy infiltrates read as possible hypostatic pneumonia. Follow-up x-ray 3 days later revealed definite improvement with less bibasilar infiltrated, now with just some minimal atelectatic changes in the left lung base. CT scan today revealed an enlarged uterus with prominent endometrial stripes, felt to be probably iatrogenic from the surgery. There was some pelvic cobwebbing, but no obvious abscess and some subcutaneous edema anterior in the abdomen with some pockets of gas, also felt to be iatrogenic. With all of these factors, infection could not be entirely excluded. No obvious evidence of thrombophlebitis was seen.

Assessment: Persistent postpartum fever with clinical evidence of endometritis initially that has improved. The patient has had good broad-spectrum antibiotic coverage and with persistent fever, the possibility of a pelvic septic thrombophlebitis must be entertained.

Diarrhea with negative *C. difficile,* possibly still related to antibiotics; also Prevacid has been shown to cause diarrhea.

Postoperative anemia—stable.

Heart murmur—likely secondary to her anemia and being immediately postpartum.

Hypokalemia, which has been difficult to normalize—-likely related to GI losses.

Plan: She has received appropriate IV antibiotic coverage for her endomyometritis and no other source of infection is identified; would recommend that anticoagulation be initiated for the possibility of pelvic septic thrombophlebitis or ovarian vein thrombosis.

Would recommend continuing the patient's current antibiotic coverage; however, because the most recent x-ray did not show significant evidence of pneumonia, the ceftriaxone could be discontinued.

Would recommend adding potassium to her IV fluids to try to correct her hypokalemia. The hypokalemia could add to her ileus.

If the patient does not improve in the next couple of days, other considerations would be to add amp or Unasyn to her regimen for possible resistant organism, such as *Enterococcus*. Also agree with continued intermittent blood cultures if she continues to spike.

Her anemia is stable, would recommend continuing to watch for now; however, if it drops or she becomes symptomatic, transfuse.

Consider echo if fever persists to rule out endocarditis.

Operative Report

Preoperative Diagnosis: Gravida 1 para 0 female at 38 weeks' gestation; prolonged rupture of membranes; prolonged second stage of labor with failure to descend

Postoperative Diagnosis: Same

Operation: Primary cesarean section, classical

Anesthesia: Epidural

Complications: Classical extension of initially low transverse incision

Findings: Viable female infant; complete placenta with three-vessel cord; normal uterus, tubes, and ovaries

Indications: This is a 26-year-old female gravida 1 para 0 who presented at 38 weeks' gestation with complaints of leaking fluid. The patient was approximately 1 cm dilated and 80% effaced at that time. She was felt to be having some leaking, although membranes could still be palpated. Therefore, artificial rupture of membranes was performed. The patient progressed very slowly in labor and required Pitocin augmentation. Over the next 24 hours, she progressed to finally complete dilation and began pushing for 3 hours. She started at approximately 0 to +1 station and progressed to + 2 or 3 station. Fetal head was seen with separation of the labia; however, after 3 hours and maternal exhaustion, she made no further progression of the fetal head over the last hour of pushing. The patient was counseled regarding the need for assistance, and forceps assistance versus cesarean section were offered. The risk and benefits of both were explained, and the patient opted for a cesarean section.

Technique: The patient was taken to the operating room and placed under epidural anesthesia. She was prepped and draped in the normal sterile fashion in dorsal supine position with leftward tilt. Pfannenstiel skin incision was made two fingerbreadths above the symphysis pubis in the midline and carried through to the underlying fascia. The fascia was incised in the midline and extended laterally with Mayo scissors. The rectus muscles were dissected off the fascia using both blunt and sharp dissection. Rectus muscles were then separated in the midline. The peritoneum was entered bluntly and extended superiorly and inferiorly. The bladder blade was inserted. The vesicouterine peritoneum was grasped with pickups and entered with Metzenbaum scissors. This was extended laterally, and the bladder flap was created digitally. The bladder blade was reinserted. The lower uterine segment was incised in a transverse fashion with a scalpel and extended laterally with blunt dissection. The infant's head was very low in the pelvis. Attempt to deliver the fetal head was difficult, and we were unable to reduce the fetal head from the vaginal canal. Nursing staff did apply pressure to the fetal head from the vaginal canal, but still was unable to be dislodged. An attempt was made to retract on the shoulders of the infant in order to dislodge the fetal head from the vaginal canal, but again this was unsuccessful. For this reason, the uterine incision was extended vertically in a classical fashion, and the feet were grasped and pulled to the uterine incision. The feet were then delivered, and the infant was delivered in a breech fashion. Nose and mouth were suctioned and cord was clamped and cut. The infant was then handed off to the waiting pediatrician.

Cord gas was obtained. The cord blood was inadvertently not obtained. The placenta was removed. The uterus was cleared of clots and debris. The uterus was exteriorized for better visualization; 0 VICRYL sutures were used to close the vertical incision in the uterus in several layers. Two layers were done initially, then the transverse portion of the incision was closed. There was a cervical extension distally, and this was also closed with 0 VICRYL sutures. Once the transverse portion of the incision was closed, attention was again turned back to the vertical incision. The uterus was returned to the abdomen and inspection of the incision appeared to be hemostatic. With all the layers being closed, the sponge, lap, and needle counts were correct × 2. The patient tolerated the procedure well and was taken to the recovery room in stable condition.

Progress Notes

Postop day 1: Patient with episode of tachycardia consistent with endomyometritis

Postop day 2: Abdomen feels distended endomyometritis, suspect ileus

Postop day 3: Endomyometritis, ileus

Postop day 4: Ileus resolved, temperature improving

Postop day 5: Continued fever, endomyometritis, internal med consult

Postop day 6: Prolonged postpartum fever with initial endometritis, probable pelvic septic thrombophlebitis—on Lovenox, postop anemia, stable; hypokalemia—improved

Postop day 7: Patient improved; will discharge home

Code Assignment Including POA Indicator

ICD-9-CM Principal Diagnosis: _____

ICD-9-CM Additional Diagnoses: _____

ICD-9-CM Procedure Code(s): _____

ICD-10-CM Code(s): _____

ICD-10-PCS Code(s): _____

Disorders of the Respiratory System

7.50. The following documentation is from the health record of a 57-year-old male patient.

Preoperative Diagnosis: Chronic right calf skin ulcer with necrosis of the bone; *E. coli* sepsis with acute respiratory failure and disseminated intravascular coagulation (DIC)

Postoperative Diagnosis: Same

Procedure: Right below-the-knee amputation

Description of Procedure: The patient was brought to the operating room and placed supine on the operating room table. The patient was placed under general endotracheal anesthesia. A tourniquet was placed on the right proximal thigh and the right lower extremity was prepped and draped in a standard sterile fashion.

A below-the-knee amputation was carried out directly below the tibial tubercle with a posteriorly based flap. The skin and soft tissue were cut sharply to bone along the line of the skin incision. Once the soft tissue was incised the tibia and fibula were provisionally cut with an oscillating saw and the remainder of the right lower extremity was removed and sent to pathology. Next, the tibia and fibula were dissected out subperiosteally proximal to the anterior portion of the skin incision and re-cut with the oscillating saw. The anterior portion of the tibia was beveled again with the oscillating saw and smoothed with a rasp. The fibular cut was beveled in a lateral to medial direction while extending posteriorly.

The nerves and blood vessels were then addressed. The anterior tibial and posterior tibial arteries, as well as the peroneal artery and attendant veins, were suture ligated with #1 Vicryl suture. The anterior and posterior tibial nerves and peroneal nerve were also identified, pulled out of the wound, cut short, and allowed to retract back into the soft tissue. In addition, large veins were identified and ligated. The tourniquet was then released for a total tourniquet time of 32 minutes and minimal bleeding was encountered. Several smaller bleeders were ligated. There was some clotting observed, which was important as the blood clotting was of significant concern preceding this operation. The wound was closed over a medium Hemovac drain with 2 limbs, with the posterior flap brought anteriorly. The fascia was closed using interrupted 1 Vicryl suture, and the subcutaneous tissue was closed using interrupted 3-0 Monocryl suture in a simple buried fashion. Staples were placed at the level of the skin in the interest of time.

After a sterile compressive dressing was placed and Hemovac drain extension and reservoir were attached and activated, the patient was awoken from anesthesia and sent to the ICU in unchanged condition.

Code Assignment Including POA Indicator

ICD-9-CM Principal Diagnosis: _____

ICD-9-CM Additional Diagnoses: _____

ICD-9-CM Procedure Code(s): _____

ICD-10-CM Code(s): _____

ICD-10-PCS Code(s): _____

Optional MS-DRG Exercise (for users with access to MS-DRG software or tables)

What is the MS-DRG assignment on this case? _____

7.51.   The following documentation is from the health record of an 80-year-old male patient.

Discharge Summary

History: The patient is an 80-year-old male with a 4- to 5-week history of pulmonary disease, apparently developing out of an acute influenzalike illness. He was admitted to his local hospital approximately 22 days ago with right middle lobe and right lower lobe alveolar filling infiltrates. Initial cultures were negative. Treatment with intravenous Ancef was not effective. The patient's hospital course was manifested by progressive pulmonary infiltrates unresponsive to erythromycin, Claforan, and Primaxin. Complications of nasogastric feeding tube placement in the right pleural space and administration of 1 L of Osmolite into the pleural space apparently occurred during hospitalization. The patient had a chest tube placed with effective removal of the Osmolite. Because of fatigue, the patient was twice placed on a ventilator but has been off the ventilator for approximately 1 week. He has become severely malnourished and was placed on TPN. Diarrhea has intervened with tube feedings. Cultures and ova and parasite findings showed *Trichomonas*. Because of failure to resolve pneumonia, malnutrition, and persistent fever, he was transferred here.

Physical Examination: The patient is a chronically-ill-appearing, thin man, responsive but unable to talk secondary to a very dry mouth. Blood pressure 144/70, pulse rate 110 per minute and regular, temperature 99.4°F, respirations 28. He is on nasal oxygen. Skin is dry. Lymph nodes are negative. Head: No deformity. Eyes: Increased bilateral purulent drainage. Sclerae are not red. Pupils round and equal. Throat very dry with caked secretions on teeth and palate. Neck is supple. Jugular venous pulse flat, carotids equal. Chest nontender. He ventilates with the left chest fairly well with scattered rhonchi. The right chest, however, showed decreased breath sounds with a line of consolidation about halfway up. Scattered rhonchi were noted above the area of consolidation. No friction rub was heard. The patient had evidence of a right pleural effusion versus right pleural thickening. Heart: PMI was at the midclavicular line. A regular rhythm was noted, no significant murmur, gallop, or rub. Abdomen: Soft and scaphoid, no organomegaly or tenderness, bowel sounds active. The patient passed a green watery stool during examination. Rectal: Slightly decreased sphincter tone, no masses were felt. Prostate was +2 enlarged, no nodules. Extremities showed no edema, clubbing, or cyanosis.

Initial Laboratory and X-Ray Findings: Blood gas on 4 L of nasal oxygen showed pH 7.48, pCO$_2$ 37, pO$_2$ 65. Initial chest x-ray showed bilateral mixed infiltrate and consolidation throughout both lungs, most prominently in the right midlung and right lung base. A left subclavian venous catheter was seen. Initial hematocrit level was 40. Within 2 days after hydration, this was noted to be 27. Sed rate 96 mm per hour. White blood cell count 16,000 with 5 bands, 73 segs, 15 lymphs, 5 monos, 2 eosinophils. Platelets 464,000. PT and PTT negative. SMA profile: Cholesterol 113, triglycerides 110, electrolytes normal except chloride of 96, CO$_2$ 34. Blood sugar 120. BUN 20, creatinine 0.8. Serum osmolality was 338. Urine osmolality was 456. Creatinine clearance was 81 mL per minute. Urinalysis was negative, except for an initial elevated specific gravity of 1.032. The patient was malnourished by low albumin and transferrin levels. IV albumin was ordered. Cryptococcal antigen of spinal fluid positive at a titer of 1:32.

Hospital Course: The day after admission on 1/9, the patient was submitted to bronchoscopy for bronchoalveolar lavage. His culture showed beta hemolytic streptococcus A, *Proteus mirabilis,* and a gram-negative bacillus that was not further identified. Legionella culture was negative. Stool showed no pathogens. Spinal tap was done with the finding of cryptococcal antigen of 1:32 in spinal fluid, the patient was started on amphotericin B for his meningitis, but he could not tolerate this and was thus switched to fluconazole. On 1/12, it became evident that the large volume of sputum he was required to mobilize and his generally weakened state resulted in increasing fatigue resulting in acute respiratory failure, such that it was necessary to transfer the patient to the ICU, intubate, and place him on ventilatory assistance. Because of continued deterioration, antibiotics were modified to include vancomycin and imipenem. Because of the inability to obtain a fully established diagnosis, the patient was submitted to right open-lung biopsy. The open-lung biopsy showed advanced fibrosis and scarring. Despite therapy with aggressive pulmonary toilet and ventilatory support, his condition continued to deteriorate. The patient experienced cardiac arrest on 1/16.

Final Diagnosis:	Pneumonia, apparently due to gram-negative bacteria
Additional Diagnoses:	Acute respiratory failure Cardiac arrest Cryptococcal meningitis Severely malnourished
Procedures:	Open-lung biopsy Ventilatory assistance

Code Assignment Including POA Indicator

ICD-9-CM Principal Diagnoses: _____

ICD-9-CM Additional Diagnoses: _____

ICD-9-CM Procedure Code(s): _____

ICD-10-CM Code(s): _____

ICD-10-PCS Code(s): _____

Optional MS-DRG Exercise (for users with access to MS-DRG software or tables)

Which of the following is the correct MS-DRG for this case? _____

a. 163, Major Chest Procedures with MCC
b. 853, Infectious and Parasitic Diseases with OR Procedure with MCC
c. 178, Respiratory Infections and Inflammations with CC
d. 003, ECMO or Tracheostomy with Mechanical Ventilation 96+ Hours or Principal Diagnosis Except Face, Mouth and Neck with Major OR

7.52. Discharge Summary

Date of Admission: 1/31

Date of Discharge: 2/3

Discharge Diagnosis: Right lower lobe pneumonia due to gram-negative bacteria, resistant to erythromycin

Admission History: This is a 56-year-old insulin-requiring diabetic female whose diabetes is out of control whom we have been following for hypertension, degenerative joint disease, aortic stenosis, and diabetic retinopathy. Over the past three days she has noted increased cough and chest congestion with a fever of approximately 102 degrees. She was found to have a right lower lobe infiltrate and was started on therapy with erythromycin. Despite initial therapy, the patient's clinical status has worsened over the past 24 hours.

Course in Hospital: Patient was admitted with the diagnosis of right lower lobe pneumonia. She was begun on intravenous ceftriaxone. Because of difficulties with venous access, patient was switched to intramuscular ceftriaxone on her third hospital day.

By 2/3 the patient was afebrile and her cough had diminished. Her blood pressure was well controlled at 140/74.

Instructions on Discharge: Follow up with me by phone in three days and in my office in two weeks. Repeat chest x-ray to be done then.

Medications

1. Calan SR 180 mg b.i.d.
2. Zestril 20 mg PO q. a.m.
3. NPH Insulin, 30 units, sub q., a.m.
4. Levoquin 500 mg PO daily × 10 days
5. Celebrex 100 mg PO b.i.d.

History and Physical

Admitted: 1/31

Reason for Admission: Physical examination on admission revealed a well-developed, acutely ill appearing black female.

History of Present Illness: A 56-year-old diabetic followed for hypertension and diabetic retinopathy. Over the past three days she has noted increased cough and chest congestion with a fever of approximately 102 degrees. She was found to have a right lower lobe infiltrate and was begun on therapy with erythromycin. Despite initial therapy, the patient's clinical status worsened over the past 24 hours and hospitalization was recommended.

Past Medical History: Hypertension, degenerative joint disease in both knees, and moderate aortic stenosis

Allergies: Dust

Chronic Medications: CalanSR 180 mg PO b.i.d., Insulin (NPH), Zestril 20 mg PO daily, Celebrex 100 mg PO b.i.d.

Family History: Notable for hypertension in mother

Social History: Noncontributory

Physical Examination

> **General Appearance:** The patient is a well-developed black female in moderate distress.
>
> **Vital Signs:** T 102, P 80, R 16, BP 150/80
>
> **Skin:** Warm and dry
>
> **HEENT:** Significant for mildly inflamed mucous membranes. Retinopathy evident in both eyes.
>
> **Neck:** Supple. Symmetrical with no bruits.
>
> **Lungs:** Coarse rhonchi bilaterally, right greater than left
>
> **Heart:** Regular rate and rhythm, positive S1, positive III/VI SEM
>
> **Abdomen:** Soft, nontender, no mass
>
> **Genitalia:** Deferred
>
> **Rectal:** Deferred
>
> **Extremities:** No edema
>
> **Neurologic:** Normal

Laboratory Data

1. EKG: NSR, widespread ST-T wave abnormalities, LV hypertrophy
2. CBC: Hgb 13, Hct 38, WBC 12.8
3. Glucose: 281
4. Urinalysis: Unremarkable
5. Sputum: Gram stain—a few WBCs, moderate gram-negative rods

Impression

1. Right lower lobe pneumonia possibly due to gram-negative bacteria
2. Diabetes mellitus on insulin—Uncontrolled
3. Hypertension—Stable
4. Degenerative joint disease—Stable
5. Moderate aortic stenosis

Plan: Admit, IV antibiotics for pneumonia. Monitor blood sugars.

Progress Notes

1/31   Patient admitted for cough associated with increased temperature with chest x-ray indicative of pneumonia. Will obtain sputum culture and begin on ceftriaxone. Will monitor blood pressure and blood sugars. Will use sliding scale to bring blood sugar into control. Patient with recent echocardiogram as outpatient that showed stable aortic stenosis.

2/1   The patient is responding well. Will request diabetic education nurse to meet with her and set up an appointment for classes following this admission.

2/2   Sputum culture reveals gram-negative bacteria as suspected. Patient's temperature is down. Patient resting comfortably. Blood sugar better.

2/3   Blood sugar with increasing control today. The importance of appropriate diet emphasized. Will discharge with p.o. antibiotics.

Code Assignment Including POA Indicator

ICD-9-CM Principal Diagnoses: _____

ICD-9-CM Additional Diagnoses: _____

ICD-9-CM Procedure Code(s): _____

ICD-10-CM Code(s): _____

ICD-10-PCS Code(s): _____

7.53.   The following documentation is from the health record of a 65-year-old male patient.

Hospital Course: This unfortunate gentleman was discharged from the hospital yesterday after being treated for several days for congestive heart failure. He presented back to the hospital within 24 hours after he developed significant respiratory discomfort and shortness of breath. He was found to be in respiratory failure and have pneumonia. The patient required intubation with subsequent mechanical ventilation in the emergency room. His x-ray showed diffuse infiltrates bilaterally, a condition also consistent with possible congestive heart failure. The patient did not have an elevated BNP. He was taken to the intensive care unit for further evaluation and treatment. It was explained to his wife and family that he was critically ill, and his survival was very guarded. The patient required blood pressure support. He was treated for pneumonia and his sputum cultures grew methicillin-resistant *Staphylococcus aureus.* He was treated with vancomycin. He had a stroke while admitted and had right-sided hemiparesis. He was found to have a left-sided internal carotid artery stenosis. He was felt not to be a surgical candidate because he was critically ill. He was placed on Bumex infusion for his congestive heart failure. His respiratory status remained very tenuous despite maximum medical management. He was placed on TPN via peripheral vein. His condition never improved despite all efforts. He remained poorly responsive, and he developed acute renal failure, as well. On day 15, it was clear that his survival was unlikely. His family asked that his ventilator support be discontinued. Shortly after, the ventilator was discontinued.

Discharge Diagnoses

Acute respiratory failure secondary to pneumonia and congestive heart failure

Cerebrovascular accident with infarction

Methicillin-resistant *S. aureus* infection

Coronary artery disease

Acute renal failure

Lung mass

Chronic obstructive pulmonary disease

Diabetes mellitus

Paroxysmal ventricular tachycardia

Hemiplegia secondary to stroke

Hyperlipidemia

Anemia

Operative Procedures

Mechanical ventilation greater than 96 hours

Packed red blood cell transfusion $\times$ 2

Placement of central venous line

Code Assignment Including POA Indicator

ICD-9-CM Principal Diagnoses: _____

ICD-9-CM Additional Diagnoses: _____

ICD-9-CM Procedure Code(s): _____

ICD-10-CM Code(s): _____

ICD-10-PCS Code(s): _____

Optional MS-DRG Exercise (for users with access to MS-DRG software or tables)

Which of the following is the correct MS-DRG for this case?

a. 189, Pulmonary Edema and Respiratory Failure
b. 291, Heart Failure and Shock with MMC
c. 207, Respiratory System Diagnosis with Ventilator Support 96+ Hours
d. 064, Intracranial Hemorrhage or Cerebral Infarction with MCC

7.54. History and Physical Exam

Present Illness: This 74-year-old male presented to the emergency room last night with complaints of increased weakness and shortness of breath. In the emergency room, he was found to be hypotensive. Blood pressure 83/42 apparently—actually that was the recording at home. In the emergency room, it was 130/80. He was afebrile, tachypneic per usual, respiratory rate of 32, and admitted with acute pneumonia. He was started on Levaquin. He has a history of purulent sputum for several days. Since admission, he feels better; tachypnea and weakness have improved. His blood pressure readings have somewhat improved. His peripheral edema improved with a diuretic.

Past Medical History: End-stage pulmonary disease, atherosclerotic heart disease and congestive heart failure, gastroesophageal reflux disease, gout, and hypothyroidism

Family History: Unremarkable

Social History: Has six children and is a widower

Physical Exam: On physical examination, blood pressure 102/70, pulse 90, respirations 28. He is pleasant, alert. Color is good. No JVD.

Chest: He has bilateral rales, which are chronic.

Heart: There is a systolic ejection murmur, grade 3, with an S4 gallop.

Abdomen: The abdomen is soft, nontender. No palpable organomegaly.

Extremities: Extremities reveal trace to +1 peripheral edema. He does have some stasis pigmentary changes. He does have clubbing of his fingers.

Musculoskeletal: No atrophic changes

Skin: Unremarkable except as noted

Neurological: He has no focal sensory or motor deficits and reflexes are physiologic.

Impressions: I suspect he probably just has purulent bronchitis and that is the cause of his deterioration. He is on Levaquin and seems to be improving. We will observe until tomorrow. If still doing reasonably well, we will let him go.

Discharge Summary

History of Present Illness: This 74-year-old male with end-stage pulmonary fibrosis was admitted via the emergency room with increased breathlessness. The admitting diagnosis was pneumonia. While here, he did not develop any significant fever.

Laboratory Studies: On admission PO_2 58, PCO_2 37, pH 7.45 on 3.5 L, his electrolytes were normal with the exception of BUN 28, creatinine 1.3, white blood cell count 8.6, hemoglobin 11.4, platelet count slightly low 117, urinalysis fairly unremarkable with trace protein, rare red and white blood cells.

Hospital Course: The patient was continued on Levaquin, which had been started 1 day previously. His chest x-ray showed decreased cardiac size from the previous examination, chronic infiltrates bilaterally, no acute infiltrates; pneumonia ruled out. Electrocardiogram showed sinus rhythm, right bundle branch block, left anterior hemiblock. He did receive intravenous diuretic and with this did achieve significant diuresis. My concern at the time of admission was the possible hypotension, which was recorded at home, but all blood pressure recordings here varied from the 100 to 130 systolic range.

Discharge Diagnosis: Probably acute bronchitis with possible mild congestive heart failure.

What are the correct code sets for this admission?

ICD-9-CM Code(s):

a. 466.0, 515, 428.0
b. 491.22, 428.0
c. 491.22, 466.0, 515, 428.0
d. 428.0, 466.0, 515

ICD-10-CM Code(s): _____

7.55. **Admission Diagnosis:** Pneumonia, hypoxemia

Discharge Diagnosis: Bilateral pneumonia, respiratory failure, dehydration, quadriplegia with old C5–C6 fracture, atonic bladder, tobacco use (2 packs of cigarettes for the past 30 years)

Disposition: The patient is being discharged to home. Her daughter stays with her full-time to care for her. She is to come to our office in one week to get a repeat chest x-ray and then further treatment with her pending results.

Hospital Course: The patient is a 50-year-old female who is a quadriplegic after a motor vehicle accident in which she suffered a C5–C6 fracture. She had a fever two days prior to admission, so we called her in a prescription for Keflex. She did not improve on this medication, and she came to the emergency room on the day of admission complaining of shortness of breath and cough. She reported a two day history of shortness of breath, fever, and cough productive of green and yellow sputum. There was no elevation in her temperature. A chest x-ray in the emergency room showed bilateral lower lobe infiltrates. She was admitted to the hospital for intravenous antibiotics for her pneumonia and treatment of her hypoxemia. Her pO_2 in the emergency room was 50 on room air. Her temperature was 102.6°F.

After admission to the hospital, the patient was placed on Biaxin, and she did become afebrile and started to feel better. Her caretaker, who is her daughter, felt that she could care for her at home. The patient is being discharged to the daughter's care.

Work-up during this admission included a glucose of 81, a BUN of 6, a creatinine of 0.5. Electrolytes were normal. Her arterial blood gases show a pH of 7.482, a pCO_2 of 33, a pO_2 low at 50, HCO_3 324, and total CO_2 was 55. Her O_2 saturation was only 88 percent on room air. She was started on handheld nebulizer treatments, and she rapidly improved.

At the time of discharge, she was breathing easy on room air. She was benefiting from her handheld nebulizer treatments, and she wants to return home.

The work-up during admission, in addition to that above, included serum electrolytes, which were normal except for a potassium level of 3.3. This was corrected with additional potassium. Her hemoglobin level on admission was 13.5. Hematocrit was 40.1, RBC was 4.40. Her MCV was 91. Her MCH was 33.6. RDW was 12.7. The urinalysis showed a moderate amount of hemoglobin but no red cells. Her chest x-ray did show a definite infiltrate in her left lower lobe and a questionable infiltrate in her right lower lobe. There is question that possibly her paraplegia may affect her ability to breathe, necessitating her seeing us for respiratory infections. The patient is discharged to home. She will be seeing Dr. Jones in two weeks after repeat chest x-ray.

Code Assignment Including POA Indicator

ICD-9-CM Principal Diagnoses: _____

ICD-9-CM Secondary Diagnoses: _____

ICD-10-CM Code(s): _____

7.56. Discharge Summary

Admit Date: 3/19/20XX

Discharge Date: 3/25/20XX

Admitting Diagnoses: Acute exacerbation of asthma, chronic obstructive pulmonary disease, acute bronchitis, hormonal replacement therapy

Discharge Diagnoses: Acute exacerbation of asthma, chronic obstructive pulmonary disease, acute bronchitis, hormonal replacement therapy

Discharge Instructions: Patient is to follow up in the office in 1 week.

Discharge Medications: Spiriva as directed daily, Pulmicort inhaler two puffs p.o. every 12 hours, Serevent Diskus one puff p.o. every 12 hours, Augmentin 500 mg p.o. 3 times a day for 6 days, prednisone 35 mg to decrease by 5 mg every day until gone.

Brief History: The patient is a 57-year-old white female who presents with an approximate 1-day history of increasing dyspnea to the point where any ambulation required increasing effort as she could not catch her breath. The patient also had mild complaints of sore throat, neck pain, and headache. She denied any fever, although a low-grade one was present on admission. The patient also admitted to a nonproductive cough.

The patient had an acute exacerbation of asthma and was admitted to observation. However, this did not clear with IV steroids, nebulizer treatments, or supportive therapy, so she was admitted for inpatient treatment of acute exacerbation of asthma with possible bronchitis and respiratory distress. During her initial 2-day stay, Z-Pak, Decadron, and albuterol and Atrovent treatments were continued because her respiratory distress did not significantly improve. The patient had increased anxiety secondary to her nebulized treatments and her medication was changed to Xopenex with some improvement.

Chest x-ray was checked on the second hospital day, and a two-dimensional echocardiogram was ordered in addition to a pulmonary consult. The patient's Zithromax was changed to Augmentin to better cover *Haemophilus influenzae* as a possibility. Inhaled steroids were added as the bronchodilators were continued. The patient's respiratory distress subsequently improved with less agitation with continued high-dose Xopenex. The two-dimensional echocardiogram was normal. The patient's respiratory condition improved with less dyspnea with her lung exam overall cleared. The patient was discharged in stable condition.

History and Physical: This is a 57-year-old female who presents with an approximate 1-day history of increasing dyspnea to the point where any ambulation required increasing effort, and she could not catch her breath. The patient stated that approximately 1 month ago some cold medication was phoned in for her, which cleared up her congestion but did not feel she totally got well. She was admitted from the emergency room to observation, but her symptoms did not resolve so she is being admitted for inpatient treatment. Patient smokes approximately one pack of cigarettes a day and denies any alcohol use.

Physical Exam

General: The patient is alert and oriented, appearing in mild to moderate respiratory distress

Lungs: Showed decreased breath sounds throughout with no wheezing present

Abdomen: Soft and nontender, with good bowel sounds present

Extremities: No cyanosis or edema

The patient is currently on 2 L of nasal cannula with O_2 saturations at approximately 92 percent. Her chest x-ray is unremarkable.

Assessment and Plan: Acute exacerbation of asthma/chronic obstructive pulmonary disease/acute bronchitis. The patient will continue with Zithromax given at 500 mg p.o. q. 24 hours. Continued on 10 mg of Decadron q. 8 hours, given albuterol as well as Atrovent treatments on a daily basis.

Hormone replacement therapy on Premarin 0.625 mg/day

Consultant Report

Reason for Consultation: Asthmatic bronchitis

Impression: Asthmatic bronchitis either representing acute exacerbation of chronic bronchitis and/or asthma. Cigarette use greater than 40-pack-years.

Recommendations: Change Zithromax to Augmentin because she has had antibiotics in the past 90 days, and there is a high incidence of resistant *H. influenzae* and streptococcal pneumonia.

Handheld steroids

Prophylactic H_2 blockers and low molecular with heparin

Check sputum for eosinophils

Cigarette cessation

Discussion: The patient has purulent bronchitis and wheezing on top of chronic daily shortness of breath and wheezing. This is compounded by at least 40-pack-years of smoking history. It is difficult to tell if this is just chronic obstructive pulmonary disease exacerbation due to infection or whether or not she has a large component of asthma. Whatever the initial diagnosis is, she would benefit with albuterol and Atrovent, inhaled steroids, and antibiotics.

On the long-term basis, she will need PFTs and a long-acting bronchodilator, Spiriva or Advair depending on the way she responds on her pulmonary function test abnormalities. Advair is recommended if the FEV1 is less than 50 percent; Spiriva would be a better choice if this is all chronic obstructive pulmonary disease.

Emergency Room Report: Chief Complaint: Shortness of breath

History of Present Illness: The patient is a 57-year-old female complaining of shortness of breath since yesterday evening. She states that breathing difficulty became very severe to the point that she felt like she could not catch her breath.

She could not walk across the room without becoming severely dyspneic. Also complaining of soreness in her neck bilaterally and of a headache.

Impression/Management Plan: Breathing difficulty with marked bronchospasm, possible fever with chills present. Rule out superimposed pneumonia. Symptoms consistent with exacerbation of asthma. Initial oxygen saturation on presentation to the emergency department 89 percent on room air.

Course in the Emergency Department: The patient received intravenous fluids, Decadron, magnesium. The patient did develop a fever in the emergency department with temperature up to 100.7°F, for which she received Tylenol. The patient received multiple nebulizer treatments in the emergency department and has persistent expiratory wheezes with somewhat labored respirations. Chest x-ray read negative for acute changes by my reading. The patient received initial dose of Zithromax in the emergency department. Decision for further treatment was made with an admission to the observation unit.

Final Diagnosis: Status asthmaticus.

What is the correct code assignment for this admission?

ICD-9-CM Code(s):

a. 493.91, 305.1, V07.4
b. 466.0, 493.22, 305.1, V07.4
c. 493.22, 305.1, V07.4
d. 493.21

ICD-10-CM Code(s): _____

7.57. Discharge Summary

Date of Admission:	12/18/XX
Date of Discharge:	12/22/XX
Admitting Diagnoses:	1. Right lung mass
	2. Postobstructive pneumonia
	3. COPD
	4. Respiratory acidosis

Procedure: Fiberoptic bronchoscopy on 12/20/XX

History of Present Illness: This 80-year-old white male was admitted with a 4-day history of increasing dyspnea, fever, and productive cough. Initial evaluation suggested a right lower lobe pneumonia based on ER data. He was known to have underlying chronic obstructive pulmonary disease, and labs verified the presence of respiratory acidosis.

Physical Examination: He presented with a temperature of 97.9, respiratory rate of 28, pulse 127, blood pressure 162/80. There were coarse crackles heard in the right base with poor air flow throughout.

Hospital Course: The patient was admitted for treatment of right lower lobe pneumonia and acute exacerbating COPD. He was initially placed on Zinacef one gram q8 hours and Solumedrol 60 mg q6 hours. He was also provided supplemental oxygen as required and supervised inhalation therapy. On the 20th, the Solumedrol was changed to Prednisone 50 mg per day and the Zinacef changed to Ceftin 500 mg po b.i.d. With that, the cough, etc., began to improve.

Further investigation in the right lower lobe abnormality via a CT scan of the chest showed a 2-cm inferior hilar mass obstructing the right lower lobe bronchi associated with post productive infiltrate and/or atelectasis. This was suspicious for right inferior hilar neoplasm. Biapical scarring was also suggested. On 12/20/XX, fiberoptic bronchoscopy was performed. Fortunately, this showed no distinct endobronchial lesion. Any obstruction was peripheral to the area visible. Washings were negative for acid-fast bacilli. Brushings showed only atypical cells. Perioperatively, the patient had some worsening of his CO_2 retention, which was transiently benefited by Bi-PAP for his sleep. He had not required this prior to this admission and his sedation has not resolved. It was felt that this was a long-term need.

Laboratory Data: During this stay, an SMA7 was done on the 18th, showing glucose 126, BUN 26, and creatinine 1. Sodium 145, Potassium 3.8, Chloride 96, CO_2 32. The most recent blood gas was on the 22nd, showing a pH 7.4, pCO_2 67, pO_2 43, on 2 L nasal cannula. Theophylline level was 15.9. Hemoglobin of 14.4 and hematocrit of 42.4. White blood cell count 14,600 with 9 percent Bands.

Discharge Summary

Disposition/Recommendations: The patient is being discharged home with plans for continued antibiotics therapy and steroid taper, and arrangements for an outpatient fine-needle aspirate of the lung abnormality.

Discharge Medications:
1. Atrovent 2 puffs inhalation q6 hours
2. Albuterol 2 puffs q4 hours while awake prn
3. Ceftin 500 mg po q12 hours for 10 more days
4. Prednisone 30 mg per day for 6 days and then decrease by 5 mg every other day until weaned

Activity and Diet: As tolerated.

As mentioned, request will be made for Radiology to arrange for an outpatient fine-needle aspiration of the lung abnormality. The patient understands that there is a risk of pneumothorax and if such occurs, he may return to the hospital for treatment of same.

Condition on Discharge: Improved.

History and Physical Exam

Date of Admission: 12/18/XX

History of Present Illness: This is an 80-year-old gentleman who presented to the emergency room last night. He had called me earlier in the evening with complaints of increasing breathlessness of about 4 days' duration. His evaluation in the emergency room suggested a right lower lung zone pneumonic infiltrate, and he did have a leukocytosis. He was admitted.

I have known this patient for approximately 3 years. For many years he has been treated for chronic obstructive pulmonary disease secondary to a long history of tobacco use. He has been oxygen-dependent for at least 3 years. In this interval, he has had 1 admission that I am aware of for exacerbation of COPD. His recent history is that of 4 days of increasing cough, purulent sputum production, and probably fever. He does describe chills and diaphoretic episodes.

Past Medical History: His past medical history is relatively unremarkable with the exception of his chronic obstructive pulmonary disease. As far as I know, he has no prior history of cardiovascular disease, stroke, or myocardial infarction.

Physical Examination: He is pleasant, alert, feels a bit more comfortable this morning. His blood pressure is 162/80, pulse 100, respirations 26. HEENT: Mouth and oropharynx are adequately hydrated. He does have a scar on his left lip at the site of corrective surgery for a harelip. Neck: Supple. There is no jugular venous distention. Chest: He does have somewhat of a pectus excavatum deformity with slight sternal retraction. He has coarse rales over his right chest laterally and posteriorly with a congested cough. Breath sounds are diminished on the left side. Heart: Regular rhythm without murmur or gallop. Abdomen: Soft, nontender. No masses. No organomegaly. Back and extremities: No clubbing, cyanosis, or peripheral edema. Distal pulses are easily palpable. Neurological: There are no focal neurological deficits.

Impression: 1. COPD. Plan: IV steroids and inhaled beta agonists.

2. Pneumonia. Plan: IV Zinacef. We will add Zithromax for community-acquired organisms.

EKG

Impression: Sinus tachycardia with premature ventricular contractions. Cannot exclude old inferior myocardial infarction, stable pattern.

Progress Notes

12/18   80 y/o admitted with 4 day hx of SOB, fever, and productive cough. #1 Pneumonia #2 COPD

12/19   CXR mass of lung neoplasm

12/19   Plan bronchoscopy

12/20   Bronchoscopy note dictated. No lesions noted. Pt. tolerated procedure well.

12/20   House Doctor: Pt. apparently very sedated after bronchoscopy –Demerol 12.5 mg and Phenergen 12.5 mg. Has now gotten 3 doses of Narcan with noticeable alertness with each dose but then drifts off to deep sleep again. V: BP 130/70, P 70 to 80s. SaO$_2$ now 95 to 97 on 2 L. Pt. opens eyes briefly with prompting but not enough to answer ?'s or follow commands. CV: RRR, Lungs: occ rales B Extremities: edema. A/P: Excessive sedation is what I suspect. Continue Narcan as needed. Will discuss with Dr. X.

12/21   S: No complaints
O: Afebrile, VSS, Lungs: poor air flow, bronchial washings neg.
A: Lung mass, post obstructive pneumonia, respiratory acidosis
P: D/C home for outpatient for FNA, scenario discussed with family

12/22   Discharged home with family.

Operative Report

Operation Performed: Bronchoscopy.

Premedication: 12.5 mg Demerol, 12.5 mg Phenergan, and 0.4 mg Atropine

Description of Procedure: The patient was taken to the endoscopy room. The nasopharynx and upper airway were anesthetized with 1 percent Xylocaine. The Olympus fiberoptic bronchoscope was introduced into the left nostril without difficulty. The nasopharynx and upper airway appeared normal. The vocal cords moved anatomically to the midline. The trachea was then entered. The carina was sharp. The right main stem bronchus was entered. There were inflammatory changes.

The bronchoscope was advanced into the right middle lobe. The mucosa was somewhat friable, but no endobronchial lesions were identified. The bronchoscope was then introduced further into the right lower lobe and brushings were obtained. The area was then irrigated with saline, and washings were recovered. The bronchoscope was then passed quickly to the left side and no endobronchial lesions were present.

The patient was monitored via blood pressure, pulse, and oximetry throughout, maintaining oximetry in the 85 to 92 range, and other vital signs were normal.

Following the procedure, the patient was given an amp of Narcan.

Impression: Bronchoscopy suggestive of inflammatory process in the right lower lobe.

Code Assignment Including POA Indicator

ICD-9-CM Principal Diagnoses: _____

ICD-9-CM Additional Diagnoses: _____

ICD-9-CM Procedure Code(s): _____

ICD-10-CM Code(s): _____

ICD-10-PCS Code(s): _____

Optional MS-DRG Exercise (for users with access to MS-DRG software or tables)

What is the MS-DRG assignment for this admission? _____

Trauma and Poisoning

7.58.   The following documentation is from the health record of a four-year-old male patient.

Case Summary: The patient is a 4-year-old male child who, at the age of 2 years, swallowed some Drano while playing in the bathroom. He was found at that time with acid burns of the mouth, throat, trachea, and esophagus. Plastic repair has been performed on the mouth and throat. He is now being admitted by a plastic surgeon for plastic reconstruction and removal of scar tissue to the trachea. The patient was admitted, prepped, and taken to surgery where the scar tissue of the trachea was removed, and plastic repair was accomplished. The patient's recovery was uneventful, and the patient was discharged in satisfactory condition 3 days postsurgery.

Which of the following code sets is correct for reporting the diagnoses of the most recent admission?

ICD-9-CM Code(s):

a. 709.2, 909.1, E929.2
b. 478.9, 909.1, 906.8, E929.2
c. 709.2, 909.5, 906.8, E864.2
d. 478.9, 909.5, E864.2

ICD-10-CM Code(s): _____

Optional MS-DRG Exercise (for users with access to MS-DRG software or tables)

What is the MS-DRG assignment for this admission? _____

7.59.   The following documentation is from the health record of a 22-year-old male patient.

Case Summary: The patient is a 22-year-old male, admitted through the Emergency Department after the motorcycle he was driving collided with an elk while driving in the mountains. It was noted that when the accident occurred the patient was driving in the mountains and not on the road. The patient was not wearing a helmet and sustained a skull fracture over the left temporal and orbital roof areas with depressed zygomatic arch on the left side. The patient was unconscious at the scene and upon examination in the ED, with a GCS score of 3: eyes, never open; no verbal response; no motor response. Left pupil was blown (fixed and dilated), indicating intracranial injury. Hypoxemia, hypotension, and cerebral edema were noted. The patient was admitted to the ICU with continuous monitoring of intracranial pressure (percutaneous). The patient experienced increasing periods of apnea and was placed on a ventilator following endotracheal intubation. The patient's family (in another state) was notified and arrived two days later. There was no improvement in the patient's status over the following five days. The patient continued to be monitored and was unconscious. Attempts to wean from ventilation were unsuccessful. Brain wave measurement showed no brain wave electrical activity. The family made the decision to discontinue life support and the life-sustaining efforts were discontinued.

Code Assignment Including POA Indicator

ICD-9-CM Principal Diagnoses: _____

ICD-9-CM Additional Diagnoses: _____

ICD-9-CM Procedure Code(s): _____

ICD-10-CM Code(s): _____

ICD-10-PCS Code(s): _____

7.60. The following documentation is from the health record of a 28-year-old female patient.

Case Summary: The patient is a 28-year-old female passenger in a motor vehicle accident with another car while traveling at high speed on the freeway. Upon arrival in the ED the patient was complaining of severe abdominal pain. CT scan revealed laceration of the liver and increasing hematoma. The patient was taken immediately to the OR, where exploratory laparotomy revealed a traumatic rupture approximately 2 cm deep. It was felt that the parenchyma could not be adequately repaired, so a right lobectomy was carried out with evacuation of the hematoma. The patient's postoperative course was stormy. The patient developed infection and dehiscence of the operative wound, necessitating return to the OR for opening and drainage of the abdominal wound. The patient was also given a 10-day course of IV gentamicin. The patient was finally able to be discharged on the 12th day postop in satisfactory condition.

Code Assignment Including POA Indicator

ICD-9-CM Principal Diagnoses: _____

ICD-9-CM Additional Diagnoses: _____

ICD-9-CM Procedure Code(s): _____

ICD-10-CM Code(s): _____

ICD-10-PCS Code(s): _____

7.61. The following documentation is from the health record of a 32-year-old male patient.

History of Present Illness: A 32-year-old male was brought to the ED via ambulance. He was the unrestrained front-seat passenger in a single-vehicle crash that occurred because of a tire blow-out at high speed; the car collided with a barricade off the highway. The patient was ejected from the vehicle and had brief loss of consciousness witnessed at the scene. Paramedics reported the following vital signs en route: BP 110/palp; heart rate 90, respiratory rate 20. A large-bore intravenous access was established, and fluids were begun.

Physical Examination
Vital signs: Unchanged
HEENT: 2-cm superficial laceration over left eyebrow
Lungs: Clear to auscultation
CV: Regular rate, S1/S2; NSR on EKG monitor
Abdomen: Mild epigastric tenderness without rebound
Pelvis: Stable, no crepitans
Extremities: No deformities
Neuro: GCS 13, nonfocal exam

Radiology: Chest x-ray, lateral C-spine, and pelvis film all are reviewed by the chief resident on call and noted to be normal. CT scan of the patient's abdomen demonstrated free intra-abdominal fluid, perisplenic hematoma, and splenic laceration. Patient remained hemodynamically stable during the scan.

Because of the patient's young age and hemodynamic stability, nonoperative management of his splenic injury was begun. The patient was admitted to the ICU for hemodynamic monitoring, serial measurement of hematocrit, and serial abdominal examinations. He was transferred to the floor on hospital day 2 and made an uneventful recovery.

Diagnoses: 1. Minor concussion with 10 minutes of loss of consciousness
2. Perisplenic hematoma and splenic laceration of capsule

Which of the following code sets for the diagnoses would be correct?

ICD-9-CM Code(s):

a. 865.11
b. 865.02, 850.9, E816.1, E849.5
c. 865.02, 850.11, E816.1, E849.5
d. 865.01, 865.02, 850.11, E816.1, E849.5

ICD-10-CM Code(s): _____

Chapter 8

Case Studies from Ambulatory Health Records

Note: Even though the specific cases are divided by setting, most of the information pertaining to the diagnosis is applicable to most settings. Even the CPT codes in the ambulatory and physician sections may be reported in the same manner. The differences in coding in these two settings may involve modifier reporting, evaluation and management CPT code reporting, and other health plan reporting guidelines unique to settings. If you practice or apply codes in a particular type of setting, you may find additional information in other sections of this publication that may be pertinent to you.

Every effort has been made to follow current recognized coding guidelines and principles, as well as nationally recognized reporting guidelines. The material presented may differ from some health plan requirements for reporting. The ICD-9-CM codes used are effective October 1, 2011, through September 30, 2012, and the HCPCS (CPT and HCPCS Level II) codes are in effect January 1, 2011, through December 31, 2011. The current standard transactions and code sets named in HIPAA have been utilized. The 2011 draft edition of ICD-10-CM was utilized.

Instructions: Assign all applicable ICD-9-CM diagnosis codes including V codes and E codes. Assign all applicable ICD-10-CM diagnosis codes including Z codes and external cause codes. Assign all CPT Level I procedure codes and HCPCS Level II codes. Assign Level I (CPT) and Level II (HCPCS) modifiers as appropriate. Outpatient healthcare settings represented in the case examples include emergency room (ER), urgent care, outpatient surgery, observation, ancillary outpatient, wound care, interventional radiology, radiation therapy, or other outpatient department. Final codes for billing occur after codes are passed through payer edits. Medicare utilizes the National Correct Coding Initiative (NCCI) edits. CMS developed the NCCI edit list to promote national correct coding methodologies and to control improper coding leading to improper payments for Medicare Part B. The purpose of the NCCI edits is to ensure the most comprehensive code is assigned and billed rather than the component codes. In addition, NCCI edits check for mutually exclusive pairs.

Cases are presented as either multiple choice or fill in the blank.

- For multiple-choice cases:
  —Select the letter of the appropriate code set.

- For the fill-in-the-blank cases:
  - —Assign up to three reasons for visit ICD-9-CM codes to describe the reason for unscheduled visits such as emergency room. Reason for visit coding is required on the UB-04 for all "unscheduled" outpatient visits.
  - —Sequence the primary diagnosis first followed by the secondary diagnoses including any appropriate V codes and E codes (both cause of injury and place of occurrence).
  - —Sequence the CPT procedure code first followed by additional procedure codes including modifiers as appropriate (both CPT Level I and HCPCS Level II modifiers).
  - —Assign HCPCS Level II codes only if instructed (case specific).
  - —Assign evaluation and management (E/M) codes only if instructed (case specific).
    - Medicare Type A Emergency Department visits are reported with CPT Level I codes 99281–99285 and critical care codes 99291 and 99292.
    - Medicare Type B Emergency Department visits are reported with Level II HCPCS codes G0380–G0384.

The scenarios are based on selected excerpts from health records. In practice, the coding professional should have access to and refer to the entire health record. Health records are analyzed and codes assigned based on physician documentation. Documentation for coding purposes must be assigned based on medical record documentation. A physician may be queried when documentation is ambiguous, incomplete, or conflicting. The queried documentation must be a permanent part of the medical record.

The objective of the cases and scenarios reproduced in this publication is to provide practice in assigning correct codes, not necessarily to emulate complete coding that can be achieved only with the complete medical record. For example, the reader may be asked to assign codes based on only an operative report; in real practice, a coder has access to documentation in the entire medical record.

The *ICD-9-CM Official Guidelines for Coding and Reporting of Outpatient Services,* published by the National Center for Health Statistics (NCHS), supplements the official conventions and instructions provided within ICD-9-CM. Adherence to these guidelines when assigning ICD-9-CM diagnosis codes is required under the Health Insurance Portability and Accountability Act (HIPAA) of 1996. Additional official coding guidance can be found in the American Hospital Association (AHA)'s *Coding Clinic* publication.

Disorders of the Blood and Blood-Forming Organs

8.1.   The following documentation is from the health record of a 39-year-old male.

Emergency Department Services

History of Present Illness: The patient is a 39-year-old African-American male who has a known history of sickle cell anemia and who presented to the emergency department with diffuse extremity pain and pain along the right inguinal area. The pains started on Friday, became a little bit better on Saturday; then improved, and again started in the past 24 hours. He denies any problems with cough or sputum production. He denies any problems with fever.

Past Medical History: See recent medical records in charts. He does have a new onset of diabetes, probably related to his hemochromatosis. He does have evidence of iron overload with high ferritins.

Review of Systems: Otherwise unremarkable except for those related to his pain. He denies any problems with fever or night sweats. No cough or sputum production. Denies any changes in gastrointestinal or genitourinary habits. No blood per rectum or urine.

Physical Examination: This is a 39-year-old African-American male who is conscious and cooperative. He is oriented $\times$ 3 and appears in no acute distress. Vital signs are stable. HEENT is unremarkable. The neck is supple. No evidence of any gross lymphadenopathy. The heart is irregular in rate without any murmurs heard. Lungs are clear to auscultation and percussion. The abdomen is soft and benign. Extremities reveal no edema. No palpable cords. He does have some tenderness along the inner aspects of his right lower extremity near the inguinal area; however, no masses were palpable and no point tenderness is noted.

He had a problem with his right inguinal area. He had evidence of pain. There was some pain on abduction of his right lower extremity. The rest was unremarkable. There was no evidence of any Holman, no palpable cords, and no masses were palpable.

Because of his sickle cell anemia, rule out the possibility of osteonecrosis of the femur. Complete x-rays of his femur and hip were carried out. However, these were both negative.

Patient is being transferred to a larger facility for treatment of his sickle cell crisis. Doppler studies should also be carried out to rule out any venous thrombosis.

Diagnoses: 1. Painful sickle cell crisis
2. Type II diabetes mellitus
3. Chronic atrial fibrillation

Condition on Discharge: Stable on pain meds

What codes would the facility report for this Medicare service? The patient met the fourth acuity level in the facility's criteria for evaluation and management in the ED.

ICD-9-CM and CPT Code(s):

a. 282.61, 789.09, 427.31, 250.00, 99285
b. 282.62, 733.42, 99284, 73550, 73510
c. 282.62, 427.31, 250.00, 73550, 73510
d. 282.62, 427.31, 250.00, 99284-25, 73550, 73510

ICD-10-CM Code(s): _____

8.2.   The following documentation is from the health record of a 66-year-old male patient.

Outpatient Hospital Department Services

History: This is a 66-year-old male who had coronary artery bypass graft in February. He did well. He was discharged home. Some time after that when he was home, he had 2 days of black stools. He mentioned it to the nurse, but I'm not sure anything was done about it. He has not had any other evidence of hematesis, melena, or hematochezia but was feeling rather weak and fatigued. He had blood work done that showed a hemoglobin of 5.7, hematocrit of 20.9, and MCV of 80. Serum iron of 8.2 percent saturation. No indigestion or heartburn. No abdominal pain of any kind. No past history of anemia or GI bleed.

Past Medical History: General health has been good.

Allergies: None known

Previous Surgeries: Coronary artery bypass graft

Medications: At the time of admission include Glucotrol, Lasix, potassium, and aspirin

Review of Systems: Endocrine: He does have diabetes controlled with medication. Cardiovascular: History of coronary artery disease with coronary artery bypass graft. No recent symptoms of chest pain or shortness of breath. Respiratory: No chronic cough or sputum production. GU: No dysuria, hematuria, history of stones, or infections. Musculoskeletal: No arthritic complains or muscle weakness. Neuropsychiatric: No syncope, seizures, weakness, paralysis, depression.

Family History: Is positive for cardiovascular disease and diabetes in his mother. No history of cancer.

Social History: The patient is married. Never smoked. Doesn't drink any alcohol. Works in a factory.

On physical examination, a well-developed, well-nourished, alert male in no acute distress. Blood pressure: 146/82. Respirations: 18. Heart rate: 78. Skin: Good turgor and texture. Eyes: No scleral icterus. Pupils are round, regular, equal, and react to light. Neck: No jugular venous distention. No carotid bruits. Thyroid is not enlarged. Trachea in the midline. Lungs are clear. Heart: No murmur noted. Abdomen is soft. Bowel sounds present. No masses, no tenderness. Liver and spleen are not palpably enlarged. Extremities: Good pulses. Trace edema of the feet.

Laboratory values show severe anemia with a hemoglobin of 5.7. Hemoccult is also positive. His iron studies showed low iron and low ferritin, consistent with chronic blood loss anemia. His B12 and folate levels were normal. His SMA-12 was essentially unremarkable.

Impression: 1. Anemia. Probably he is anemic after bypass and then had stress gastritis with a little bit of bleeding and has never recovered from that. No evidence of acute or active bleeding at this time. The patient is stable. Possibility of occult malignancy or active peptic ulcer disease does exist.
2. Arteriosclerotic heart disease of native vessel, stable

Recommendations: Admit patient as an outpatient for blood transfusion. Patient is being transfused. He should have an esophagogastroduodenoscopy and colonoscopy, possible biopsy, or polypectomy, which has been explained to the patient along with potential risks and complications including bleeding, transfusion, perforation, and surgery. These tests will be scheduled as soon as possible.

Discharge Note

Final Diagnoses: 1. Severe blood loss anemia; weakness
2. Type II diabetes mellitus
3. History of coronary artery disease status post coronary artery bypass graft

The patient received three units of packed red blood cells, leukoreduced, CMV negative. He felt better, with subsidence of his shortness of breath, and his weakness improved. His last hemoglobin was 8.4, with a hematocrit of 27.7.

The patient was scheduled for EGD to rule out peptic ulcer disease and colonoscopy to rule out occult malignancy in 1 week. The patient will be discharged home, and he will have a clear liquid diet. He is to call for any problems. He will continue with his home medications, and he was placed on ferrous sulfate, one tablet twice a day.

What codes are reported for this outpatient encounter? The facility purchases its blood from the blood bank.

ICD-9-CM, CPT, and/or HCPCS Code(s):

a. 280.0, 792.1, 414.01, 250.00, V45.81, V17.49, 36430, P9051 (3 units)
b. 285.9, 780.79, 36430, P9051 (3 units)
c. 280.0, 578.1, 414.01, 250.00, V45.81, V17.49, 36430
d. 285.9, 792.1, 414.01, 250.00, V45.81, V17.49, P9051 (3 units)

ICD-10-CM Code(s): _____

8.3. The following documentation is from the health record of an 87-year-old female patient.

Emergency Department Services

History: The patient is an 87-year-old white female brought to the ED because of pleural effusion, urinary tract infection, and dehydration. She had been taking medication. She lives at the nursing home and has been doing fairly well. Today she was found to be weak and not eating well. Then she was sent to the emergency room for evaluation and found to have pleural effusion and dehydration, urinary tract infection, also thrombocytopenia with petechial hemorrhage. She was found to have a platelet count of 77,000.

Past History: She has a history of cholecystectomy.

Social History: She is a retired woman. No smoking, no drinking, no allergies.

Family History: Noncontributory

Systemic Review: Otherwise normal

Physical Examination: Today reveals blood pressure is 163/62. Pulse of 80. Respirations of 15. Temperature of 98.6°F. General condition of the patient showed chronically ill, confused, disoriented. No jaundice, no cyanosis. No pallor, no edema. The patient has dehydration +3. Scalp and skull are normal. There was a bluish color around the eyes and petechial hemorrhage at the eyelid and conjunctiva. Ears, nose, and throat are normal. Neck showed normal cervical spine. The neck veins are flat. No bruits of the carotid arteries. The trachea is midline. Thyroid gland cannot be palpated. Lymph glands cannot be palpated. Chest shows normal contour. The breasts are normal. Movement of the chest equal on both sides. There is dullness of the chest with some rales and rhonchi. Heart shows apex beat is at the fifth intercostal space, left midclavicular line. No diffuse precordial pulsation, no thrill. Heart rate is 80, regular, with premature ventricular contraction, no murmur. Back is normal. Abdomen showed normal contour, soft, nontender, no guarding, no rigidity. Liver, spleen, and kidneys cannot be palpated; no mass is palpable. Bowel sounds are positive. No fluid thrill. No shifting dullness. No bruits of the abdominal vessels. Extremities show no clubbing of the fingers. No varicose veins. No phlebitis. Hematoma of the right hand. Peripheral pulses are normal. The deep tendon reflexes are normal. Babinski sign is negative.

Laboratory Studies: Hematocrit was 43, white count 9,000 with 82 percent neutrophils, and the platelet count 77,000. The MCV was 102. Creatinine was 1.7. Bilirubin was 1.7. The alkaline phosphatase was 122. AST 498, ALT 493, and albumin 3.6. The prothrombin time was 18 seconds; the PTT was 25 seconds. The chest x-ray showed a right pleural effusion.

Impression: 1. Urinary tract infection
2. Dehydration
3. Pleural effusion from congestive heart failure
4. Primary thrombocytopenia with petechial hemorrhage
5. Type II diabetes mellitus

Plan of Treatment: The patient will be stabilized and started on IV fluids. Also will start IV antibiotic for urinary tract infection. Patient will be transferred at the family's request to a larger facility. A consultation with hematology will be arranged, and a transfusion of platelets may be indicated.

What are the appropriate diagnosis codes for this service?

ICD-9-CM Code(s):

a. 599.0, 276.51, 428.0, 287.5, 250.00
b. 599.0, 276.51, 428.0, 511.9, 287.5, 250.00
c. 599.0, 276.51, 428.0, 287.30, 250.00
d. 599.0, 276.51, 428.0, 511.9, 287.30, 782.7, 250.00

ICD-10-CM Code(s): _____

8.4. The following documentation is from the health record of a 39-year-old female patient.

Hospital Outpatient Department Services

This 39-year-old female was diagnosed with breast cancer 2 years ago. At that time she had a mastectomy performed, with no evidence of metastases to the lymph nodes. About 8 months ago, metastases were discovered in her liver. The patient was given chemotherapy. She has been losing weight and developing increased fatigue. Patient was referred to hospice care program, with a life expectancy of 4 to 6 months. Progressive weight loss due to loss of appetite led to cachexia and program of home intravenous hyperalimentation. Progressive, unrelenting abdominal pain led to chronic use of analgesics. Patient is awake, alert, and desires to spend more time with family. Progressive weakness and dropping hemoglobin led to the decision to transfuse the patient every 2 weeks with 2 units of packed cells. Patient is stable and more comfortable on this regimen.

She is coming into the outpatient department now for transfusion.

Diagnosis: History of breast cancer, current liver metastases, anemia in neoplastic disease and due to chemotherapy.

What are the correct diagnosis codes assigned in this case?

ICD-9-CM Code(s):

a. 285.22, 285.3, 197.7, V10.3, E933.1
b. 285.9, 197.7, V10.3, E933.1
c. 197.7, 285.22, V10.3, E933.1
d. 285.9, 197.7, V10.3

ICD-10-CM Code(s): _____

Disorders of the Cardiovascular System

8.5.   The following documentation is from the health record of a 60-year-old male patient.

Outpatient Hospital Diagnostic Services

A 60-year-old man was given a stress test for recent left arm pain that occurred with exercise the day before. His only medication was Dyazide 1 daily. He was exercised by the Bruce protocol for a duration of 6 minutes, 2 seconds using the treadmill. Maximum heart rate achieved was 137; 85 percent maximum predicted was 136. His blood pressure during the stress test went up to 182/80. He denied any arm pain with the exercise. He did have 2 mm of ST depression at a point of maximum exercise in 2, 3, AVF, but these were all upsloping. Also in V5, V6, he had 1.4-mm ST depression, also upsloping.

Following exercise he was placed at rest. At about 1 minute, 45 seconds post exercise, his STT waves changed. He had STT wave depression with T-wave inversion in the interior and V5 and V6 leads. The patient remained asymptomatic throughout, with no arrhythmias. His blood pressure dropped to a low of 38 systolic over 0 at 6 minutes post exercise and remained low for several minutes. During this time period, an IV was started and D5 1/2 normal saline at 200 cc/hour was given to elevate the blood pressure. IV started at 12:30 and stopped at 13:20. The patient remained pain-free during this episode and felt fine during the entire episode. At the 10-minute mark, the T-wave inversion started resolving, and the STT waves returned to normal.

Upon consultation with Dr. Jones at Magic Memorial, the patient was advised to report for a cardiac catheterization to rule out ischemic heart disease.

Which codes are reported by the hospital for this outpatient service?

Note: The cardiologist is not employed by the hospital reporting the test.

In addition to the IV infusion codes, which codes are reported by the hospital for this outpatient service?

ICD-9-CM and CPT Code(s):

a. 786.50, 796.3, 93015
b. 729.5, 796.3, 93015
c. 414.8, 458.29, 93017
d. 729.5, 458.9, 93017

ICD-10-CM Code(s): _____

8.6.   The following documentation is from the health record of a patient who received hospital outpatient surgical services.

Preoperative Diagnosis: Hypertensive cardiovascular disease with end-stage renal disease and congestive heart failure

Postoperative Diagnosis: Same

Procedure: Placement of AV fistula with Gore-Tex graft of the right forearm for dialysis access

Description: After placement on the operating table, the patient was premedicated with .05 mg of Versed. The right arm was prepped and draped in the usual sterile fashion. Following the infiltration of 1 percent lidocaine, a transverse incision was made just beyond the antecubital fossa. Dissection was carried down, the basilic vein and artery were identified and mobilized, and Silastic loops were placed. Another incision was then made, just above the wrist. After the area was infiltrated with lidocaine, a 6-mm Gore-Tex graft was tunneled through the loop. Anastomosis to the artery was accomplished after the patient received 2,000 units of IV heparin. End-to-side anastomosis was accomplished with 6-0 and 7-0 Prolene sutures. The end areas were interrupted and the edges approximated with running sutures. On removal of the clamps, excellent blood flow was evident. Anastomosis was deemed satisfactory. Venous anastomosis was then accomplished with 6-0 and 7-0 Prolene sutures. Flushing and back-bleeding were allowed prior to completion of the anastomosis. Upon completion, excellent flow was evident through the vein. After a period of observation with no bleeding, both wounds were closed with subcutaneous 3-0 VICRYL in a running fashion, and the skin was closed with 4-0 Prolene sutures. Dressings were applied and the patient returned to the outpatient recovery area in stable condition.

Which of the following is the correct code set?

ICD-9-CM and CPT Code(s):

a. 404.92, 36830
b. 404.93, 585.6, 428.0, 36830
c. 585.6, 428.0, 401.9, 36821
d. 404.93, 36821

ICD-10-CM Code(s): _____

8.7.   The following documentation is from the health record of a patient who received hospital outpatient diagnostic services.

Preoperative Diagnosis: Angina

Postoperative Diagnosis: Patent coronary arteries and grafts, ASHD present

Procedure: Right and left heart cath with coronary angiography

The patient was brought to the cath lab in a fasting state. The right groin was prepped and draped in the usual sterile fashion. After local anesthesia was administered, sheaths were placed percutaneously into the right femoral artery and vein. IV heparin 3,000 units were given.

Using a thermodilution catheter, right heart pressures were measured, and thermo-dilution cardiac outputs and AV oxygen differences were obtained. A pigtail catheter was inserted into the left ventricular cavity, and simultaneous left ventricular pressures were measured. A pullback was obtained across the aortic valve.

Using a 7R4 catheter, angiography was performed of the right coronary artery and both vein grafts. A 7L4 was used for angiography of the left coronary artery. Additional attempts were made to image the vein graft to the right coronary artery with a right coronary artery bypass catheter. The pigtail catheter was reinserted, and left ventricular angiography and aortic root angiography were performed. The patient tolerated the procedure well and returned to the recovery room in good condition.

Which codes are assigned for this service?

ICD-9-CM and CPT Code(s):

a. 414.00, 413.9, V45.81, 93461
b. 414.01, 414.02, 93453, 93460
c. 414.00, 413.9, V45.81, 93453, 93462
d. 414.01, 414.02, 413.9, V45.81, 93461

ICD-10-CM Code(s): _____

8.8. This 21-month-old male presents to the Emergency Department with nausea and vomiting since 10 pm last night, at least 8 times, which is nonbloody but bilious. Temp of 39.8 since last night. He has a history of Tetralogy of Fallot, s/p repair 2 months ago. He has known immunodeficiency, laryngomalacia, and a gastrostomy tube. After examination, working differential diagnoses are acute gastroenteritis, bacteremia, or possible septicemia. Symptoms similar to episode about 1 month ago that was determined to be bacteremia with G-tube site infection. The patient is treated with Zofran 2 mg IV, followed by Ceftriaxone 600 mg IV. The patient is discharged after resolution of vomiting and fever. Diagnosis listed as acute gastroenteritis.

Assign the correct codes for the facility services provided today.

ICD-9-CM Code(s): _V13.65_

a. 279.3, 558.9, 748.3, V13.69, V15.1, V44.1
b. 558.9, 790.7, V15.1, V44.1
c. 787.01, 558.9, V44.1
d. 787.03, 780.60, 558.9, 745.2, V15.1, V44.1

ICD-10-CM Code(s): _____

8.9. A 69-year-old patient was hit by a car, causing intra-thoracic trauma and hemorrhage. The patient was taken directly from the Emergency Department to the operative suite where the chest was opened and hemorrhage was controlled, but the patient's heart stopped. Open heart massage was performed but the patient expired before the patient could be admitted.

Assign the appropriate CPT code(s) and any required modifier(s) to report this service.

a. 32110-CA
b. 32110, 32160
c. 32160-CA
d. 32110-CA, 32160-CA

8.10. This 63-year-old male patient presents to the ED by ambulance after collapsing while mowing the lawn at home. He has a diminished level of consciousness but says that he had palpitations and lightheadedness followed by apparent syncope. His wife saw him fall and immediately called 9-1-1. He has a prior history of MI 3 years ago and coronary atherosclerosis of the native vessels. His vital signs on presentation show hypotension with a heart rate of 110. His EKG shows arrhythmia. While on the heart monitor the patient's rhythm changes to ventricular fibrillation. 150-J biphasic cardioversion shock is performed, following standard advanced cardiac life-support protocols. Arrhythmia continues following cardioversion, and the patient arrests. CPR is performed, and the patient is resuscitated.

The physician documents: 35 minutes of critical care provided, exclusive of the time spent performing cardioversion, for a patient with acute ventricular tachycardia, ventricular fibrillation, prior MI, coronary atherosclerosis of native vessels, and cardiac arrest, successfully resuscitated.

What are the correct diagnosis and procedure codes for this patient?

ICD-9-CM and CPT Code(s): _____

ICD-10-CM Code(s): _____

8.11. The following documentation is from the health record of a patient who received hospital outpatient radiology department services.

Preoperative Diagnosis: Left carotid aneurysm, internal extracranial portion

Postoperative Diagnosis: Same

Procedure: Left carotid artery test occlusion

Procedure Description: With the patient properly prepared and draped in sterile fashion, a 6-French sheath was inserted in antegrade fashion into the right femoral artery. A diagnostic catheter was inserted coaxially through the sheath and used to select the left internal carotid artery. An exchange 018 wire was placed through the catheter and then the catheter was removed. A 6 mm × 2 cm balloon catheter was threaded over the wire and positioned with the balloon across the lumen of the proximal left internal carotid artery. The balloon was inflated to 0.5 atmosphere while slowly injecting contrast through the end of the balloon around the wire. Complete stasis of the carotid artery was documented. Neurologic testing was performed for 5 minutes. The patient was placed on heparin prior to this procedure, and a 5,000-unit bolus was administered in the left carotid artery just prior to balloon inflation. Another 1,000 units of heparin were slowly administered through the tip of the balloon over a 5-minute period, along with saline. Only a small amount of total fluid was administered, and contrast was found to be static in the carotid artery during the entire period. After 5 minutes, the balloon was deflated and the patient was sent to the recovery area in good condition.

What is the correct code assignment?

ICD-9-CM and CPT Code(s):

a. 437.3, 36100, 37204, 75894
b. 442.81, 36620
c. 442.81, 36100, 37204, 75894
d. 442.81, 61626, 36100, 75894

ICD-10-CM Code(s): _____

8.12. The following documentation is from the health record of a cardiac catheterization patient.

Procedures Performed: Left heart catheterization.

Coronary angiography.

Right coronary artery mid in-stent restenotic lesion.

Percutaneous transluminal coronary balloon angioplasty.

Placement of intracoronary stent.

Right coronary artery-distal stent edge lesion.

Percutaneous transluminal coronary balloon angioplasty.

Placement of intracoronary stent.

Adjunct use of intravenous Aggrastat infusion.

Complications: None.

Indication: This is a 70-year-old white male with known history of hyperlipidemia, TIA, and coronary artery disease status, post PTCA with stent placement of the mid right coronary artery on July 27, 20XX, who presented with recurrence of chest pain. The stress MIBI cardiac scan performed on January 29, 20XX, revealed proximal inferior wall perfusion defects extending to the LV apex.

Diagnostic Angiography: After obtaining informed consent, the patient was brought to the cardiac catheterization laboratory in a fasting state. The bilateral femoral areas were prepped sterilely in the standard fashion, and ECG monitoring was established. Using the modified Seldinger technique, arterial access was obtained in the right femoral artery.

The #7 French Cordis JL-4 HF and JR-4 HF catheters were used to perform the diagnostic coronary angiography. The left main artery was large and essentially normal. The left anterior descending artery was moderate-sized, long, and wrapped around the apex without significant lesion. The first diagonal branch artery was large, bifurcated, and essentially normal. The second diagonal branch artery was small-sized and normal. The left circumflex artery was large and had 40 to 50 percent ostial stenosis. The first and second obtuse marginal arteries were small and normal. The right coronary artery was dominant and had 90 to 95 percent multifocal in-stent restenosis in the mid artery. There was also 60 to 70 percent distal stent edge stenosis in the early distal right coronary artery. The PDA and PLB arteries were normal.

Procedure: Mid right coronary artery (RCA) in-stent restenosis and distal stent edge lesions: Following the diagnostic coronary angiography, Aggrastat 16.1 cc IV bolus was then given to the patient with continuous infusion at rate of 14 cc/ hour for 50 minutes. Heparin, 5,400-unit IV bolus, was also given to the patient to control ACT around 200 to 300 seconds. After this, a #8 French Cordis JR-4/ side hole guiding catheter was used to engage into the ostium of the right coronary artery. After baseline angiography was performed, a Guidant 0.014 inch Hi-Torque floppy extra support guidewire was then advanced out of the guide into the RCA. The guidewire was then advanced across the mid RCA in-stent restenotic lesion and positioned in the distal PLB artery without difficulty. After this, an NC Ranger balloon, 2.75 mm in diameter by 22 mm in length, was advanced over the guidewire into the mid RCA in-stent restenotic lesion. The balloon was positioned across the lesion and inflated twice at 18 atmospheres and 20 atmospheres for 60 seconds, respectively. The patient had transient chest pain and ST-T wave elevation in the inferior leads.

Following this, the balloon was then advanced further to cross the distal stent edge lesion in the early distal right coronary artery and inflated at 10 atmospheres for 60 seconds. Repeat angiogram still revealed some residual narrowing at the distal stent edge lesion. After this, the balloon was then exchanged out for a BX Velocity, 2.75 mm × 8 mm, coronary stent that was advanced to deploy cover in the distal stent edge lesion at 12 atmospheres for 15 seconds; however, the stent did not overlap with the mid RCA previously stented segment. Repeat angiogram revealed a small dissection at the distal RCA in the gap between the old and the new coronary stent. The operator then elected to deploy another short stent to cover the dissection. The second BX Velocity, 2.75 mm × 8 mm, coronary stent was then advanced to position to cover the dissection, overlapping with the mid RCA and distal RCA stented segment. The stent was then successfully deployed at 12 atmospheres for 30 seconds. Follow-up angiogram revealed good luminal dilatation in the distal RCA stented segment; however, there was increased renarrowing within the mid RCA in-stent restenotic lesion with irregular border. The operator decided to deploy another stent to cover within the mid RCA in-stent restenotic lesion. The third BX Velocity, 2.75 mm × 18 mm, coronary stent was then advanced to position within the mid RCA in-stent restenotic lesion and successfully deployed at 14 atmospheres for 30 seconds. After this, the stent balloon was used to post dilate sequentially within the entire mid RCA and distal RCA stented segment at 10 atmospheres and 12 atmospheres for 3 minutes of total duration.

Final orthogonal angiogram revealed no residual stenosis in the overlapping stented mid- and distal RCA in-stent restenotic lesion and distal stent edge lesion. There was no angiographic evidence of dissection or thrombus. Flow to the distal vessel was TIMI grade 3. Plavix, 375 mg, was given to the patient after the stent deployment. At this point, it was elected to conclude the procedure. Balloon, wires, and catheters were removed. The hemostatic sheaths were sewn in place. The patient was transferred back to the ward in stable condition.

Conclusions: 1. Significant multifocal in-stent restenotic lesion in the mid RCA with distal stent edge lesion in the distal RCA.
2. Successful percutaneous transluminal coronary balloon angioplasty and placement of three overlapping coronary stents (BX Velocity 2.75 mm × 18 mm, 2.75 mm × 8 mm, and 2.75 mm × 8 mm) in the mid RCA in-stent restenotic lesion and distal stent edge lesion in the early distal right coronary artery.

What are the correct diagnosis and procedure codes for this patient?

ICD-9-CM First-Listed Diagnosis: _____

ICD-9-CM Additional Diagnoses: _____

CPT Code(s): _____

ICD-10-CM First-Listed Diagnosis: _____

ICD-10-CM Additional Diagnoses: _____

8.13. **Emergency Services:**

Chief Complaint: Cardiac Arrest

HPI: The 37-year-old female was found on the floor of her bathroom by her husband. She was in full arrest and he started CPR immediately. She could have been down as long as 20 minutes prior to him finding her. The EMTs took over CPR when they arrived some 20 minutes later and applied AED. They intubated her with a 7.5 ET—the cords were visualized and taped at 24 cm. Good breath sounds bilaterally after intubation.

The EMTs administered 1 mg EPI and 1 mg Atropine—no response and ECG was still in asytole.

Physical Exam upon Arrival: The patient was unconscious and apneic and pulseless. Skin: Purple from just above the clavicle and skin was cool and dry. HEENT: Pupils fixed and dilated. Neck: No JVD or trachea deviation. Chest: clear and equal bilateral sounds with intubation. Abdomen: Distended and tight. Extremities: Flaccid and cool.

Emergency Physician's Note: This 37 y/o white female arrived by ambulance in full arrest. Epi and bicarb were given on the way to the hospital. Two leads showed agonal asystole rhythm.

A high dose of epi 5 mg was given IV and shock with 360 joules $\times$ 2—no response. A total of 4 amp of bicarb and 4 high dose epi given with intervening defib at 360 joules. No response. Her pupils were fixed and dilated on arrival—has full neck and chest venous stasis. The endo tube was aerating both lungs. Blood gases revealed:

Ph 6.909, PO_2 57, HCO_3 9.9, Base 22.4, O_2 sat 64%, PCO_2 49

The patient arrived at 11:10 and the code was called at 11:45. Patient never had any pulse or spontaneous electrical activity.

Which of the following codes represent the services provided for this patient?

ICD-9-CM and CPT Code(s):

a. 427.5, 782.5, 92950, 92960, 99291, J0171
b. 427.5, 92950, 92960, 99291, J0171
c. 427.5, 782.5, 92950, 92960, 99291
d. 427.5, 99291, J0171

ICD-10-CM Code(s): _____

Disorders of the Digestive System

8.14. The following documentation is from the health record of a 86-year-old female patient.

Preoperative Diagnosis: Paraesophageal hernia

Postoperative Diagnosis: Paraesophageal hernia

Procedure: Laparoscopic reduction of paraesophageal hernia

Indication: The patient is a pleasant, 86-year-old female who presented with an acute onset of hematemesis. Endoscopy was performed, which revealed a large portion of the patient's stomach in her chest. The condition was discussed with the patient and her family. The options of open versus laparoscopic repair of her hernia were discussed. The patient and her family understood the risks versus benefits, as well as potential complications of both procedures, and elected to undergo the laparoscopic procedure. Based on the presence of multiple other chronic illnesses, the patient and family have signed a Do Not Resuscitate order as of today.

Procedure Description: After consent was obtained, the patient was taken to the operating room and placed supine on the operating table. After adequate general endotracheal anesthesia, the patient's abdomen was prepped and draped in the usual surgical fashion. Initial entry was gained through an infraumbilical elliptical incision. Cut down technique was used. A 5-mm trocars was inserted. A pneumoperitoneum was then obtained. Two additional 5.0 mm trocars were placed—one in the left epigastric region and another in the left upper quadrant. The initial 5.0-mm infraumbilical trocar was replaced with a 12-mm trocar. A 10-mm 30 degree scope was used throughout the procedure for visualization.

The stomach was then grasped with the soft bowel grasper and reduced from the chest in a hand-over-hand fashion. There were dense attachments of the stomach to the superior portion of the hernia sac in the chest. These were carefully taken down with the harmonics shearers. This allowed for good mobilization of the stomach and return of the stomach to the abdomen. The hernia sac was resected and sent to Pathology. The 1.0 cm defect of the diaphragm around the esophagus was repaired with mesh implantation.

The abdomen was then inspected for hemostasis which was noted to be pristine. The laparoscopic trocars were removed and the CO_2 insufflation was released. The skin incisions were closed with Monocryl, benzoin, and Steri-strips and followed by sterile Band-Aids. The patient tolerated the procedure well. She was awakened, extubated, and taken to the recovery room in satisfactory condition.

What codes will be reported for the outpatient care of this Medicare patient?

ICD-9-CM and CPT Code(s):

a. 578.0, 553.3, V49.86, 43281
b. 553.3, 49652
c. 553.3, V49.86, 43282
d. 578.0, 553.3, 43659

ICD-10-CM Code(s): _____

8.15. A patient reported to the ambulatory surgery department at the request of her general surgeon.

Operative Report:	Hospital Outpatient Surgery Department
Preoperative Diagnoses:	1. Inguinal hernia 2. Postcolorectal resection for CA
Postoperative Diagnosis:	Same
Procedure:	Right inguinal herniorrhaphy

Description of Procedure: Under general anesthetic, an incision was made over the anterior wall of the inguinal canal, which was opened. The cord was isolated, taking care to protect the nerve. The hernia sac was seen, which has direct hernia on the medial aspect of the wound. This was reduced and held in place using mesh that was stapled into place with a hole being made for the cord. The anterior wall of the inguinal canal was then closed with VICRYL, a hemostasis was achieved, and the wound closed with skin clips. Following this, the attention was turned to a screening colonoscopy, which was performed to the ileocecal valve without difficulty. Ascending, transverse, and descending colon were normal. There was no true evidence of diverticula. The sigmoid was normal, and a retroflex view of the rectosigmoid anastomosis in the rectum shows no gross abnormalities. The patient tolerated the procedure well and will be followed up in the office.

Which code set is reported by the facility for this outpatient surgery?

ICD-9-CM and CPT Code(s):

a. 550.90, 562.10, V10.05, 49505-RT, G0105
b. 550.90, V76.51, V10.06, 49505-RT, 45378
c. 550.91, V76.51, V10.05, 49505-RT, 49568-RT
d. 550.90, V10.06, 49520-RT, 45330

ICD-10-CM Code(s): _____

8.16. The following documentation is from the health record of a 70-year-old Medicare patient who received hospital outpatient services.

Operative Report

History and Indications: The patient is a 70-year-old female who previously underwent a cholecystectomy but presents again with similar pain in the right upper quadrant in the presence of disturbed liver function studies.

Procedure: ERCP sphincterotomy and stone extraction. The Olympus Video side-viewing duodenoscope was atraumatically introduced into esophagus and advanced with slide-by technique into the stomach. The gastric mucosa was normal. The pyloric channel was normal and easily intubated. The first and second parts of the duodenum were visualized. The ampulla appeared normal. Initial cannulation with a precurved catheter revealed a normal pancreatic duct. A single injection was made into the pancreas. Repositioning was accomplished with the assistance of a straight 0.035 guidewire, and free cannulation and injection of the papilla of Vater was accomplished. Full visualization of the common duct was obtained, revealing a large multifaceted free-floating stone within the proximal duct. The intrahepatic biliary system appeared normal. The extrahepatic biliary system appeared dilated. An exchange was made with the 20-millimeter sphincterotome and a sphincterotomy was performed with perfect hemostasis. The duct was then swept with a 15-millimeter stone extraction balloon, and the stone was pulled into the duodenal lumen. The duct was "swept" two more times with negative results. Additional spot and overhead films were obtained to confirm clearance of all stone material. The procedure was terminated with the patient in satisfactory condition, and she was returned to the recovery area.

Assessment: Choledocholithiasis associated with obstruction.

Which code set will be submitted for this Medicare patient for the services described?

ICD-9-CM and CPT Code(s):

a. 574.50, 43262, 43273
b. 574.50, 43262, 43264
c. 574.51, 43262, 43264, 43273
d. 574.51, 43262

ICD-10-CM Code(s): _____

8.17. The following documentation is from the health record of a 65-year-old male who received hospital outpatient GI laboratory services.

Endoscopy Record

Preoperative Diagnosis: Guaiac positive stools

Postoperative Diagnosis: Multiple colon polyps, diverticulosis

Procedure: Total colonoscopy with biopsy and polypectomy

Indications: This is a 65-year-old male who was found to have guaiac positive stools on a routine exam; no change in bowel habits or appreciable weight loss.

The patient was brought to the endoscopy suite and placed in the left lateral decubitus position. 50 mg of Demerol and 2 mg Versed were administered. Digital rectal exam was performed, which was normal. Olympus colonoscope was inserted and passed under direct vision. A large polyp was seen immediately at 20 cm. This appeared to be pedunculated and approximately 1.5 cm long. Scope was passed all the way to the cecum and then slowly withdrawn. Cecum, ascending colon, hepatic flexure, transverse colon all appeared normal except for fairly extensive diverticula in the cecum and scattered throughout the rest of the sets. At the splenic flexure at 80 cm, there was a lesion, which was biopsied with a hot biopsy probe. At 60 cm, there was another small polyp, which was cauterized at the base with the probe and excised. At 20 cm, the pedunculated rectal polyp was snared and removed. The exam of the base revealed complete excision. The rest of the sigmoid and the rectum were unremarkable.

The pathology report showed mucus polypoid tissue at 80 cm and adenomatous polyps at 60 cm and 20 cm.

Which of the following code sets should be reported?

ICD-9-CM and CPT Code(s):

a. 211.3, 211.4, 562.10, 45385, 45384-59, 45380-59
b. 211.3, 569.0, 45384
c. 211.3, 569.0, 45385, 45384-59, 45380-59
d. 792.1, 211.3, 569.0, 562.10, 45385, 45384

ICD-10-CM Code(s): _____

8.18. This is the health record of a patient treated in Ambulatory Surgery

Significant Findings: This patient is an 84-year-old male with complaint of recurrent left inguinal hernia with associated discomfort. The original surgery on this patient was 2 years ago and the patient wraps his abdomen without physician's order. This in fact is increasing the discomfort in his abdominal. He currently denies any urological or GI problems. The physical examination revealed a very pleasant senior citizen in minimal distress. HEENT were normal. Chest/heat revealed no rales or rhonchi. Skin: warm and dry to the touch although he does have an eczematous rash on the upper chest which has not been diagnosed previously. He admits to using some type of OTC cream for this. His inguinal area is significant for a healed scar in the left groin area which today shows a significant and reducible bulge. There was a smaller hernia on the right side.

Laboratory Findings: Electrolyte panel was within normal limits. Bleeding time acceptable at 2 minutes. His white count was 12,500. HB was 14 and HCT 43 with a normal differential. Urinalysis showed the following results: Dark yellow, cloudy urine with evidence of pyuria. RBCs 2; WBC 10; pH6 Potassium 15. Findings suggest early UTI.

Two view chest x-ray was normal with some moderate cardiomegaly and healed rib fractures.

Admitting Diagnosis: Recurrent left inguinal hernia and initial right inguinal hernia

Postoperative diagnosis was the same.

Procedure: Laparoscopic repair of recurrent left inguinal hernia and right inguinal hernia

Description of Procedure: The patient was taken to the Ambulatory Surgery suite where he was prepped and draped in the usual manner and placed in the supine position on the table. Monitoring equipment was attached and he was given general anesthesia for a laparoscopic repair of a recurrent left inguinal hernia and an initial right inguinal hernia.

Trocars were inserted for laparoscopy and the hernias repaired. A piece of 3 × 5 mesh was trimmed to fit the defect in the left inguinal hernia and was placed down in the inguinal canal. It was tacked down using interrupted sutures. A unilateral repair of the initial right hernia was done.

The procedures were performed without any complications. The patient was sent to PACU where he was monitored for several hours. The incisions remained dry and there was no evidence of any unusual swelling in the inguinal areas. The IV was discontinued and the patient was discharged to home. He was given a Lortab prescription and advised to return to the hospital if any complications should occur. The patient was given 1,000 mg of Ampicillin Sodium IM for UTI.

Which codes will be reported for this ambulatory surgery service?

ICD-9-CM and CPT Code(s):

a. 550.93, 49650, 49651, J0290 × 2
b. 550.92, 49650, 49651, 49568
c. 550.93, 49650, 49651
d. 550.91, 550.90, 49650-50, J0290 × 2

ICD-10-CM Code(s): _____

8.19.   The following documentation is from the health record of a 40-year-old female patient.

Emergency Department Services

HPI: This is a 40-year-old female with a 3-year history of diarrhea and a 1-year history of epigastric discomfort. She had a CT scan with a mass on the tail of the pancreas, as well as gastrin level greater than 1,000 while taking Prilosec. She has been amenorrheic for the past 4 months.

The patient presents to the ED with severe diarrhea and dehydration after discontinuing medications to allow for a repeat gastrin level off medications to eliminate the compounding effect of Prilosec on gastrin levels. Unfortunately, she was unable to stay off medication long enough, and she developed severe diarrhea with dehydration and a creatinine greater than 3, and she was admitted to observation services. Gastrin level is 1,023 with VIP of 290.

Patient was rehydrated and orally treated with 200 mEq of potassium. The patient had significantly elevated calcium, which normalized with rehydration. Vitamin D level is pending, and PTH level also has returned elevated, concurrent with a calcium of 9.9. MRI of the abdomen has revealed multiple lesions in the liver with a density consistent with metastatic malignancy. Additionally on the MRI, a 6-cm pancreatic mass was noted at the tail of the pancreas.

This scenario is most consistent with multiple endocrine neoplasia syndrome (MEN-1) with parathyroid hyperplasia leading to hypercalcemia when dehydrated. Most likely, the recent normal calcium is due to a concurrent hypovitaminosis D, which is, in turn, secondary to chronic diarrhea. Dostinex has been initiated today at 0.25 mg 2 times a week. Most likely she has MEN-1 given the current pancreatic and pituitary evidence of adenoma.

She is transferred to Memorial Hospital for CT-guided biopsy of a possible adenocarcinoma and to rule out the possibility of MEN-1.

Discharge Diagnoses:
1. Pancreatic and pituitary adenomas with multiple lesions on the liver with questionable metastasis
2. Probable carcinoid syndrome (MEN-1)
3. Hypercalcemia while dehydrated with normalization on rehydration
4. Severe chronic diarrhea with hypokalemia and hypomagnesemia
5. Amenorrhea

Discharge Medications:
Prevacid 30 mg, one p.o. b.i.d.
Magnesium oxide 400 mg, one p.o. t.i.d.
Sandostatin ampules 0.5 amp of 1 mg per amp every 8 hours
Trazodone 50 p.o. q. h.s. p.r.n. insomnia
Darvocet N 100 mg p.o. q. 4–6 hours p.r.n.
Dostinex 0.5 mg 1/2 tab every Wednesday and Saturday

Which of the following is the correct code set for this observation service?

ICD-9-CM Code(s):

a. 237.4, 573.8, 275.42, 276.51, 787.91, 276.8, 275.2, 626.0
b. 211.6, 227.3, 197.7, 275.42, 276.51, 787.91, 276.8, 275.2, 626.0
c. 235.5, 237.0, 197.7, 275.42, 276.51, 787.91, 276.8, 275.2, 626.0
d. 237.4, 573.8, 259.2, 275.42, 276.51, 787.91, 276.8, 275.2, 626.0

ICD-10-CM Code(s): _____

8.20. The following documentation is from the health record of a 57-year-old male patient.

Hospital Outpatient Department Services

Diagnoses: 1. Lung cancer
2. Chemotherapy with Taxol and carboplatin with dexamethasone
3. Type II diabetes with neuropathy and nephropathy, uncontrolled
4. Hyperlipidemia
5. Hepatomegaly

This patient is a 57-year-old male who presents to the outpatient department for chemotherapy, which has been complicated by his diabetes because it has been difficult to control. He had surgery for lung cancer in September and has now undergone chemotherapy with Taxol and carboplatin, including dexamethasone as part of his chemo and prophylaxis for nausea. He has done very well with the chemotherapy. His diabetes is complicated by neuropathy and nephropathy. Dr. Johnson consulted with the patient to manage his diabetes. He has been on 70/30 insulin, 25 units in the morning and 15 units in the evening, for over 1 year. His hepatomegaly has enlarged from the last time that I saw him. I question whether this is fatty infiltration due to poor diabetes control, or whether there is now some involvement with metastatic carcinoma.

Taxol and carboplatin were infused today, followed by dexamethasone; see infusion sheet. The patient appears to have tolerated the chemotherapy well.

Laboratory Data: Sodium 128, potassium 5.5, chloride 89, CO_2 34, BUN 13, creatinine 0.8, glucose 210, calcium 9.4, WBC 9.8, hemoglobin 11.6, hematocrit 34.3, platelets 277,000

Plan: One difficulty here is the cyclic nature of his treatment regimen, likely to produce major shifts in his glucose, which is already difficult to control. The patient will need to monitor his glucose levels closely and follow up with Dr. Johnson. The patient has instructions to call in to Dr. Johnson's nurse on a daily basis for the next week. He is to follow up with me for further chemotherapy next week.

Which of the following is the correct code set combination for this outpatient visit?

ICD-9-CM Code(s):

a. 162.9, 250.62, 357.2, 250.42, 583.81, V58.67, 272.4, 789.1
b. V58.11, 250.62, 250.42, V58.67, 272.4, 789.1
c. V58.11, 162.9, 250.62, 357.2, 250.42, 583.81, V58.67, 272.4, 789.1
d. 162.9, 250.02, V58.67, 272.4, 789.1

ICD-10-CM Code(s): _____

Disorders of the Genitourinary System

8.21. The following documentation is from the health record of a 22-year-old male patient who received hospital outpatient surgery services.

A patient with chronic benign hypertension and stage V chronic kidney disease requiring chronic dialysis, replacement of a permanent Quinton catheter, and the formation of an arteriovenous graft in the left forearm. Following heparinization, the anastomosis was performed, which resulted in a good pulse, but no thrill. The vein was then explored where an area of stenosis was found. This was opened and a dilator passed, but no more than 2-mm diameter was possible. Therefore, the anastomosis was taken down, a tunnel formed, and a 4 × 7 Impra graft used. The graft originated at the antecubital fossa, which was opened transversely. The vein here was about 4 mm, so there were no problems passing a dilator. The graft was then anastomosed over a distance of approximately 5 mm, resulting in good flow. Wounds were closed in layer fashion with 3-0 VICRYL for deep tissues and continuous suture of 6-0 Prolene.

Following completion of the graft, the patient was reprepped and draped for the changing of the Quinton catheter. Following administration of local anesthesia, an incision was made high in the neck close to the point of insertion in the internal jugular. A guidewire was then tunneled centrally through the existing catheter. The old Quinton catheter was removed and an obturator placed. Then a peel-away introducer was inserted easily. The wounds were then closed and a confirmatory x-ray obtained for placement. This showed the Quinton catheter extended well into the internal jugular. Dialysis was provided the same day.

Which of the following code sets will be assigned for this?

ICD-9-CM and CPT Code(s):

a. 585.6, 401.1, 36830, 90935
b. 403.90, 36825, 90935
c. 403.11, 585.5, 36830, 36581-59
d. 403.11, 585.6, 36830, 36581-59, 90935

ICD-10-CM Code(s): _____

8.22. The following documentation is from the health record of a patient who received hospital radiology department services.

A patient who has had his bladder removed due to carcinoma without recurrence is ordered to have a radiology procedure to evaluate the patency of his ileal conduit, including a ureteropyelography using contrast media. The chief complaint and reason for service line in the progress note is blank. The entire procedure is performed in the radiology suite with the radiologist's impression of "normal functioning ileal conduit."

Which of the following procedure codes should be reported for the UB-04 in this case? Do not assign ICD-9-CM Volume III procedure codes.

ICD-9-CM and CPT Code(s):

a. V55.6, V45.74, V10.51, 50684, 74425
b. V55.2, V10.51, 74425
c. 596.8, 188.9, 74425
d. Contact the ordering physician to obtain a diagnosis before coding this encounter.

ICD-10-CM Code(s): _____

8.23.   The following documentation is from the health record of a 47-year-old female.

Hospital Outpatient Surgery Services

Preoperative Diagnosis: Menorrhagia, failure of conservative treatment

Postoperative Diagnosis: Same

Procedure: Hysteroscopy with biopsy, dilatation and curettage

Diagnosis: Menorrhagia

Anesthesia: General

Indications: The patient is a 47-year-old multigravida female with increasing irregular vaginal bleeding. The uterus is very tender, and ultrasound reveals no specific adnexal masses. A Pap smear shows some chronic inflammatory cells and cervicitis. Bleeding has not been controlled in the past month with conservative therapy; thus, the patient is admitted for dilatation and curettage, and a hysteroscopy and biopsy will be carried out.

Technique: Under general anesthesia, the patient was prepped and draped in the usual manner with Betadine, with her cervix retracted outward. Secondary uterine prolapse was noted with minimal cystocele, large rectocele, enterocele, and moderate cervical erosions. The vaginal vault appeared to be clear, as did both adnexa. However, the uterus was thought to be slightly enlarged. Sound was passed into the intrauterine cavity after the cervix was found to be 8 cm deep. The cervix was dilated with Hegar dilators up to #5. The 5-mm Wolff scope, with normal saline irrigation, was then inserted. An inspection of the endocervical canal showed no abnormalities.

Upon entering the uterine cavity, some irregular shedding of the endometrium was noted. Endometrial shedding was noted more to be the patient's left cornu area than the right. The contour of the cavity appeared to be normal; no bulging masses or septation were noted. The Wolff scope was removed, and the cervix was further dilated with Hegar dilators up to #12. A medium-sharp curette was inserted into the uterine cavity and the uterus was curettaged in a clockwise manner, with a moderate amount of what appeared to be irregular proliferative endometrium being obtained.

Again, the contour of the cavity appeared to be normal. Endometrial biopsies also were taken. The patient was transferred to the recovery room in good condition.

Pathology report reveals secretory proliferative endometrium without additional abnormalities noted.

Which of the following code sets will be reported?

ICD-9-CM and CPT Code(s):

a. 626.2, 618.4, 618.6, 616.0, 58558
b. 626.2, 58558
c. 626.2, 618.4, 618.6, 616.0, 58100, 58120
d. 618.4, 618.6, 616.0, 58558

ICD-10-CM Code(s): _____

8.24.   **Chief Complaint:**   Persistent hematuria

History of Present Illness: This is an 83-year-old white female with a 5-day history of gross hematuria. Patient contacted her family physician several days ago. He prescribed antibiotics but the problem is unresolved. The patient does not have a history of urinary tract infections and has never experienced hematuria prior to this episode. Patient had an IVP earlier today which disclosed relatively normal upper urinary tracts but some filling defects in the urinary bladder.

Her current medications include lanoxin for congestive heart failure, iron supplements, and one baby aspirin daily. She does have a history of long-standing CHF.

Allergies: NKA

Past Surgical/Medical History: Patient has had three normal pregnancies and 2 spontaneous abortions completed by dilation and curettage. The patient has a history of bunionectomy and comminuted wrist fracture following a fall several years ago. Generally, she is in good health.

Social/Personal History: Patient neither smokes nor drinks. She does consume several cups of caffeine each day in the form of coffee and hot tea.

Family History: Unremarkable from a urological standpoint.

Review of System: The ROS is unremarkable. The patient denies weight or gain, no shortness of breath or chest pain. No change in bowel habits, no nausea or vomiting. Patient has experienced no problems with gait or sensation and has no discernable pain.

Physical Examination: The patient is a well-nourished, slightly overweight, well-developed female. HEENT: Unremarkable. EOM are full and conjunctivae are normal. Neck: No lymphadenopathy, no enlargement of the thyroid. No bruits heard in the carotids bilaterally. Chest/lungs: Clear to A&P, no rales or rhonchi heard. Breasts: No lumps or adenopathy in the axillary area. Abdomen: No pain or tenderness. GU: External genitalia and pelvic examination do not reveal any obvious problems.

Procedure: Cystourethroscopy with resection of single bladder tumor

Anesthesia: General

Preoperative Diagnosis: Gross hematuria

Postoperative Diagnosis: Bladder tumor

Technique: The patient was placed in the modified dorsolithotomy position, prepped and draped in the usual manner. General anesthesia was attained. A urethroscopy was carried out with Foroblique lens. A 28-French resectoscope sheath with obturator was inserted into the bladder. Transurethral resection of the approximately 2.1-cm bladder tumor was performed and the specimen sent to pathology. Because of the suspicion for bladder carcinoma, fulguration of the surrounding bladder mucosa was performed. There did not appear to be any induration of the bladder mucosa with carcinoma. Instruments were withdrawn and a 20-French Foley catheter inserted. The patient was transported to PACU in stable condition.

Pathology Report

Tissue Submitted: Bladder tumor

Gross Findings: Received in formalin and labeled with the patient's name and "bladder tumor" are 2 irregular segments of soft, rubbery, pink-tan tissue ranging from 0.6 × 0.3 × 0.3 to 1.2 cm × 0.9 × 0.04 cm.

Microscopic Findings: There appears to be evidence of a papillary lesion with thickened epithelium and nuclear pleomorphism. There may be a minimal degree of infiltration into the lamina propria but extensive infiltration is not noted and none of the muscularis is involved with tumor.

Pathological Findings: Papillary transitional cell carcinoma of the urinary bladder.

Which of the following would be reported for this encounter?

ICD-9-CM and CPT Code(s):

a. 188.9, 599.71, 52000, 52235
b. 233.7, 599.71, 52214
c. 188.9, 599.71, 52235
d. 188.9, 52214, 52235

ICD-10-CM Code(s): _____

8.25. Ambulatory Surgery Operative Report

Preoperative Diagnosis:	Cervical dysplasia and right vaginal wall cyst.
Postoperative Diagnosis:	Cervical intraepithelial dysplasia I and right vaginal wall cyst
Procedure:	Cervical laser ablation; I&D of vaginal wall cyst; EUA.

History: The patient is a 28-year-old nulligravida who has had a history of PAP smears showing slight dysplasia. A colposcopy was done 2 weeks ago which showed a significant amount of erythematous, angry-looking areas. At that time it was noted that she had a sebaceous cyst of the right vaginal wall. Patient has type I diabetes mellitus but this seems to be under control with no significant complications. Preop lab work demonstrated sugar levels at 105, HGB 12.9, HCT 42, and BUN 12. Heart and lung exam were within normal limits.

Description of Procedure: The patient was taken to OP surgery where she was placed in the dorsal lithotomy position and prepped and draped in the usual manner. Induction of general anesthesia was successful. The perineum was cleansed with betadine. An EUA was performed and revealed a large right vaginal wall cyst measuring approximately 4 × 6 cm. There appeared to be significant cervical dysplasia although no masses were palpable. The uterus appeared within normal limits.

A speculum was placed into the vagina which allowed the cervix and vaginal wall to be well visualized. A 4-mm incision was made into the center of the vaginal cyst using electrocautery. A thick sebaceous substance oozed from the cyst. The contents of the cyst were thoroughly expressed.

Two areas of significant dysplasia around the cervical os were noted. The area of cervical dysplasia was ablated 8 cm deep using a CO_2 laser at 40 watts. The surrounding area was brushed using a 20-watt laser. Good hemostasis was observed during the procedure. The speculum was removed from the vagina and the patient was sent to PACU in stable and good condition. Blood loss was minimal.

Pathological Findings: CIN 1 and sebaceous cyst of the right vaginal wall.

Which of the following represents correct coding for this service?

ICD-9-CM and CPT Code(s):

a. 233.1, 57420
b. 622.10, 57023, 57513
c. 622.11, 57420, 57513
d. 622.11, 623.8, 57513, 57010

ICD-10-CM Code(s): _____

Infectious Diseases/Disorders of the Skin and Subcutaneous Tissue

8.26.   The following documentation is from the health record of a 62-year-old female patient.

Hospital Outpatient Surgery Services

The patient is a 62-year-old female who has been in generally good health until last month, when she developed a crusty lesion inside the left naris. She initially treated it with Vicks ointment. When it failed to heal, she decided to seek medical attention. Her primary care physician biopsied this lesion, and the pathologic diagnosis was squamous cell carcinoma of the left internal nasal ala. She is posthysterectomy (10 years) for endometrial carcinoma. She has smoked $1^{1}/_{2}$ packs of cigarettes each day for the past 40 years.

The patient presented to the outpatient surgery center of the hospital for wide excision of the left internal nasal alar lesion, which is less than .5 cm in diameter. This procedure included a full-thickness resection in the middle and posterior thirds of the lateral cartilage, along with vestibular skin and mucous membrane. Nasal reconstruction was required to provide an acceptable cosmetic appearance following excision. A flap graft composite reconstruction was utilized for primary closure of the defect that was left following excision, using donor tissue from the right arm and requiring primary closure of a 2-cm graft.

Which of the following code sets is appropriate for this case?

ICD-9-CM and CPT Code(s):

a. 173.3. V10.42, 30118, 30400
b. 160.0, V10.42, 305.1, 30150, 15760
c. 160.0, 15760, 30150
d. 173.3, V10.42, 305.1, 14060

ICD-10-CM Code(s): _____

8.27. The following documentation is from the health record of a 44-year-old female patient.

Hospital Outpatient Surgery Services

Preoperative Diagnosis: Extensive superficial partial-thickness wounds to the abdomen, secondary to poor wound healing; status post abdominoplasty

Postoperative Diagnosis: Same

Operation: Split-thickness skin graft

History: This is a 44-year-old white female who underwent abdominoplasty for morbid obesity in October 20XX and had poor wound healing after the procedure. The patient underwent several debridement and presently has an extensive superficial, partial-thickness abdominal wound that is granulating well, but it was felt the patient would benefit significantly from split-thickness skin graft to decrease wound pain and decrease convalescence time.

Details of Procedure: The patient was taken to the operating room and prepared and draped in the usual sterile fashion, preparing the donor site of the right thigh as well as abdominal superficial partial-thickness wound. First, two donor grafts were taken with the Brown dermatome, adjusted to a #10 blade, 10:1000-of-an-inch size. The grafts were placed over the abdominal superficial partial-thickness wound in the abdomen after it was prepared by a sharp debridement with Bard-Parker #10 blade. The graft was scored with a #10 blade Bard-Parker in a meshing fashion. The graft was then sewn into place with multiple 5-0 VICRYL sutures. The wounds as well as the donor site were then covered with an Owens dressing. Sutures were placed, and the Owens was reinforced with wet saline cotton balls and with a fluff dressing. The stents were then tied in place and covered with a pressure dressing of Elastoplast, while the donor site received wet-to-dry dressing with ABD burn pad taped into place. The patient was extubated in the operating room. All needle and sponge counts were correct, and the patient was taken to the PAR in stable condition.

Pathology Report: None

Which of the following code sets is correct for this case?

ICD-9-CM and CPT Code(s):

a. 998.59, E878.8, 15100
b. 998.59, 15002, 15100
c. 998.83, E878.8, 15100, 15002
d. 998.83, 278.01, 15200

ICD-10-CM Code(s): _____

8.28.   The following documentation is from the health record of a patient who received hospital outpatient surgery services.

Preoperative Diagnoses: 1. Biopsy-proven malignant melanoma, Clark Level I, right shoulder
2. Neoplasm on left heel

Postoperative Diagnosis: Same

Operations: 1. Wide excision of malignant melanoma, Clark Level I, right shoulder with wide undermining, rotation, and advancement flap reconstruction

2. Excision of left heel 2 cm × 1 cm × .5 cm pigmented neoplasm, rule out dysplasia vs. malignant melanoma, with wide undermining, rotation, and advancement flap reconstruction

Description of Procedure: The patient was placed on the operating table in the prone position with the back and left heel prepped and draped in sterile fashion. Utilizing 1 percent Xylocaine with epinephrine, a block of the two sites was performed.

The right shoulder lesion was outlined with Brilliant Green in the lines of relaxation, excised in full-thickness fashion down to the fascial level. Undermining over the fascial level was then performed with rotation flaps elevated into position and sutured deeply at the fascial level with #5-0 PDS interrupted, #6-0 PDS, superficial dermis, and #6-0 PDS running intracuticular on the skin. Total area slightly over 10.2 sq cm.

Attention was then turned to the left heel where the pigmented neoplasm was outlined with Brilliant Green, excised in full-thickness fashion, and closed at the fascial level with #4-0 PDS interrupted and 4-0 black nylon interrupted on the skin.

The patient tolerated the procedure quite well and was taken to the recovery room.

Pathology Report

Preoperative Diagnosis: Melanoma right shoulder and lesion left heel

Postoperative Diagnosis: Same

Macroscopic: Specimen 1: Received in formalin, labeled "melanoma right shoulder; biopsy proven Clark Level I" is one ellipse of tan skin, 5 × 1.3 × 1.8 cm. In the center is a healing pink ulcer, 0.6 × 0.4 cm.

The specimen is serially sectioned, and the central lesion is totally submitted in multiple cassettes.

Specimen 2: Received in formalin, labeled "lesion left heel" is one ellipse of tan skin, 1.8 × 0.9 × 0.4 cm. In the center is a brown macular lesion that covers much of the center of the specimen. The specimen is totally submitted in multiple cross sections.

Microscopic and Summary

Specimen 1: Right shoulder excision. Healing ulcer of skin overlying eschar. There is mild scarring and focal foreign body response.

Specimen 2: Left heel. Compatible with a giant pigmented dysplastic nevus.

Which of the following code sets would be reported for this ambulatory surgery?

ICD-9-CM and CPT Code(s):

a. 172.6, 216.7, 14001, 15002
b. 216.7, 216.6, 14000
c. 216.6, 238.2, 14001, 11606, 11423
d. 172.6, 238.2, 14001, 11423-59, 12041

ICD-10-CM Code(s): _____

8.29.   The following documentation is from the health record of a patient who received hospital outpatient surgery services.

Preoperative Diagnosis:	Nevus of the left auricle
Postoperative Diagnosis:	Nevus of the left auricle
Operation:	Excision of nevus, left auricle, with reconstruction with full-thickness skin graft, postauricular area

Description of Procedure: The patient was brought to the operating suite and placed under satisfactory general anesthetic using an indwelling endotracheal tube. The left ear and postauricular areas were prepped with Betadine.

A total of 6 cc of 1 percent Xylocaine with 1:200,000 adrenalin were utilized during the procedure. The lesion measured about 6 mm and was superficially infiltrating at its margins with some variegated color being present as well. The lesion was at a 2 o'clock position on the auricular helix. Margins of about 5 mm were made around the lesion. The tissues were submitted for permanent section.

The resulting defect could not be closed primarily. The postauricular incision was outlined for development of postauricular skin graft centered at the level of the cephaloauricular groove. The graft measured about 8 mm × 10 mm in its form and was elliptical in its orientation. The resulting defect postauricularly was closed in layers with 4-0 VICRYL to the subcutaneous layer and 4-0 nylon in an interrupted fashion to the skin.

The skin graft was placed and sutured in place with 4 sutures peripherally with 4-0 silk and then was tied over bolster sutures of 4-0 silk with a bacitracin-impregnated section of sponge rubber. The patient is to avoid contact sports and to keep a prescription for Duricef 250 mg twice a day for 10 days. A prescription for Cap elixir with codeine 1 to 2 tsp, 8 oz was also given. The patient is to be followed up in approximately 1 week in the office.

Pathology Report

Tissues/Specimen: Skin of external ear, nevus of left auricle

Clinical History: Left ear nevus

Gross Description: "Nevus left auricle" consists of small 4-mm fragment of skin. Entire specimen submitted.

Microscopic: Sections show the specimen to consist of an ellipse of skin showing a benign compound nevus. There is no evidence of malignancy.

Which of the following code sets will be reported for this service?

ICD-9-CM and CPT Code(s):

a. 216.8, 15240, 15004, 12051
b. 216.2, 15260, 11442
c. 173.2, 15260, 11442
d. 216.2, 14060

ICD-10-CM Code(s): _____

8.30.   The following documentation is from the health record of a male patient who received emergency department services (Type A provider-based emergency room).

ED Report

A patient who is a known heroin addict is brought in significant distress to the emergency room by friends. His genitalia are covered with many lesions. Due to his IV drug habit and sexual preference, he is at risk for HIV exposure and hepatitis. He has experienced febrile jaundice for 3 days. He is unable to provide a medical history, but the physician is able to get some information from his girlfriend. Although severely ill, he is not comatose. Medical decision making was stated to be of high complexity. The ER acuity system used by the hospital for medical visits indicated a Level IV service.

Physical examination reveals multiple excoriations covering the penis and scrotum with fluid-filled blisters. The patient is jaundiced and in significant distress. The last "fix" was 3 hours ago per the girlfriend, and the patient has been using heroin daily for the past 2 months. A number of laboratory tests were run, and it was determined that the patient should be transferred to a tertiary care center for definitive treatment and an infectious disease consultation and substance abuse rehabilitation when stable.

The physician's dictated report that details the test results shows the following diagnostic assessment:

1. Herpes simplex virus-2 infection, culture confirmed, severe outbreak
2. Hepatitis suspected, pending laboratory results for type, abnormal liver function studies confirmed; febrile jaundice × 3 days
3. HIV seropositive; recommend Western blot to confirm
4. High-risk lifestyle; sexual habits and drug addict

Which of the following code sets will be reported in addition to chargemaster-reported codes?

ICD-9-CM and CPT Code(s):

a. 054.10, 782.4, 790.6, 042, 99284
b. 054.19, 573.3, 795.71, 305.51, V69.8, 99214
c. 054.13, 054.19, 070.1, 790.6, 795.71, 305.51, V69.2, 99284
d. 042, 305.51, 070.1, 99291

ICD-10-CM Code(s): _____

Behavioral Health Conditions

8.31.   The following documentation is from the health record of a 26-year-old male.

Hospital Outpatient Services

On 1/15, a 26-year-old white male was admitted after being transferred from the outpatient evaluation service with severe homicidal and suicidal ideation. Admitting diagnosis was severe major depressive disorder with psychotic features. Pharmacological treatment was initiated, and suicide precautions were instituted. After a thorough diagnostic evaluation, the risks and benefits of ECT were reviewed. Due to the severity of the psychotic episode and the patient's delusional state, it was determined that ECT was warranted. Extensive efforts were made to secure informed consent from the patient, and a course of ECT was begun.

On 1/23, the psychiatrist reviewed the patient's status noting any changes in his physical condition and his response to the treatment. He performed a problem-focused interval history, a problem-focused examination, and medical decision making of low complexity. At this visit, the psychiatrist again reviewed the treatment options and confirmed the patient's continued consent for ECT. Subsequently on 1/23, the fourth treatment of ECT was administered via placement of a stimulus electrode frontotemporally. Sufficient electrical stimulus was applied to produce an adequate ictal response. A generalized seizure was monitored via EEG. EKG, blood pressure, and pulse remained acceptable throughout. Postictal observation was notable for cardiac arrhythmia, which subsided without sequelae. The patient tolerated the procedure well and was returned to his inpatient room in good condition.

He was discharged to a group home on 1/25 and returned to the hospital as an outpatient for his final planned ECT treatment. Again, sufficient electrical stimulus was applied to produce an adequate ictal response. A generalized seizure was monitored via EEG. EKG, blood pressure, and pulse remained acceptable throughout. Postictal observation was notable for cardiac arrhythmia, which subsided without sequelae. The patient tolerated the procedure well and was held in observation for 4 hours posttreatment, then discharged to the care of his group home supervisor in good condition.

Which of the following code sets is reported for the 1/25 outpatient hospital service?

ICD-9-CM and CPT Code(s):

a. 296.24, 90870
b. 296.24, 90870, 95812, 93040
c. 296.24, 298.9, 90870, 99211-25
d. 296.24, 90870, 95812, 93040, 99234-25

ICD-10-CM Code(s): _____

8.32. The following documentation is from the health record of a 56-year-old man.

Emergency Department and Hospital Observation Services

Final Diagnosis: Chronic schizophrenia, paranoid type with acute exacerbation; improved, compensated congestive heart failure

Pertinent Laboratory Results: Electrolyte panel within normal limits. Digoxin level was 0.6, hemoglobin A1C 6.5, triglycerides 138, CBC unremarkable. TSH 1.3, urinalysis negative. EKG showed normal sinus rhythm.

Assessment: This is a 56-year-old male who presented to the Emergency Room with his sister after decompensating at a hotel where he thought people were trying to get into his apartment, and he continued to decompensate with his paranoia and persecutory-type delusions, so that she felt he needed evaluation for hospitalization. Psychiatric consultation was initiated with Dr. Brown.

Recently, his personal physician has been switching his medications from Zyprexa to Seroquel to Risperdal, and then he started Prolixin. We requested and reviewed his records, and it appears he did quite well on Risperdal, so he went back to taking that, and he was titrated up to 30 mg q. h.s. of Risperdal and 100 mg of trazodone. These 2 medications helped significantly to eliminate his delusions and paranoid ideation. He was admitted to observation status and slept peacefully for 6 hours. His sister reported that he is doing the best that she has seen him in quite some time, and we were conversing at the time of discharge. After consultation with this psychiatrist about the change in medication, the patient was released in the custody of his sister to follow up with his personal physician next Tuesday.

Pertinent Findings on Mental Status at Discharge: Patient spent 45 minutes in the final examination. Behavior is cooperative, fair eye contact. Speech is of normal rate and volume. Not rapid or pressured. Mood euthymic, affect appropriate. Thought process is goal directed, decreased paranoid ideation. Negative for racing thoughts and flight of ideas. Thought content: He denies signs of active psychosis, denies current suicidal or homicidal intent. Insight and judgment improved. Impulse control is fair.

Prognosis: Fair. The main problem is that the patient did not respond well to medication changes. He did do well with the changes we made, but his mental illness may be exacerbated if his medical conditions are not well controlled or if he is noncompliant with dosages.

Aftercare Recommendations: The patient will be discharged to his sister's care and will be followed by his personal psychiatrist, Dr. X. Social services will follow the patient from his hometown.

The hospital acuity system used showed this to be a Level 4 ER service. Which of the following code sets is correct for reporting this service?

ICD-9-CM and CPT Code(s):

a. 295.34, 428.0, 99201
b. 295.32, 99283
c. 295.34, 428.0, 99284
d. 295.84, 99234

ICD-10-CM Code(s): _____

8.33. The following documentation is from the health record of a female patient who received psychiatrist treatment services in a hospital outpatient–based clinic.

XX/XX/XX 6:20 p.m. Dialectical behavior therapy (DBT), individual therapy—1:1 × 45 minutes at 5 p.m.

Subjective/Objective: Patient and I reviewed diary card and target hospitalizable behaviors and increased skills to stay out of the hospital and complete the outpatient program. Target goals 1 through 3 were reviewed today. Patient did not engage or act on urges for self-harm and urges for suicide after self-injurious behavior on XX/XX/XX. We focused on reinforcing skills of emotion regulation, highlighting times she used these while at work and with family members. Suicidal ideation today was minimal with sense of increased willingness to learn to apply skills. Discussed need to address ETOH dependence because patient notes increased risk of suicidal ideation with ETOH use. She identifies "fear" of "running in panic" will be what keeps her from staying with chemical dependency (CD) program. We addressed treatment plan (see below) to increase skills associated with CD treatment follow-through as well as structuring environment to "keep me in CD treatment."

Assessment: Major depressive disorder, recurrent; posttraumatic stress disorder, ETOH dependent; borderline personality disorder. Continued suicidal risk; patient has had some success over urges but is now coping well with the outpatient treatment where she receives therapy four times a week.

Plan: Patient and I identified targeting emotion regulation and distress tolerance in individual therapy to increase control over urges for suicidal thoughts, as well as follow-through with substance abuse treatment. Extended structuring continues with increased resources for managing son's behavior at home. Patient wants family meeting to orient family to DBT to increase chance they will be supportive of her treatment after discharge as opposed to disparaging, which, according to the patient, has increased her emotional vulnerability leading to increased suicidal urges. I gave times I would be available for a family meeting.

Addendum: Patient now has few suicidal urges and wants to do target behaviors. She reviewed skills with me to "get through" the rest of her week at home and at work. She notes that level of urges right now is manageable for her, and she believes she is improving.

Which of the following code sets is correct for reporting the outpatient services provided to this patient?

ICD-9-CM and CPT Code(s):

a. 296.20, 309.81, 303.92, 301.83, 300.9, 90819
b. 296.30, 309.81, 303.90, 301.83, 300.9, 90845
c. 296.30, 309.81, 303.90, 301.83, 90818
d. 296.30, 309.81, 303.90, 301.83, 300.9, 90818

ICD-10-CM Code(s): _____

8.34. The following documentation is from the health record of a 45-year-old female patient.

Mental Health Clinic Visit (Facility Services)

The 45-year-old patient is seen today for 20-minute medication review in the Community Mental Health Center. Patient continues to be somewhat elevated in her mood with some evidence of grandiosity but overall is goal directed and seems to be doing reasonably well with her subchronic schizophrenia in the structured setting. Patient currently is now off Seroquel and will continue to transition from oral Prolixin to Prolixin Decanoate. She did receive Prolixin Decanoate 12.5 mg IM on XX/XX/XX. When I try to decrease her oral Prolixin dosage, we notice some more increased grandiosity as well as more impulsive behavior and more thought disorganization, so on XX/XX/XX we increased her Prolixin back to 5 mg q. h.s. orally. On seeing her today, she seems to be improving somewhat on that. Her appetite and sleep pattern were fine over the weekend. She had no evidence of aggressive behavior. I decided at this time to maybe increase her Prolixin Decanoate to 25 mg IM every 2 weeks, and that will start today. Will continue with the oral Prolixin for a period of time and then will be able to eliminate that. There is a meeting with her family this upcoming Wednesday, and we'll discuss patient's care and how they feel she is doing and also discuss discharge and aftercare planning if that's appropriate.

Mental Status Exam: Appearance: The patient is a female who looks her stated age. Behavior: Cooperative, fair eye contact. Speech: Normal rate and volume. Mood slightly elevated. Affect less labile. Thought process: More goal directed. Negative for racing thoughts, flight of ideas. Thought content: Has delusional belief system, but it has decreased in intensity. No evidence of auditory, visual, or olfactory hallucinations. Denies current suicide or homicide intent. Insight: Judgment remains impaired. Impulse control improving.

Impression: Axis I: Schizophrenia, paranoid type, acute exacerbation
Axis II: None known
Axis III: Hypercholesterolemia; currently on Lipitor

Plan: At this time will continue on the Prolixin Decanoate but increase to 25 mg IM every 2 weeks. Will continue with the oral Prolixin at 5 mg q. h.s.

Which of the following is the correct code set for reporting this clinic service?

ICD-9-CM and CPT Code(s):

a. 295.33, 272.0, 90862
b. 295.30, 272.0, 90862
c. 295.30, 272.0, 90862, 99231
d. 295.33, 272.0, M0064, 99231

ICD-10-CM Code(s): _____

8.35. The following documentation is from the health record of a female patient who received services in a community mental health center.

Reason for Encounter: The patient has not had any self-injurious behavior or behavioral problems this past week except that she has used marijuana, which she endorses. Today we discussed her treatment, and overall she is happy with the DBT program and her chemical dependency program. She and I discussed future care and the need for her to get away from her current living arrangements.

Counseling/Coordination of Care: We reviewed how her DBT is going and what skills she could use when she has high urges to use marijuana. We also discussed that I would be doing periodic drug screenings.

Response to/Complications of Current Medications: None. The patient is happy with her medications as they are.

Examination:	WNL	Abnormal
General appearance	X	
Muscle strength/tone, gait		
Speech		
Thought process	X	
Associations/psychosis		
Suicidal/homicidal ideation	X	
Judgment and insight	X	
Attention span/concentration		
Orientation	X	
Recent and remote memory	X	
Fund of knowledge	X	
Mood and affect	X	

Assessment of Current Status: The patient appears to be stabilizing; however, she does appear to have a need for ongoing chemical dependency treatment and support, perhaps on an inpatient basis if the outpatient treatment plan fails to control relapses.

Diagnosis: Borderline personality disorder; major depression, recurrent; cannabis dependence

Plan: Continue DBT and chemical dependency treatment. The social worker and the patient should begin to work on alternative living arrangements because the patient is exposed to substance abuse in the current living arrangements and has conflicts with others living in the same apartment. We will not be changing any medications at this time.

Session Time: 25 minutes

Over 50 percent Counseling/Coordination of Care? ___ Yes _x_ No

History: Problem focused

Examination: Problem focused

Decision Making: Straightforward

Which of the following code sets is correct for reporting this clinic visit with a psychiatrist?

ICD-9-CM and CPT Code(s):

a. 301.83, 296.30, 304.31, 99214
b. 301.83, 296.30, 304.30, 99212
c. 301.83, 296.30, 304.30, 90805
d. 301.83, 296.30, 304.31, 90805

ICD-10-CM Code(s): _____

Disorders of the Musculoskeletal System and Connective Tissue

8.36. The following documentation is from the health record of a 39-year-old male patient.

Hospital Outpatient Surgery Services

Operative Report

Preoperative Diagnosis: Right quadriceps tendon rupture

Postoperative Diagnoses: Right quadriceps tendon rupture

Procedure Description: The patient was brought to the operating room and after the instillation of a satisfactory spinal anesthesia, the right lower extremity was appropriately prepared and draped in the usual sterile fashion. A midline incision was made and centered over the patella and carried down to the quadriceps mechanism. Medial and lateral dissection was carried out to expose the retinaculum, which was torn approximately 2 cm laterally and medially. There was a direct avulsion of the quadriceps tendon off the patella. The quadriceps tendon and patellar surface were freshened. Three holes, center, mid lateral, and mid medial, were marked. Following this, a #5 Ethibond and #2 fiberwire were placed in the quadriceps mechanism both medially and laterally, beginning in the midportion with a Krackow suture. Following this, 3 drill holes were made longitudinally from superior to inferior through the patella and a suture passer was used to retrieve the ends of the suture. When these were secured, the quad tendon was brought down into the patellar bed. Following this, #2 Ethibond retinacular sutures were added from the superolateral and superomedial junction of the patella laterally and medially. These were then tightened. As they were tightened, the sutures in the patella were securely tightened as well. The retinacular sutures were then tightened. Supplemental 2-0 Vicryl anteriorly into the quad tendon and patellar soft tissue and retinaculum was then accomplished. This knee could be flexed to about 30 degrees before there was significant tension on this quadriceps tendon. Therefore, we will be holding him in extension. Following this, a thorough irrigation was accomplished. The subcutaneous was closed with interrupted 2-0 Vicryl and the skin closed with skin clips. A sterile dressing and a knee immobilizer were placed. The patient tolerated the procedure well and was taken to the recovery room in satisfactory condition.

Which of the following is the correct code assignment?

ICD-9-CM and CPT Code(s):

a. 844.9, 27385-RT
b. 844.9, 27430-RT
c. 844.8, 27658-RT, 27685-RT
d. 844.8, 27664-RT

ICD-10-CM Code(s): _____

8.37. The following documentation is from the health record of a 47-year-old male patient.

Hospital Outpatient Surgery Services

Operative Report

Preoperative Diagnosis: Torn medial meniscus and DJD right knee

Postoperative Diagnosis: Large flap tear, posterior horn, medial meniscus; chondral loose bodies; significant degenerative arthritis right knee

Operation: Arthroscopy of the right knee with partial medial meniscectomy; arthroscopy of the right knee, with removal of chondral loose bodies

Procedure Description: This 47-year-old male was taken to the operating room and placed in the supine position. General anesthesia was accomplished without complication. Evaluation under anesthesia of the right knee showed it was stable with a negative Lachman's test and firm end point. Negative anterior and posterior drawer, stable to varus and valgus testing. A tourniquet was placed on the midright thigh. The right leg was prepped and draped free in the usual sterile manner. Tourniquet inflated to 325 mm Hg. There were loose bodies throughout the knee, which were flushed and removed. The patient had a large flap tear of the posterior horn of the medial meniscus that was unstable. He underwent a partial medial meniscectomy with small basket forceps and small synovial resector removing the torn portion of the meniscus, leaving about a 2-mm rim posteriorly and then saucerizing this to smooth margins anteriorly. The anterior cruciate ligament and posterior cruciate ligament were normal. The lateral compartment could not be entered because of significant arthritis medially. The knee joint was thoroughly irrigated and the portals closed with interrupted 3-0 nylon mattress sutures. Sterile dressing was applied. No complications occurred. The tourniquet was deflated after 20 minutes. The patient went to the recovery room in stable condition.

Which of the following is the correct code assignment?

ICD-9-CM and CPT Code(s):

a. 717.2, 717.6, 715.96, 29881-RT
b. 717.43, 718.16, 29881-RT, 29874-RT
c. 844.8, 717.6, 29881-RT, 29877-RT
d. 717.2, 715.96, 29881-RT, 29874-RT

ICD-10-CM Code(s): _____

8.38. The following documentation is from the health record of a 68-year-old male patient.

Hospital Outpatient Surgery Services

This patient presented to the podiatrist for surgical evaluation at the request of the primary care physician. After surgery was completed, a copy of the evaluation and operative report was sent to the primary care office.

Preoperative Evaluation: This 68-year-old male of Italian descent presents with degenerative arthritis and bunion formation. On 6/30/XX, patient was sent by Dr. Brown for bunionectomy evaluation. A problem-focused history was conducted followed by an expanded problem-focused examination.

Impression: Painful left foot due to: (1) Bunion with degenerative joint disease in the toes. (2) Metatarsus primus varus. (3) Hammer toe, second digit. (4) Elongated metatarsal, second digit, left.

Plan: Surgery scheduled for 8:00 a.m. 7/12/XX, at the Hospital

Procedures: Keller bunionectomy; Austin bunionectomy; arthroplasty, second digit; and excision of the metatarsal head, second digit, left foot

Operative Report: The patient was placed in the semisupine position where Dr. Graybeard administered spinal anesthesia. After prepping and draping the patient in the usual aseptic manner and under ankle hemostasis, the left foot was approached. A dorsal linear incision was performed medial to the extensor hallucis longus tendon. Incision was carried through the skin and subcutaneous tissue and extended from midshaft metatarsal to distal proximal phalanx. The superficial fascia was separated from the deep fascia using sharp and blunt dissection techniques. An inverted L-capsulotomy was performed and sharp capsular periosteal dissection was performed with a #15 blade to expose the first metatarsal and base of the proximal phalanx. The medial eminence was resected with a micro-oscillating saw.

Next, attention was directed to the base of the proximal phalanx, where the Keller procedure was performed. One third of the proximal phalanx was resected and excised in toto.

Attention was next directed to the head of the first metatarsal where an Austin osteotomy was performed in the usual manner with screw fixation. The area was flushed with copious amounts of antibiotic flush. The capsular periosteal layer was next closed with 3-0 VICRYL. The subcutaneous tissue was reapproximated with 4-0 VICRYL.

Attention was next directed to the second digit and MPJ area, where a dorsal curvilinear incision was performed. The incision was deepened and the PIPJ was exposed. A transverse incision was performed through the capsular periosteal tissue at the PIPJ. Medial and lateral capsulotomies were performed, exposing the head of the proximal phalanx. The head of the proximal phalanx was resected and excised in toto.

Attention was next directed to the second MPJ. The incision at this area was deepened. A dorsal linear capsulotomy was performed and the head of the second metatarsal was resected and excised in toto. The surgical sites were next flushed with copious amounts of antibiotic flush. The second digit was noted to be aligned without pressure on the neurovascular structures.

Next, a .45 K-wire was placed percutaneously into the hallux distal to proximal. Capsular periosteal closure was next performed with 3-0 VICRYL. Subcutaneous closure was performed with 4-0 VICRYL. The skin was closed in 4-0 nylon. Postop anesthesia consisted of 17 cc 5.0 percent Marcaine plain and 1 cc of Decadron 4 mg/mL. Next, the sterile dressing was applied, which consisted of Betadine ointment, 4 × 4 gauze, and 4-inch Kling. The tourniquet was released, and the patient was returned to recovery in stable condition.

Which of the following is the correct code assignment for this outpatient procedure?

ICD-9-CM and CPT Code(s):

a. 727.1, 735.4, 99242-25, 28202, 28285
b. 727.1, 715.97, 754.52, 735.4, 754.59, 28299-TA, 28285-T1
c. 735.4, 754.52, 28296
d. 727.2, 715.97, 754.52, 735.4, 754.59, 28296-TA and 28292-TA-59, 28285-T1

ICD-10-CM Code(s): _____

8.39. The following documentation is from the health record of a patient who received hospital outpatient surgery services.

Preoperative Diagnosis: Deep laceration, left hand with extensive tendon disruption of the fourth and fifth digits, secondarily of the third digit, middle finger; open fracture with chip fracture from the MCP joint of the fifth digit; open fracture of the middle phalanx of the index finger

Postoperative Diagnosis: Deep laceration, left hand with extensive tendon disruption of the fourth and fifth digits, secondarily of the third digit, middle finger; open fracture with chip fracture from the MCP joint of the fifth digit; open fracture of the middle phalanx of the index finger

Operation: Extensive tendon repair, fourth and fifth digits, third digit longitudinally, index finger second digit with extensor hood, and debridement; open fracture middle phalanx; and intra-articular laceration of fourth and fifth digit

Anesthesia: Intravenous Bier block

The patient was brought to the operating theater and anesthetized with a Bier block. We explored the wound, and the joint capsule to fourth and fifth was excised into the joint. The superior pole of the articular surface of the distal metacarpal on the fifth digit was avulsed, and we excised this because it was impregnated with a lot of dirt.

The tendon of the extensor indices communis to the fifth digit was lacerated. The extensor indices proprius ulnarly was still intact. The extensor hood over the MCP joint of #4 was torn, as was the capsule. The extensor tendon along the central hood of the third digit was torn longitudinally and the point was spared. The index finger had a longitudinal tear of the extensor hood in the central portion of the midphalanx, with the lateral band on the radial side torn. The wound was copiously irrigated with bacitracin saline with a pulsatile lavage. The joint surface of the fourth and fifth were irrigated. The open fracture of the fifth digit was removed. The open fracture of the middle phalanx of the index was debrided and irrigated.

We then began the definitive repairs. We sutured the joint capsule of the fourth and fifth with a 4-0 VICRYL continuous. We sutured the extensor digitorum communis tendon to #5 with 5-0 Prolene and to #4 over the central hood, over the MCP joint with a 5-0 Prolene continuous. The extensor tendon of the third or middle finger was sutured longitudinally, and a lateral band on the radial side was repaired with a 5-0 VICRYL. The longitudinal tear, which was really a split or a double split, was sutured with over-and-over 5-0 VICRYL as well. We then increased her incision in an S-shaped fashion over the index finger to expose the central hood, which was torn, and lateral on the radial aspect, which was torn as well. This was repaired with 5-0 VICRYL, and the main extensor hood was repaired with 5-0 Prolene simple sutures. We then irrigated again with a liter of bacitracin pulsatile figure-of-8 mattress sutures, alternating with simple sutures. A bulky dressing was then applied, with a volar slab with the hand in the position of function, extension of the wrist, extension of the MCP joint, flexion of the PIP, and DIP of 30 degrees. The patient then had the tourniquet deflated fully and was sent to the recovery room in good condition.

Which of the following is the correct code assignment? Report the codes a hospital outpatient surgery department would report for this hand surgery. Do not assign E codes.

ICD-9-CM and CPT Code(s):

a. 882.1, 817.1, 26418, 26735, 26746, 11012
b. 842.12, 817.0, 26746-F4, 11010-F1, 11012-F4
c. 842.12, 817.1, 26418–F1, 26418–F2, 26418–F3, 26418–F4
d. 882.2, 816.11, 26418–F1, 26418–F2, 26418–F3, 26418–F5, 11010–F1, 11012–F4

ICD-10-CM Code(s): _____

Neoplasms

8.40.   The following documentation is from the health record of a patient who received hospital outpatient surgery services.

Operative Report

Preoperative Diagnosis: Lesion, right forehead

Postoperative Diagnosis: Basal cell carcinoma, right forehead

Procedure: Excision of 1.0-centimeter lesion involving the right forehead

Technique: The skin and subcutaneous tissue around the forehead lesion were infiltrated with 0.5% Marcaine with 1:100,000 epinephrine. A total of 1.5 cc was used. The patient was then prepped and draped in the usual sterile fashion.

Microscopic excision was carried out. A 2.0-mm margin of resection was planned around the lesion. Long suture was placed on the superior margin and a short suture was placed on the inferior margin. The tissue was excised and sent for frozen section, which returned with a diagnosis of basal cell carcinoma with clear margins.

The site was closed with interrupted 5-0 plain gut. The patient was sent to the recovery area in good condition. No complications. Blood loss was 1 cc.

Which codes will be reported for this service?

ICD-9-CM and CPT Code(s):

a. 173.31, 11641
b. 173.31, 11642
c. 239.2, 11441
d. 239.2, 11442

ICD-10-CM Code(s): _____

8.41. The following documentation is from the health record of an 88-year-old female patient.

Hospital-Based Oncology Department Services

This 88-year-old white female is here to rule out the possibility of myeloma. She has been followed by Dr. Black as an outpatient and has sustained a 13-lb weight loss over a 6-week period. She seemed to stabilize at a weight of 82 lb but has recently dropped an additional 2 pounds. She is experiencing recurrent pain in the chest. Three weeks ago, she was treated by Dr. Black for a sinus infection, and sinus films showed lytic lesions of the skull, as well as the left maxillary sinus.

The patient had a left radical mastectomy 38 years ago for carcinoma of the breast without recurrence. The right breast is atrophic and without masses. Laboratory tests are attached and without noteworthy comments, except for urinalysis culture revealing over 100,000 *Escherichia coli*. A bone scan shows multiple areas of increased bony uptake and two areas of increased rib uptake and present healing osteoporotic fractures. There are multiple areas of increased uptake throughout the bony skull, suggestive of progressive metastatic disease or perhaps myeloma.

This is a delightful elderly woman who has markedly abnormal bone films and severe osteoporosis. General appearance of the bone is metastatic malignancy, supported by the weight loss history. Myeloma is consistent with her symptoms, but a normal sed rate and relatively normal globulin level are somewhat contradictory of that diagnosis. Certainly light chain myeloma is a possibility. In addition, some other metastatic disease, including the previous breast cancer, could give this appearance, but that seems unusual. I have never seen recurrent breast cancer this late (38 years).

Pertinent studies have been ordered, but I believe it would also be worthwhile to do Beta II microglobulin, which may be helpful in confirming myeloma. The UTI due to Shiga toxin-producing *E. coli* is being treated with antibiotics. Additional x-rays of the lateral skull and long bones have also been ordered. In addition, I performed a bone marrow aspiration today from the left posterior iliac crest.

At this point, my recommendation is to wait and see what the additional tests show. If we can determine that this is a myeloma, then it would be worth treating her with an alkylator-prednisone combination. In terms of any other metastatic disease, there is little we can do short of palliative radiation therapy. If this looks like recurrent breast cancer, then it may be useful to try tamoxifen. I would probably do that at any rate, if the carcinoma is further collaborated in any fashion by the bone marrow biopsy or other studies.

I cannot make any more definitive recommendations at this point. When I return next week and we see the studies ordered, we will go from there.

Procedure Note

Bone Marrow Biopsy Results: Metastatic poorly differentiated carcinoma and hyperplastic marrow with decreased iron stores

Comment from Pathologist: The features of the tumor do not suggest a definite site or origin. The most common tumors causing extensive lytic lesions of the bone are breast carcinoma, lung carcinoma, and renal cell carcinoma. With regard to the patient's previous history of breast cancer, although late recurrence has been described after more than 20 years, 38 years is an extreme interval.

Which of the following are assigned for the services performed on this date of service?

ICD-9-CM and CPT Code(s):

a. 203.01, 199.1, 38221
b. 198.5, 199.1, 733.19, 733.00, V10.3, 599.0, 041.43, 38221
c. 199.0, 27299
d. 198.5, 203.01, 174.9, 38221

ICD-10-CM Code(s): _____

8.42.   The following documentation is from the health record of a female patient who received hospital outpatient surgery services.

Operative Report

A 52-year-old female presented with abdominal pain and change in bowel habits. A barium enema suggested a diverticular stricture, so a sigmoidoscopy was performed in the clinic, finding a stricture at 25 cm. The patient was then scheduled for exploratory laparoscopy in the hospital outpatient surgical center to treat the stricture.

Preoperative Diagnosis: Stricture of the sigmoid colon, rule out carcinoma

Postoperative Diagnosis: Carcinoma of the sigmoid with invasion into adjacent tissue and suspected metastasis to the liver

The patient was brought to the surgical suite, and an NG tube was placed in the stomach and a Foley catheter in the bladder. She was placed in the lithotomy position and routine prep and draping were performed. A small incision was made in the right upper quadrant directly into the peritoneal cavity with CO_2. Once we had a good tent, we examined the peritoneal cavity and could not really see the liver because we were too close to it, but one view suggested surface lesions. After placement of the three cannulas (12 mm in the RUQ, 10 mm LLQ, and 5 mm in LUQ), we mobilized the sigmoid off the pelvic gutter and dissected down towards the bladder. She had undergone a previous hysterectomy, but there were no adhesions. We could not get the small bowel to easily come up out of the pelvis, and lesions were evident surrounding the colon, so biopsies were taken. We then used a colonoscope through the rectum and advanced to 25 cm where we saw, not a stricture, but carcinoma, and biopsies were taken for pathologic evaluation. Complete evaluation of the colon was performed with no other pathology found. The surgery was discontinued, the trocars removed, and the patient returned to recovery in stable condition. The patient will undergo evaluation and consultation with oncology before further treatment is undertaken.

Pathology report confirms invasive adenocarcinoma, moderate to poorly differentiated, of the sigmoid colon with extension to the pericolic adipose.

Which codes are assigned to this surgery?

ICD-9-CM and CPT Code(s):

a. 153.3, 197.4, 49329
b. 153.9, 49321-74, 45380-59
c. 197.4, 153.3, 197.7, 49321, 45380
d. 153.3, 198.89, 49321, 45380

ICD-10-CM Code(s): _____

8.43. The following documentation is from the health record of a female patient who received hospital outpatient surgery services.

Operative Report

Preoperative Diagnosis: Vulvar lesion

Postoperative Diagnosis: Carcinoma in situ of the vulva

Operative Procedure: Vulvectomy

Indications for Procedure: This 74-year-old patient was found to have a suspicious-looking lesion on her vulva. Medically, she is diabetic, has Parkinson's disease, and is obese. On the day of surgery, her cardiac, pulmonary, and mental status were adequate.

Operative Findings: On the posterior vulva was a vulvar lesion which was superficially ulcerated and extended along the posterior vaginal introitus involving the perineum. The urethra was normal. The bladder was negative for tumor. The vaginal mucosa and remainder of the vulva appeared without any lesions.

Description of Operation: The patient received general anesthesia, was intubated and placed in the dorsal lithotomy position. A pelvic examination was performed. A vaginal prep with Betadine was done and she was draped for a vaginal procedure.

An incision was made transversely along the perineum halfway between the vaginal introitus and the rectum. The skin was dissected towards the vaginal introitus bilaterally and posteriorly. The lesion was then excised with a good margin at the posterior vagina and laterally, along the vulva. Dimensions were approximately 4 cm $\times$ 3 cm $\times$ 1 cm in a triangular shape. Bleeding points were either ligated with 3-0 Vicryl or cauterized with electrocautery. The specimen was submitted for pathology evaluation with a suture marker designating the rectal margin.

The vaginal mucosa, which was undermined for at least 2 cm, was approximated to the perineal skin by interrupted 2-0 Vicryl sutures. The entire wound was closed in this way. The patient tolerated the surgical procedure well and left the operating room in satisfactory condition.

Tissue Consultation Report

Preoperative Diagnosis: Vulvar lesion

Postoperative Diagnosis: Carcinoma in situ of the vulva

Specimen: #1. Vulvar lesion with anal margin

Gross Description: #1. Received in formalin labeled "vulvar lesion and margin tag" is a roughly triangular-shaped fragment of tissue covered on one surface with wrinkled pink-white focally hair-bearing skin and on the other surface with fibrous pink tissue. There is a suture at one apex. The specimen measures 3.5 × 2.5 cm. with a thickness that ranges from 0.3 to 0.4 cm. The surface is slightly hypopigmented and slightly rough and granular in some areas. The margins are inked. A portion of the margin containing the suture is additionally marked with yellow ink. A line diagram is drawn. The specimen is sectioned and entirely submitted in eight cassettes.

Microscopic Description: #1. The specimen consists of squamous mucosa. In the center of the specimen, there is epithelial hyperplasia with markedly abnormal maturation extending from the basal layer to the surface. The surface is composed of compact hyperkeratosis. The abnormal cells display nuclear enlargement, hyperchromasia, a disorganized growth pattern, and increased mitotic figures, many of which are abnormal. Invasive squamous cell carcinoma is not identified.

Diagnosis:

#1. Vulvar lesion, including anal margin, excision:

Carcinoma in situ (vulvar epithelial neoplasia VIN III), with clear margins

Which of the following code sets is assigned?

ICD-9-CM and CPT Code(s):

a. 239.5, 250.00, 332.0, 278.00, 57410, 56620
b. 624.02, 250.00, 332.0, 278.00, 56630
c. 233.32, 250.00, 57410, 11626, 12042
d. 233.32, 250.00, 332.0, 278.00, 56620

ICD-10-CM Code(s): _____

Disorders of the Nervous System and Sense Organs

8.44.   The following documentation is from the health record of a 22-year-old male patient who received hospital outpatient surgery services.

Operative Report

A patient injured his foot using a razor-sharp garden hoe while gardening in his yard at his home and severed the superficial branch of the external plantar nerve and the flexor digiti minimi brevis tendon in his left foot. The patient experienced loss of sensation on the outer side of the fifth toe and across the side of the foot, so a neurology consultation was requested, and the patient was taken directly to surgery. Following exploration of the wound and identification of the nerve avulsion, a repair of the nerve was undertaken using a nerve graft from the sural nerve. A lateral incision was made on the lateral malleolus of the ankle. The nerve was identified and freed for grafting, and the proximal and distal sural nerve endings were anastomosed. The wound was dissected, and the damaged area of the nerve was removed. The innervation of the external digital nerve was restored by suturing the 1.5-cm graft to the proximal and digital ends of the damaged nerve, using the operating microscope. Tenoplasty was performed on the tendon injury, and the wound closed in layers.

Which of the following would be correct? Do not assign evaluation and management service codes for the ER visit or consultation service.

ICD-9-CM and CPT Code(s):

a. 956.5, E920.4, E849.0, 64831, 28200
b. 892.2, 956.5, E920.4, E849.0, 64891, 28202
c. 892.2, 956.5, E920.4, E849.0, 64890-LT, 28200-LT
d. 956.5, 64890-LT, 28200-LT

ICD-10-CM Code(s): _____

8.45. The following documentation is from the health record of a patient who received hospital outpatient surgery services.

Preoperative Diagnosis:	Reflex sympathetic dystrophy
Postoperative Diagnosis:	Same
Operation:	Right stellate ganglion block #1
Location:	Outpatient Pain Clinic Surgery Center
Anesthesia:	Local with conscious sedation

Details: The patient was placed in the supine position to start the IV in his left hand for the sedation of 4 mg of Versed. Then he was positioned using a shoulder roll with the neck extended. Betadine was used for preparation. Following local anesthesia, a #22, 1.5-cm needle was introduced paratracheally at the level of the cricoid cartilage towards the stellate ganglion. Ten cc of .05 percent Marcaine with epinephrine 1:200,000 was injected, and the patient tolerated this very well. There was no paresthesia, heme, or CSF detected. The patient swallowed copiously during the procedure, but we were able to obtain an adequate block, with the patient's right hand temperature changing from 90.1 to 93 °F following the block. He was moved to the outpatient recovery area where he tolerated fluids and nutrition and was able to be discharged home to his caregiver.

Assign the correct diagnosis and procedure codes. Do not assign HCPCS Level II codes for the drug(s) injected.

ICD-9-CM Diagnosis Code(s): _____

Procedure Code(s): _____

ICD-10-CM Code(s): _____

8.46.   The following documentation is from the health record of a 48-year-old female patient.

Emergency Department Services

This is a 48-year-old female presenting to the ER in the middle of the night with a complaint of unexpected right-sided weakness. It occurred during sleep, and the patient awoke and found it difficult to use her right dominant arm or leg. She denies fever, shortness of breath, cough, headache, or other symptoms, and related that she was asymptomatic until this occurred.

Medication: Glucophage for type II diabetes mellitus control. Has never used oral contraceptives.

Allergies: None.

Habits: Tobacco, one pack per day; social use of alcohol.

Family History: Positive for early stroke in maternal grandmother at 52; father deceased at 53 due to lung cancer.

Physical Exam: Patient is alert and oriented times three. HEENT: Pupils are round, regular, equal, and reactive to light and accommodation. Extraocular muscles are intact. Oral mucosa moist and pink. Decreased nasolabial fold on the right side and slight drooping of the angle of the mouth on the right. Neck supple, without lymphadenopathy, carotid bruit, or thyromegaly. She has impaired speech. Chest: Negative. Cardiovascular: Negative. Abdomen: Benign. Neurologic: Mild paralysis evident. Cranial nerves II through XII intact. Marked decrease in power and tone on the right side when compared to the left. Decrease in sensation on the right compared to the left. She has no visual disturbances or vertigo.

CT scan without contrast shows a small infarction in the left basal ganglia near the internal capsule. This is a small to medium-size arterial embolism causing the stroke.

Plan: Will transfer for further neurologic consultation to University Medical Center for lab work per Dr. Smith on the neurology service. MRI, carotid Doppler, and two-dimensional echocardiogram were ordered to be completed there also.

Acuity Level: IV

Which of the following code set combinations will be used for reporting this ER visit for the facility?

ICD-9-CM and CPT Code(s):

a. 436, 99284-25, 70450
b. 434.91, 99283, 70470
c. 434.91, 342.90, 784.59, 305.1, 250.00, V17.1, 99284–25, 70450
d. 436, 342.90, 784.59, 305.1, 250.00, V17.1, 99284, 70470

ICD-10-CM Code(s): _____

8.47. The following documentation is from the health record of a 35-year-old female patient.

Hospital Outpatient Surgery Services

Operative Report

Preoperative Diagnosis: Right trigeminal neuralgia

Postoperative Diagnosis: Right trigeminal neuralgia

Operation: Right radiofrequency coagulation of the trigeminal nerve

Indications: This is a 35-year-old lady with intractable trigeminal neuralgia causing her considerable pain and inability to eat or speak, and who was referred for treatment of her affliction. Indications, potential complications, and risks were explained to the patient and family.

Operative Procedure: After the patient was positioned supine, intravenous sedation with propofol was administered. Lateral skull x-ray fluoroscopy was set. The right cheek was infiltrated dermally with Xylocaine, and a small nick in the skin 2.5 cm lateral to the corner of the mouth was made with an 18-gauge needle. The radiofrequency needle with 2-mm exposed tip was then introduced using the known anatomical landmarks and under lateral fluoroscopy guidance into the foramen ovale. Confirmation of the placement of the needle was done by the patient grimacing to pain and by the lateral x-ray. The first treatment, 90 seconds in length, was administered with the tip of the needle 3 mm below the clival line at a temperature of 75 °C. The needle was then advanced further to the midclival line and another treatment of similar strength and duration was also administered. Finally, the third and last treatment was administered with the tip of the needle approximately 3 cm above the line. The cerebrospinal fluid was noted. The needle was removed. The patient tolerated the procedure well and had adequate tearing and corneal sensation and had reduction, if not complete cure, of her pain by the end of the procedure.

Which of the following code sets is correct?

ICD-9-CM and CPT Code(s):

a. 350.1, 64600, 77003
b. 350.1, 64610, 77003
c. 350.1, 64610
d. 350.1, 64605

ICD-10-CM Code(s): _____

8.48.   The following documentation is from the health record of a 32-year-old male patient.

Preoperative Diagnosis:	Phantom limb pain
Postoperative Diagnosis:	Phantom limb pain
Procedure:	Right lumbar sympathetic block

Findings: This patient underwent a right below-the-knee amputation approximately 7 months ago for osteosarcoma of the fibula. The patient received 3 rounds of chemotherapy following the surgery as well as rehabilitation. He presented to the office 3 months ago with some significant phantom pain which was initially managed with medication. The medications, however, are providing minimal relief and he continues to have severe pain in the foot area. Surgery was held off until the stump could achieve healing, which it has. The stump does look generally good with some small areas of irritation. Lidoderm patches are used on the stump for sensitivity issues. He is seen today for injection of Marcaine and epinephrine into the L2 space in hopes of providing more relief for the pain.

Description of Procedure: The young man was positioned prone on the operating table with a block under the abdomen. The L2 spinous process was identified. A 20-gauge spinal needle was advanced through the skin to the spinal process so that the needle is lying on the anterolateral aspect of the L2 body. The appropriate location was confirmed by US prior to the injection. Twenty mL of Marcaine and epinephrine was slowly injected into the spinal space. The patient was raised into the upright position and allowed to relax. He indicated that he felt well and that there was no pain at that time. The patient was cautioned to be careful and I discussed the possibility of continuing with oral medications although a repeat block is certainly an option if the pain returns. He was sent home in good condition.

Which of the following is the correct code assignment for this outpatient surgery?

ICD-9-CM and CPT Code(s):

a. 353.6, V10.81, 62311
b. 353.6, 729.5, V49.75, V10.81, 62311
c. 353.6, V49.75, V10.81, 0230T
d. 353.6, V49.75, 170.7, 0230T

ICD-10-CM Code(s): _____

8.49.   The following documentation is from the health record of a 33-year-old female patient.

Hospital Outpatient Surgery Services

Operative Report

Preoperative Diagnosis:	Left frontal lesion
Postoperative Diagnosis:	Left frontal lesion
Operation:	Stereotactic biopsy of left frontal lesion

Indications for Procedure: The patient is a 33-year-old female transferred to the university neurosurgical service for outpatient treatment from Blank Memorial

Hospital, where she is an inpatient. She presents with neurologic deterioration, nausea, neck pain, and headache. A CT and MRI revealed a left frontal cystic mass. It was recommended that the patient undergo stereotactic biopsy and aspiration. The risks and benefits of the procedure were explained in detail to the patient and her family, who requested the procedure be performed, and the patient returned to Blank for further therapy.

Procedure: The patient was first taken to the CT suite, where a stereotactic halo was placed on the patient's head with the four-pin system using local anesthesia. The stereotactic CT was then performed, and the patient was transported to the operating room. The patient was placed on the operating room table in the supine position. General endotracheal anesthesia was smoothly induced. The left frontal area was then clipped and shaved, and the area was then prepped and draped in the usual sterile fashion. The stereotactic arm was then brought into the field and placed on the stereotactic ring. The localizing arm and the pointer were used to mark the left frontal area for skin incision. The area was then infused with 1 percent lidocaine with epinephrine, and a 2-cm skin incision was created in the left frontal region. The self-retaining retractor was placed, and hemostasis was obtained. The pointer was again used to mark the spot on the skull to make the burr hole, and a perforator was used to create a left frontal burr hole. The dura was coagulated and incised using a #15 bladed knife. The pia was then also coagulated and nicked with a #11 blade knife. The biopsy needle was then placed into the stereotactic localizing arm. The coordinates were dialed into the arm, and the biopsy needle was advanced to the appropriate depth. Upon entering the lesion, 25 cc of yellowish fluid was withdrawn from the cyst. The fluid was sent for cytology and bacteriology. The biopsy needle was then removed, and the incision was irrigated with bacitracin irrigation. The self-retaining retractor was then removed, and the incision was closed using #00 Dexon for the galea and staples for the skin. Estimated blood loss was 15 cc. No transfusion was given. The sponge, needle, and instrument counts were reported as correct at the end of the case. The patient was removed from the stereotactic halo ring. She was allowed to wake up and was extubated and taken to the recovery area. She will be transferred by ambulance back to Blank as soon as she has recovered from the anesthesia.

Assign the correct CPT codes for this procedure.

Code(s): _____

8.50.   The following documentation is from the health record of a patient seen for retinal detachment.

Ophthalmologic Procedure—Nervous/Sense

Surgery Date: 04/20/XX

Preoperative Diagnoses: 1. Retinal detachment, left eye.
2. Vitreous hemorrhage, left eye.
3. Traumatic iritis, left eye.

Postoperative Diagnoses: 1. Retinal detachment, left eye.
2. Vitreous hemorrhage, left eye.
3. Traumatic iritis, left eye.

Operative Procedures:	1. Scleral buckle, left eye.
	2. Pars plana vitrectomy, left eye.
	3. Air fluid exchange, left eye.
	4. Endolaser, left eye.
	5. Injection of 16% C3F8 gas, left eye.
Anesthesia:	General.

Indications: The patient presents with count-fingers vision in the left eye 4 days after blunt trauma to the left eye caused by a punch. B-scan revealed moderate vitreous hemorrhage and retinal detachment with tear at 4:30 with macula off.

Description of Procedure: After informed written consent was obtained, patient was brought to the operating room and prepped and draped in the usual sterile fashion after he was induced under general anesthesia. Speculum was placed in the left eye. A 360-degree peritomy was performed with a 0.12 forceps and Westcott scissors. Each quadrant was dissected bluntly with the curved Stevens scissors. Muscles were looped with a muscle hook and threaded with a 2-0 silk and then isolated with 2-0 silk. Quadrants were inspected and found to be pathology-free. Then a Gill knife and corneal dissector were used to perform scleral buckle procedure, 1 belt loop in each quadrant, 3 mm posterior to the muscle insertion, 3 mm long and 3 mm wide. The 41-band was threaded through each belt loop and under each muscle and tied with a Watzke sleeve superonasally. A standard 20-gauge pars plana vitrectomy was then performed with sclerotomies placed 3.5 mm posterior to the limbus with an MVR blade. The first sclerotomy placed was inferotemporal, and the trocar was used to place the cannula. Infusion line was screwed into place and turned on after it was visualized in the vitreous cavity. Other two cannulas were placed with trocars, and the BIOM viewing system was used to perform a complete vitrectomy. Tears were noted not only at 4:30, but also at the 5 o'clock that were out near the vitreous base, and there was a large tear running radially along the edge of the detachment and traction of vitreous from 6:30 all the way past the equator and about 3 disc diameters from the optic nerve head. After vitreous was removed, air fluid exchange was performed to flatten the retina and endolaser was performed 360 degrees and around the tears. Air was exchanged for 16% C3F8 gas and sclerotomies were tied with 7-0 VICRYL, as was the conjunctiva. Retrobulbar block was given, a total of 6 cc of a 50/50 mixture of 2 percent lidocaine and 0.75 percent Marcaine. Maxitrol and atropine were applied to the eye. The eye was patched with a soft pad followed by a hard pad. The patient left the room awake in a stable condition and will follow up tomorrow morning at 8 a.m.

Which of the following is the correct code assignment for this outpatient surgery?

ICD-9-CM and CPT Code(s):

a. 361.02, 379.23, 364.3, 67108
b. 361.9, 379.23, 364.3, 67108
c. 361.02, 364.3, 67108
d. 361.02, 379.23, 364.10, 67107, 67036

ICD-10-CM Code(s): _____

8.51. The following documentation is from the health record of a 17-year-old admitted for endoscopic sinus surgery.

Preoperative Diagnosis: Nasal septal deviation, hypertrophic inferior turbinates, nasal airway obstruction, and chronic frontal, ethmoid, and maxillary sinusitis with sinus polyposis.

Postoperative Diagnosis: Same

Procedure: Nasal/sinus endoscopy, surgical, with frontal sinus exploration, right.
Nasal/sinus endoscopy, surgical, with frontal sinus exploration, left.
Nasal/sinus endoscopy, surgical, with anterior and posterior ethmoidectomy, right.
Nasal/sinus endoscopy, surgical, with anterior and posterior ethmoidectomy, left.
Septoplasty.
Nasal/sinus endoscopy, surgical, with maxillary antrotomy and polypectomy, right.
Nasal/sinus endoscopy, surgical, with maxillary antrotomy and polypectomy, left.
Submucous resection of inferior turbinate, right.
Submucous resection of inferior turbinate, left.

History: The patient is a 17-year-old Caucasian male presenting with a history of chronic nasal obstruction and chronic sinusitis. He has been refractory to conservative therapy. Preop evaluation reveals an obvious gross nasal septal deformity, with hypertrophic inferior turbinates, causing bilateral nasal airway obstruction. His preop CT scan confirms these findings, along with evidence of polypoid degeneration involving the maxillary, ethmoid, and frontal sinuses. The recommendations for septoplasty with endoscopic sinus surgery were given to the patient and his mother. All benefits, risks, alternate therapies, and expected outcomes were discussed. Consent form signed. The patient presents at this time for this procedure.

Details of Procedure: The patient was taken to the operating suite and placed in the supine position. General anesthesia with endotracheal intubation was carried out by the Department of Anesthesia. Following adequate anesthesia, the table was turned.

Further preparation of the nasal cavity was carried out in the usual manner. Following this, the patient was properly draped and the procedure begun.

A #15 blade was used to make a Killian incision into the left aspect of the mucoperichondrium. A mucoperichondrial and mucoperiosteal flap was then developed. The cartilaginous septum was detached from the maxillary crest and from the bony septum, and a portion of reflected bony septum causing obstruction was taken down with a Gorney scissors and a biting Takahashi forceps. The large bony spur coming out the maxillary crest was then taken down with a curved chisel and mallet technique. Bone fragments were removed with a biting forceps. Following this, the cartilaginous septum was allowed to swing to the midline and attention was turned to the endoscopic portion of the procedure.

The zero-degree endoscope was inserted into the left nasal cavity and brought up to the head of the left middle turbinate. The left middle turbinate was medialized.

An infundibulotomy incision was made, followed by uncinectomy. The maxillary antrum was then entered. The antrotomy opening was widened with the Xomed straight shot microdebrider. Polypoid tissue encountered in the left maxillary sinus was then visualized and evacuated with a series of biting forceps. Following this, the debrider was used to gain access to the anterior, then the posterior, ethmoid air cells, removing diseased mucoperiosteal tissue along the way. The nasal frontal recess was then identified. Polypoid tissue in this region was evacuated. The nasofrontal duct was then cannulated. Further disease around the duct was removed with the debrider. Following these maneuvers, submucous resection of the left inferior turbinate was then carried out. Next, attention was turned to the opposite maxillary, ethmoid, and frontal sinuses. Identical procedures and findings were noted here. Submucous resection of the right inferior turbinate was then carried out.

The middle turbinates were then sutured in the midline, utilizing 4-0 VICRYL on a PS2 cutting needle. Silastic splints, Merocel sinus and nasal packs were then placed. The oral cavity was then suctioned of all blood and debris. The patient tolerated these procedures well. He was turned back over to the Department of Anesthesia, and was taken to the recovery room in satisfactory condition.

Report of Surgical Pathology

Final Diagnosis: Nasal sinus mucosa with septal bone and cartilage
Mild chronic allergic sinusitis; nasal bone and cartilage showing
no specific gross abnormality specimen(s)
Nasal septum—with sinus products
Clinical diagnosis: recurrent sinusitis

Gross Examination: Received are multiple portions of somewhat mucinous mucosa accompanying bits of platelike, wedge-shaped, and sail-shaped bone and cartilage. The latter present no specific gross abnormalities. The mucosa has an estimated aggregate volume of 2 cc and is submitted for histologic processing (1 block).

Microscopic Examination: Sections disclose edematous sinonasal mucosa with mild chronic inflammation, basement membrane thickening, and a somewhat mucinous epithelium. The inflammatory infiltrate is dominantly lymphoplasmacytic with foci of eosinophilic admixture. There is no evidence of squamous metaplasia or dysplasia.

Select the correct code set to report for this patient.

ICD-9-CM and CPT Code(s):

a. 470, 478.0, 519.8, 473.0, 473.2, 473.1, 471.8, 31276-50, 31255-50, 30140-50-59, 30520, 31256-50
b. 470, 478.0, 519.8, 473.0, 473.2, 473.1, 471.8, 31276, 31255, 30140, 30520, 31256
c. 470, 478.0, 519.8, 461.0, 461.1, 461.2, 471.8, 31276-50, 31255-50, 30520, 31256-50
d. 470, 478.0, 519.8, 461.0, 461.1, 461.2, 471.8, 31276-50, 31255-50, 30140-50-59, 30520, 31256-50

ICD-10-CM Code(s): _____

Newborn/Congenital Disorders

8.52. The following documentation is from the health record of a 3-year-old child.

Hospital-Based Clinic Outpatient Services

Parents bring their 3-year-old boy, who was born with hydrocephalus, to the pediatric neurology clinic at University Hospital to have the child evaluated by the pediatric neurologist and have his VP shunt lengthened to accommodate a growth spurt. Their pediatrician requested a consultation to evaluate the shunt and replace the peritoneal catheter if needed. Outpatient surgery had been previously scheduled tentatively pending this evaluation for the afternoon.

The catheter used in the shunt was removed and replaced in the outpatient surgery suite following a follow-up consultation, which included a detailed interim history, a detailed examination, and medical decision making of moderate complexity. Findings documented in the consultation include "Assessment: Shunt valve malfunction requiring replacement." The VP shunt valve was replaced, along with a new peritoneal catheter in a longer length.

Which of the following code sets will be reported for this service?

ICD-9-CM and CPT Code(s):

a. V53.01, 62230
b. 996.2, 742.3, 62230
c. 742.3, V53.01, 62225
d. 742.3, 62230

ICD-10-CM Code(s): _____

8.53. The following documentation is from the health record of a 4-week-old baby.

Emergency Department Services

A 4-week-old baby is rushed to the hospital after the parents found her cyanotic. While in the ER, she suffered respiratory arrest followed by cardiac arrest and was given cardiopulmonary resuscitation. The baby was born at 36 weeks, with a birth weight of 2400 g. Her current weight is 2700 g. An emergency intubation was performed, and then she was placed on a ventilator and transferred to the neonatal intensive care unit at the university hospital across town for monitoring and further workup. The ER physician provided 1 hour and 20 minutes of critical care, not including the cardiopulmonary resuscitation. His final diagnosis for the ER service is "Hypoxia with respiratory failure in a preterm infant—etiology unknown."

Which of the following code sets (diagnoses and CPT codes) will be reported for the hospital emergency room encounter?

ICD-9-CM and CPT Code(s):

a. 770.84, 765.19; 765.28, 99285
b. 770.84, 779.85, 427.5, 765.18, 765.28; 99291, 92950, 31500
c. 770.84, 779.85, 765.18; 99468, 92950
d. 770.84, 779.85, 427.5, 765.18, 765.28; 99291

ICD-10-CM Code(s): _____

Pediatric Conditions

8.54. The following documentation is from the health record of a female patient who received clinic services.

Chief Complaint: Spina bifida clinic follow-up visit

History: The patient is a 12-year-old girl with T11-12 spina bifida and shunted hydrocephalus. She also has neurogenic bladder and neurogenic bowel and is status post congenital scoliosis, repaired with rodding. When I saw her last, she also complained of some right-sided lower abdominal pain but that resolved shortly after her last visit. Today, she denies headache, nausea, vomiting, diarrhea, any change in bowel or bladder function, upper extremity weakness, cognitive changes, or difficulties swallowing or chewing. Mother has requested a modular wheelchair with hand rails, platforms, and switchback, which I ordered today.

Examination: Normocephalic. Shunt catheter is taut over the right clavicle. Heart regular rate and rhythm. Lungs clear to auscultation. Abdomen has positive bowel sounds. She has some tenderness in the right lateral latissimus area around the inferior border of her scapula. It does not appear to be point tender. It appears to be either musculoskeletal or tendon tenderness. Upper body strength is 5/5. Grip is excellent. There is no weakness noted at all. Lower extremity, she is 0/5. Her skin is clean and dry. She has multiple healed scars on her back from various surgeries. Her toes are clean and dry with no breakdown. Perineal area is clean and dry.

Diagnoses:
1. 12-year-old girl with T11-12 spina bifida and shunted hydrocephalus
2. Neurogenic bladder and bowel
3. Status post scoliosis repair with rodding

Disposition: Continue current catheterization. Keep next week's appointment with Neurology to assess VP shunt.

Which is the correct diagnosis code set for this clinic service?

ICD-9-CM Code(s):

a. 741.02, 596.54, 564.81, 737.30, 996.2
b. 741.02, 596.54, 564.81, V45.2, V13.68
c. 741.90, 596.54, 331.4, 737.30
d. 741.92, 596.54, 564.81, V45.2, V13.68

ICD-10-CM Code(s): _____

Conditions of Pregnancy, Childbirth, and the Puerperium

8.55. The patient is seen in the Women's Clinic in this Ambulatory Surgery center:

Admission Diagnosis: First trimester intrauterine pregnancy in a patient desiring suction evacuation followed by laparoscopic tubal ligation.

Procedures Performed: Suction evaluation of products of conception; bilateral tubal fimbriectomy.

Indications for Procedure: This is a 37-year-old gravida 5, para 3, ab 1 who desires termination of her current pregnancy followed by a tubal ligation. Two of her children were born with significant congenital deformities and she is concerned about the possibility that this will occur with the current pregnancy. She has discussed this at length with her husband and wishes to proceed with the surgeries.

Past history includes three vaginal deliveries and one spontaneous abortion. No other significant past medical or surgical history to date. There are no mitigating factors in her family history. Patient has a history of tobacco use but quit smoking 4 years ago. She does not drink alcohol or use illegal drugs.

Review of Systems: HEENT: negative; cardiorespiratory: negative; GI: negative; GU: deferred

Physical Examination revealed a well-nourished, well-developed female of 37 years. She is presenting today for abortion and tubal ligation. Vital signs include temperature of 98.5 and blood pressure of 110/75 in her left arm. HEENT: normal. Breasts: Normal with no masses or lumps palpable. Heart and lungs are normal to percussion and auscultation and no rales or rhonchi are heard. Her abdomen is soft without tenderness or masses. Her pelvic examination confirms a first trimester pregnancy.

Consent for the procedures was obtained after a thorough discussion of the risks of each of the surgeries and the combination of surgeries. The possibility of occurrence of complications including death were explained and all questions answered.

Description of Procedure: The patient was anesthetized, prepped, and draped in a normal sterile fashion for a vaginal procedure. The cervix was stablilized with a Lahey clamp and the uterus sounded to 10 cm. The internal os accommodated a #8 Hegar dilator and the uterine contents were vaccumed out until no more evidence of products of conception was noted. A light curettage of the uterine wall revealed no additional fetal remnants. The dilator was removed and attention turned to the tubal ligation. Through four strategically placed trocars, the contents of the abdominal/pelvic cavities were examined and no abnormalities noted. Sufficient insufflation had been achieved. Attention was turned to the right fallopian tube which was cut with a curved Kelly and clamped and fulgurated then tied with #1 chromic. The left fallopian tube was dissected in a similar manner. The trocars were removed and the patient tolerated the procedure well. There was blood loss of approximately 100 ml. The patient was sent to PACU in excellent condition.

Pathological Findings: Tissue submitted consisted of products of conception and portions of the right and left fallopian tubes.

Gross examination revealed pieces of irregularly shaped placenta and fetal tissue. Two grossly identifiable pieces of fallopian tubes each about 18 mm in length and 6 mm in diameter were examined.

Final Diagnoses based on Pathological Findings: Products of conception; fallopian tubes.

The patient was allowed to go home after being given her discharge instructions including a return visit to the physician's office in 2 weeks.

What is the correct code assignment for this outpatient surgery?

ICD-9-CM and CPT Code(s): _____

ICD-10-CM Code(s): _____

8.56. The following documentation is from the health record of a 33-year-old woman who received hospital observation services.

Observation Patient

Admit Note: 2/28/XX, 07:30

This is a 33-year-old G2, P0, estimated delivery date of 2/28 and estimated gestational age of 40 weeks. She presents for induction secondary to gestational DM. She has required insulin since 28 weeks with adequate control. PNL: O positive, rubella immune. PE: AVSS, abdomen FH 40 cm, EFW 3800–4000 g. Cervix is closed/50 percent/-3/post/ceph. Plan is for Prostin EZ induction and insulin infusion when in active labor.

Progress Note: 2/28/XX, 09:15

Patient is having uterine contractions every 3 to 8 minutes. Cervix is 1 cm/100 percent/floating. Patient does not want to start Pitocin yet. Feels that she is in labor. FHR reactive, baseline 120s with accelerations.

Progress Note: 2/28/XX, 19:25

Patient's uterine contractions have resolved. Cervix unchanged. Discussed options, would like to go home to sleep and return in a.m. for Pitocin induction. Discharged home for tonight to sleep. Admit in a.m., start IV Pitocin as per protocol, start insulin drip, clear liquid diet.

Which of the following is the correct code set for this outpatient encounter?

ICD-9-CM and CPT Code(s):

a. 648.81, 250.01, V58.67, 99235
b. 648.83, 250.81, 99235
c. 648.83, V58.67, 99235
d. 648.83, 790.29, V58.67, 99235

ICD-10-CM Code(s): _____

8.57. The following documentation is from the health record of a female patient who was seen in the Emergency Department.

Emergency Department Record

This is a 30-year-old G2 P1 female who is 13 weeks pregnant who came in following a motor vehicle crash today. The patient was a passenger in the vehicle and appeared unhurt at the scene. She accompanied her daughter, who had obvious injuries, to the ED in the ambulance. During the initial exam of the child, this patient became lightheaded and had mild abdominal cramping. She was triaged and care began for her. She has had passage of 2 clots since the initial cramping episode. Pregnancy was confirmed as intrauterine on ultrasound at 7 weeks. There has been no dizziness, no syncope, and no other complaints on review of systems. She has a history of a left-sided conductive hearing loss following several childhood illnesses. The patient has a poor obstetrical history with pre-term labor during her first pregnancy.

Vital Signs: 37.0. 78, 18, 132/73, 98%. Alert and oriented × 3. HEENT is generally normal with significant hearing loss demonstrated on the left. Chest is clear to auscultation bilaterally. Heart shows RRR. Back is normal. Normal bowel sounds, nontender and nondistended. + VB from cervical OS. No POC seen. Musculoskeletal does show tenderness over the right olecranon and proximal ulna on palpation. Motion is slightly painful but full. Neuro, Nodes and Skin are all normal. Fetal heart tones are appropriate for gestational age. On re-exam after two hours of bedrest, VB appears to have stopped. Fetal heart tones continue to be strong. Patient's VS are stable.

Thirty-year-old female with threatened AB and contusion to right elbow, status post MVA, restrained passenger. Doubt ectopic given positive IUP on ultrasound. She is anxious to join her daughter at her bedside and agrees that she will be re-seen here if she has any further symptoms. Agrees that nurses on pediatric floor will monitor her closely, and they are alerted to the situation. She will be seen by her OB tomorrow AM if she is not seen here in the ED later today.

Assign the correct codes for this encounter.

ICD-9-CM and CPT Code(s): _____

ICD-10-CM Code(s): _____

8.58. The following documentation is from the health record of a 36-year-old female patient.

Hospital Outpatient Surgery Services

Preoperative Diagnosis: Left ectopic pregnancy

Postoperative Diagnosis: Same

Anesthesia: General

Operation: Diagnostic laparoscopy
Left salpingostomy with removal of ectopic pregnancy

Rationale for Surgery: This patient is a 36-year-old gravida III, para I, AB I, at 9 weeks gestation, who has a positive pregnancy test with left adnexal mass that is a gestational sac with FHTs, and left ectopic pregnancy diagnosis was made. She was admitted at this time for laparoscopy with removal of this left ectopic pregnancy. We did talk about possibly sacrificing the tube on that side if we did get into problems with bleeding. This patient has a history of pelvic adhesions with blocked right tube. She is aware that we may have to sacrifice the left tube and that essentially she would be unable to become pregnant in all probability if we're not able to save the tube. She is also aware of the risks and benefits of surgery, including hemorrhage, bowel and bladder injury, and infection.

Procedure: With the patient in the lithotomy position and under satisfactory general anesthesia, the abdomen and perineum were prepped and draped in the usual manner. A weighted speculum was placed in the vaginal vault. The anterior lip of the cervix was grasped with a single-toothed tenaculum. The uterus was sounded to about 9 cm, and it was retroverted. The endocervical canal was dilated with Pratt dilators, and the Zumi uterine manipulator was placed and the bulb insufflated with approximately 8 cc of air. A red rubber catheter was placed to gravity and attached to the Zumi uterine manipulator. Attention was then turned to the abdominal area, where a small skin incision was made with a scalpel. A large trocar was placed in the direct insertion technique, and pneumoperitoneum was established without difficulty. It is noted she did have some blood in the cul-de-sac. The right tube and ovary looked grossly within normal limits except the fimbriated end on the right was somewhat blunted. The ectopic pregnancy was really at the fimbriated end and had a small clot that was extruded from the fimbriated end. She also had the ovarian cyst on that side, which was not complicating this pregnancy. It was opened and drained. She also had a peritubular cyst, which I left intact. I isolated the ectopic pregnancy and then made a small cut using the needle coagulator over the ectopic pregnancy and extruded this with the needle nose forceps. Had some oozing along the fimbriated end. I did put Avitene in this area and then topped it with some Surgicel. We watched it for several minutes, and it seemed to control the small amount of oozing. We irrigated the pelvic region with copious amounts of irrigation and then aspirated it. We again checked the operative field, and it seemed to be dry. We watched it as we deflated the abdominal pressure. I then removed all the instruments, used .25 mg of Marcaine injection at the injection sites, and closed the incisions with staples. Vaginal instruments were removed. She was taken to the recovery room in good condition. Estimated blood loss approximately 50 cc. Sponge and needle count was correct × 2. Patient did tolerate the procedure well and left the operating room in good condition.

Which of the following is the correct code set for this outpatient surgery?

ICD-9-CM and CPT Code(s):

a. 633.20, 620.2, 59121, 49320
b. 633.10, 620.2, 620.8, 59150, 58662
c. 633.10, 620.2, 58673, 49320
d. 633.20, 654.43, 58673, 58662

ICD-10-CM Code(s): _____

Disorders of the Respiratory System

8.59.   A patient is respirator-dependent and has a tracheostomy in need of revision due to redundant scar tissue formation surrounding the site. Under general anesthesia and establishing the airway to maintain ventilation, the scar tissue is resected, and then repair is accomplished using skin flap rotation from the adjacent tissue of the neck. What codes will be used to report this procedure, which was performed in the hospital outpatient surgical department?

ICD-9-CM Diagnosis Code(s): _____

CPT Code(s): _____

ICD-10-CM Code(s): _____

8.60. The following documentation is from the health record of a 72-year-old female patient.

Hospital-Based Clinic Services

This 72-year-old female presented to the hospital-based urgent care clinic with a chief complaint of recurrent epistaxis for 3 days prior to admission. The bleeding occurred in the right nostril. She also complained of weakness and dizziness when standing. At the last clinic visit, hematocrit was 35, and this morning it is 27. Her past medical history is positive for COPD, with a negative surgical history.

A right anterior limited nasal pack was placed in the clinic treatment room. Because of the weakness and dizziness, we decided to admit the patient to an observation bed. In the evening, the anterior pack required replacement with extensive cauterization in the right nares because of refractory bleeding. Due to falling hematocrit, two units of packed red cells were transfused for the blood-loss anemia resulting. The next morning, the patient was still experiencing some bleeding around the anterior nasal pack. For this reason, she was taken back to the treatment room, and a posterior nasopharyngeal pack in the right nares was placed by another physician. No further bleeding occurred throughout the day, and the patient was discharged to home healthcare follow-up following pack removal.

Which of the following should appear on the UB-04 claim for the outpatient services rendered to this Medicare patient?

Note: The facility purchases its blood from the blood bank.

ICD-9-CM and CPT Code(s):

a. 784.7, 30901-RT, 30903-RT, 30905-RT, 36430-RT
b. 784.7, 280.0, 496, 30901-RT, 30901-RT-76, 30905-RT-77, P9021
c. 784.7, 285.9, 30901-RT, 30903-RT-59, 30905-RT-77, 36430-RT, P9021 (two units)
d. 784.7, 280.0, 496, 30901-RT, 30903RT-59, 30905-RT-59, 36430-RT, P9021 (two units)

ICD-10-CM Code(s): _____

8.61. The following documentation is from the health record of a 66-year-old male patient.

Emergency Department Services

The patient is a 66-year-old male who presented to the Emergency Department with a 2-day history of severe shortness of breath, nonproductive cough, and slight fever. His medical history includes non-small cell lung cancer in the right middle lobe, 2 months post completion of radiation therapy. Surgery was contraindicated because of atrial fibrillation and long-term use of Coumadin. The Oncologist documented that chemotherapy was not indicated in this case and felt that the tumor was eradicated. The patient also has been plagued with dermatitis over the radiation port area on the right lateral chest wall following the 2nd radiation treatment. The skin showed no infection on exam. A 2-view chest x-ray showed consolidation in the right lower lobe of the lung.

The physician diagnosed pneumonitis as an aftereffect of radiation therapy and prescribed both the inhaled corticosteroid, Beclomethasone Dipropionate, and long-term oral corticosteroids on a tapering dose.

Which of the following represents correct coding for this service, including the chargemaster-assigned codes?

ICD-9-CM and CPT Code(s):

a. 486, 692.3, V10.11, E879.2, 71010
b. 508.0, 692.82, 427.31, V58.61, V10.11, E879.2, 71020
c. 508.0, 990, E926.5, 162.4, 427.31, V58.69, 71030
d. 508.1, 692.82, 162.4, 427.31, V58.69, E926.5, 71020

ICD-10-CM Code(s): _____

8.62.   The following documentation is from the health record of a patient who received hospital outpatient surgery services.

Operative Report

Preoperative Diagnosis:	Chronic sinusitis
Postoperative Diagnosis:	Sinusitis of the maxillary, ethmoid, and sphenoid sinuses
Procedure:	Bilateral endoscopic sinusotomies, anterior and posterior ethmoidectomies, and sphenoidotomy, with debris removal in all sites

EBL: <100 cc

Description of Operation: The patient was placed in the supine position after appropriate preparation, draping, and induction of endotracheal anesthesia. The nose was cocainized and injected with Xylocaine 2 percent with 1:100,000 epinephrine.

The endoscope was then used to examine the maxillary sinus structures on the left side. There were several polyps present, and these were carefully injected with Xylocaine 0.5 percent with 1:200,000 epinephrine and removed. The maxillary sinus opening was identified by blunt dissection and was then opened, and with various rongeurs, the tissue was débrided. We then started through the posterior of the middle meatus region involving the ethmoid floors. Care was taken to preserve the parietal mucosa while performing the ethmoidectomies; then we proceeded posteriorly and entered into the sphenoid posteriorly and inferiorly. Gelfilm was folded and placed in the areas involved.

Attention was then directed to the right side in similar fashion. Again, polyps were removed from the maxillary sinus. The uncinate was prominent and was resected, and more polyps were debrided. We then identified the maxillary sinus opening on the right and opened it in a satisfactory manner. We then proceeded anterior through posterior ethmoidal cells into the sphenoid cavity posteriorly, opening and removing large amounts of polypoid mucosa, polyps, and some mild purulence. When this was completed to our satisfaction, Gelfilm was folded and placed. The posterior throat was suctioned clear, and the patient was awakened and taken to recovery in good condition.

Which codes will be reported for this ambulatory surgery service?

ICD-9-CM and CPT Code(s):

a. 473.9, 31256-50, 31287
b. 473.0, 473.2, 473.3, 471.8, 31256-50, 31287–50
c. 473.0, 473.2, 473.3, 471.8, 31255-50, 31267–50, 31288–50
d. 473.0, 473.2, 473.3, 471.8, 31255, 31267

ICD-10-CM Code(s): _____

Trauma and Poisoning

8.63. The following documentation is from the health record of a 25-year-old female patient.

Emergency Department Services

A 25-year-old female fell off of her horse in the morning, sustaining an injury and fracture of the spinal cord and vertebra at the C4 level. The patient was brought to the nearest ED by ambulance in a full-body air splint. CT scan revealed the injury to be a complete injury to the spinal cord (tetraplegia). The patient was having some difficulty breathing, and after endotracheal intubation, ventilator support was initiated. Vital signs were unstable in the ED. The patient had no feeling below the level of the injury. The patient was closely monitored throughout her stay in the ED. Later that day, when it was thought that she was stable enough for transport, she was transferred to the neurosurgical intensive care unit at the teaching hospital downtown for definitive treatment at the fracture site.

Critical care services were provided according to the acuity system. The ED physician who managed this patient recorded extensive progress notes, which included the specific time he spent with the patient on and off throughout the day. Times noted included the following: 0800–0900, 1000–1030, 1100–1115, 1300–1315, 1500–1600.

Which of the following sets of codes would be appropriate for facility reporting of this ED service in addition to the CT scan, 72125, assigned via the chargemaster?

ICD-9-CM and CPT Code(s):

a. 805.04, 344.01, E828.2, 99291, 31500
b. 805.04, 344.01, E828.2, 99291, 31500
c. 806.01, E828.2, 99291, 31500
d. 806.01, E828.2, 99291, 31500, 22305

ICD-10-CM Code(s): _____

8.64. The following documentation is from the health record of a male patient with a hand injury.

Hospital Outpatient Surgery Services

Preoperative Diagnosis: Open fracture, shaft of the middle phalanx of the left small finger, on the oblique

Postoperative Diagnosis: Open fracture, shaft of the middle phalanx of the left small finger, on the oblique with disruption of collateral ligament and extensor tendon

Procedure: Irrigation and debridement, open reduction of fracture, repair of extensor tendon and lateral collateral ligament, left small finger

Indications: This 42-year-old man sustained this injury at his single-family home while using a powered hedge trimmer which slipped. The medial ligament, soft tissue, and skin are intact. Because of this wound, the patient was brought to the operating room today.

Description: Two grams of Ancef were administered prior to the start of the case. The patient was identified by site of surgery, by direct communication with the patient, and by consent form. Following induction of general anesthesia, the left upper extremity was prepped and draped in the usual manner. A tourniquet was placed. Attention was first directed to the wound, and the margins of the wound were trimmed of devascularized tissue. There was a significant amount of debris in the wound. It was debrided of bone chips using the operating microscope and lavaged with 4 liters of Kantrex saline solution. Following this, the oblique fracture of the middle phalanx was approximated over a metal pin using fluoroscopic guidance. This provided excellent alignment of the fracture and appropriate positioning of the finger. The extensor tendon was repaired with acceptable extension being achieved. The lateral collateral ligament was repaired and the PIP joint was again stable. The wound was closed using 4-0 nylon suture, apposing his soft tissues. The tourniquet was released. Tourniquet time was 40 minutes. Vascularization appeared adequate. Sterile bandage of bacitracin, Adaptic, 2 × 2s, and a tube gauze bandage were applied. Estimated blood loss was minimal during the procedure.

Which of the following code sets is appropriate for this service?

ICD-9-CM and CPT Code(s):

a. 816.00, 26756-F4, 13131-F4
b. 816.01, E920.1, 11012, 26735-F4
c. 816.11, E920.1, E849.0, 26735-F4
d. 816.11, E920.1, E849.0, 26756-F4, 26418-F4, 26540-F4, 11012, 13131

Note: E codes E000.8 and E016.1 would be appropriate to use as well.

ICD-10-CM Code(s): _____

8.65.   **Emergency Department Visit**

HPI: This white female, aged 28 years old, was brought to the emergency room by her friends after she took approximately 60, 15 mg Dalmane, approximately 100, 7.5 mg Tranxene and several glasses of wine. This was done out of sight of the friends. They noticed that the patient became very drowsy and unable to ambulate. She got up from the sofa to go to the kitchen when she fell and hit her forehead on the corner of the table. There is a 2.2-cm laceration on the forehead which is bleeding profusely. The patient admitted to the friends what she had done and they brought her to the hospital immediately. She actually appears to be alert but somewhat combative. Her speech is slurred but she is oriented as to time, date, and place. There is a question of exactly how many pills she took.

Past Medical/Surgical History: Patient is gravida 3, para 1, AB 2. Her most recent spontaneous abortion occurred a little more than a month ago and she has been very depressed since the miscarriage.

Social History: Patient is married with one small child. She married quite young at age 16. She smokes about 1 pack per day and usually drinks very little alcohol. She works as a teacher's aide.

Family History: Her mother is deceased from complications of diabetes. Her father died of colon cancer complicated by cirrhosis of the liver. The father was an alcoholic. No family history of mental illness.

Review of Systems: A very brief ROS was taken. Cardiovascular: patient has no trouble with SOB, dyspnea or exertion, palpitations, or chest pain.

Neuropsychiatric: Patient did have postpartum depression following the birth of her child. This was mild to severe and she continues to seek outpatient treatment for it. The Tranxene was prescribed by her psychiatrist. The depression was exacerbated by her recent miscarriage.

Vital Signs: BP 130/50 and P 95.

Services Provided: 1. Patient underwent gastric lavage to remove all pills that she ingested. Following this the patient's forehead wound was sutured with single layer closure. The wound was debrided prior to suturing.

The patient's husband arrived at the hospital and the patient was released to his care to be admitted to the local mental health hospital for suicide prevention.

What codes are reported for this emergency department service?

ICD-9-CM and CPT Code(s): _____

ICD-10-CM Code(s): _____

8.66. Emergency Department Services

This 17-year-old girl was a passenger on a motorcycle and was thrown from the back of the motorcycle when they hit a hole in the road. She was thrown onto the side of the road and sustained multiple contusions and reported pain in her left forearm and ribs. Patient was taken to x-ray to have the hand and ribs examined. While waiting for the results, the nurse cleaned an abrasion on her left knee, on her left cheek, and on the scalp. She had a 1.1-cm. laceration on her right palm which the physician examined. It was debrided to remove a significant amount of dirt, gravel, and even wood chips. It was then copiously washed with sterile water. The physician examined the palm and was able to suture it using single layer 3.0 chromic sutures.

X-ray results showed a non-displaced fracture of the distal one-third of the ulna. The radius was not involved. A long-arm plaster cast was applied to the arm. There were no injuries sustained to the ribs. There appears a large ecchymosis to the right upper quadrant but there is no flank tenderness or swelling of the organs.

The patient is given a prescription for Lortab 1 q. 6 hrs. p.r.n. and told to see her family physician in the morning.

What codes are reported for this emergency department visit?

ICD-9-CM and CPT Code(s): _____

ICD-10-CM Code(s): _____

Chapter 9

Case Studies from Physician-based Health Records

> **Note:** Although the specific cases are divided by setting, much of the information pertaining to the diagnosis is applicable in most settings. Even the CPT codes in the ambulatory and physician sections may be reported in the same manner. The differences in coding in these two settings may involve modifier reporting, evaluation and management CPT code reporting, and other health plan reporting guidelines unique to settings. If you practice or apply codes in a particular type of setting, you may find additional information in other sections of this publication that may be pertinent to you.
>
> Every effort has been made to follow current recognized coding guidelines and principles, as well as nationally recognized reporting guidelines. The material presented may differ from some health plan requirements for reporting. The ICD-9-CM codes used are effective October 1, 2011, through September 30, 2012, and the HCPCS (CPT and HCPCS Level II) codes are in effect January 1, 2011, through December 31, 2011. The current standard transactions and code sets named in HIPAA have been utilized. The 2011 draft edition of ICD-10-CM was utilized.
>
> **Instructions:** Assign all applicable ICD-9-CM diagnosis codes including V codes and E codes. Assign all CPT Level I procedure codes and HCPCS Level II codes. Assign Level I (CPT) and Level II (HCPCS) modifiers as appropriate. Final codes for billing occur after codes are passed through payer edits. Medicare utilizes the National Correct Coding Initiative (NCCI) edits. CMS developed the NCCI edit list to promote national correct coding methodologies and to control improper coding leading to improper payments for Medicare Part B. The purpose of the NCCI edits is to ensure the most comprehensive code is assigned and billed rather than the component codes. In addition, NCCI edits check for mutually exclusive pairs.
>
> Cases in this workbook are presented as either multiple choice or fill in the blank.
>
> - For multiple-choice cases:
>   —Select the letter of the appropriate code set.
> - For fill-in-the-blank cases:
>   —Sequence the primary diagnosis first followed by the secondary diagnoses including appropriate V codes and E codes (both cause of injury and place of occurrence).
>   —Sequence the primary CPT procedure code first followed by additional procedure codes including modifiers as appropriate (both CPT Level I and HCPCS Level II modifiers).

—Assign HCPCS Level II codes **only if instructed** (case specific).

—Assign evaluation and management (E/M) codes **only if instructed** (case specific).

The scenarios are based on selected excerpts from health records. In practice, the coding professional should have access to and refer to the entire health record. Health records are analyzed and codes assigned based on physician documentation. In physician practice, valuable information for coding purposes is available on the superbill; however, documentation for coding purposes must be assigned based on medical record documentation. A physician may be queried when documentation is ambiguous, incomplete, or conflicting. The queried documentation must be a permanent part of the medical record.

The objective of the cases and scenarios reproduced in this publication is to provide practice in assigning correct codes, not necessarily to emulate complete coding, which can only be achieved with the complete medical record. For example, the reader may be asked to assign codes based on only an operative report; in real practice, a coder has access to documentation in the entire medical record.

The *ICD-9-CM Official Guidelines for Coding and Reporting of Outpatient Services*, published by the National Center for Health Statistics (NCHS), supplements the official conventions and instructions provided within ICD-9-CM. Adherence to these guidelines when assigning ICD-9-CM diagnosis codes is required under the Health Insurance Portability and Accountability Act (HIPAA) of 1996. Additional official coding guidance can be found in the American Hospital Association (AHA)'s *Coding Clinic* publication.

Anesthesia Services

9.1.   A neonatal patient is brought to the operating room for repair of complete transposition of the great arteries under cardiopulmonary bypass. The infant is in critical condition and may not survive. Assign the correct diagnosis codes and CPT codes to report the administration of anesthesia, including physical status, Level I and II modifiers, and qualifying conditions for this procedure.

ICD-9-CM and CPT Code(s):

a. 745.10, 00562–AA–23, 99100
b. 745.11, 00561–AD–P5, 99140
c. 745.10, 00561–AA–P5
d. 745.19, 00563–AA–P5, 99100, 99140

ICD-10-CM Code(s): _____

9.2.   A patient came into the pain clinic for management of chronic neck and shoulder pain after a car accident one year ago. The vehicle she was driving struck a bus on a country road. The pain extended down into her left hand, and the patient had difficulty lifting or moving anything with that hand. She also reported inability to sleep well due to pain. Her attending physician requested that Dr. Jones, a pain specialist, take over the care for her pain. Dr. Jones performed a brief history and expanded problem-focused physical exam with medical decision making of low complexity. He and the patient discussed the injection of Marcaine and steroids into the cervical plexus for relief. The patient agreed to this plan, and after consents were signed, the injection was performed. The patient noted approximately 40 percent relief in pain almost immediately. Dr. Jones requested that the patient come back in one week and again in two weeks for another injection.

Diagnosis: Cervicobrachial syndrome, due to auto accident one year ago.

Assign the correct diagnosis and CPT codes (including E/M) for this scenario.

ICD-9-CM and CPT Code(s):

a. 723.3, 907.3, E929.0, 99201, 64413
b. 907.3, 723.3, E929.0, 99242, 64413
c. 723.3, 907.3, E929.0, 99212, 64415
d. 907.3, E929.0, 99245, 64490

ICD-10-CM Code(s): _____

9.3. A 55-year-old patient is brought into the operating room for elective decompression of the median nerve for carpal tunnel syndrome. She is in excellent health otherwise. The surgeon places an Esmarch bandage on the arm, and the arm is exsanguinated. A tourniquet is then placed and the surgeon administers Bier block anesthesia.

Tourniquet time was approximately 50 minutes. Assign the ICD-9-CM diagnosis code and CPT surgical and anesthesia codes with any applicable modifiers.

ICD-9-CM and CPT Code(s):

a. 354.0, 64719
b. 354.0, 64722–47
c. 354.0, 64721–47
d. 354.1, 64721, 01810

ICD-10-CM Code(s): _____

Disorders of the Blood and Blood-Forming Organs

9.4. A 32-year-old female has recently had surgery for melanoma of the right arm, Clark level IV. She had no other signs of metastasis or adenopathy. Under general anesthesia, a sentinel node biopsy of the deep axillary nodes was performed with a gamma counter probe. An injection of isosulfan blue dye was performed and the nodes followed carefully to the single bright-blue node. This node was excised and sent for frozen section, which proved to be negative for melanoma. Before the procedure, the radiologist performed a lymphoscintigraphy. Which of the following code sets would the surgeon report? (Do not report supplies.)

ICD-9-CM and CPT Code(s):

a. 173.69, 38525
b. 172.6, 38525, 38792
c. 172.6, 38525, 38792–51, 78195
d. 172.9, 38525, 38790–51

ICD-10-CM Code(s): _____

9.5.   The following documentation is from the health record of a male patient.

History: This is a 66-year-old male who had a coronary artery bypass graft in February. He did well. He was discharged home. Some time after that when he was home, he had two days of black stools. He mentioned it to the nurse, but I'm not sure anything was done about it. He has not had any other evidence of hematemesis, melena, or hematochezia but was feeling rather weak and fatigued. He had blood work done, which showed a hemoglobin of 5.7, hematocrit of 20.9, MCV of 80. Serum iron of 8, 2 percent saturation. No indigestion or heartburn. No abdominal pain of any kind. No past history of anemia or GI bleed.

Past Medical History: General health has been good.

Allergies: None known

Previous Surgeries: Coronary artery bypass graft

Medications: At the time of admission include Glucotrol, Lasix, potassium, and aspirin

Review of Systems: Endocrine: He does have diabetes, controlled with medication. Cardiovascular: History of coronary artery disease with coronary artery bypass graft. No recent symptoms of chest pain or shortness of breath. Respiratory: No chronic cough or sputum production. GU: No dysuria, hematuria, history of stones, or infections. Musculoskeletal: No arthritic complaints or muscle weakness. Neuropsychiatric: No syncope, seizures, weakness, paralysis, or depression.

Family History: His mother had cardiovascular disease and diabetes. No history of cancer.

Social History: The patient is married. Never smoked. Doesn't drink any alcohol. Works in a factory.

On physical examination, a well-developed, well-nourished, alert male in no acute distress. Blood pressure 146/82. Respirations 18. Heart rate 78. Skin: Good turgor and texture. Eyes: No scleral icterus. Pupils are round, regular, equal, and react to light. Neck: No jugular venous distention. No carotid bruits. Thyroid is not enlarged. Trachea in the midline. Lungs are clear. No heart murmur noted. Abdomen is soft. Bowel sounds present. No masses, no tenderness. Liver and spleen are not palpably enlarged. Extremities: Good pulses. Trace edema of the feet.

Laboratory values show severe anemia with a hemoglobin of 5.7. Hemoccult is also positive. His iron studies showed low iron and low ferritin, consistent with chronic blood loss anemia. His B_{12} and folate levels were normal. His SMA-12 was essentially unremarkable.

Impression: 1.   Anemia. Probably he is anemic post bypass and then had stress gastritis with a little bit of bleeding and has never recovered from that. No evidence of acute or active bleeding at this time. The patient is stable. Possibility of occult malignancy or active peptic ulcer disease does exist.
   2.   Arteriosclerotic heart disease of native vessel, stable

Recommendations: Admit patient as an outpatient for blood transfusion. Patient is being transfused. He should have an esophagogastroduodenoscopy and colonoscopy, possible biopsy or polypectomy, which has been explained to the patient along with potential risks and complications, including bleeding, transfusion, perforation, and surgery. These tests will be scheduled for a later date.

Discharge Note

Final Diagnosis: Severe blood loss anemia, weakness, diabetes mellitus, history of coronary artery disease status post coronary artery bypass graft.

The patient received three units of packed red blood cells; he felt better with subsidence of his shortness of breath and his weakness improved. His last hemoglobin was 8.4, with a hematocrit of 27.7.

The patient was scheduled for EGD to rule out peptic ulcer disease and colonoscopy to rule out occult malignancy in one week. The patient will be discharged home, and he will have a clear liquid diet. He is to call for any problems. He will continue with his home medications, and he was placed on ferrous sulfate one tablet twice a day.

What diagnosis codes are reported for this hospital outpatient encounter reported by the physician?

ICD-9-CM Code(s):

a. 280.0, 792.1, 414.01, 250.00, V45.81
b. 285.9, 780.79
c. 280.0, 578.1, 414.01, 250.00, V45.81
d. 998.11, 285.1, 792.1, 414.01, 250.00, V45.81

ICD-10-CM Code(s): _____

Disorders of the Cardiovascular System

9.6.   A patient who is six weeks post anterior MI with congestive heart failure has been taking Lanoxin and is experiencing nausea and vomiting and profound fatigue. The evaluation and treatment were focused on adjustment of medication only. Blood levels show 4 ng/mL. Which of the following diagnosis codes will be reported?

ICD-9-CM Code(s):

a. 972.1, E858.3, 787.01
b. 410.12, 428.0
c. 787.01, 780.79, E858.3
d. 787.01, 780.79, E942.1, 410.12, 428.0

ICD-10-CM Code(s): _____

9.7.   The following documentation is from the health record of a female patient.

History: This is a 70-year-old female who had noted exertional tachyarrhythmia described as palpitations, diaphoresis, and presyncope. She had noted no frank syncopal episodes. Prior to this admission, she had been on Lopressor, Norpace, and Lanoxin in combination but was still experiencing breakthrough atrial flutter.

Hospital Course: Upon admission, the patient underwent echocardiography. This revealed moderate left ventricular dysfunction, mild to moderate aortic regurgitation, mild mitral regurgitation, and the left atrium proved to be within the upper limits of normal. At that time, it was recommended that the patient begin on amiodarone therapy due to drug refractory atrial flutter. Pulmonary function test and thyroid function test were also performed. Thyroid function test results proved within normal limits. Pulmonary function test results revealed normal lung volumes with mild loss of alveolar capacity. Amiodarone loading continued. The patient was taken to the electrophysiology lab, and overdrive pacing was attempted. This was unsuccessful. The patient therefore underwent direct-current external atrial cardioversion and at that time converted to normal sinus rhythm. The patient was discharged with a scheduled follow-up in 1 month.

Final Diagnoses: 1. Drug refractory atrial flutter
2. Successful cardioversion to normal sinus rhythm

Which of the following is the correct code assignment?

ICD-9-CM and CPT Code(s):

a. 429.9, 424.0, 92961
b. 429.9, 394.1, 33240
c. 427.32, 394.1, 429.9, 33211
d. 427.32, 396.3, 429.9, 92960

ICD-10-CM Code(s): _____

9.8.   The following documentation is from the health record of a 66-year-old male patient.

Discharge Summary

Admission Date: 6/19/XX

Discharge Date: 6/28/XX

History of Present Illness: This patient is a 66-year-old male admitted on 6/19 because of unstable postinfarct angina. He underwent cardiac bypass surgery here 15 years ago. He did well until 1989, when he developed angina and underwent angioplasty here. On 6/9, he was awakened by severe chest pain and was taken to a nearby community hospital where he was found to have a small anterior wall myocardial infarction with the CPK only slightly elevated. He had cardiac catheterization performed at that time. Because of this small infarction, he was referred here for consideration for further surgical intervention. He was discharged from the hospital on 6/16. On 6/19, as the patient was walking from the car to the office, he developed significant chest pain and was therefore admitted to rule out further infarction.

Documentation of recent cardiac catheterization showed that complete left heart catheterization, left ventricular cineangiography, coronary arteriography, and bypass visualization were performed. The left ventricle showed severe anterior hypokinesis, although it did still move. The left main coronary artery was narrowed by about 70 percent. The bypass to the circumflex looked good, but the bypass to the left anterior descending had a very severe stenosis in the body of the graft. There was a very large, marginal circumflex artery that had an orificial, 80 percent stenosis. He was thought not to be a candidate for angioplasty but bypass surgery instead.

Surgical Procedure: Using extracorporeal circulation, the left internal mammary artery was anastomosed to the left anterior descending coronary artery, and a venous graft was placed from the aorta to the marginal circumflex. It was found that the old venous graft to the main circumflex was in excellent condition with very soft, pliable walls so that the vessel was left intact. There were no complications of this surgery. His postoperative course was singularly uncomplicated. He never had any arrhythmia problems; his wounds healed nicely. He had a tiny left pleural effusion that never needed to be tapped. He was walking about the ward participating in the cardiac rehab program at the time of discharge.

Discharge Instructions: Discharge medications will simply be aspirin grains 5 q.d., Tylenol with Codeine 1 or 2 p.r.n. for pain, Lopressor 50 mg a day, and Colace, as necessary. He was instructed to contact his private physician upon return home for resumption of his medical care. He is to call me here at the medical center if there are any questions or problems that he wishes to discuss.

Discharge Diagnoses:
1. Unstable angina (intermediate coronary syndrome)
2. Recent incomplete, anterior wall myocardial infarction
3. Coronary atherosclerosis, three vessel
4. Successful double-bypass surgery

What are the correct codes for this admission?

ICD-9-CM and CPT Code(s):

a. 414.01, 414.05, 410.12, 411.1, 33517, 33533, 33530
b. 414.01, 414.05, 410.12, 411.1, 33510, 33533
c. 414.00, 414.05, 410.11, 411.1, 33530
d. 414.01, 414.05, 410.12, 412, 33518, 33530

ICD-10-CM Code(s): _____

9.9.   The following documentation is from the health record of an 85-year-old female patient.

Admission Date: 12/10/XX

Discharge Date: 12/22/XX

Discharge Diagnoses:
1. Acute pulmonary edema with congestive heart failure
2. Myocardial infarction ruled out
3. Chronic obstructive pulmonary disease
4. Pneumonia
5. Senile dementia

History of Present Illness: This 85-year-old female was admitted via the emergency room from the nursing home with shortness of breath, confusion, and congestion. There was no history of fever or cough noted. Patient has a history of senile dementia and COPD. Prior to admission, the patient was on the following medications: Prednisone, Lasix, Haldol, and Colace.

Physical Examination: Blood pressure 140/70, heart rate of 125 beats per minute, respirations were 30, temperature of 101.4°F. The eyes showed postsurgical eyes, nonreactive to light. The lungs showed bilaterally bibasilar crackles. The heart showed S1 and S2, with no S3. The abdomen was soft and nontender. The extremities showed leg edema. The neurological exam revealed no deficits, and she was alert × 3.

Laboratory Data: ABGs were 7.4, PO_2 of 63, CO_2 of 43, bicarbonate 26, saturation of 89. Hemoglobin 11.7, hematocrit was 31.5, platelets of 207,000. Sodium 139, chloride 107, potassium 4.4, BUN 42, creatinine 1.2. The EKG was unremarkable.

Hospital Course: Basically, this patient was admitted to the coronary care unit with acute pulmonary edema, rule out myocardial infarction. Serial cardiac enzymes were done, which were within normal limits, therefore ruling out myocardial infarction. A chest x-ray performed on the day of admission confirmed congestive heart failure and pneumonia. The patient was started on Unasyn and tobramycin for the pneumonia, which improved. The congestive heart failure, however, was not improving with administration of Lasix. The patient was not taking foods and liquids well and, at the family's request, she was labeled DNR. On hospital day 12, she was found without respirations, with no heart sounds, and pupils were fixed. She was pronounced dead by the physician, and the family was notified.

Which of the following answers demonstrates the correct ICD-9-CM code assignment?

ICD-9-CM Code(s):

a. 428.0, 486, 496, 290.0, V49.86
b. 428.0, 518.4, 486, 496, 290.0
c. 428.0, 410.91, 486, 496, 290.0, V49.86
d. 518.4, 428.0, 486, 496, 290.0, V49.86

ICD-10-CM Code(s): _____

9.10. Dr. Hiram performs an endovascular repair of a very long aneurysm of the descending thoracic aorta, with placement of two distal extension components due to the extensive length of the aneurysm. The left subclavian artery was not covered during this procedure. Assign the appropriate CPT code(s) to report this procedure.

a. 33880
b. 33779
c. 33881
d. 33881, 33883, 33884

9.11. Ms. Jones has a pseudoaneurysm of her left iliac artery that has developed proximal to an area of occlusion. She is admitted to Community Hospital for iliac artery endovascular revascularization and repair. She undergoes a percutaneous transluminal balloon angioplasty of the area of occlusion, with placement of a drug-eluting stent, and an endovascular repair of the pseudoaneurysm using ilio-iliac tube endoprothesis. An endovascular ultrasound is performed after the procedure to assure patency of the vessel. Assign the appropriate CPT code(s). You do not need to assign modifiers for this exercise.

    a. 34900, 37221, 37250
    b. 34900, 37221
    c. 37221
    d. 34825, 37221, 37250

9.12. In the cardiac catheterization laboratory of Big City Hospital, Dr. Hart performed a PTCA on a patient's right coronary artery, with placement of a drug-eluting stent. He also performed a PTCA of the left circumflex coronary artery and placement of two stents. The patient had undergone a complete diagnostic cardiac catheterization at an outlying hospital the previous day, so complete cardiac catheterization was not performed. Dr. Hart performed the procedure via femoral artery cutdown without left heart catheterization. Assign the appropriate CPT codes and HCPCS Level II modifiers that Dr. Hart would use to report these procedures. You do not need to assign CPT Level I modifiers for this exercise.

CPT and HCPCS Level II Code(s):

    a. 92980-RC, 92981-LC
    b. 92982-RC, 92984-LC, 92980-RC, 92981-LC × 2
    c. 93455, 92980-RC, 92981-LC
    d. 93455, 92982-RC, 92984-LC, 92980-RC, 92981-LC × 2

9.13. This is a progress note from the office records of a physician's office:

Chief Complaint: Chest pains in a 44-year-old man

HPI: Patient indicates that he woke up this morning with what he thought was indigestion but as the morning progressed he began to have some intermittent chest pains. He comes to the office for check-up.

Past Medical History: Patient has open angle glaucoma, mild hypertension, and DJD. He does smoke a pack of cigarettes per day. In light of his family history, I have repeatedly suggested that the patient attempt a smoking cessation regime. I have offered prescription meds but patient refuses.

Family History: Patient's father died at age 43 of myocardial infarction. His older brother has had one minor MI at age 51.

Vital Signs: BP 163/78; pulse 89; respirations 17.

Physical Examination:

HEENT: Glaucoma, diagnosed 8 months ago, is in control. He last saw his ophthalmologist just about 3 weeks ago. I will continue to monitor in between visits with the specialist.

Pulmonary: Chest is clear to percussion and auscultation. No rales or rhonchi heard. Hiatal hernia noted.

Abdomen: Obese. No gross hepatosplenomegaly. Bowel sounds are normal.

Extremities: Pedal edema in the lower extremities. There did not appear to be any lesions or open wounds on the lower extremities. Patient complained of some pain in the right knee. He has a history of a right knee replacement some 10 years ago. I see no obvious abnormalities with the knee but if it continues to cause him discomfort he should see an orthopedist.

Cardiovascular: Heart sounds were regular. No murmurs or ectopic beats heard.

Plan: Because of the patient's hypertension and family history of myocardial infarctions, the chest pains are extremely worrisome. I have arranged for the patient to have a cardiac catheterization today. He was instructed to report to the hospital immediately.

What codes would be recorded for this office visit?

ICD-9-CM Code(s): _____

ICD-10-CM Code(s): _____

9.14.   Operative Report

Preoperative Diagnoses: Atrial fibrillation with sick sinus syndrome.

Postoperative Diagnoses: Atrial fibrillation with sick sinus syndrome.

Procedure: Insertion of Medtronics N rhythm dual chamber pulse generator pacemaker, model number P1501DR with atrial and ventricular leads under fluoroscopic guidance.

Anesthesia: 1% Xylocaine local with sedation.

Estimated Blood Loss: Minimal.

Comment: This is an elderly gentleman with atrial fibrillation and sick sinus syndrome who had a dual chamber pacemaker placed with a screw-in atrial lead in the operating room. During the time of implantation, the permanent lead parameters were recorded in the patient's permanent medical record and the entire procedure was performed under fluoroscopy. The patient has been on Coumadin for several years but blood loss was minimal. The patient tolerated the procedure well.

Procedure: The patient was taken to the operating room and placed on the table in supine position. After adequate intravenous sedation was given, the left chest wall was prepped with DuraPrep and draped with sterile drapes in the usual fashion. After infiltration with 1% Xylocaine, an oblique incision was fashioned inferomedial to the deltopectoral groove. The incision was deepened to the skin and subcutaneous tissue to the pectoralis fascia where a pocket was fashioned inferiorly for the pulse generator. Through the wound, two Seldinger wires were placed uneventfully into the left subclavian vein with the patient in Trendelenburg and these were then exchanged for dilator and breakaway sheaths through which were introduced a tinned-tipped ventricular lead advanced to the central circulation under fluoroscopic guidance with the tip brought to rest in the apex of the right ventricle until satisfactory parameters were obtained in this location and the lead was then secured to the chest wall with three interrupted #2-0 Ethibond sutures. More medially, the dilator and breakaway sheath in this position was then replaced with a screw-in type pre-formed, J-shaped atrial lead advanced in the septal circulation under fluoroscopic guidance with the tip implanted in the right atrium with the screw-in device until satisfactory parameters were obtained in this location. This lead was secured to the chest wall in a similar fashion. The two leads then firmly connected to the pre-programmed Medtronics pulse generator model as noted above, which was placed into the previously fashioned subcutaneous pocket with the leads coiled beneath it. The subcutaneous tissues were irrigated with Ancef saline and the superficial subcutaneous tissues were closed over the top of the pacemaker leads with interrupted #3-0 Polysorb suture and the skin closed with running inverted, interrupted subcuticular #4-0 Biosyn followed by application of a Bioclusive dressing. Sponge, needle, and instrument counts were reported to be correct $\times$ 2 at the termination of the procedure. The patient tolerated the procedure well and left the Operating Room in satisfactory condition.

What are the correct codes for this outpatient surgery?

ICD-9-CM and CPT Code(s):

a. 427.41, 427.81, 33202, 33213
b. 427.41, 427.81, 33212, 33217
c. 427.31, V58.61, 33201
d. 427.31, 427.81, V58.61, 33208

ICD-10-CM Code(s): _____

Disorders of the Digestive System

9.15.   This is the documentation from the record of a patient seen in the outpatient surgery suite.

Procedure: Upper GI endoscopy

Indications: Heartburn

Complications: No immediate complications

Procedure: After obtaining informed consent, the endoscope was passed under direct vision. Throughout the procedure, the patient's blood pressure, pulse, and oxygen saturations were monitored continuously. The Olympus GIF-Q160 gastroscope (Serial No. 2306352) was introduced through the mouth, and advanced to the third part of the duodenum. The upper GI endoscopy was accomplished without difficulty. The patient tolerated the procedure well.

Findings: Biopsy of esophageal mucosa with a cold forceps was performed for histology, evaluation for microscopic esophagitis, and evaluation to rule out Barrett's Esophagus.

Diffuse mildly erythematous mucosa with no bleeding was found in the gastric antrum. Biopsies were taken with a cold forceps for histology. Biopsies were taken with a cold forceps for Helicobacter pylori testing.

The examined duodenum was normal. Biopsy with a cold forceps was performed for histology, evaluation of celiac sprue, evaluation of celiac disease, and evaluation of chronic inflammation.

Impression: GERD.

Mild antral gastritis/gastric mucosal abnormality characterized by erythema. Normal examined duodenum. This was biopsied.

Recommendations: – Continue present medications.

                – Use sucralfate tablets at 1 gram PO QID.

                – Telephone endoscopist for pathology results.

                – Await pathology results.

Which codes would the physician use to report these services?

ICD-9-CM and CPT Code(s):

a. 530.81, 535.40, 43239
b. 530.81, 535.50, 43239
c. 530.81, 535.40, 43202, 43605, 44010
d. 530.81, 535.40, 43239

ICD-10-CM Code(s): _____

9.16. A 48-year-old man came in to the emergency department complaining of vomiting material resembling coffee grounds several times within the past hour. He has abdominal pain and has been unable to eat for the past 24 hours. He is dizzy and lightheaded. Two stools today have been black and tarry. While in the emergency department, he vomited bright-red blood and some material resembling coffee grounds. A nasogastric tube was inserted by the ED physician and attached to suction. An abdominal exam showed a fluid wave consistent with ascites. CBC and clotting studies were drawn. A detailed history and physical exam with high-complexity medical decision making were documented. A GI consultant was called and the patient was taken to Endoscopy for further evaluation of upper GI bleeding. Diagnosis:

Hematemesis, rule out esophageal varices; blood loss anemia, acute; ascites.

Which of the following is the correct diagnosis and CPT procedure code assignment for the independent ED physician?

ICD-9-CM and CPT Code(s):

a. 578.0, 285.1, 789.59, 99285, 43752
b. 578.0, 789.00, 780.4, 99284-25, 91105
c. 789.51, 578.0, 280.0, 99284, 43752
d. 578.0, 285.1, 789.59, 99284-25, 43752

ICD-10-CM Code(s): _____

9.17. This 35-year-old man has had a history of diverticulosis with frequent bleeding in the past. He came in to have a colonoscopy and rule out any other pathology, such as carcinoma. During the colonoscopy, severe diverticulosis was noted. This is definitely the cause of the bleeding. Also noted were a polyp at the splenic flexure and a polyp in the transverse colon. The polyp at the splenic flexure was removed by hot biopsy, and the second polypectomy was done by snare technique. The polyps were both classified as adenomatous with no signs of malignancy. What are the correct codes for this case?

ICD-9-CM and CPT Code(s):

a. 562.12, 211.3, 45385, 45384-51 or 45384-59
b. 211.3, 562.10, 578.1, 45384
c. 562.12, 211.3, 578.9, 45385
d. 562.12, 211.3, 45384

ICD-10-CM Code(s): _____

9.18. The patient had a laparoscopic Nissen fundoplasty performed for gastroesophageal reflux with esophagitis. He also has Barrett's esophagus. These conditions have not been responding to conservative treatment, and the patient wishes to undergo surgery at this time. The patient has also had many instances of treatment for chronic cholecystitis. It has been decided to pursue a laparoscopic cholecystectomy at the same time that the fundoplasty is done. Which of the following is the correct code assignment?

ICD-9-CM and CPT Code(s):

a. 530.81, 530.85, 47562, 43289-51
b. 530.11, 530.85, 574.10, 43327, 47600-52
c. 530.11, 530.89, 575.11, 43326
d. 530.11, 530.85, 575.11, 43280, 47562-51

ICD-10-CM Code(s): _____

9.19.   The following documentation is from the health record of a 58-year-old male patient:

Preoperative Diagnosis:	Diverticular disease of left colon Non-continuity of bowel
Postoperative Diagnosis:	Diverticular disease of left colon
Operation:	Laparoscopic left colon resection with coloproctal anastomosis Laparoscopic splenic flexure mobilization
Anesthesia:	General endotracheal, Marcaine 0.5% local
Estimated Blood Loss:	20 cc.

Indications: This 58-year-old male presents back to the operating room four months after his sigmoid colon perforation due to diverticular disease. A temporary ostomy was performed, along with sigmoidectomy at that time. In the interim, the patient has undergone a colonoscopy identifying additional diverticular disease in the left colon. Upon discussion with him, we plan today for reanastomosis of the bowel but also additional colon resection on his left colon in light of this additional disease. The risks, benefits, and alternatives of the procedure are explained, and he is agreeable.

Gross Findings: Appropriate splenic flexure mobilization was completed to allow for advancement of the colon down to the rectal stump providing a tension-free anastomosis.

Description of Procedure: The patient was placed in a supine position after sterile prep and drape was complete. Marcaine was infiltrated in the area of about 1.0 centimeters around the midline incision site and blunt dissection was then done, including sharp dissection to the fascia. This was then opened and entrance was gained into the abdomen. #11 port was placed and CO_2 insufflation was then obtained. Additional ports were placed for laparoscopic approach to the procedure. With the aid of a ligature, the splenic flexure was completely mobilized. After completion of this, additional mobilization was done for the colon. The rectal stump was identified easily with the Prolene sutures that were utilized for its location, placed on the last procedure. After adhesions were taken out of this area, the ostomy on the left side of the abdomen was then excised with sterile technique and dissection was done about the subcutaneous tissues to the fascia freely mobilizing the colon. Advancement of the left colon was then done outside of the abdomen and a pursestring device was then used to fire across the proximal portion of the left colon; this bowel was then sent to Pathology. A 25 mm EEA device was then utilized and its anvil was placed at the end of the colon. This was then placed back into the abdomen and towel clips were used to temporarily approximate the skin allowing pneumoperitoneum to exist.

Next, re-evaluation of the rectal site was done with the assistance of the surgical assist. Advancement of the EEA device was then done in the rectum, and this trocar was advanced through the anterior portion of the rectum. The phenol end of the device was then attached to the trochar and approximation of the tissues was then done. Minimal tension and no twist were appreciated on the anastomosis. Once it was fired, two donuts were appreciated. Irrigation and aspiration was done revealing minimal blood loss with the procedure.

C02 pneumoperitoneum was then released into the air and additional irrigation was done at the old ostomy incision site. This fascia was re-approximated with one Vicryl suture and the other port sites 10 mm or larger were re-approximated with 0-Vicryl suture. All incisions were closed with Vicryl and the ostomy site was also closed with skin clips in light of the higher chance of infection. The patient tolerated the procedure well and went to the recovery room in stable condition.

Which of the following is the correct CPT code assignment?

a. 44207, 44213
b. 44207, 44213, 44620
c. 44227
d. 44626

9.20. The following documentation is from the health record of a 33-year-old female patient.

History and Physical

The patient is scheduled for surgery today.

Chief Complaint: Anal pain with bleeding

History of Present Illness: This is a 33-year-old woman with a 2-year history of anal pain and bleeding, which has been markedly worse lately. Has been on stool softener and sitz baths; symptoms have not improved. She presents for ligation of internal hemorrhoids.

Past History: General health is good. There are no major medical illnesses. She has had a tubal ligation in the past.

Family History and Review of Systems: Otherwise noncontributory

Physical Examination: HEENT: Grossly intact. Neck: Supple. Chest: Clear. Heart: Regular rate and rhythm. Abdomen: Soft, without mass, tenderness, or organomegaly. Anal exam: There is marked posterior tenderness and pain.

Impression: Bleeding, prolapsed internal hemorrhoids, not responding to conservative therapy

Recommendations: Internal rubber band ligation. The procedure has been explained in detail to the patient, and she understands and accepts.

Operative Report

Preoperative Diagnosis: Internal prolapsing hemorrhoids

Postoperative Diagnosis: Same

Surgery Performed: Proctosigmoidoscopy, rubber band ligation of the internal hemorrhoids, done with an anoscope

Procedure: The patient was placed on the operating table in a sitting position. The patient was placed in prone jackknife position and the buttocks were retracted. Proctosigmoidoscopy was then carried out to 20 cm and was normal except for the anal findings mentioned above. The proctoscope was withdrawn, and the anus was prepped and draped in antiseptic fashion. A field block with Marcaine 0.25 percent was then placed. The anoscope was inserted. There was a prolapsing hemorrhoid in the anterior midline. This was rubber-band ligated above the dentate line by applying two bands. In the posterior midline, there was another hemorrhoid, which was banded in the same manner. Bleeding was checked, and none was noted.

The patient was taken to the recovery room in stable condition. Blood loss was negligible. Counts correct; no drains.

Which of the following is the correct code assignment?

ICD-9-CM and CPT Code(s):

a. 455.2, 46221, 45300-51, 46600-51
b. 455.2, 46221, 46221-59, 45300
c. 455.0, 46945, 45300
d. 455.8, 46083, 45300-51, 46600-51

ICD-10-CM Code(s): _____

Evaluation and Management (E/M) Services

9.21. **Physician Encounter:** A primary care physician in the patient's very small hometown sees the patient and recommends a partial lumpectomy for a 0.9-cm lesion in the right breast. The general surgeon completes a very thorough preoperative evaluation and refers the patient to a general surgeon in a neighboring, much larger community, for the actual removal of the lump. The PCP asks that the general surgeon perform the lumpectomy only. The patient has the lumpectomy and returns back home to the care of the primary care physician. How would the surgeon's service be coded? The primary care practitioner's (PCP)?

a. Surgeon: 19120-52; PCP: 19120
b. Surgeon: 19120-54; PCP: 19120-55-56
c. Surgeon: 19101-54; PCP: 19120-55-56
d. Surgeon: 19101-54; PCP: 19120, 99213

9.22. Dr. Bill admitted a patient to observation after seeing him in the emergency department with severe nausea, vomiting, and dizziness from dehydration. IVs were started, and the plan was to hydrate the patient and discharge him to home the next morning. The patient, however, had not improved enough the next day (day two) and was kept an additional 24 hours. On day three, the patient was discharged home.

Assuming documentation guidelines have been met, choose the correct sequence of CPT procedure E/M codes for Dr. Bill's observation service coding.

a. 99219, 99231, 99217
b. 99219, 99224, 99217
c. 99283, 99219, 99217
d. 99283, 99231, 99217

9.23. Dr. Smith sent a patient to observation care at the local hospital following his visit to the nursing facility. The patient was admitted for observation to rule out stroke due to a change in mental status. The next morning, Dr. Smith left town, and his partner, Dr. Johnson, admitted the patient to inpatient care because of sudden worsening symptoms. The patient expired later the same day. Assuming documentation guidelines were met, how would E/M services for these two physicians be coded?

    a. Dr. Smith: 99315, 99219; Dr. Johnson: 99236
    b. Dr. Smith: 99219; Dr. Johnson: 99217, 99236
    c. Dr. Smith: 99219; Dr. Johnson: 99236
    d. Dr. Smith: 99315, 99222; Dr. Johnson: 99238

9.24. An 85-year-old patient of Dr. Smith's was brought to the clinic from her home after her family failed to get her to respond to their phone calls. She was poorly nourished, dehydrated, and confused. Dr. Smith admitted her to the hospital to stabilize her, then discharged her to a nursing facility the next day. Assuming that all documentation guidelines for each level of service have been met, assign the correct CPT codes for Dr. Smith's services to the hospital and nursing home.

    a. 99214, 99222, 99239, 99305
    b. 99222, 99239, 99305
    c. 99214, 99235, 99305
    d. 99222, 99305

9.25. Dr. Donahue had an elderly Hispanic male come to his office for an initial visit. The patient had multiple medical problems and had not had any care for at least 10 years. The patient brought his 12-year-old granddaughter to interpret; however, she was of minimal assistance due to her unfamiliarity with medical terms and problems. Dr. Donahue's nurse called the local hospital and requested the services of their Spanish-speaking interpreter. By putting the interpreter on speakerphone, Dr. Donahue was able to finish his examination of the patient, prescribe medications, and give instructions for follow-up care. He documented a comprehensive history, a physical examination, and medical decision making that was moderate. He spent an additional 50 minutes counseling and coordinating the care of this patient, for a total of 95 minutes of care.

Assign the correct CPT code for Dr. Donahue's services.

    a. 99204, 99354
    b. 99205, 99354, 99355
    c. 99205, 99354
    d. 99204

9.26. The following documentation is from the health record of a 56-year-old female.

Preventive Medicine Visit

This patient is a 56-year-old female who comes in today for a complete physical, which is covered by her insurance company. Patient is known to me, although has not been in to see me since last year.

Past Medical History: 1. History of proctosigmoiditis, probably ischemic, treated 1/93
2. History of TAH-BSO for endometriosis
3. History of NSVD × 2
4. History of correction of bunion and hammer toe, 1996

The only concern that she has is some problems with headaches in the frontal area in the morning. The headaches seem to be worse fairly consistently in the morning. She has also had some problems with hips aching, and her eyes occasionally have been a little blurry. Other than that, she has no other concerns on ROS. She has no jaw claudication, joint pains, etc.

Family History: Her mother died of CVA and colon cancer at age 76. Her father died of heart disease at age 80.

Social History: She has been married for 25 years. She has two children and is a homemaker. She does not smoke or drink. Her husband is a farmer.

Allergies: No known allergies

Medications: ASA, Premarin, Caltrate

ROS is otherwise entirely unremarkable.

Physical Exam: She appears to be in no acute distress.

HEENT:	Head is normocephalic. PERRLA: Fundi benign. TMs are clear. Pharynx is negative. There is no temporal artery tenderness.
Neck:	Without adenopathy or thyromegaly
Lungs:	Clear
Heart:	Showed a normal S1, S2, with regular rate and rhythm and no murmur
Breasts:	Without masses. Self breast examination was taught and encouraged on a monthly basis. Axillary is unremarkable.
Abdomen:	Soft and nontender with no hepatosplenomegaly present
Genitalia:	External genitalia normal. Cervix was absent. Vaginal Pap smear was done. Bimanual exam revealed an absent uterus and nonpalpable ovaries. Rectal exam was normal.
Neurological:	Exam intact

Assessment: 1. Headaches, exact etiology not clear. I am going to check her sed rate. If that is normal, then will proceed with CT scan of the head.
2. Routine physical

I will write to her with the test results. If she does not hear from me in two weeks, she will give me a call. Otherwise, I will see her right after her head CT.

Assign the correct codes for this visit:

ICD-9-CM and CPT Code(s):

a. V72.31, V76.47, V45.77, 99396, 784.0, 99213-25
b. V70.9, 99396, 784.0, 99213
c. V76.2, V76.47, V45.77, G0101, Q0091, 784.0, 99213-25
d. 784.0, V72.31, V76.47, V45.77, 99214

ICD-10-CM Code(s): _____

9.27. The following scenario involves a female patient in the intensive care unit.

Hospital Emergency Visit

Subjective: I was called regarding endotracheal tube cuff leak and copious secretions suctioned through ETT. N/G sounds not heard in stomach per nurse, though no evidence by exam that N/G was withdrawn partially. Anesthesia called in. Patient is very afraid of losing airway.

Objective: Vital signs stabilized. Endotracheal tube replaced by anesthesia and verified with good bilateral breath sounds. There are a few mild right expiratory rhonchi. Cor 50s to 60s. O_2 saturation remained in the 90s.

Assessment:
1. Respiratory failure: Holding own; chest x-ray ordered
2. Congestive heart failure: Retaining fluid despite increased diuretics
3. Nutrition: Improved
4. Heart: Remains in normal sinus rhythm
5. Atelectasis and pneumonia: Now afebrile, still needs frequent pulmonary toilet
6. INR 1.9

Critical Care Time: 2 a.m. to 3 a.m.—Emergent

Plan:
1. Transfer to ICU
2. Increase Coumadin
3. Continue respiratory care and IV antibiotics
4. Increase diuresis: She is above her dry weight

Determine the correct E/M code(s) for the ER physician for this scenario.

a. 99233
b. 99291, 99292
c. 99233, 99354
d. 99291

9.28. The following documentation is from the health record of a male patient.

Well Child Check—Newborn

This 4-day-old male patient is seen in clinic today for his routine well check following release from the newborn nursery with his first-time mom. He is spitting up much of his feedings and also is not latching on as well as he had been for the first 2 days. His weight is down 6 ounces to 6 pounds, 2 ounces and he is again below his birth weight. Remainder of the exam is normal.

The mom is advised to reinstitute supplemental bottle feedings with pumped breast milk. She will see the lactation nurse this afternoon in the Woman's Care Center for additional counseling on feeding problems. The patient will be seen again tomorrow in follow-up. If spitting up continues after appropriate latch response is achieved and it's not related to excess air intake, will discuss switching to formula feeds.

Diagnosis: Normal newborn with feeding problems

Determine the correct code assignment for this physician's services.

ICD-9-CM Code(s):

a. V20.2, 779.31
b. V20.2, 783.21
c. V20.31
d. V20.31, 779.31

ICD-10-CM Code(s): _____

9.29.   Office Visit

Chief Complaint: Patient claims he has no problem swallowing, no shortness of breath, or chest pains.

Past Medical History: Patient has hypertension and hyperlipidemia. Patient is taking atenolol, lovastatin, and cimetidine.

Social History: Patient is married and was in the military for 25 years until his health problems necessitated an honorable discharge.

The patient is a 51-year-old African-American male who has long-standing hyperlipidemia and hypertension. He has a history of esophageal dilatation for swallowing difficulties. Today he denies any SOB or chest pains. He mentions that his reflux is much improved on the cimetidine. I will schedule a follow-up EGD for three months. The patient is severely overweight but he is not motivated to lose weight. He does not restrict his diet in any way and refuses to engage in any sort of physical activity. His morbid obesity is of no concern to the patient. Nor is the possibility of stroke or MI.

Vital signs today show a slightly elevated blood pressure of 145/89, heart rate of 100 beats per minutes, and a weight of 267. Patient has gained 3 pounds since his last appointment 2 months ago.

However his physical examination today is relatively normal. His GERD is much improved on the cimetidine so we will continue that and do a repeat EGD in 3 months. Patient is moderately depressed although can't really find a cause. He did suffer a setback at work 6 months ago and this seems to be contributing to his depression. I will put him on a trial of Celexa until his next visit to see if this will help with the depression.

History is of detailed level; examination is comprehensive; MDM moderate complexity.

Which of the following answers best reflects the code assignment for this encounter?

ICD-9-CM and CPT Code(s):

a. 272.4, 278.00, 530.81, 311, 401.9, 99204
b. 272.4, 278.00, 530.81, 311, 401.9, 99214
c. 272.4, 278.01, 530.81, 311, 401.9, 99214
d. 272.4, 278.00, 530.81, 311, 401.9, 99213

ICD-10-CM Code(s): _____

Endocrine, Nutritional, and Metabolic Diseases and Immunity Disorders

9.30. A 13-year-old male patient is being evaluated in the children's clinic for growth problems. He is 4'1" and does not exhibit any signs of puberty or secondary sexual characteristics. His parents wonder if the necrotizing enterocolitis that he had at birth is the cause of his short stature. Other than his short stature, the patient seems in normal health. Blood tests indicated a deficiency of growth hormone. The patient returned to the clinic for follow-up of test results and parents were given the option of starting him on growth hormone treatments. Diagnosis on the second visit is HGH deficiency. Give the codes for both the first and second visits.

ICD-9-CM Code(s):

a. First visit: 259.4, 259.0; second visit: 253.3
b. First visit: 783.43, 259.0; second visit: 253.3
c. First visit: 259.0; second visit: 253.4
d. First visit: 259.4; second visit: 253.4

ICD-10-CM Code(s): _____

9.31. An 18-year-old female was referred to an endocrinologist by her family doctor with symptoms of a right-sided neck mass that is increasing in size. A thyroid ultrasound completed today shows a complex cystic structure in the right lobe of the thyroid with recent hemorrhage of the thyroid. There was also a small thyroid nodule located in the left lobe.

The endocrinologist requests a surgical consultation for treatment options because of the likelihood of a re-bleed if the thyroid is drained and a potential for malignancy, given the two areas of concern in the thyroid.

Which of the following is the correct diagnostic code set for this visit to the endocrinologist?

ICD-9-CM Code(s):

a. 240.9
b. 241.0, 246.2
c. 241.0, 246.3
d. 241.0, 246.2, 246.3

ICD-10-CM Code(s): _____

9.32. The following documentation is from the health record of a 69-year-old female.

HPI: The patient is a 69-year-old female with a large pituitary tumor found after lymph node biopsy that demonstrated lung cancer. The lung cancer is apparently non–small cell adenocarcinoma. This is being followed by Dr. Smith who is planning chemotherapy, I believe, for the future. The pituitary gland appears to be nonfunctioning. She underwent transphenoidal surgery 3 days ago and is doing well without complaints.

Physical Exam: Vital signs normal. General: Elderly white female in no acute distress. HEENT: Normocephalic and atraumatic. Pupils are equal, round, and reactive to light. Lids and conjunctivae are normal. Throat unremarkable. No blurred vision. Lungs: Clear, but with decreased basilar breath sounds. Cardiac: Regular rate and rhythm without any murmurs. Abdomen: Positive bowel sounds. Soft and nontender, without hepatosplenomegaly. Extremities: Negative; no edema. Neuro: Oriented × 3. Cranial nerves II–XII intact.

Lab Data: WBC 6.9, hemoglobin 12.1, hematocrit 36.2, platelets 314,000

Glucose 116, BUN 9, creatinine 0.7, sodium 134, potassium 3.9, Chloride 85, CO_2 26, calcium 8.2

Assessment and Plan: Pituitary tumor, status post resection. Currently on steroids, 50 mg q. 8 hours. Wean to 20 mg in the morning and 10 mg in the evening starting tomorrow. Recommend follow-up in 2 weeks with Dr. Smith; he will further evaluate that. We will watch urine output and look for any evidence of diabetes insipidus.

Which of the following is the correct code set for this physician?

ICD-9-CM Code(s):

a. 227.3, 162.9, V77.1
b. 194.3, 162.9
c. 239.7, 162.9, 253.5
d. 239.7, 162.9

ICD-10-CM Code(s): _____

Disorders of the Genitourinary System

9.33.   This is the documentation from the record of a patient admitted to the hospital.

Chief Complaint: Gross hematuria, headache, dizziness, feeling lousy.

HPI: Patient is a 39-year-old white male with C5-6 quadriplegia managed with a suprapubic tube for urinary diversion. He was in the hospital about three weeks ago and at that time had a cystoscopic examination, biopsy of polypoid cystitis, bled for a day or two but that seemed to clear up. He awoke this morning, had some mild gross hematuria which progressed throughout the day, started passing clots and then developed headache, feeling lousy. He was seen in the ER and found to have a blood pressure of 168 systolic and bradycardia and was felt to be having autonomic dysreflexia as a manifestation of his bladder distension. His bladder was irrigated; blood pressure promptly fell back into the 98 range. He is admitted at this time for control of his gross hematuria.

Past Medical History: He has had a penile implant for condom catheter drainage. He has also had tracheostomy in the past, chest tubes on the left side, and a suprapubic tube. Current medication includes Ditropan, Vitamin C, and Metamucil.

Allergies: Penicillin caused a rash.

Social History: Does not smoke, drinks occasionally. He is disabled but currently attending school.

Family History: Both parents are living and well.

Review of Systems: Negative except for HPI

Physical Examination:

General:	Shows a cooperative male in no acute distress.
Skin:	Warm and dry.
HEENT:	Pupils are equal, round, reactive to light and accommodation. Pharynx is clean.
Lungs:	Clear
Heart:	Regular without murmur or gallops.
Abdomen:	Soft. There is a suprapubic tube present.
Genitalia:	Penis has a small implant in it. Testes are down bilaterally without induration.
Rectal:	Shows a normal size prostate. No rectal masses are appreciated.
Neurological:	Shows C5-6 quadriplegia, limited use of arms and hands, decreased triceps musculature.
Neck:	Regular

Impression: Gross hematuria secondary to cystitis, probable urinary tract infection, autonomic dysreflexia, C5-6 quadriplegia, and catheter dependence.

Discharge Summary

Admission Diagnoses: Gross hematuria, suprapubic catheter dependent, quadriplegia, autonomic dysreflexia, anemia secondary to hematuria.

Discharge Diagnoses: Same

Transfusion: Two units packed cells

Laboratory values on admission: His admitting HGB was 13.2; later that evening it had fallen to 9.8 and the patient received two units. The next morning his HGB was 11.3 but again the following morning it had fallen to 9.3. His BUN was 18, creatinine 0.6.

Hospital Course: Patient was admitted, started initially on intermittent catheter irrigations. He had persistent problems with clotting and then a Foley catheter was inserted per urethra and the patient was placed on a continuous irrigation with prompt clearing of his urine. He was also treated with oral Amicar. At the time of discharge, even though the patient's HGB was 9.3, the patient declined further transfusion and wished to be discharged.

Which of the following code sets (excluding E&M) would be reported for this hospital admission?

ICD-9-CM and CPT Code(s):

a. 599.71, 280.0, 344.04, 337.3, 596.54, 599.0, 51700, 36430
b. 599.71, 280.0, 344.03, 337.3, 596.54, 599.0, 51700, 36430
c. 599.71, 280.0, 344.04, 337.3, 596.54, 51700, 51702, 36430
d. 599.71, 280.0, 344.04, 337.3, 51700, 51702, 36430

ICD-10-CM Code(s): _____

9.34. A patient has a transrectal ultrasound-guided placement of prostatic radiation palladium seeds with a cystoscopy for localized adenocarcinoma of the prostate.

Procedure Description: The patient was given general anesthesia, placed in the lithotomy position, and prepped and draped in sterile fashion. The bladder was drained, and 100 cc of half contrast and half saline were placed into the bladder. The scrotum was then draped up out of the way. The BUK 7.5 MHz transrectal ultrasound probe was then introduced into the rectum, and the prostate was imaged. The probe was placed into the stabilization bar mechanism. We then centered the prostate image on the template screen and established our base image. Stabilization needles were then put into position. We then passed the needles using a perineal approach at the corresponding positions to the corresponding depth, using ultrasound and fluoroscopy for guidance. After satisfactory placement of all the needles, the ultrasound probe and needles were removed. A total of 60 palladium seeds were put in place. We had good distribution of the seeds and good images on the ultrasound. Using the #22 French cystoscope, a cystoscopy was performed, and the bladder was fully inspected with the 30- and 70-degree lenses without notable findings. The bladder demonstrated no tumors, lesions, or other abnormalities, there were no seeds present, and there was very minimal bleeding. The bladder was drained and the patient was taken to the recovery room in stable condition.

Which of the following code sets would be reported for this service in addition to the HCPCS Level II supply codes for the implants and contrast used? The procedure was performed in the cancer center.

ICD-9-CM and CPT Code(s):

a. 233.4, 55875, 52000, 77763, 76965, 76000-59
b. 185, 55875, 77778, 76965, 76000-59
c. 185, 55875, 77787, 76872, 77790
d. 185, 52000, 77762

ICD-10-CM Code(s): _____

9.35. A female Medicare patient is scheduled for breast biopsy of a palpable lump in the right breast. In the left breast is a much smaller lesion as shown on mammography and identified by a radiological marker. An excisional biopsy is performed on both sides. The specimen on the right is diagnostic for breast malignancy with clear margins, while the small lesion in the left breast is found to be only fibrocystic disease without evidence of malignancy.

Which of the following is reported for the physician services? The procedure is completed at the hospital surgery center.

ICD-9-CM and CPT Code(s):

a. 611.72, 610.1, 19120-50
b. 174.9, 610.1, 19125-50, 19290-50, 19120-50
c. 174.9, 610.1, 19120-RT, 19125-LT-51, 19290-LT-51
d. 174.9, 610.2, 19120, 19125-59, 19290-59

ICD-10-CM Code(s): _____

9.36. The following documentation is from the health record of a 48-year-old female patient.

Surgical Procedure

The patient is here for office hysteroscopy. She has a long history of dysfunctional bleeding. She is known to have multiple fibroids. Recent ultrasound did demonstrate normal appearing ovaries but several large fibroids, the largest of which is 5 cm in diameter.

After informed consent and taking the preop medication, the patient was sterilely prepped. We then injected her with a total of 12 cc of 2% Lidocaine without Epinephrine. We then performed an office hysteroscopy using a uterine sound. The uterus sounded to 8 cm. We then dilated the cervical OS with Pratt dilators. The hysteroscope was placed with good visualization of all portions of the endometrium. We were able to identify both tubal ostium. There was a very large fibroid posterior that does press in on the endometrium and occupies much of it. This is not a pedunculated endometrium and is intramural. There are other fibroids that also affect the cavity size and shape, but again these are intramural fibroids and not accessible through the hysteroscope. D&C was performed without difficulty and the patient tolerated the procedure well. Instrument, needle, and sponge count were correct.

I advised the patient to see how her symptoms proceed in the next few months. Her last FSH level was 30, suggesting a perimenopausal state. She does understand that the fibroids should shrink in size or at least remain the same once she is menopausal. However, if she feels her bleeding problems are persistent, we may have to consider hysterectomy. The patient will follow up in three or four months and will document her bleeding.

Which diagnosis and CPT procedure codes does the surgeon assign?

ICD-9-CM and CPT Code(s):

a. 626.8, 218.1, 58558
b. 626.8, 218.9, 57800, 58558
c. 627.0, 218.9, 58558, 58120
d. 627.0, 218.1, 58558

ICD-10-CM Code(s): _____

9.37. The following documentation is from the health record of a female patient.

Operative Report

Preoperative Diagnosis: Cystocele, urinary stress incontinence

Postoperative Diagnosis: Incomplete cystocele, urinary stress incontinence

Operation: Monarch trans obturator tension free suburethral sling and anterior repair of cystocele

Indication: The patient is an 80-year-old G4, P4, status post hysterectomy done for benign reasons, now with a cystocele and urinary stress incontinence. I presented her with options and she wished to proceed with the surgical correction.

Description of Procedure: The patient was taken to the operating room suite and anesthesia was administered. The patient was placed into the dorsal lithotomy position and her vagina, perineum, and inner thighs were prepped and draped in the usual fashion for a sling procedure. A Foley catheter was placed into the urinary bladder and then a weighted speculum was placed into the vagina.

A small mid-urethral vaginal incision was then made to a distance of approximately 2.0 cm. Dissection was carried out beneath the vaginal mucosa up toward the inferior edge of the pubic bone. The notch along the internal edge of the ischiopubic ramus was palpated on the patient's left side and then a small stab wound incision was made. This was repeated in the same fashion on the patient's right. The Monarch helicopasser was now placed into the incision on the patient's left and then a guiding finger placed through the vaginal incision until the tip of the Monarch passer was palpated. The Monarch passer was now guided around the ischiopubic ramus and through the vagina incision keeping direct contact with the surgeon's finger. The Monarch sling was attached to the passer and the passer rotated out and through, bringing the Monarch sling through the incision. Using the opposite Monarch passer on the patient's right side, this was repeated in a similar fashion, again guiding the passer with the surgeon's finger in direct contact throughout. The other end of the Monarch sling was then attached and the Monarch helicopasser brought back out through the obturator foramen. Now with the two ends of the sling still attached to the Monarch passers on each side, the sling was positioned using the alignment marks on the sling. It was placed and then the helicopassers cut from the sling. Now the plastic sheaths were withdrawn and the sling placed without tension. The mesh was then cut at subcutaneous level adjacent to the lateral skin incisions.

Once that was done, attention was turned to the cystocele. A longitudinal injection with 1% Lidocaine was made. Vaginal mucosa was dissected away from the cystocele. Anterior repair was performed by placing purse string sutures of 2-0 Vicryl to correct for the cystocele, and the excess vaginal tissue was trimmed away. The vaginal mucosa was repaired with a locking stitch of 0-Vicryl. The lateral skin incisions were reapproximated using DermaBone tissue adhesive. The patient was returned to the supine position. She was then awakened and transferred to the recovery room in stable condition.

Which of the following code sets is reported for the surgeon for this hospital-based ambulatory surgical service?

ICD-9-CM and CPT Code(s):

a. 618.2, 57288
b. 618.2, 625.6, 57240, 53440
c. 618.2, 625.6, 57240, 57288
d. 625.6, 57288

ICD-10-CM Code(s): _____

9.38.   The following documentation is from the health record of a male patient.

Operative Report

A patient with an elevated prostate-specific antigen (PSA) of 35.7 comes to the surgery center for a transrectal, ultrasonic-guided (TRUS) prostate biopsy.

Technique: The patient is placed in the Sims position with the left side down. The anus was generously lubricated with 2 percent Xylocaine jelly. The ultrasound probe was then introduced and scanning initiated. A great deal of calcification was noted in the outer margin of the central zone. The area proximal and anterior to the calcifications was hypoechoic but may have been influenced by the stones. There was very thin peripheral zone tissue available. Three needle biopsies were taken from each side, starting in the periphery and working toward the midline and trying to biopsy anterior to the stones on the more medial biopsies from each side.

The pathology report confirmed carcinoma in situ of the prostate.

Which codes will be reported for this service? The facility bills for the technical and professional components and also reports procedure codes for radiologic procedures for reimbursement. Do not include surgical supplies in this example.

ICD-9-CM and CPT Code(s):

a. 185, 55700
b. 233.4, 790.93, 55705, 76872
c. 185, 790.93, 602.0, 55700, 76872, 76942
d. 233.4, 602.0, 55700, 76872, 76942

ICD-10-CM Code(s): _____

Infectious Diseases/Disorders of the Skin and Subcutaneous Tissue

9.39. A 53-year-old male is seen in the office for a skin problem on the left shin. It started two days ago as mild redness and has developed into an area of severe itching, is swollen with dark red blotches, and has an area of open weeping. The patient has Type II diabetes mellitus, diabetic peripheral vascular disease, and a previous MRSA infection. A detailed history and a comprehensive examination are documented.

The physician diagnoses cellulitis of the left leg and obtains cultures from the open area. To speed the start of treatment, the physician administers one dose of 300 mg Clindamycin IV push at the office before sending the patient to the observation unit at the hospital for continued doses of antibiotic every 6 hours for the next 48 hours. The patient's primary insurance is Blue Cross.

Which of the following code sets is appropriate for physician reporting of these services? Do not code laboratory services.

ICD-9-CM and CPT Code(s):

a. 686.9, V12.04, 250.00, 443.81, 99214, 96372
b. 682.6, V02.54, 250.70, 443.81, 99214, 96374, S0077
c. 682.6, V12.04, 250.70, 443.81, 99215, 96374, S0077
d. 891.1, V02.54, 250.70, 443.81, 99215, 96372, J3490

ICD-10-CM Code(s): _____

9.40. The following documentation is from the health record of a 73-year-old male patient.

Physician Office Record

This 73-year-old male slipped and fell while carrying a pane of glass. He was changing an outside window at his single-family home. He sustained three lacerations—one on his left ankle, one on his right ankle, and one on his left hand.

Left ankle: 3.5-cm laceration, involving deep subcutaneous tissue and fascia, was repaired with layered closure using 1 percent lidocaine local anesthetic.

Right ankle: 4.2-cm laceration was repaired under local anesthetic with a single-layer closure.

Left hand: 2.5-cm laceration of the dermis was repaired with simple closure using DERMABOND tissue adhesive.

Assessment: Wounds of both ankles and left hand requiring repair.

Plan: Follow-up in 10 days for suture removal. Call office if there are any problems or complications.

What are the correct diagnosis and CPT procedure codes?

ICD-9-CM and CPT Code(s):

a. 891.0, 882.0, E920.8, E849.0, E013.9, 12004
b. 891.1, 882.0, 12002, 12032-51
c. 894.0, 12032, 12002, supply code for the DERMABOND adhesive
d. 891.0, 882.0, E920.8, E849.0, E000.8, E013.9, 12032, 12002-51, G0168

ICD-10-CM Code(s): _____

9.41. An operative report provides the following information.

Preoperative Diagnosis:	Ductal carcinoma in situ of the right breast
Postoperative Diagnosis:	Ductal carcinoma in situ of the right breast
Procedure:	Right needle-localized lumpectomy

Indications: The patient is a 68-year-old woman who was noted to have abnormal calcifications at roughly the 6 o'clock position of the areola. These were biopsied and found to be ductal carcinoma in situ. She was inclined to proceed with needle-localized lumpectomy. The risks of bleeding, infection, poor wound healing, and unappealing cosmetics were discussed. The possibility we could find invasive carcinoma was also discussed. The need for postoperative radiation therapy was also discussed. She was well aware of the possibility of positive margins which would lead to further surgery or a mastectomy.

Procedure Description: The patient was initially taken to the Center for Breast Diagnostics where the radiologist placed a needle at the inferior aspect of the breast. The patient was then taken to the Operating Room. General anesthesia was administered. SCDs were placed. A curvilinear incision was made on the inferior aspect of the areola. This was taken down to the subcutaneous tissue. Flaps were raised in each direction for approximately 2 cm and taken down to the chest wall. A long stitch was placed medially, a short stitch superiorly.

The specimen was removed. The cavity was then thoroughly irrigated. 0.25% Marcaine was used for local anesthesia. The subcutaneous tissue was then approximated using 3-0 Monocryl. The skin was approximated using 4-0 Monocryl in a running subcuticular fashion. A sterile dressing was applied. The patient tolerated the procedure well and was taken to the Recovery Room.

What is the correct code set for the services of the surgeon?

ICD-9-CM and CPT Code(s):

a. 174.0, 19290, 19301
b. 174.9, 19290, 19125
c. 233.0, 19125
d. 233.0, 19301

ICD-10-CM Code(s): _____

9.42. The following documentation is from the health record of a patient who received outpatient surgical services.

Operative Report

Preoperative Diagnosis:	Full-thickness burn wound to anterior left lower leg
Postoperative Diagnosis:	Same
Operation:	Split-thickness skin graft, approximately 35 cm; preparation of the wound
Anesthesia:	General

Procedure: The left lower leg was prepped and draped in the usual sterile fashion. The ulcer, which measured approximately 8 × 4 to 4.5 cm, was debrided sharply with Goulian knife until healthy bleeding was seen. The bleeding was controlled with epinephrine-soaked lap pads. Split-thickness skin graft was harvested from the left lateral buttock area approximately 4.5 to 5 cm × 8 cm at the depth of 14/1000 of an inch. The graft was meshed to 1 to 1.5 and placed over the prepared wound. This was stabilized with staples, and then Xeroform dressings and dry dressings, wrapped with gauze and finally immobilized in a posterior splint. The donor site was covered with Xeroform and dry dressings.

What is/are the correct procedure code(s) reported by the physician for this procedure performed in the hospital outpatient surgical suite?

a. 15220, 15221-51, 15002-51
b. 15100
c. 14021, 15002-51
d. 15100, 15002-51

9.43.   The following documentation is from the health record of a patient who received outpatient surgical services.

Operative Report

Preoperative Diagnosis:	Basal cell carcinoma of the forehead
Postoperative Diagnosis:	Same
Procedure:	Excision of basal cell carcinoma with split-thickness skin graft

The patient was given a local IV sedation and taken to the operating room suite. The face and left thigh were prepped with pHisoHex soap. The cancer was outlined for excision. The cancer measured approximately 2.5 cm in diameter. The forehead was infiltrated with 1 percent Xylocaine with 1:1,000,000 epinephrine.

The cancer was excised and carried down to the frontalis muscle. The area of the excision measured 5 × 4 cm in total. A suture was placed at the 12 o'clock position. The specimen was sent to pathology for frozen section.

Attention was then turned to the skin graft. A pattern of the defect was transferred to the left anterior thigh using a new needle. A local infiltration was performed on the thigh. Using a free-hand knife, a split-thickness skin graft was harvested. The thigh was treated with Tegaderm and a wraparound Kerlix and ACE wrap. The skin graft was applied and sutured to the forehead defect with running 5-0 plain catgut.

Xeroform with cotton soaked in glycerin was sutured with 4-0 silk. A sterile dressing was applied. The patient tolerated the procedure well with no complications or blood loss.

What are the correct codes reported by the physician for this procedure performed in the hospital outpatient surgical suite?

ICD-9-CM and CPT Code(s):

a. 195.0, 15120
b. 173.31, 15120, 11646
c. 173.31, 15100, 11646
d. 195.0, 15004, 15120

ICD-10-CM Code(s): _____

9.44.   The physician sees an established patient in the office. She is a 2-year-old girl with a two-day history of fever to 100.5 degrees, fuzziness, fatigue, and headache. She also has been complaining for five days of pain in the left buttock with an area that is swollen and red as of today, with no known injury. She is a known asthmatic. A detailed history is obtained. Physical exam reveals a 4 cm × 4 cm abscess over the left upper buttock that is fluctuant and red, as the only finding on a comprehensive exam. Laboratory done in the office today reveals: Elevated WBC on the automated complete CBC with differential and an abnormal automated urinalysis with microscopy. A moderate level of medical decision making is used.

After obtaining consent, the physician and the staff observer prepare the patient for conscious sedation in the procedure room. The physician injects 5 cc of 2% Lidocaine as anesthetic and incises the abscess with a #11 blade straight scalpel. 10 cc of pus is drained and the area is packed with Iodoform gauze. Culture and sensitivity of the drainage is sent to an outside laboratory for evaluation. Total intra-service time was 30 minutes. The patient was given Ceftin 300 mg b.i.d. for 10 days to treat both the UTI and the abscess and will return to clinic in two days for a wound check.

What are the correct diagnosis and CPT procedure codes for the services provided?

a. 599.0, 682.5, 780.60, 493.90, 99214-25, 99143, 10061, 99000
b. 599.0, 682.5, 780.61, 99215, 99143, 10061, 36415, 85025, 85009, 81001
c. 599.0, 682.2, 99214, 99144, 10060, 99000, 36415, 85025, 81003
d. 599.0, 682.5, 493.90, 99214-25, 99143, 10060, 99000, 36415, 85025, 81001

ICD-10-CM Code(s): _____

9.45. Office Progress Note

Chief Complaint: The patient presents today for removal of a scalp cyst.

HPI: This patient has had a cyst present in the scalp for the last several months. She has been monitoring it as instructed but feels that it has grown significantly in the months since her last appointment.

Physical Exam: The original lesion was approximately 1.5 cm but today seems to have grown to approximately 2.0 cm. The cyst rests in the frontal lobe close to the hairline—patient is beginning to feel very awkward in public.

Procedure: After obtaining informed consent from the patient, I injected the periphery of the cyst will 2% buffered lidocaine. The hair around the scalp was carefully shaved leaving a clear field. A linear incision was made through the scalp and the cyst was removed followed by lavage to the wound. The contents of the cyst appeared to be clear with no pus or infection. 2-0 nylon was used to approximate the edges and to maintain hemostasis. The area was treated with an antibiotic ointment and a bandage was carefully placed on the wound site.

Patient is instructed to not shower or wash her hair for 2 days and to put ice on the wound 20 minutes at a time throughout the next 24 hours. She will be seen in 1 week for removal of sutures.

Assign the correct codes for this office visit:

ICD-9-CM and CPT Code(s): _____

ICD-10-CM Code(s): _____

9.46. This is the documentation from the record of a patient presenting with a mass in the right breast.

Chief Complaint: Mass in the right breast

Past Medical History: No serious illnesses. She has had a tubal ligation. She has had an appendectomy. She has had an exploratory laparotomy.

Systemic Review: She does have headaches. She has had abdominal pain and has to get up at night to urinate. Her menses are usually every 28 days and last 7 days. She has four children who are living and well. She has had three miscarriages.

Family History: There is cancer, epilepsy, diabetes, and heart attacks in the family.

Social History: She does not smoke and takes a rare social drink. She is a housewife, married and lives with her family.

History of Present Illness: This 31-year-old white female is admitted with the chief complaint of a nodule in her right breast and a lump in her left axilla. She has had this lump for several months but it is getting larger, was tender for a while, but is no longer tender. She had a mammogram which suggests a benign process in the right breast but there are concerns about the lesion in the axilla.

Physical Examination:

Blood Pressure 108/78; Pulse 68; Respirations 16

HEENT:	Head and neck are normal. Eyes—pupils are round, regular and equal. Reactive to light and accommodation. EOM are normal. Sclera—white. Conjunctiva—pink. Oral cavity is within normal limits. Tympanic membranes are clear bilaterally.
Neck:	No venous distention; no palpable thyroid.
Chest:	Clear to A&P. Breath sounds are normal and no rales are heard.
Cardiac:	The apex beat is in the fifth interspace, midclavicular line. Normal sinus rhythm is present and no murmurs are heard.
Abdomen:	Soft. No masses, tenderness, or palpable organs. Peristalsis is present and normal.
Breasts:	There is a nodule about 1.5 to 2 cm at the lower border of the areola in the right breast. There is a fairly large lymph node in the left axilla.
Extremities:	No edema. No deformity.
Pelvic:	Not done as she had one last week with a PAP and these were all ok.
Diagnosis:	Lesion of the right breast; nodule in the left axilla.

Laboratory: The urine was negative; HGB was 13.8; HCT 39.8; WBC was 4,900 and 46 polys.

Operative Record

Preoperative Diagnosis:	Nodule of the right breast; lymphadenitis left axilla.
Postoperative Diagnosis:	Same
Operation Performed:	Excision of nodule of the right breast and excision of 3 or 4 lymph nodes in the left axilla.

Findings: The patient was found to have at least 1 large lymph node and 2 or 3 small lymph nodes deep in the left axilla and these were all excised. She had a nodule, sort of like an oval nodule, at the areolar skin junction of the right breast. This was about 2 cm × 1 cm.

Operative Note

Under satisfactory general anesthesia, the patient is in the supine position and both breasts and left axilla were prepared with Hibiclens and draped with sterile drapes. A semi-lunar incision was made at the skin, areolar junction of the right breast. Subcutaneous tissue was divided, bleeding points were picked up with hemostats and ligated with 4-0 sutures. The nodule was excised by sharp dissection and bleeding points were again ligated with 4-0 Vicryl. The breast tissue was closed with interrupted 2-0 Vicryl sutures in a figure-of-eight manner. The skin and subcutaneous tissue were closed with continuous 4-0 sutures. The wound was cleansed with Hibiclens and a sterile Opsite dressing and sterile pressure dressings were applied. Incision was made at just about the apex of the axilla on the left side and the subcutaneous tissues were divided; bleeding points were picked up with hemostats and ligated with 4-0 sutures. Superficial lymph nodes were picked up with Allis forceps and dissected free and after we got these all dissected and free and the bleeding controlled we found another larger lymph node, much deeper, and this we excised by sharp dissection and bleeding points carefully ligated. Following this the deep tissues were closed with interrupted 2-0 Vicryl sutures. Subcutaneous tissues were closed with continuous 4-0 sutures. Sterile dressings were applied. The patient withstood the procedures well and returned to PACU in good condition.

Pathological Findings: Sections labeled as specimen "A" consist of portions of fibrofatty breast tissue containing duct ectasia, small cyst formation, and aprocrine metaplasia. Sections labeled as "B" reveal the large ovoid structure and the small fragment of homogenous gray-tan tissue to consist of lymph nodes. The large lymph node shows some evidence of follicular hyperplasia with abundant mitotic and phagocytic activity. Lymphocytes are also noted in the surrounding fibrous capsule. The small lymph nodes contain general lymphoid-like tissue.

Pathological Diagnoses: 1. RT Breast Nodule: Mild fibrocystic disease

2. LT Axillary Nodule: Lymph nodes containing hyperplasia. The large lymph node has signs of toxoplasmosis but this can not be determined without further testing.

What codes are reported for this physician service?

ICD-9-CM and CPT Code(s):

a. 610.1, 289.3, 19120-RT, 38525-LT, 38500-LT
b. 610.2, 130.9, 19120-RT, 38525-LT, 38500-LT
c. 610.2, 289.3, 19100-RT, 38525-LT
d. 610.1, 289.3, 19101-RT, 38525-LT, 38500-LT

ICD-10-CM Code(s): _____

Behavioral Health Conditions

9.47. A patient was brought to the emergency department by her mother after she was found to be groggy after an intentional overdose of a "handful" of aspirin approximately one-half hour before. The mother thought the bottle was almost empty. The patient was beginning to experience dizziness and loud ringing of the ears. The physician inserted a gastric tube and lavage was performed. The patient was stabilized in the ED, during which time bleeding studies and urinalysis were completed. A detailed history and physical examination were performed, and medical decision making was of moderate complexity. The diagnosis was suicide attempt with unknown quantity of aspirin, dizziness, and tinnitus. A psychiatric consult was arranged, and the patient was transferred to the psychiatric hospital by ambulance.

What are the correct diagnosis and CPT codes for this visit?

ICD-9-CM and CPT Code(s):

a. 965.1, 780.4, 388.30, E950.0, 99284-25, 43753
b. 965.1, 780.4, E980.0, 99284
c. 780.4, 388.30, E935.3, 99284-25, 43752
d. 780.4, 388.30, 965.1, E935.3, 99284, 43752

ICD-10-CM Code(s): _____

9.48. A 20-year-old patient was brought into the emergency department in nearly comatose condition following an evening of drinking beer and vodka with friends. Vital signs were depressed. A blood-alcohol level was measured, which was reported as 0.38. The patient had vomited several times before passing out. There was a 1-cm laceration on the patient's eyebrow. This was treated with a Steri-Strip. The patient was stabilized in the ED for one and a half hours and admitted to intensive care by the Internal Medicine physician on call. Documentation in the ED record supports a level 5 ED visit. Diagnosis was alcohol poisoning, acute alcohol intoxication, and 1-cm laceration, right eyebrow.

What is the correct ICD-9-CM and CPT code assignment?

a. 303.00, 980.9, 99291, 99292
b. 980.9, 305.00, 99285-25, 12011
c. 980.0, 305.00, 873.42, E860.0, 99285
d. 980.0, 303.00, 99291, 12011

ICD-10-CM Code(s): _____

9.49. The following documentation is from the health record of a 22-year-old female patient.

Date of Admission: 02/10/XX

Date of Evaluation: 02/12/XX

Amount of Time of Evaluation: The patient participated in a direct interview for 40 minutes.

Sources of Information: The patient participated in a 40-minute direct interview. Patient's commitment documents from ABC facility were also reviewed. Patient's records from Dr. S. were also reviewed.

Chief Complaint: "I came here because someone was hurting me, and they thought that I wasn't eating enough and that I was throwing up too much."

History of Present Illness: The patient is a 22-year-old female with a past history of anorexia nervosa and attention deficit disorder. She was committed after a six-week stay at ABC. Her parents brought her to this facility after her mother noticed that she was fasting and vomiting and was not sleeping. Her mother also noted that she was more weak than usual and was only able to work her job for one or two hours rather than a full day. It was also noticed that she was losing track of time, appearing confused, fearful, and angry. Patient notes that, prior to admission, she was actually sleeping fairly normally for her, about five hours of sleep per night, though she does agree that she was eating rather little and vomiting because of some abuse that was troubling her. On admission, she was noted to be withdrawn and refused to talk to staff and was very tearful. Later that day, however, she did not remember this incident of being tearful. On admission she was noted to be 84 pounds at a height of 5 feet. She at that time admitted to vomiting as much as three times a day and that she had to have her teeth resurfaced due to purging. At ABC facility, staff noted she was hoarding condiments in her room and was also noted to purge in front of staff during her stay there. The patient, however, does not think that her purging was due to an eating disorder; rather, she thinks that it was due to stress and anxiety over a previous abuse. Previous records reveal potassium levels as low as 2.0. She states that the low potassium is due to a kidney disorder; however, a nephrologist thought that the low potassium was most likely due to her purging behavior. Her weight at discharge from ABC was 85.5 pounds. Patient notes that her sleep has not been disrupted prior to her hospital stay. She states that she usually gets about five hours of sleep per night, which is normal for her. She notes that her appetite has been decreased for the past several months because of stress regarding prior abuse. She denies any thought racing or excessive energy for the past several months. She also denies any suicidal thoughts or behaviors. She also denies any obsessive-compulsive actions. She denies feeling hopeless or depressed.

Chemical Dependency History: Patient denies any current or previous use of alcohol or drugs.

Current Prescribed Medications: Claritin 10 mg p.o. q. d.; potassium chloride 20 mEq t.i.d. to q. i.d. p.r.n. hypokalemia; Dexedrine SR 40 mg t.i.d.

Past Psychiatric History: Patient has a history of problems with eating disorders that goes back to the age of 14. Over the past eight years she has been involved in a variety of treatment programs. She was first treated in an inpatient setting at the age of 14. She was subsequently hospitalized at the age of 15, age 16 $\times$ 2, and age 17. From the age of 17 to 18 she was placed in foster care. She has attempted suicide three times in her life. Each time the attempt was made by trying to overdose on her asthma medication, theophylline. She has been hospitalized five times for hypokalemia. She notes that she currently sees a psychiatrist and a psychologist as an outpatient. In the past, she has exhibited some features of self-injurious behavior. She burned a cross into her arm at age 13. She also has a past history of scratching her arm.

Family Psychiatric History: She notes that her younger sister attempted to overdose one time in the past and that her father has been treated for depression with ECT, which was successful.

Mental Status Examination: The patient is a petite, too-thin young female who appears younger than her stated age of 22. She is clean, well groomed, and dressed in jeans and a large hooded sweatshirt. Her general behavior is noted to be normal and appropriate throughout the interview. She is cooperative throughout our question-and-answer session. Her mood is somewhat subdued, and she seems slightly anxious. Her affect is rather flat throughout the interview. No abnormal movements are noted during the interview. Her speech is fairly soft and rather monotone in nature. Speech is noted to be of normal speed. Stream of mental activity is normal and appropriate. The form of thought processes appears to be normal without any tangential thinking. Thought content appears to be normal as well. She denies delusions, hallucinations, and suicidal or homicidal ideation at present. She does not seem to be impulsive in her speech or thought processes throughout the interview. She does seem to have some insight into her illness in that she is able to name her illness as anorexia. She states that her weight now is OK. Her judgment, concentration, and orientation all appear to be within normal limits. Recent and remote memory appears intact. Her general fund of knowledge is above average. Her calculations, abstractions, proverbs, and similarities are all within normal limits. Estimated IQ would be 120 based on educational background and verbal skills. The patient does not appear to be dangerous or suicidal at present.

Biopsychosocial Discussion and Discussion of Differential Diagnosis: The patient is a 22-year-old female with a past history of anorexia and subsequent hypokalemia. She notes that recent exacerbation in her anorexia and vomiting seems to be due to stress over abuse in the past by a physician with whom she had previous professional contact and subsequently became friends. She has limited insight into her eating disorder in that she is able to name it as anorexia now. In the past, however, she has denied the existence of an eating disorder. In the past, she has had suicidal attempts. However, at this time she does not appear to be depressed and does not indicate any suicidal thoughts or plans. At this time, she does not indicate feeling particularly anxious but, rather, regards her main symptom as stress. She states that her only fear right now is that of being in the hospital for her first commitment. She appears to have a long history of hospitalizations for her eating disorder and subsequent hypokalemia. Her family history does appear to have a history of mental illness, with depression in her father and a suicide attempt by her younger sister. She also was noted to have burned a cross into her arm as a young child, as well as a history of scratching her arm. There is a possibility that she has a personality disorder with borderline features. Though she does not seem to be in danger of suicide right now or hurting others, it is felt that because of her history of severe hypokalemia and history of anorexia, as well as purging behavior, she will require a long-term inpatient hospitalization for her safety.

Admitting Diagnosis

Axis I:	1. Anorexia nervosa, purging type
	2. Attention deficit hyperactive disorder
Axis II:	Personality disorder with predominant borderline features
Axis III:	1. History of hypokalemia
	2. Asthma
	3. Hypokalemic periodic paralysis (per patient report)

Axis IV:	Severe with stresses incurred due to previous abuse
Axis V:	Current GAF—50 to 60

Prognosis: Guarded due to her history of multiple hospitalizations for her eating disorder

Strengths:
1. Patient is very intelligent.
2. Patient is enrolled in school and has had a high level of education.
3. Patient has a therapeutic relationship with her therapist and psychiatrist as an outpatient.
4. Patient's weight is near her target weight already.
5. The patient has some insight into her eating disorder.

Problems:
1. Patient lacks a deep insight into her eating disorder.
2. Patient clings to a diagnosis of hypokalemia periodic paralysis, which she claims is a kidney disorder that she has. Nephrologist cannot corroborate this theory.
3. Patient has a high rate of recidivism in the hospital system for treatment of her eating disorder.

Short-Term Goals:
1. Patient will identify and discuss high-risk situations.
2. She will listen.
3. She will demonstrate four alternative coping skills to purging.
4. She will seek out assistance from staff before acting on urges to purge.
5. Patient will identify triggers.
6. Patient will be able to discuss short- and long-term consequences of her eating disorder.
7. Patient will complete a crisis plan to control purging urges.
8. Patient will maintain personal safety by not engaging in purging.
9. Patient will maintain her current weight or increase that weight to 90 lb.

Long-Term Goals:
1. Patient will reduce the frequency of purging.
2. Patient will complete community passes without reports of purging in preparation for transition to home.
3. Patient will develop the ability to control impulses and demonstrate strategies to deal with dysphoric moods.
4. Patient will maintain her current weight or increase that weight.
5. Patient will maintain normal potassium levels and will not require supplemental potassium treatment.

Biopsychosocial Treatment Plan:
1. Because of her anorexia nervosa and possible personality disorder, she would likely benefit from a referral to dialectical behavior therapy.
2. She would also benefit from a referral to the eating disorders group.

3. Because of her history of hypokalemia, we will regularly monitor her potassium level and treat accordingly with supplemental potassium.
4. We will weigh her three times a week in order to monitor her progress here. We will expect that she maintain her current weight or increase it.
5. She will be allowed initially to go to the cafeteria on her own and choose what she eats, assuming that her weight stays at her current level or increases.
6. She will be started at level B privileges.

Discharge Criteria:
1. She will maintain or increase her weight during her stay here.
2. She will maintain normal potassium levels during her stay here.
3. She will participate in dialectical behavior therapy as well as the eating disorders group.
4. She will reduce the frequency of her purging behaviors while here.
5. She will complete community passes without reports of purging in preparation for transition to home.

Estimated Length of Stay as Per UM Norms: 45 days

Which of the following is the correct code set for reporting this physician's service?

ICD-9-CM and CPT Code(s):

a. 307.1, 314.01, 301.83, 493.90, V17.0, 90801
b. 301.1, 314.01, 301.83, 276.8, 493.90, 359.3, 90801
c. 307.1, 314.01, 301.83, 493.90, V17.0, 99223
d. 301.1, 314.01, 301.83, 276.8, 493.90, 359.3, 99223

ICD-10-CM Code(s): _____

Disorders of the Musculoskeletal System and Connective Tissue

9.50.   The following documentation is from the health record of a patient having surgery on facial trauma.

Preoperative Diagnosis: Complicated left facial fracture

Postoperative Diagnosis: Complicated left facial fracture

Operation:
1. Open reduction internal fixation of comminuted left tripod fracture
2. Open reduction internal fixation of left lateral orbital wall telescoped fracture
3. Endoscopic exam of left orbital floor

Findings: A comminuted fracture involving the left tripod and mid face. There were two fractures in the left lateral orbital rim with a central fragment telescoped in the lateral orbital wall. The Zygoma was depressed and rotated. There was a comminuted fracture of the distal zygomatic arch. The orbital floor showed a nondisplaced fracture. There is no evidence of orbital herniation into the antrum. Several mucosal lacerations of the lateral antral wall.

Description of Procedure: After an adequate induction, the oral cavity was examined. The occlusion was deemed class I, thus an oral intubation was performed. The patient's face was prepped with Betadine paint, ophthalmologic. The patient was draped in the usual manner. The original laceration over the left zygoma was opened. There was some serosanguineous fluid expressed. The wound extended to the large zygomal fragment.

A sublabial incision was made from the right piriform aperture to the left zygomaticomaxillary buttress. This incision had previously been injected with 1% Lidocaine with 1:100,000 Epinephrine. The incision was taken to the face of the maxilla and then all soft tissue was elevated off the piriform aperture, the anterior maxilla, zygomaticomaxillary buttress, and zygoma. The left lateral orbital wall was also skeletonized through the previous laceration, which was extended superiorly into the left brow. At this point, a Carol Gerard screw was placed in the left zygoma, and the zygoma was reduced into its native position. The telescoped fragment in the left lateral orbital wall was also reduced. The zygomaticomaxillary buttress fracture was identified and found to be reduced in its native position.

The following plates were placed: On the left lateral orbital rim, a 2 mm orbital rim plate was placed with six 6 mm × 2 mm diameter screws. On the left zygomaticomaxillary buttress, an L-shaped plate was placed using four 6 mm screws × 1.5 mm in diameter.

The nasal cavity was examined and a simple reduction was performed. There appeared to be slight medial displacement of the nasal bones. The orbital floor was examined endoscopically. All the antral contents of devitalized mucosa and old blood was debrided. There was no evidence of fat herniation into the antrum, but there appeared to be a few small nondisplaced fractures with gentle palpation of the globe.

All the areas were then copiously irrigated. The left lateral orbital incision was then closed in layers with 4-0 Vicryl and 5-0 plain gut. Sublabial incision was closed with interrupted 3-0 Chromics.

Total blood loss 10–20 cc. No complications. The patient emerged and was sent to recovery in stable condition.

Which CPT code(s) is/are assigned to the surgical services?

a. 21365-LT
b. 21315-LT, 21365-LT
c. 21365-LT, 31292-LT
d. 21315-LT, 21365-LT, 21406-LT, 31237-LT

9.51. The following documentation is from the health record of a patient having orthopedic surgery on the leg.

Operative Report

Preoperative Diagnosis: Left distal femur osteosarcoma

Postoperative Diagnosis: Left distal femur osteosarcoma

Operation: 1. Resection of left distal femur

2. Prosthetic reconstruction of the left knee

3. Osteotomy of the left femur

4. Femoral artery exploration

Anesthesia: General

Estimated Blood Loss: 500 ml. The patient received 4 units of packed RBCs.

Complications: None

Indications for Procedure: The patient is a 23-year-old female who was diagnosed with a left distal femur osteosarcoma on biopsy and has undergone preoperative chemotherapy. Risks, benefits, complications, and alternatives of resection and reconstruction were discussed with her, and consent was obtained.

Description of Procedure: The patient was seen in the preoperative area and a history and physical examination were performed. Consents were reviewed. She was taken to the operating room and given general anesthesia. She received preoperative antibiotics, and a Foley catheter was placed. Both legs were prepped and draped out. An external incision was made on the anteromedial aspect of the left thigh, extending towards the anterior aspect of the proximal tibia, including excision of the previous biopsy tract.

Dissection was carried down to the subcutaneous tissue leaving a cuff of healthy tissue on the biopsy tract, and also a cuff of muscle was left. Dissection was carried subvastus, elevating the muscle but leaving the fat and other loose tissue including fascia on the tumor. Medially the vastus medialis was elevated off the medial septum. Dissection was carried further subvastus as well as laterally. The patella was preserved. Distally the subpatellar tendon fat pad was left with the knee to be resected. Following dissection, an Osteotomy site was located further laterally and proximally at 16 cm from the articular surface of the femoral condyle. This was based on the recent MRI. An osteotomy was performed, parts of the posterior cortex were curetted, and marrow was removed and passed off to the pathologist for evaluation. Both of these were read on frozen sections as being normal and not containing any malignant tissue.

With these findings known, the remaining posterior attachments to the femur were dissected/transected. The femoral artery extending towards the popliteal space was carefully explored and retracted, and any branches of the tumor were either clipped or suture ligated. The tumor was dissected and the resection was carried out under tourniquet at 270 mmHg.

The tourniquet was let down and hemostasis was achieved with Bovie cautery, vascular clips, or suture ligations. The wound was slightly irrigated. The specimen was sent off to the pathologist for evaluation. The tibial surface was reamed and trial implants were placed. The femoral canal was reamed to 15 mm, which gave satisfactory chatter suggestive of a good fit. A 15-mm-diameter, 150-mm-long stem was placed into the femur with various length trials. A regular femoral condyle was chosen along with a regular tibial component. Following adequate leg length, which gave us satisfactory soft tissue tensioning and rotation as well as the ability to close the wound and patella tracking, but also about 1 extra cm length on the left side, the appropriate components were chosen. The tibial plastic component was cemented into place. An uncemented 150-mm-long, 15-mm-diameter stem with the components in place was gently impacted into the femur and was checked under fluoroscopy. It was noted to be satisfactorily placed. After placement of the bushings, the hinge, and the bumper, the components were reduced. The soft tissue tension was adequate and the vessels seemed to be without any undue stress, and adequate pulsation of the femoral artery was present extending down to the popliteal space. With these findings, patella tracking was again checked and noted to be satisfactory. The wound was thoroughly irrigated, 2 drains were placed, and the various layers were reapproximated with either #1 Ethibond, #1, 0, or 2-0 Vicryl sutures, and then the skin was closed with 4-0 Monocryl. Steri-strips were applied, and the dressings were applied as well as the knee immobilizer with a slight flexion of the knee.

Postoperatively, the foot showed adequate blood flow with a palpable dorsalis pedis pulse. The patient was extubated. She will be admitted for postoperative pain control as well as rehabilitation and discharged when stable.

Which of the following is the correct code assignment for the services of the surgeon?

ICD-9-CM and CPT Code(s):

a. 170.7, 27360, 27447, 35741, 27448, 76000
b. 170.7, 27365, 27445, 35721, 27448-59, 76000-26
c. 238.0, 27329, 27445, 27448-59, 76000-26
d. 239.2, 27360, 27447, 27448, 76000

ICD-10-CM Code(s): _____

9.52. The following documentation is from the health record of a 42-year-old male patient.

Physician Office Record Entries

Hospital Copy: History and Physical

Admitting Diagnosis: Herniation of intervertebral disc, L5–S1 right side

Present Medical History: Patient is a 42-year-old Native American male who initially developed problems with his back in July of this year. He was treated with anti-inflammatory agents and started on an exercise program; his condition improved enough to return to work. About 1 month ago, he had recurrence of pain, which has become steadily worse in the past week. He noticed some numbness of his right foot, primarily the toes and right heel. The patient was initially evaluated by his family physician and is now admitted to the orthopedic service for microdiskectomy after MRI revealed herniation and protrusion of the disc encroaching on the nerve root.

Past Medical History: Patient denied any known allergies or drug sensitivities. He has been taking Advil on a p.r.n. basis. Also takes Lotensin 10 mg daily for hypertension and has a history of incomplete bundle branch block, hyperlipidemia (no meds), hiatus hernia with gastroesophageal reflux.

Previous Surgeries: Tonsillectomy as a child and also tendon repair to the right hand in 1989. Does state that he injured his kidney in a motorcycle accident at age 21 years and was hospitalized with viral pneumonia in 1983.

Family History: Father is 62 years with heart disease and hypertension problems. Mother is 64 years and in good health, without significant illness. Three siblings, all in good health.

Social History: Patient is employed full-time at the Harley-Davidson dealership. At the present time, he is divorced and has one child who lives with her mother. He does not smoke, is sexually active, and admits to sporadic alcohol use.

Review of Systems

HEENT: Patient denies any unusual problems with headaches and dizziness, or visual or hearing difficulty. Cardiorespiratory: Denies chest pain; does have occasional asthma symptoms with some wheezing but does not use medications. Hypertension for 2 years, well controlled on medication. Gastrointestinal: Denies distention, diarrhea, and constipation. Genitourinary: Negative. Musculoskeletal: See present complaint.

Physical Examination: Reveals a well-developed, well-nourished male in no acute distress. Does have a hard time sitting due to pain on the right side. Height 6'1", weight 210 lb, blood pressure 122/90, pulse 72, respiration 20. Skin is clear, normal temperature and texture. HEENT: Head normal cephalic. Pupils are round, equal, and reactive to light accommodation. Canals are clear. Tympanic membranes, nose, and throat are clear of infection. Neck: Supple, thyroid negative. No adenopathy, no distomegaly or carotid bruits. Chest: Symmetrical, lungs clear to P & A. Heart: Normal sinus rhythm, no thrills or murmurs. Abdomen: Soft, no tenderness or masses. No organomegaly. Normal male genitalia. Extremities: Normal development. Patient does have tenderness in the area of the right sciatic knot and in the lower lumbar area on the right side. Has positive leg raising and some decrease in the deep tendon reflexes on the side.

Impression: Herniation of intervertebral disc at L5–S1 right side

Plan: Microdiskectomy tomorrow morning

Operative Report

Preoperative Diagnosis: Herniated nucleus pulposus, right

Postoperative Diagnosis: Same

Operation: Right L5–S1 diskectomy with minifacetectomy foraminotomy

Complications: None

Indications: The patient is an otherwise healthy 42-year-old Native American male who has had 6 months of disabling right leg pain. He has tried extensive physical therapy, nonsteroidal anti-inflammatory drugs, and an epidural injection, without relief. He has a positive straight leg-raising test on the right side and an absent ankle jerk. MRI scan confirms the disk herniation at L5–S1 on the right side.

Description of Procedure: The patient was brought to the operating room, and general anesthesia was administered in the usual fashion. He was positioned in the prone position onto a well-padded Andrews frame. All pressure points were well padded. The back was prepped and draped in a sterile fashion. He received 1 g of Ancef prior to the beginning of the case, along with 30 mg of IV Toradol.

Initially, an x-ray was checked that showed we were at the L4–5 interspace, so we went down one level. A 3/4 skin incision was made in the midline of the lumbar sacral spine, and this was carried down to the subcutaneous tissue. The fascia over the L5–S1 lamina was then dissected away. The paraspinal muscles were then elevated above the lamina, and a laminotomy was performed in between L5 and S1. The superior facet of S1 was undercut using a Kerrison rongeur. The S1 nerve root was well visualized and this area was protected throughout the procedure. Following this, a foraminotomy was performed over the top of the S1 nerve root. The S1 nerve root was then gently retracted medially, and a very large extrusive disk fragment was pulled out from underneath the S1 nerve root. The annulotomy that had been made from the disc herniation was then explored, and no further fragments could be found. The wound was thoroughly irrigated with a bacitracin solution. Gelfoam and thrombin were placed over the top of the dura, and the deep fascia was closed with interrupted 0 VICRYL sutures. The subcutaneous tissue was closed with 2-0 VICRYL suture, and the skin was closed with 4-0 VICRYL suture. Benzoin and Steri-Strips were applied to the wound. The patient was returned to recovery in stable condition. EBL 10 cc.

Pathologic Diagnosis: Intervertebral disc L5–S1 resection, herniated nucleus pulposus

Which of the following is the correct code assignment for physician service? Code for surgical services only.

ICD-9-CM and CPT Code(s):

a. 722.52, 401.9, 63047
b. 722.73, 401.9, 63030
c. 722.10, 63047
d. 722.10, 401.9, 63030

ICD-10-CM Code(s): _____

9.53. The following documentation is from the health record of a male patient.

Operative Report

Preoperative Diagnosis: 1. ACL deficient, right knee
2. Medial and lateral meniscal tear, right knee

Operation: 1. Examination under anesthesia, right knee
2. Arthroscopic-assisted anterior cruciate ligament reconstruction, right knee
3. Partial medial and partial lateral meniscectomy

Anesthesia: General

Complications: None

The patient was identified and taken to the operating room and general anesthesia administered. The patient's lower extremity was examined under anesthesia. The patient had evidence of +2 Lachman and +2 pivot shift. After examination under anesthesia, the right lower extremity was prepped and draped in the usual sterile fashion. Routine arthroscopic portals were placed. Examination of the patellofemoral joint was fairly unremarkable. Coming down the medial gutter and the medial compartment, there was a complex tear of the posterior horn of the medial meniscus. Using a combination of basket and 4.2 shaver, partial medial meniscectomy was carried out. This resected about 50 percent of the posterior horn of the medial meniscus. There was a horizontal cleavage component remaining that was stable to probing; it was left alone. Intercondylar notch revealed a complete tear of the anterior cruciate ligament. Going to the lateral compartment, there was a flap tear of the posterior horn of the lateral meniscus, and, again utilizing the lateral meniscus, partial lateral meniscectomy was carried out. This resected about 30 percent of the posterior horn. At this point, the scope was removed from the knee. We did make a longitudinal incision based upon the tibial tubercle medially. This was carried down through the skin and down the subcutaneous tissue. We readily identified the hamstring tendon and harvested the gracilis and semitendinosus. These were taken to the back table and a #2 ETHIBOND leader was placed on the leading edge, and the graft was doubled over for quadruple graft. The scope was placed back into the knee. Notchplasty was performed. Subsequently, we made a tibial tunnel utilizing the Arthrex tibial guide referenced off the posterior cruciate ligament. We then made a femoral tunnel, again utilizing the Arthrex femoral guide referenced off the posterior cortex. Both of these were 8-mm tunnels. We subsequently placed the graft on the knee, and we fixed it on the femoral side with 8 × 23 Arthrex bioabsorbable screw. Visualization of the graft revealed no evidence of impingement, no roughing on the medial aspect of the lateral wall. We subsequently held the knee in just short of full extension with appropriate amount of tension and fixed it on the tibial side with an 8 × 28 Arthrex bioabsorbable screw. Examination after placement of the graft revealed a negative Lachman and negative pivot shift. Multiple intraoperative photos were obtained. At the end of the procedure, subcutaneous tissue was closed with 2-0 VICRYL, the skin with running 2-0 nylon, and portals with 3-0 nylon. Sterile dressing was placed followed by ACE wrap and total thigh and knee immobilizer. The patient tolerated the procedure well, and there were no complications.

Assign the correct codes for this case.

ICD-9-CM Primary (First-Listed) Diagnosis: _____

ICD-9-CM Additional Diagnoses: _____

CPT Procedure Code(s): _____

ICD-10-CM Code(s): _____

9.54. The following documentation is from the health record of a patient admitted for a right total hip.

Preoperative Diagnosis:	Right hip osteonecrosis, Ficat stage IV
Postoperative Diagnosis:	Right hip osteonecrosis, Ficat stage IV
Procedure Performed:	Right total hip arthroplasty
Blood Loss:	350 cc
Complications:	None .

Implants Used:
1. DePuy Articul/EZE femoral head 28 mm + 1.5, lot #1169939
2. DePuy large AML femoral component, 150 mm long, 45-mm offset, lot #YDZCV1000
3. DePuy hole eliminator, lot #YH9DH1000
4. DePuy pinnacle acetabular liner 28 mm, lot #X69AR1000
5. DePuy cancellous bone screw 25 mm long, lot #X2BEN1000
6. DePuy acetabular cup 36 mm, lot #X60CK1000

Indications for Operation: The patient is a 54-year-old man who is presented with long-standing right hip pain secondary to osteonecrosis. Nonsurgical treatment was unsuccessful. After risks, benefits, and alternatives of the surgery were explained to the patient, informed consent was obtained for this procedure.

Details of Procedure: Patient was taken back to the operating room and placed on the operating table in a supine position. After induction of general anesthesia, the patient was placed in the left lateral decubitus position and the left lower extremity was prepped and draped in usual sterile manner. Lateral incision was made over the greater trochanter. This incision was approximately 15 cm long. It was carried down through subcutaneous tissue to the iliotibial band, which was incised longitudinally. The gluteus medius was identified and split in line with its fibers down to the level of the greater trochanter. The gluteus medius was then split. This ran along with greater trochanter and was lifted anteriorly off the greater trochanter in line with vastus lateralis as well. These structures were dissected off of the greater trochanter. The gluteus minimus was exposed and its tendon was transected longitudinally as well. Capsule was delineated just lying underneath the gluteus adducted and placed in a sterile bag as it was dislocated. The neck was cut with an oscillating saw. Retractors were placed inferiorly, posteriorly along the acetabulum, as well as superiorly. The acetabulum was then debrided off the remaining capsular and labral tissue as well as ligamentaries. The acetabulum was then reamed starting with a 49-mm reamer and reamed sequentially in 1-mm increments to 55; 56 was trailed and it was deemed to be appropriate. Version was checked at each sequential reaming. The 56-mm acetabular component was then inserted and hammered into place. Trial liner was placed. The limb was then placed in the bag and the medial aspect of the greater trochanter was cut with the use of a box cutter. The femoral canal was then reamed sequentially and increments to a 13.5. The lateral side cutter was then used to cut out the cancellous bone from the calcar. A small broach was replaced with 13.5 large broach. The head component was placed and was trailed. The hip was deemed to be too tight. Intraoperative x-ray was obtained and demonstrated the femoral neck cut to be insufficient. The hip was dislocated. The trial head and neck were removed and the femur was then reamed further distally. The calcar planar was used to take down the femoral neck cut. The broach was placed prior to calcar planning often reaming the femoral canal sufficiently, the 13.5 large broach did in fact sink further end of the canal and after the hip was reduced it was deemed to be both stable and not in too much tension. The hip was then dislocated. The broach was removed as well as the trial liner. The true liner was then placed as well as the femoral stem component. Femoral head was placed and the hip was located. Tension was deemed to be adequate. The hip was tested and position of instability was deemed to be stable. The wound was copiously irrigated to sterile saline. The minimus was repaired with interrupted #0 VICRYL sutures. The medius was reapproximated with running #0 VICRYL sutures as well as drill holes placed into greater troch and #5 Tycron sutures. The IT band was repaired with interrupted #0 VICRYL sutures and subcutaneous tissue was repaired with interrupted #2-0 VICRYL sutures. The skin was closed with staples. Sterile dressings were applied. The patient was extubated and recovered in a holding area uneventfully.

Code the orthopedic surgeon's code sets.

ICD-9-CM and CPT Code(s): _____

ICD-10-CM Code(s): _____

Neoplasms

9.55.   The patient is a four-year-old male with acute lymphocytic leukemia who has had a fever for the last 24 hours. It has been nine days since his last chemotherapy, which was his first. A comprehensive history is documented. On examination, the skin over his Hickman site is extremely red and starting to break down. No other abnormal findings are noted in the comprehensive exam. Labs show that the patient is not neutropenic. The physician lists the diagnoses as: ALL not in remission, infected Hickman. The patient is given 770 mg of Ceptaz over 10 minutes through a new peripheral IV site and admitted for continued treatment. Medical decision making is moderate.

What code set is reported for the services of the emergency physician?

ICD-9-CM and CPT Code(s):

a. 204.00, 996.62, 780.60, 99284-25, 96374
b. 204.00, 999.31, E878.2, 99284
c. 208.00, 996.69, 780.61, 99285
d. 208.00, 999.31, 99285-25, 96374

ICD-10-CM Code(s): _____

9.56.   A patient with a chronic cough and shortness of breath is scheduled for a pleural biopsy following a chest x-ray that revealed a significant mass in the left lower lobe of the lung. Due to the position of the mass, a pleural biopsy is planned rather than a bronchoscopic biopsy.

Following the administration of local anesthetic in the interventional radiology suite of the hospital, a pleural biopsy needle is passed over the left side of the ribs. Fluoroscopic guidance is used to guide needle placement into the mass, so that tissue is obtained for pathologic evaluation.

Which of the following code sets would the physician assign for this procedure if carcinoma of the lung is diagnosed?

ICD-9-CM and CPT Code(s):

a. 162.9, 32400, 77002
b. 786.09, 786.2, 32405
c. 162.5, 32405, 77002-26
d. 162.5, 786.09, 786.2, 32405, 77002-26

ICD-10-CM Code(s): _____

9.57.   A patient with hemoptysis, hoarseness, and chronic cough was scheduled for an outpatient flexible fiberoptic laryngoscopy including a biopsy of the cricoid. Procedure: Patient was taken to operating outpatient suite #2. IV sedation was administered at 1300 and topical anesthetic spray was applied. Next, a flexible fiberoptic laryngoscope was introduced. Biopsies were taken from multiple sites of the affected areas. The pathology report states "metastatic carcinoma of the arytenoid cartilage and the posterior commissure and well-differentiated carcinoma of the cricoid and extrinsic larynx." The operative note states suspected involvement of the thyroid cartilage with primary malignancy believed to be from the esophagus. The patient experienced an increase in blood pressure after the biopsies were obtained, and the procedure was discontinued at 1316. An esophagoscopy will be scheduled after the patient's blood pressure is stabilized.

Which of the following code sets would the physician report?

ICD-9-CM and CPT Code(s):

a. 197.3, 199.1, 796.2, 31576, 99144
b. 161.8, 198.89, 401.9, 31510
c. 150.9, 197.3, 197.3, 197.3, 197.3, 997.1, 31576-53
d. 150.9, 161.8, 796.2, 31576, 99144, 99145

ICD-10-CM Code(s): _____

9.58. A Medicare patient with a personal history of colon cancer, considered to be at high risk for recurrent disease, presents to the office for a screening colonoscopy. The gastroenterologist also examines the anastomosis sites following a previous hemicolectomy.

Procedure: The patient was prepped in the usual fashion, followed by placement in the left lateral decubitus position. I administered 3 mg of Versed. Monitoring of sedation was assisted by a trained RN.

A colonoscopy to the terminal ileum was performed with lesions found just beyond the splenic flexure, which were biopsied. In the sigmoid colon, two polyps were found and excised by hot biopsy forceps.

The pathology report showed the descending colon lesions to be a recurrence of the malignancy and the polyps to be adenomatous.

Which of the following code sets would be reported for the procedure performed in the office?

ICD-9-CM and CPT Code(s):

a. 153.2, 45384
b. 153.2, 211.3, 45384, 45380-59
c. V67.09, V10.05, 153.2, G0105, 45384-59
d. 153.9, V10.05, V45.89, 45384, 45380

ICD-10-CM Code(s): _____

9.59. The following documentation is from the health record of a 23-year-old female patient.

Preoperative Diagnosis:	Osteochondroma of the right scapula
Postoperative Diagnosis:	Same
Procedure:	Excision of osteochondroma of right scapula

Indication: This 23-year-old female has noticed a growing lump coming out of the back of her right scapula over the past year. It has become unsightly and recently has become tender, especially when it's bumped. CT scan has shown a pedunculated osteochondroma coming off the scapula, right at the base of the spine on the medial border. There is no thickened cartilage cap, and simple excision should be adequate.

Findings: Classic osteochondroma of right scapula

Specimen Sent: Osteochondroma

Description of Procedure: After induction of adequate general anesthesia and appropriate timeout, the patient was positioned on her left side with the right side uppermost. The right upper extremity was prepped and draped in the standard fashion with the arm free in the field. We marked out a 4-cm incision over the medial border of her right scapular spine and made this incision through the skin and subcutaneous tissues down to the fascia. I could palpate the osteochondroma easily. We worked our way down through the fascia and separated a 3-cm-wide section of trapezius over the bump, which let us see the pseudocapsule over the bump. We then dissected bluntly down around the osteochondroma to its base, where we could feel that it was right at the takeoff of the scapular spine. The osteochondroma had a well-defined pedunculated stem as we had seen from the CT scan, and with the 3/4-inch osteotome, we went around part of it and were able to come from the other side and separate it from the scapula. There were a couple of rough edges, which were rongeured and smoothed, and then we bone waxed the stalk of the osteochondroma. We removed the excess bone wax. The osteochondroma was inspected and the cartilage cap was seen to be intact. We then infiltrated the bone in the local area with 0.5% Marcaine with epinephrine, of which about 6 mL stayed in the wound. We also infiltrated the skin edges. We then closed the trapezius muscle with three 2-0 mattress sutures after a copious round of irrigation and cauterizing a few little bleeders. The subcutaneous tissue was then approximated with 2-0 inverted mattress Vicryl sutures, and the skin was closed with 3-0 running subcuticular Prolene. The wound was then dressed in two layers with a 4×4 and Tegaderm on the first layer and a bulky dressing on the top, which can be taken off in a couple of days. The patient was then awakened and taken to the recovery room in satisfactory condition.

Which of the following will be reported for the surgical service?

ICD-9-CM and CPT Code(s):

a. 170.4, 23182
b. 170.4, 23190
c. 213.4, 23140
d. 213.4, 23190

ICD-10-CM Code(s): _____

9.60. The following documentation is from the health record of a 78-year-old male patient.

Preoperative Diagnosis: Need for permanent venous access

Postoperative Diagnosis: Same

Description of Procedure: Placement of Infuse-A-Port, right subclavian vein

The patient is a 78-year-old Hispanic male with widely disseminated metastatic colon carcinoma under chemotherapy management. His oncologist has requested placement of a permanent venous access catheter.

The patient was brought to the operating room and placed in the supine position. The initial request was for placement in the left subclavian vein. However, after cannulation of the vein and injection of contrast, there was not adequate flow to allow passage of the guidewire through the vein into the superior vena cava. Therefore, the left-sided procedure was aborted.

The right subclavian vein was cannulated without difficulty, and the guidewire was passed centrally down into the superior vena cava. The location was confirmed with fluoroscopy. A subcutaneous pocket and tunnel were then created for the port. The port was placed just above the pectoral fascia. The dilator and peel-away catheter and sheath were passed off the guidewire into the subclavian vein. The sheath was peeled away, and the catheter that had been previously trimmed to the appropriate length and flushed with heparinized saline was passed through the sheath into the subclavian vein. The sheath was peeled away, and hemostasis was achieved. The port was sutured into the pocket with 3-0 Dexon. The 2.5-cm wound was irrigated with saline and closed in layers with 3-0 Dexon subcutaneously followed with 4-0 Dexon subcuticular for the skin. Steri-Strips were applied with sterile dressing and tape. Following the procedure, a chest x-ray in the holding area revealed no pneumothorax and the catheter in excellent position.

Which of the following code sets would the surgeon report for this ambulatory surgical service performed at the hospital?

ICD-9-CM and CPT Code(s):

a. 199.0, 153.9, 36561, 36556-59
b. 153.9, 36563, 36410-53
c. 199.0, 153.9, 36561, 36410-59
d. V58.81, 199.0, 153.9, 36561, 12031

ICD-10-CM Code(s): _____

9.61.   The following documentation is from the health record of a patient with a lesion on the left calf.

COMPREHENSIVE VISIT

History

Referring Doctor:	Primary care physician
Chief Complaint:	Lesion lt. calf
History of Present Illness:	4 to 5 yr. HX pigmented lesion posterior lt. calf. Lesion changed (divided into 2, became rough). Pt. saw primary care physician and lesion was biopsied. Path positive for malignant melanoma in situ. Pt. referred for wide re-excision.
Medications:	Indural 40 mg 2 qd, Norvasc 5 mg 1 qd, Lasix 80 mg 2 qd, Potassium 20 meq 2 qd
Allergies:	Septra
Medical History:	Wears glasses, high BP
Surgery:	Tonsillectomy 1945, partial hysterectomy 1963, lumpectomy rt. breast 1965, lumpectomy rt. breast 1967

Physical

HT:	5'1"
WT:	147

TEMP:	
BP:	160/72
P:	64
R:	
General:	NDWF
HEENT:	No bruits or JVD
Heart:	RSR without murmur
Extremities:	Lt. posterior calf recent biopsy site—greater than 1-cm-diameter defect—dermal based
Diagnosis:	Melanoma in situ, lt. posterior calf
Plan:	Will need wide local excision with STSG to excision site. Donor site—thigh or hip.

Select the correct codes for this physician.

ICD-9-CM Code(s):

a. 172.7
b. 232.7
c. 232.7, 172.7
d. 172.7, 709.9

ICD-10-CM Code(s): _____

Disorders of the Nervous System and Sense Organs

9.62. A patient presents to the neurology clinic for assessment of apraxia at the request of her primary care physician. The patient has a history of CVA and has expressive aphasia. She is unable to carry out purposeful movements, even though she has normal muscle tone and coordination. A full assessment is performed using the Boston Diagnostic Aphasia Examination including interpretation and report (one hour). The consulting neurologist conducts a detailed history and examination, performs medical decision making of low complexity, and dictates a complete report to the requesting physician, along with the finding of the aphasia assessment.

Which of the following code sets is reported for this service?

ICD-9-CM and CPT Code(s):

a. 438.11, 438.81, 99203, 96105
b. 784.3, 784.69, 99244
c. 438.81, 99243
d. 438.11, 438.81, 99243-25, 96105

ICD-10-CM Code(s): _____

9.63.   This 35-year-old female patient was admitted with the diagnosis of cerebral aneurysm. The following procedure was performed: intracranial aneurysm repair by intracranial approach with microdissection, carotid circulation. The patient continued to improve with no residual defects. During the hospital stay, she did experience postoperative pneumonia due to *Pseudomonas.*

In addition to the E/M codes submitted by the office, what other codes are assigned?

ICD-9-CM and CPT Code(s):

a.   437.3, 61700
b.   430, 482.1, 61700, 69990-51
c.   437.3, 997.3, 482.1, 61700, 69990
d.   747.81, 997.3, 61703, 69990

ICD-10-CM Code(s): _____

9.64.   A patient presents to the neurology clinic for a consultation with a neurologist for intention tremors with periodic muscle weakness in the upper body.

Short-latency somatosensory-evoked potential studies were conducted immediately following a comprehensive history, comprehensive neurologic examination, and decision making of moderate complexity. Both arms and the head and trunk were tested. The results of the interpretation of the tests state "Rule out MS," and a report was sent to the requesting physician stating that a diagnosis of multiple sclerosis could not be ruled out at this time and further testing would be undertaken at a later date. Which of the following is correct?

ICD-9-CM and CPT Code(s):

a.   333.1, 728.9, 99244-25, 95925, 95927-51
b.   340, 99245-25, 95927
c.   333.1, 728.9, 99204, 95925, 95927-51
d.   728.9, 781.0, 99244-25, 95927

ICD-10-CM Code(s): _____

9.65.   A Medicare patient has a persistent pain syndrome of the low back and leg subsequent to an automobile accident five years ago in which he sustained back injuries. The patient is brought to the outpatient surgery center nerve block area and is premedicated so he is relaxed enough to be positioned appropriately. The sacral area is prepped with Betadine and a 25-gauge needle, followed by a 22-gauge needle, and is placed under lidocaine anesthesia in the caudal space. The area is injected with 29 cc of solution containing 150 cc of Xylocaine and 16 mg of Decadron LA. The patient remained in good condition in the block room and the recovery area.

Which of the following procedure code sets is reported?

a.   64449
b.   62319
c.   62311
d.   62311, 77003

9.66. This 45-year-old patient has been followed for left ear conductive hearing loss. It was decided to proceed with surgery to correct the condition. The postoperative diagnosis is left ear otosclerosis. During the procedure, a markedly thickened stapes footplate was observed; however, the eustachian tube was intact, and there was normal mobility of the malleus and incus. The left ear stapedectomy with drillout of the footplate proceeded uneventfully. During recovery, the patient experienced atrial fibrillation. This was felt to be due to the surgery because the EKG was normal during the preoperative evaluation. The patient was admitted to the hospital from the outpatient surgical area, and a consultation was requested from the cardiologist.

With the exception of E/M codes, what are the correct diagnosis and procedure codes for physician reporting?

ICD-9-CM and CPT Code(s):

a. 387.9, 997.1, 427.31, 69661-LT
b. 387.9, 69661-LT
c. 387.9, 427.31, 69661-LT
d. 387.9, 69660-LT

ICD-10-CM Code(s): _____

9.67. The following documentation is from the health record of a patient seen in the ambulatory surgery center.

Chief Complaint: Bilateral decrease in vision especially in the right eye.

History of Present Illness: The patient is a 62-year-old woman who has had very poor vision in her right eye for some time which was the result of a cataract and is finding increasing difficulty with reading and watching television because of a cataract developing in the other eye at this time.

Allergies: Sulfa

Family History: She has a brother who had a retinal detachment.

Social History: She denies smoking or drinking alcohol.

Review of Systems: Neuro: Negative. Eye, ear, nose and throat: Bilateral decrease in vision as well as occasional sinus problems. Cardiovascular: Negative except for a very long history of hypertension. HTN is well controlled when the patient takes her meds. She tends to be somewhat noncompliant with taking her medication for high blood pressure. Patient states "I really don't need the little pills for my blood pressure." Pulmonary: She does have COPD which is well controlled on her medications. GI: History of liver biopsy in the past—reason unknown. GU: Occasional frequent urination and she does have a history of kidney stones in the past. Gynecologic: Negative. Endocrine: Negative. Hematologic: Patient has a history of a platelet disorder for which she had a splenectomy several years ago. Skin: Negative.

Physical Examination:

Vital Signs:	BP 145/76; Pulse 72; Respirations 16
Neck:	Negative
Cardiovascular:	S-1, S-2 without murmur, gallop, or rub
Chest:	Clear to A&P. Characteristic for patient with history of COPD
Abdomen:	Negative
Extremities:	Shows 1+ pedal edema
HEENT:	Bilateral cataracts
Impression:	Bilateral cataracts, right eye greater than left. Plan: Cataract extraction with implant in the right eye.

Operative Report

Preoperative Diagnosis: Cataract right eye

Postoperative Diagnosis: Same

Procedure: Extracapsular cataract extraction with implantation of a 16 Diopter posterior chamber lens (a Sinskey style posterior chamber lens) in the ciliary sulcus.

Operative Note: A honan balloon was placed in the right eye for 30 minutes at 35 mm of Mercury pressure. The patient was then prepped and draped in the usual fashion and an O'Brien block and a retrobulbar injection of Marcaine and Lidocaine and Wydase were performed on the right. The lid speculum was inserted, superior rectus suture was placed. A fornix-based flap was made, limbal hemostasis was obtained with bipolar cautery. A corneal groove was made with a 64 Beaver blade and a microsharp entered the anterior chamber. Healon was injected into the anterior chamber and an anterior capsulotomy was performed. The wound was enlarged with corneal scleral scissor to the right and to the left and 8-0 silk 10 o'clock and 2 o'clock sutures were placed. Nucleus expression was performed without difficulty and temporary sutures were tied. Site irrigation aspiration was performed and Kratz scratcher was used to polish the posterior capsule. The 16 Diopter implant was inspected, irrigated and Healon placed on the implant and in the anterior chamber. The implant was then inserted beneath the iris at 6 o'clock into the sucus avoiding the capsule. The superior Haptic was then placed beneath the iris at 12 o'clock. The lens was rotated to approximately 9 and 3 o'clock positions with excellent centration. The peripheral iridectomy was performed. The wound was closed and the superior rectus suture was removed. Ointment was placed on the eye followed by a patch and shield.

How would the physician report his services for this outpatient surgery?

ICD-9-CM and CPT Code(s):

a. 366.1, 401.9, 496, V15.81, 66984-RT
b. 366.9, 401.9, 496, V15.81, 66984-RT
c. 366.9, 401.9, 496, V15.81, 66985-RT
d. 366.9, 401.9, 496, 66984-50

ICD-10-CM Code(s): _____

Newborn/Congenital Disorders

9.68. The following documentation is from the health record of a newborn infant.

Newborn Care

Delivery Note: 11/20/XX, 2300. Called to provide pediatric standby during delivery for suspected nuchal cord. Mother G2, P1. Onset of labor 0730 with normal progression. Entered stage 2 labor at 2100. Fetal monitor showed occasional decelerations. Spontaneous rupture of membranes at 2110, fluid was clear. Noted to have nuchal cord at time of delivery. Otherwise uneventful course.

O: Initial Apgar score 8/9. Weight 3,340 g. Approximate gestational age 38 weeks.

General: Pink with lusty cry. HEENT: Normal, moderate molding, minimal caput. Spine intact. Lungs: Clear bilaterally. Cardiovascular: No murmur noted, capillary refill less than 2 seconds.

Assessment: Normal full-term newborn, noted to have nuchal cord with occasional decels, otherwise uneventful delivery.

Plan: No further intervention at this time. Transferred to newborn nursery for routine newborn care and monitoring.

Progress Note: 11/21/XX, 0630

Subjective: Female newborn, gestational age 39 3/7 wks. Product of full-term pregnancy, NSVD, SROM epidural anesthesia, sl nuchal cord. Initial Apgar score 8/9.

Mother is 32-year-old G2 P1. Pregnancy was significant for maternal hypothyroidism and vanishing twin syndrome. See delivery note for labor course. EDC 24 Nov, initial prenatal care at 10 3/7 wks. Maternal labs: Blood type O positive, ABS neg, Rub immune, VDRL nonreactive, HIV neg, GBS neg, 1hr GTT 82, HBsAg neg, GC/Chlm neg.

Objective: Birth wt 7 lb 6 oz, head circ 14″, length 19 3/4″, head: normocephalic, fontanelles soft nonbulging. Mild caput, moderate molding. Skin: Pink and warm. Eyes: + red reflux × 2, PERRL. ENT: Nares patent, palate intact. TMs clear bilaterally. Lungs: Bilateral breath sounds equal, no accessory muscle use noted. Cardiovascular: Regular rate and rhythm, no murmur appreciated. Well-perfused, normal pulses. Capillary refill less than 2 seconds. Abdomen: Normal active bowel sounds, soft, no masses, three-vessel cord. No erythema or discharge at umbilical stump. Genitalia: Normal female, minimal engorgement, anus patent. Neuro: Lusty cry, good suck, reflexes: + rooting, + morrow, + grip, + Babinski reflex present bilaterally. Skeletal: Clavicle is intact. Spine: No dimples or defects noted. Hips: Normal range of motion, no click noted.

Assessment: Healthy, full-term infant. No defects noted.

Plan: Continue routine newborn care and monitoring. Hearing screen ordered. Check bili, ABO, CBC, and Coombs given Rh+ mother. Continue breast feeding, no supplemental feeding at this time.

Discharge Exam: 11/22/XX, 1000

Subjective: 2 d/o female infant. Breast feeding q. 2 h.r., 10 min ea breast; mother denies diff with latching on (+ breast fed previous infant), + lusty cry when hungry, easily consoled. + Wet diapers q. 2–3 hours, + meconium diapers × 3 since birth.

Objective: Wt 7 lbs 1.5 oz, afebrile throughout admission

See Newborn D/C Pe Form

Laboratory: Coombs neg, blood type B neg, bili 12, HTC 37, hearing screen pass, initial PKU pending

Assessment: Normal, healthy term infant, s/p SVD

Plan: D/C to home. Continue breast feeding. Follow up in clinic for wt check and repeat bili in 3 days. Hep B and 2nd PKU in 2 weeks. RT ER for temp >100.5°F, no wet diapers > 12 hours, lethargy, or resp distress. Education given to parents regarding use of car seat, + verbalized understanding.

Which of the following CPT code sets accurately represents the physician's services for this newborn hospital stay?

	11/20	11/21	11/22
a.	99460	99462	99238
b.	99460, 99464	99462	99238
c.	99460, 99360	99233	99238
d.	99464	99232	99238

9.69.   The following documentation is from the health record of a two-year-old boy.

Patient Name: Johnny Jones

CC: Routine checkup

HPI: Johnny is 2 1/2 years old and has Down syndrome and a ventricular septal defect, surgically corrected. Mother reports he is pulling at his ears and has been running a temp of 99 to 100°F in the past two evenings. Tylenol liquid has been effective in fever resolution according to mother. Development is coming along as expected. Walks with an ataxic gait but does not run. One-word speech pattern. No two-word sentences yet. Appetite is good. Child appears happy, well groomed, and well nourished. Mother reports no specific behavior or social-adjustment concerns.

Past History: Normal SVB, 8 lb 5 oz, 24″ long. Heart surgery at 7 months. No known allergies. No medication at this time. Takes daily multivitamins.

Social: Lives at home with mother, father, and older brother. Receives physical, speech, and occupational therapy services from area education services in the home on a periodic basis.

Review of Systems: See patient data sheet and pediatric growth profile chart, not remarkable other than notation concerning recurrent ear infections. No cyanotic episodes, difficulty breathing, or other cardiac symptoms reported. Johnny had a follow-up visit to the cardiologist last month and his findings were reviewed; no significant problems. No voiding or digestive complaints by mother. Child still in diapers. All other systems negative (see detailed history).

Physical Exam: Weight 27 lb, Height 36″. HEENT: Both ears positive for redness and otitis media with effusion evident on the left, eyes PERRLA, nose slightly congested clear discharge, neck supple without adenopathy. Throat slightly red. Temperature 99.6°F, blood pressure 108/82, R 15, P 72. Heart regular rate and rhythm; lungs clear to auscultation and percussion, no rales or wheezing. Abdomen soft without tenderness.

Extremities negative. (Detailed)

Assessment: Acute serous otitis media and slight throat infection, likely viral. Inject Bicillin L-A, 600,000 units and follow-up appointment in 3 days. No immunizations needed at this time. Fifteen additional minutes spent in counseling the mother concerning developmental expectations, reviewing cardiologist findings, and answering questions about future cardiac risks.

Which of the following code sets is assigned for reporting the pediatrician's services?

ICD-9-CM and CPT Code(s):

a. 381.01, 462, 758.0, V45.89, 99214, 96372, J0561
b. V20.2, 381.01, 462, 758.0, V45.89, 99392, 99214-25
c. 381.01, 462, 99214, 96372
d. 758.0, V45.89, 99213, J0561

ICD-10-CM Code(s): _____

9.70. The following documentation is from the health record of a 10-year-old boy.

Preoperative Diagnosis: Status post palatoplasty, history of bilateral incomplete cleft palate with recurrent tonsillitis

Postoperative Diagnosis: Same

Operation: Second-stage palatoplasty with attachment of pharyngeal flap and incidental tonsillectomy

Indications: A 10-year-old patient scheduled for revision of palatoplasty with incidental tonsillectomy requested by pediatrician due to repeated infections

Description of Procedure: The patient was prepped and draped in normal sterile fashion. A midline incision was made through the soft palate, exposing the posterior pharyngeal wall. A flap was then taken by incising the mucosa, submucosa, and underlying muscle, and securely sutured to the soft palate.

Bilateral tonsillectomy was then performed by grasping with a tonsil clamp and capsule dissection. Bleeders were controlled with electrocautery and gauze packing. Sponge and instrument counts were taken and correct, and the patient was transferred to the recovery room in good condition. Follow-up in the office in 3 days.

Which of the following code sets will be reported?

ICD-9-CM and CPT Code(s):

a. 749.04, 42225, 42825
b. 749.04, 474.00, 42225
c. 749.04, 474.00, 42225, 42825-51
d. V50.8, 749.04, 474.00, 42200, 42826-51

ICD-10-CM Code(s): _____

9.71.   The following documentation is from the health record of a 10-month-old baby.

Hospital Outpatient Services

A 10-month-old boy is seen in the Gastroenterology Lab to insert a gastrostomy tube. The child pulled out his previous G-tube during the night. He is being followed for congenital cytomegalovirus infection and GERD with erosion of the esophagus. Conscious sedation is provided by the anesthesiologist. The gastroenterologist positions the patient and probes the site with a catheter, injects contrast medium into the tract for assessment, and maneuvers a wire through the tract into the stomach under fluoroscopic guidance. The physician advances the gastrostomy tube over the wire and into position and then secures the device internally and externally. The system is put to gravity drainage and a sterile dressing is applied.

Which of the following code sets is reported by the pediatric gastroenterologist?

ICD-9-CM and CPT Code(s):

a. 536.49, 079.99, 530.81, 49440
b. 536.41, 771.1, 530.81, 530.89, 43760, 76000-26
c. V55.1, 530.81, 530.89, 771.1, 49450
d. V55.1, 530.81, 079.99, 49450, 76000-26

ICD-10-CM Code(s): _____

Pediatric Conditions

9.72.   A three-year-old child was brought to the emergency department after inhaling a peanut. The child had a brassy cough that was not present prior to the incident. X-rays showed congestion in the lungs but no obvious foreign body in the larynx. The child was given Versed intravenously and placed on a papoose board. The ED physician could see the peanut on indirect laryngoscopy but could not grasp it with multiple attempts. An ENT specialist took the patient to surgery for removal under anesthesia. An expanded, problem-focused history, problem-focused physical exam, and medical decision making of low complexity were documented.

Give the correct CPT codes for reporting the independent ED physician's service.

a. 99281-25, 31505
b. 99281-25, 31511
c. 99282, 31505
d. 99281, 31511

9.73.   The patient is a five-week-old male infant brought in by ambulance after the mother called 9-1-1. The baby was taking a bottle feeding normally and suddenly was blue in the face, appeared to stop breathing, and went limp. Breathing returned spontaneously as the mother moved the baby into various different positions but was still reportedly labored. A comprehensive history was obtained. A comprehensive physical exam in the emergency department revealed only mild tachycardia and increased work of breathing. The patient was transferred to the local pediatric hospital for continued evaluation, with a diagnosis of apparent life threatening event, cyanosis, apnea, rule out respiratory syncytial virus infection, rule out asphyxia by aspiration.

Which of the following diagnoses will be reported?

ICD-9-CM and CPT Code(s):

a. 770.83, 079.6, 933.1, E911, 99284
b. 782.5, 786.03, 799.82, 99285
c. 799.82, 99285
d. 782.5, 799.82, 99291

ICD-10-CM Code(s): _____

9.74. The following documentation is from the health record of a boy with a fracture.

Office Visits

3/31 Office Visit (Primary Care Physician)

S: Peter was playing basketball today, fell, and hurt his wrist.

O: Tenderness and swelling of the wrist, especially the volar aspect. There is a slight abrasion over the swelling. X-ray shows a fracture of the ulnar styloid and possibly the distal radius. There is some question of dorsal displacement of the epiphysis. Short arm cast is applied for comfort measures.

A: Fracture of the ulnar styloid

P: I am going to have the orthopedist look at the x-ray and obtain a consult to determine if reduction is necessary. Return to clinic in 2 days for ortho appt, sooner if problems.

4/1 Office Visit (Primary Care Physician)

S: Peter has pain inside his cast.

O: We thought this was pressure, so I split the cast and it really didn't relieve the pain much at all. I asked him what was hurting about it, and he said it was hurting further up his arm. Then he told me that at the time he had the injury he noticed a great big bulge there. He thought it was the bone poking through, pushed on it, and it sort of went down by itself. His x-ray clearly shows there is no bony injury at that area, but that he has the fracture down by the epiphyseal plate. This is probably a torn muscle.

A: Torn muscle left arm with fracture

P: Keep the appointment with ortho tomorrow. In the meantime, symptomatic care, and we left the cast split because it is probably going to have to be removed for adequate exam tomorrow anyway.

4/2 Office Visit (Primary Care Physician)

S: Peter injured the left wrist playing basketball. He is right-hand dominant. He is currently in a short arm cast, which had been split previously because it was a bit too snug. With the cast he has wrist in extension at least 15 degrees despite the fact that he has the epiphyseal plate fracture with slight posterior displacement of the distal fragment of about 4 mm. He has seen the orthopod in consultation, who felt that this did not require further reduction.

O: He has intact CMS today. Cast is removed, and he is placed in a short arm cast with anterior flexion of about 10 degrees with very slight ulnar deviation. The position of the distal epiphysis of the radius appears to be about the same as it was on the original x-rays taken 1 week ago. This position alignment should be quite satisfactory.

A: Distal radial fracture, Colles' type, with ulnar styloid fracture

P: We will continue with the short arm cast for a duration of 6 weeks. He is to return to see me in 2 weeks for repeat x-ray through the cast and follow up sooner if any problems.

Which of the following is the correct code set to report these visits with the primary care physician?

ICD-9-CM and CPT Code(s):

a. 3/31: 813.43, 25600, A4580
   4/1: 813.43, 840.9, 99024
   4/2: 813.44, 99024, A4580
b. 3/31: 813.43, 29075, A4580
   4/1: 840.9, 813.43, 99213
   4/2: 813.44, 25600, A4580
c. 3/31: 813.43, 25605, A4580
   4/1: 840.9, 813.43, 99213
   4/2: 813.44, 29075, A4580
d. 3/31: 813.43, 29075, A4580
   4/1: 840.9, 813.43, 99213
   4/2: 813.44, 25605, A4580

ICD-10-CM Code(s): _____

9.75.   The following documentation is from the health record of a 14-year-old male patient.

Admission Date:	2/2/XX
Discharge Date:	2/3/XX
Admission Diagnosis:	Peritonsillar abscess
Discharge Diagnoses:	1. Peritonsillar abscess
	2. Chronic tonsillitis
	3. Mononucleosis
	4. Type I diabetes

Reason for Hospitalization: This patient is a 14-year-old white male with a history of right peritonsillar abscess in December who presented with a 4- to 5-day history of progressively increasing sore throat. He had previously been started on amoxicillin as an outpatient, but the severity of his symptoms increased. He presented to the ER on 2/2 with findings consistent with a peritonsillar abscess.

Hospital Course: He was admitted and started on IV Unasyn. Blood glucose levels were drawn and showed only slight hypoglycemia, no doubt as a result of decreased intake due to throat pain. Insulin dosage was adjusted accordingly. An ENT consult was performed, and I&D was recommended. An endocrinology consult was obtained, and he was cleared for surgery. The patient was taken to the operating room that same day. An I&D of the right peritonsillar abscess was performed with a unilateral right tonsillectomy, given his history of recurrent peritonsillar abscesses. The patient was continued on IV antibiotics overnight. The following day, the patient reported significant improvement in his throat pain. He was noted to be afebrile. His Monospot was positive and consistent with acute infectious mononucleosis. Blood glucose levels were adequate. Later, on 2/3, he was seen by the surgeon, who thought he was doing well from a surgical standpoint. The patient was tolerating p.o. well, and the decision was made to discharge the patient home later that same day.

The patient is in satisfactory condition at the time of discharge. Discharge medications include Roxicet p.r.n. for throat pain, Augmentin, and insulin.

He was instructed to comply with a soft diet until further follow-up. Extra time was spent reviewing his insulin regimen and making adjustments (35 minutes with patient and family). Additionally, he was educated about activity restrictions, including no vigorous exercise or contact sports for the next 3 to 4 weeks because of his mononucleosis. The patient was instructed to follow up with the surgeon in 2 weeks.

Which of the following code sets is correct for reporting the attending physician's services on the day of discharge?

ICD-9-CM and CPT Code(s):

a. 475, 474.00, 075, 250.01, 99239
b. 475, 474.00, 075, 250.81, 99238
c. 475, 075, 250.01, 99238
d. 475, 474.0, 075, 250.81, 99239

ICD-10-CM Code(s): _____

Conditions of Pregnancy, Childbirth, and the Puerperium

9.76.   The following documentation is from the health record of a female patient.

Discharge Summary

Admission Date: 03/12/XX

Discharge Date: 03/23/XX

Discharge Diagnoses:
1. Term intrauterine pregnancy, delivered, single liveborn
2. Maternal obesity
3. Iron deficiency anemia
4. Retained placenta
5. Endometritis

Procedures Performed: Right paramedian episiotomy, low outlet forceps vaginal delivery, repair of right paramedian episiotomy with repair of partial fourth-degree extension, manual removal of placenta 3/13/XX. Dilatation and suction curettage 3/22/XX.

Hospital Course: This patient presented at 39 weeks' gestation with rupture of membranes of clear fluid. She was not in active labor, her cervix was unfavorable for induction. She was initially managed expectantly, and oxytocin was used to facilitate labor. She progressed throughout the active phase of labor without complications. The fetal evaluations were reassuring throughout the labor process.

The fetal head presented on the perineum in the OA position; because of maternal exhaustion and inability to allow further descent because there was a single nuchal cord released, low outlet forceps were placed after right paramedian episiotomy was performed, and the fetal head was delivered without difficulty. Upon delivery, there was a partial fourth-degree extension just through the anal mucosa. There was retained placenta and manual extraction was required. The episiotomy was repaired by using 000 VICRYL suture, closing the rectal mucosa.

The postpartum course was complicated by the patient developing endometritis. The patient was placed on IV antibiotics and showed some sign of improvement with a dropping white blood cell count; however, her temperature continued to spike. An initial ultrasound revealed some intrauterine products that appeared to be retained placenta. The following day, however, she passed these retained products without difficulty, and her bleeding subsided. Her temperature, however, continued to develop intermittent fever, the antibiotics were switched to the IV, and she again showed a good clinical response with decreased uterine tenderness. Because of the fever continuing, however, a follow-up ultrasound was performed, and no placental products were appreciated. However, there were some clots and unidentifiable tissues still remaining in the intrauterine cavity. Thus, a dilatation and curettage was performed on 3/22/XX, and some amniotic membranes were removed, which appeared to be infected. There were no placental products noted in the curettage.

After removal of the amniotic membrane, her temperature defervesced, and she remained afebrile throughout the remainder of the hospitalization. On discharge, she was tolerating a regular diet, ambulatory without complaints, very scant vaginal spotting, and on oral antibiotics.

It should be noted that because of the excessive blood loss she was given two units of transfused blood to maintain hemoglobin levels from 8 to 9. She was asymptomatic with this hemoglobin, and thus was placed on iron and Colace therapy throughout the remainder of her hospitalization.

Discharge Medications: Include iron sulfate, Colace, and Augmentin

Which of the following is the correct code set, presuming this physician provided the antepartum and postpartum care?

ICD-9-CM and CPT Code(s):

a. 667.02, 670.02, 664.31, 663.31, V27.0; 648.22, 280.0, 59400, 59160-78
b. 667.04, 670.02, 664.31, 663.31, V27.0; 648.22, 280.0, 59400, 59300-51, 58120-78
c. 667.02, 664.31, 663.31, V27.0; 59400, 59300, 59160
d. 667.04, 670.02, 664.31, V27.0; 59400, 58120

ICD-10-CM Code(s): _____

9.77.   The following documentation is from the health record of a female patient.

Anesthesia: IV sedation by CRNA, combined with paracervical block

Preop DX: Anembryonic gestation

Operation: Suction curettage

Postop DX: Anembryonic gestation

History: Problem list includes G4, P2, L2, and missed abortion. Patient has asthma with medications including albuterol p.r.n.

Findings: The laminaria that had been placed in the office yesterday had dilated the cervix, which easily fit a #20 Hanks dilator. The uterus sounded 12 cm. The uterus was 10-week size. There was a moderate amount of tissue obtained from the uterine cavity.

Procedure: Under satisfactory intravenous medication, the patient was prepped and draped in the dorsolithotomy position. A speculum was placed. Paracervical block was administered. The laminaria was removed. Using a #9 rigid curved Vacurette, curettage was performed. There was good clamping down effect of the uterus. The intrauterine contents were expelled. There were no complications of the procedure. There was a satisfactory amount of bleeding following the procedure. Estimated blood loss was negligible.

Path report demonstrates histological sections of the uterine contents, which show multiple chorionic villi. This is accompanied by fragments of decidualized tissue and gestational-type endometrium. These histological findings represent products of conception.

Which of the following code sets would be reported for this procedure?

ICD-9-CM and CPT Code(s):

a. 632, 493.90, 59820, 59200-51
b. 630, 493.90, 59870
c. 631, 59856, 59200
d. 631, 493.90, 59820

ICD-10-CM Code(s): _____

Disorders of the Respiratory System

9.78. A patient is seen in the office with increasing shortness of breath, weakness, and ineffective cough. This patient is seen frequently for this chronic condition. Orders were given for a chest x-ray and lab work. Antibiotics were also prescribed. This patient already is on oxygen at home. The physician will try to manage this patient at home, according to his wishes. A detailed history was done with an expanded problem-focused exam and medical decision making of moderate complexity. Diagnoses were listed as acute respiratory insufficiency and acute exacerbation of COPD. Which of the following is the correct code assignment?

ICD-9-CM and CPT Code(s):

a. 491.21, 518.82, 99214
b. 518.81, 491.21, 99213
c. 518.82, 491.21, 99203
d. 491.21, 99214

ICD-10-CM Code(s): _____

9.79. A patient has recurrent polyposis with right pansinusitis and left anterior polyposis with blocked maxillary ostiomeatal units on both sides. The surgeon performs a bilateral intranasal sphenoethmoidectomy and maxillary antrostomy with polypectomy.

The patient was placed under general anesthesia and appropriately prepped and draped. The nose was anesthetized with cocaine flakes, 200 to 300 mg, and topical adrenaline 1:1000. A large polyposis on the right side was removed to gain access for more vasoconstriction using a Robert's snare. Injections of Xylocaine and epinephrine were also used, and the procedure was essentially the same on both sides.

On the left side, there was extensive scarring of the middle turbinate, so through-cutting punches were used to open up the ethmoidectomy bilaterally. While manipulating the left middle turbinate, there was a small CSF leak noted at the junction of the turbinate with the equivaform area. No instrumentation had been done in this area, and it was only a slitlike small leak. This was packed with topical Gelfoam and topical thrombin with Gelfoam at the end of the case and held onto the pack. The nasal antral windows were opened bilaterally and were cannulated, using the right-angle ethmoid curet until palpation showed the natural ostium of the maxillary sinus. The uncinate process was still there from the previous surgery, and this was removed with back-biting forceps and opened into the maxillary sinus widely.

Both sphenoides were widely opened. There was an adhesion from the head of the middle turbinate to the nasal septum on the left side, and this was lysed. A Cottle speculum and the through-cutting forceps were used throughout the case as well as the 1.7-power-magnification operating microscope. The patient had a moderate bout of bleeding bilaterally that was controlled with towel clip pledgets of 1:10,000 of adrenaline. Silastic splints were placed on both sides of the nose to prevent adhesions and were sewn in with 4-0 Prolene sutures. Expandable foam packs were then placed and expanded with 1 g and 10 cc of Ancef. The procedure was then terminated with estimated blood loss at 300 cc for the entire case. The patient tolerated the procedure well and there were no CSF leaks found at the end of the procedure.

Which diagnosis and procedure codes are assigned for this procedure performed in the outpatient surgical department of the hospital?

ICD-9-CM and CPT Code(s):

a. 473.8, 471.8, 349.81, 31201-50, 31051-50, 31020-50
b. 473.8, 471.8, 998.2, E870.0, E849.7, 31201-50, 31051-50, 31020-50
c. 478.19, 473.8, 31267-50, 31288-50, 31254-50
d. 473.8, 471.8, 998.11, 998.2, E870.0, E849.7, 31090-50

ICD-10-CM Code(s): _____

9.80. A patient with bilateral partial vocal cord paralysis requires removal of the arytenoid cartilage to improve breathing. Following a temporary tracheostomy, a topical anesthetic is applied to the oral cavity, pharynx, and larynx, and the laryngoscope with operating microscope is inserted. After adequate visualization is established, the arytenoid cartilage is exposed by excision of the mucosa overlying it. The procedure is performed in the outpatient surgery center of the hospital. Which diagnosis and procedure codes are going to be reported for this procedure?

ICD-9-CM and CPT Code(s):

a. 478.33, 31561, 31600
b. 478.30, 31560
c. 478.33, 31561
d. 478.33, 31560, 69990

ICD-10-CM Code(s): _____

9.81. A 54-year-old male patient with bronchial carcinoma, right lower lobe, has an obstructed bronchus in the right lower lobe of the lung. The pulmonologist views the airway using a bronchoscope introduced through the oral airway following administration of conscious sedation. Thirty minutes of moderate sedation services were performed. The obstruction is identified with the assistance of fluoroscopic guidance. A laser probe is introduced through the bronchoscope to eradicate the obstruction and relieve the stenosis. The procedure was performed in the physician's clinic/surgery center. What codes are reported for physician services for the procedure performed at the outpatient ambulatory surgery center?

ICD-9-CM and CPT Code(s):

a. 162.5, 31641, 99144
b. 162.5, 31641, 76001
c. 239.1, 31640, 99144-51
d. 239.1, 31641, 99144, 76001

ICD-10-CM Code(s): _____

9.82. A 78-year-old-patient is scheduled for a transbronchial needle aspiration biopsy with fluoroscopic guidance for a lung mass. Following the administration of conscious sedation by the anesthetist, the patient experiences a run of atrial fibrillation, and the physician elects to terminate the procedure before the biopsy is obtained. The procedure is done in the hospital's same-day surgery department.

Which of the following shows correct code assignment for physician services?

ICD-9-CM and CPT Code(s):

a. 239.1, V64.1, 31629, 76000
b. 786.6, 427.31, 31629-52
c. 786.6, 427.31, V64.1, 31628-53
d. 786.6, 427.31, V64.1, 31629-53

ICD-10-CM Code(s): _____

9.83. A patient is admitted to have a thoracoscopic lobectomy performed. The patient has a malignant neoplasm of the left lower lobe. Because of extensive pleural effusion, the physician was unable to complete the endoscopic procedure. They converted to an open technique, and a successful lobectomy was performed. What are the correct procedure codes?

a. 32480, 32663-53
b. 32663, 32480
c. 32480
d. 32484, 32663-52

9.84. The following documentation is from the health record of a two-year-old boy seen in the pediatric clinic.

Chief Complaint: Difficulty breathing.

History of Present Illness: Patient is a two-year-old black male with a one-day history of difficulty breathing and a cough. No fever or chills. He otherwise has been acting normally.

Past Medical History: Unremarkable. No history of asthma.

Medications: Over-the-counter cough medicine.

Allergies: None.

Physical Examination
General: Alert, playful black male in no apparent distress.
Vitals: Temperature 98.5°F; pulse 125; respiration 28; blood pressure 95/64.
Head, Ears, Eyes,
Nose, and Throat: Conjunctivae clear. Pupils are equal and reactive to light.
                        Tympanic membranes normal. Oropharynx negative.
Neck: Supple without adenopathy.
Heart: Regular. No murmurs or gallops noted.

Lungs:	Breath sounds equal bilaterally with mild wheezing. Minimal retractions.
Abdomen:	Benign.

Diagnosis: Acute bronchitis with bronchospasm.

Disposition and Plan: The patient was given two breathing treatments and his wheezing cleared. He was no longer retracting. He was discharged home on albuterol syrup 3/4 teaspoon q 8 hours; Amoxil 250 mg per 5 mL one teaspoon three times a day. Follow-up in two to three days with primary care physician. Return if worse.

Which of the following is the correct code set for this physician?

ICD-9-CM Code(s):

a. 466.0
b. 466.0, 519.11
c. 519.11
d. 466.19

ICD-10-CM Code(s): _____

Trauma and Poisoning

9.85. An adult patient is seen in the emergency department after sustaining second- and third-degree burns of the chest and both upper and lower arm after pulling a pan of boiling soup out of the microwave onto his right side while cooking dinner at home. The burn size was documented as 18 cm × 24 cm on the chest, and 26 cm × 8 cm on the right arm. The chest burn was full thickness and the arm burn was partial thickness. The total size was estimated to be about 11% third degree of the total body surface area. Due to the associated pain, local anesthesia, including IM Demerol, was administered. The wound was debrided, and a sterile dressing was applied. The patient was transferred to a local burn unit for further treatment.

What are the correct code assignments for this procedure as reported and billed by the ED physician, who performed a detailed medical history, performed an expanded problem-focused physical examination to rule out other injuries, and rendered moderately complex medical decision making before undertaking the burn care?

ICD-9-CM and CPT Code(s):

a. 942.32, 943.29, 948.10, E924.0, E849.0, E015.2, E000.8, 99283-25, 16030
b. 942.32, 948.00, E924.0, E000.8, 16025
c. 942.23, 942.33, E924.0, E015.2, 99284, 16025
d. 942.22, 943.20, 948.10, E924.0, 11000, 11001

ICD-10-CM Code(s): _____

9.86. A motorcyclist is brought into the emergency department after a motorcycle accident. The ED physician confirms an open tibia (proximal) fracture and performs extensive debridement of gravel, glass, and other matter, down to and including part of the muscle, at the site of the fracture in preparation for surgery. The orthopedic surgeon then takes the patient to surgery to perform the reduction of the fracture, and the patient is subsequently admitted to the hospital.

In addition to the evaluation and management service, what is the correct code assignment for the ED physician's services?

ICD-9-CM and CPT Code(s):

a. 823.10, E819.2, 27535, 11011-51
b. 823.12, E819.2, 11043
c. 823.10, E819.2, 11011
d. 823.90, E819.2, 27535, 11043-51

ICD-10-CM Code(s): _____

9.87. A 35-year-old patient was a passenger on a motorcycle involved in an accident and sustained three severely broken ribs and a fractured femur. Chest x-ray showed a 45 percent collapse of the left lung and air in the pleural space. The patient complained of increasing shortness of breath and was cyanotic. A chest tube was inserted into the third intercostal space by the emergency department physician. A subsequent chest x-ray showed marked improvement to only 5 percent collapse. The patient was thoroughly evaluated by the ED physician for possible internal injuries. The ED physician documented a comprehensive history, comprehensive physical examination, and complex medical decision making. The final diagnosis was tension pneumothorax; fractured femur, midshaft; and multiple rib fractures. The patient was taken to surgery by the on-call orthopedic surgeon to care for the fractured femur sustained in the accident.

Which of the following is the correct code set for reporting the ED physician's services?

ICD-9-CM and CPT Code(s):

a. 512.0, 821.01, 807.03, E819.3; 99284-25, 32551
b. 860.0, 821.01, 807.03, E819.3; 99285-25, 32551
c. 860.0, 821.00, 807.09, E819.3; 99285, 32422
d. 512.0, 821.00, 807.09, E819.3; 99284, 32422

ICD-10-CM Code(s): _____

9.88. A patient was seen in the emergency department for an intentional overdose of barbiturates and acetaminophen. The patient was stabilized medically and transferred to the psychiatric unit for further treatment.

Excluding External Cause Status, Activity, and Place of Occurrence codes, what diagnosis codes would be reported by the ED physician?

ICD-9-CM Code(s):

a. 965.4, E950.0
b. 968.3, E950.4
c. 969.3, E938.3, 965.4, E950.0
d. 967.0, E950.1, 965.4, E950.0

ICD-10-CM Code(s): _____

9.89. A patient arrived in the emergency department in full cardiopulmonary arrest following a gunshot wound to the chest. He was intubated, and large-bore IVs of lactated Ringer's solution were started in each arm. A STAT type and cross-match was ordered, along with six units of PRBCs. Dr. Jones, a private trauma surgeon, was on call and was present in the ED when the patient arrived. The patient's chest was opened, and cardiac massage was begun. Despite all efforts at resuscitation, the patient expired of massive blood loss after approximately 85 minutes in the ED.

What CPT codes will be reported by Dr. Jones?

a. 99291, 99292, 32160, 31500
b. 99291, 99292, 32160
c. 99291, 99292, 31500-51
d. 99291, 32160, 31500

9.90. A surgeon performs an evacuation of an epidural hematoma. The physician incises the scalp and peels it away from the area to be drilled. After drilling a burr hole in the cranium and identifying the hematoma via CT scan, the hematoma is decompressed and bleeding is controlled. The hematoma is located outside the dura just under the periosteum. The scalp is repositioned and sutured into place. The patient tolerates the procedure well and is sent to recovery.

What is the correct code set for physician reporting of this procedure?

ICD-9-CM and CPT Code(s):

a. 852.40, 61154
b. 853.00, 61108
c. 852.40, 61156
d. 853.00, 61156

ICD-10-CM Code(s): _____

9.91. The following documentation is from the health record of a 19-month-old with a burn.

Preoperative Diagnosis: Full-thickness burn with deep necrosis and limb loss involving bilateral lower extremities and posterior buttocks area

Postoperative Diagnosis: Full-thickness burn with deep necrosis and limb loss involving bilateral lower extremities and posterior buttocks area and a small portion of the left flank

Procedure Performed: Cultured skin placement to bilateral lower extremities and right buttock with autografting to bilateral buttocks and left flank and a small portion of the left stump. Total area covered was 1,030 cm^2, of which 720 cm^2 was cultured skin.

Anesthesia: General

Estimated Blood Loss: 100 mL

IV Fluids: 250 mL of Normosol
140 mL of blood
350 mL of Pitkin

Urine Output: 42 mL

Indications for Procedure: The patient is a 19-month-old male who has undergone multiple excision and grafting procedures in the past for a 72 percent total body surface area (TBSA) burn (50% third degree). He most recently underwent removal of allograft on his bilateral extremities and buttocks area in preparation for skin grafting today. He also has a small area on his left flank where he has not received grafting in the past for which he will also receive skin if sufficient skin is available. His grandmother is present and knows the initial attempt will be to see if the cultured skin is sufficient to cover everything without donor site. However, given the recent fact that 900 cm^2 was reduced to 700 cm^2 and 20 cm^2, this may not be sufficient and the donor site will then be taken from the scalp and lower abdomen. The grandmother is aware of risks and we are proceeding today.

Description of Procedure: After successful induction of general anesthesia, time out for patient identification and surgery planned, the patient was placed in the supine position. His dressings were removed to level of the red rubber catheter.

A 0 Prolene was placed into the bilateral stumps in order to allow for easy access to the lower extremities with elevation. The dressings were removed down and revealed a nice healthy base. Hemostasis was obtained using Epinephrine-soaked laparotomy pads as well as electrocautery. Cultures were taken from the left lower extremity for the cultured skin study as well as biopsies from the past autograft of the lower abdomen and cultured skin. The cultured skin was placed in serial fashion along each of the lower extremities with coverage attained with all but a small portion of the left lower extremity stump. Three pieces remained which will be placed on the abdomen, but since donor site will be necessary, the skin was then harvested from the upper scalp and lower abdomen after Pitkin infiltration using the Padgett dermatome at a thickness of 0.015 inches. Once complete, this was meshed

2:1 and the donor sites were covered with Kaltostat and dry gauze. The patient was then flipped into the prone position. Dressings were removed and patient was re-prepped and draped and then the final dressing lying over the base was removed revealing a nice healthy base. Hemostasis was obtained again with electrocautery and Epinephrine-soaked laparotomy pads. When complete, the meshed skin was placed over the defect and the remaining three pieces of cultured skin on the right upper buttock area. These were all secured with surgical staples and covered with a layer of fine mesh gauze, burn gauze, red rubber catheters, burn gauze and a spandex stent. A small piece of skin was placed onto the left flank where Bacitracin and sterile nonadherent dressing was used as coverage due to the small size. The patient was then returned to the supine position with no shearing of the cultured skin. The distal area on the left stump was covered with meshed graft with a final dressing being attained using a layer of fine mesh gauze, burn gauze, red rubber catheter, burn gauze, and Ace wrap for the right lower extremity, then a Spandex stent for the left lower extremity in order to keep the upper thigh protected and avoid maceration.

Which codes does this surgeon assign?

ICD-9-CM and CPT Code(s):

a. 945.50, 942.44, 942.43, 11100-59, 15150, 15151, 15152 × 7, 15100, 15101 × 3
b. 945.50, 942.49, 11100-59, 15150, 15151, 15152 × 7, 15100, 15101 × 3
c. 945.50, 942.44, 942.43, 11100, 15150, 15151, 15152 × 7, 15100, 15101 × 3
d. 945.50, 942.44, 942.43, 11100-59, 15150, 15151, 15152, 15100, 15101 × 3

ICD-10-CM Code(s): _____

Part IV
Coding Challenge

Chapter 10

Coding Challenge: Nonacute Settings; ICD-10-CM and ICD-10-PCS Code Sets; CPT Modifiers, HCPCS Level II Modifiers

Note: Even though the specific cases are divided by setting, most of the information pertaining to the diagnosis is applicable to most settings. If you practice or apply codes in a particular type of setting, you may find additional information in other sections of this publication that may be pertinent to you.

Every effort has been made to follow current recognized coding guidelines and principles, as well as nationally recognized reporting guidelines. The material presented may differ from some health plan requirements for reporting. The ICD-9-CM code sets utilized are the 2011 codes that are in effect October 1, 2011, through September 30, 2012. The ICD-10-CM/PCS code sets utilized are the 2011 draft codes published in 2011, and the HCPCS (CPT and HCPCS II) codes are in effect January 1, 2011, through December 31, 2011. The current standard transactions and code sets named in HIPAA have been utilized, which require ICD-9-CM Volume III procedure codes for inpatients.

Instructions: Assign all applicable codes appropriate for the setting for the case studies presented. Some of the cases provide multiple-choice answers, and the reader must select the appropriate code set. In other instances, the reader is expected to assign codes without any prompts.

The scenarios are based on selected excerpts from health records without reproducing the entire health record. However, in practice, the coding professional should have access to the entire health record. Health records are analyzed and codes are selected only with the physician's complete and appropriate documentation available. According to coding guidelines, codes are not assigned without physician documentation.

The objective of the cases and scenarios reproduced in this publication is to provide practice in assigning correct codes, not necessarily to emulate actual health record analysis. For example, the reader may be asked to assign codes based only on an operative report or discharge summary. Labeled excerpts are used as source documentation for coding skill practice.

Home Health

10.1.   A patient is being followed for postoperative care after surgery for a bleeding gastric ulcer. What code would be assigned in M0230?

    a. V code for aftercare of surgery
    b. Bleeding gastric ulcer
    c. Traumatic wound of abdomen
    d. None of the above

10.2.   This 85-year-old female lives alone. She recently was in the hospital with aspiration pneumonia. There are infiltrates still present on the chest x-ray, and home healthcare is focused on the treatment of the pneumonia. She also has type II diabetes mellitus. She had partial colectomy last year for acute diverticulitis. What diagnosis would be reported in M0240?

    a. Aspiration pneumonia
    b. Diverticulitis
    c. Diabetes mellitus
    d. Acute diverticulitis and diabetes mellitus

10.3.   This patient had colon resection because of carcinoma of the transverse colon. He has skilled nursing services for management of the surgical wound, which has a surgical drain not scheduled to be removed for several days. He lives alone and has right hemiplegia after a stroke. What code is reported in M0230?

    a. 438.20
    b. 153.1
    c. V58.42
    d. V58.31

10.4.   A 72-year-old female patient recently had rectal resection for rectal cancer. She is scheduled for radiation and chemotherapy treatments. Home health services will provide visits four times per week to teach colostomy care and assess compliance with medication. What coding is the best?

    a. M0230: V58.42; M0240: 154.1, V55.3
    b. M0230: V55.3; M0240: 154.1, V58.42
    c. M0230: 154.1; M0240: V55.3, V58.42
    d. M0230: V55.3; M0240: V10.06, V58.42

10.5.   What code is assigned for a patient who had prostate cancer two years ago? He underwent a proctectomy and received chemotherapy. He has had no treatment in the past year. How is the cancer reported in M0240?

    a. 185
    b. V10.46
    c. V16.42
    d. The status of the cancer would not be reported.

10.6. This 80-year-old female patient recently had cholecystectomy for chronic cholecystitis and cholelithiasis. She developed postoperative infection and is being seen for monitoring of antibiotics, vital signs, and observation of the wound, with frequent surgical wound dressing changes. What code is assigned in M0230?

   a. 998.59
   b. V58.31
   c. 879.2
   d. 574.10

10.7. Patient is status post total hip replacement secondary to localized osteoarthritis and was experiencing problems with ambulation and gait following hip surgery. The patient was discharged with home health services twice weekly. Home care was ordered for wound care. The patient also received physical therapy for gait training and strengthening to increase the patient's ability to ambulate. How should this encounter be coded? **Note:** Include codes for M0230, M0240, and M0246 (if applicable). _____

10.8. The patient is a 75-year-old man with chronic stasis ulcer of the leg, but he also has two diabetic toe ulcers at this time. Patient has chronic lower extremity edema, CHF, HTN. He has daily caregivers through the Medicaid program. The nurse is seeing him four times per week to change leg dressings (using Polymem and covering with stretch bandage), monitor/adjust medications, teach medication management, teach caregivers to provide a low-sodium diet, and keep leg elevated. The nurse hopes to teach a neighbor to change the dressing at least once per week. Physical therapy is ordered every other week for exercise, transfer training, and gait training. Patient ambulates minimally, only with close assistance and a walker. He needs assistance with all ADLs. What codes are assigned? **Note:** Include codes for M0230, M0240, and M0246 (if applicable). _____

10.9. A 69-year-old right-handed woman is discharged from the hospital four days after a left modified radical mastectomy for breast cancer. Her only medications are oral tamoxifen and pain medications. She is scheduled to begin chemotherapy in the next two weeks. Skilled nursing is prescribed for management of the surgical wound, including dressing changes. The surgical drain is not scheduled to be removed for several days. The patient lives alone and has residual dysfunction of her right arm due to monoplegia after a stroke. The nurse will also supervise the patient's performance of the exercises ordered to improve her shoulder range of motion on the affected side and to monitor for the development of lymphedema in her arm. What codes are assigned? **Note:** Include codes for M0230, M0240, and M0246 (if applicable). _____

10.10. Section I of the *Official Guidelines for Coding and Reporting* must be followed for:

   a. Hospital inpatients
   b. Physician services
   c. Home health agencies
   d. All of the above

10.11. A 74-year-old patient was discharged from the hospital after surgical amputation of the right foot due to diabetic osteomyelitis. The patient has type II diabetes. She was admitted to home healthcare for wound care consisting of assessment for signs and symptoms of a wound infection, instructing the patient and her husband on wound care, and surgical wound dressing changes. She will also receive physical therapy to improve her gait. What codes are assigned? **Note:** Include codes for M0230, M0240, and M0246 (if applicable).

_____

10.12. An 89-year-old man fell in his home, sustaining a right hip fracture. An open reduction with internal fixation was performed six days ago. The patient was discharged home, where his daughter now cares for him. The patient does not bear weight on the right lower extremity but can perform supervised pivot transfers with contact guard assistance in and out of bed. The physician orders the agency to provide physical therapy for gait training and exercise three times per week for five weeks. What codes are assigned? **Note:** Include codes for M0230, M0240, and M0246 (if applicable). _____

10.13. What code(s) is/are assigned for a patient receiving home care after a kidney transplant?

   a. V58.44
   b. V58.44, V42.0
   c. 585.6
   d. V42.0

10.14. How many categories are there for skin disorders in the HH-PPS?

   a. One
   b. Two
   c. Three
   d. Four

ICD-10-CM and ICD-10-PCS

Introduction

HIM professionals across the country will lead the transition from ICD-9-CM to ICD-10-CM and ICD-10-PCS. In preparation they need to take steps to become experts on how ICD-10-CM and ICD-10-PCS differ from ICD-9-CM. Coding professionals will need to become proficient in coding with the ICD-10 systems. The following exercises are designed to increase your familiarity with ICD-10-CM and ICD-10-PCS.

Selected sections of the code sets are included with the exercises where possible. Current drafts of the ICD-10-CM index and tabular volumes are available on the Web site for the National Center for Health Statistics (NCHS). You may download the volumes at http://www.cdc.gov/nchs/icd/icd10cm.htm.

The current draft of both the ICD-10-CM and ICD-10-PCS coding system and Official Coding Guidelines are available on the Web site for the Centers for Medicare and Medicaid Services (CMS). You may access this information at http://www.cms.gov/ICD10/.

ICD-10-CM

10.15. A myocardial infarction is considered acute for _____ weeks according to the ICD-10-CM *Official Guidelines for Coding and Reporting*.

    a. 2
    b. 4
    c. 6
    d. 8

10.16. Which of the following conditions is not represented by a code from the J44 category?

    a. Asthma with chronic obstructive pulmonary disease
    b. Chronic bronchitis with emphysema
    c. Chronic emphysematous bronchitis
    d. Emphysema

10.17. ICD-10-CM codes will be utilized by all healthcare settings to assign diagnosis codes.

    a. True
    b. False

10.18. What would be the appropriate ICD-10-CM code for lumbar stenosis?

    a. M48.00
    b. M48.06
    c. M48.07
    d. M48.26

10.19. Assign the appropriate ICD-10-CM diagnosis code(s) for cataract due to hypoparathyroidism.

    a. E88.9, H28
    b. H28
    c. E20.9, H28
    d. H28, E20.9

10.20. Assign the appropriate ICD-10-CM diagnosis code for aspiration pneumonia due to inhalation of food.

    a. J15.9
    b. J69.0
    c. J18.9
    d. J69.1

ICD-10-PCS

10.21. ICD-10-PCS is based on a seven-character alphanumeric code. The meaning of each individual character changes according to the needs of the clinical section.

a. True
b. False

10.22. Recall that the first character of an ICD-10-PCS code specifies the section within ICD-10-PCS. Using the list of ICD-10-PCS sections provided below, identify the first character that would be assigned to the following procedures.

Sections of ICD-10-PCS

0	Medical and surgical
1	Obstetrics
2	Placement
3	Administration
4	Measurement and monitoring
5	Extracorporeal assistance and performance
6	Extracorporeal therapies
7	Osteopathic
8	Other procedures
9	Chiropractic
B	Imaging
C	Nuclear medicine
D	Radiation oncology
F	Physical rehabilitation and diagnostic audiology
G	Mental health
H	Substance abuse treatment

a. _____ Cranioplasty
b. _____ Cholecystectomy
c. _____ Gait training
d. _____ Computerized tomography, spine
e. _____ Application of lower extremity pressure dressing
f. _____ Acupuncture

10.23. Using the list of ICD-10-PCS root operations provided below, identify the root operation used to describe each of the procedures in items a through k.

ICD-10-PCS Medical and Surgical Root Operations

0	Alteration	H	Insertion
1	Bypass	J	Inspection
2	Change	K	Map
3	Control	L	Occlusion
4	Creation	M	Reattachment
5	Destruction	N	Release
6	Detachment	P	Removal
7	Dilation	Q	Repair
8	Division	R	Replacement
9	Drainage	S	Reposition
A	Alteration	T	Resection
B	Excision	U	Supplement
C	Extirpation	V	Restriction
D	Extraction	W	Revision
F	Fragmentation	X	Transfer
G	Fusion	Y	Transplantation

a. _____ Kidney transplant

b. _____ Total nephrectomy

c. _____ Diagnostic bronchoscopy

d. _____ Lithotripsy, bladder stone

e. _____ Varicose vein stripping

f. _____ Fallopian tube ligation

g. _____ Face lift

h. _____ Pyloromyotomy

i. _____ Adhesiolysis

j. _____ Adjustment of hip prosthesis

k. _____ Urinary catheter change

10.24. Match the approach term with the correct definition.

ICD-10-PCS Character-Approach

0   Open

3   Percutaneous

4   Percutaneous endoscopic

7   Via natural or artificial opening

8   Via natural or artificial opening endoscopic

F   Via natural or artificial opening with percutaneous endoscopic assistance

X   External

Definitions

a. _____ Entry, by puncture or minor incision, of instrumentation through the skin or mucous membrane and any other body layers necessary to reach the site of the procedure.

b. _____ Entry of instrumentation through a natural or artificial external opening to reach the site of the procedure.

c. _____ Cutting through the skin or mucous membrane and any other body layers necessary to expose the body site of the procedure.

d. _____ Entry of instrumentation through a natural or artificial external opening to reach and visualize the site of the procedure, and entry, by puncture or minor incision, of instrumentation through the skin or mucous membrane and any other body layers necessary to aid in the performance of the procedure.

e. _____ Entry, by puncture or minor incision, of instrumentation through the skin or mucous membrane and any other body layers necessary to reach and visualize the site of the procedure.

f. _____ Entry of instrumentation through a natural or artificial external opening to reach and visualize the site of the procedure.

g. _____ Procedures performed directly on the skin or mucous membrane and procedures performed indirectly by the application of external force through the skin or mucous membrane.

10.25. Using the definitions listed in item 10.24 above, match the following:

Procedure
a. ____ Total abdominal hysterectomy
b. ____ Needle biopsy of the pancreas
c. ____ Endotracheal intubation
d. ____ Arthroscopy

Approach
1. Via natural or artificial opening
2. Open
3. Percutaneous endoscopic
4. Percutaneous

10.26. What is the correct ICD-10-PCS code for a total right knee arthroplasty with insertion of total knee prosthesis? _____

ICD-10-CM/PCS Application Exercise

10.27. You are a coding professional at General Medical Center. One of your responsibilities includes responding to requests for coded data. Facility data in the registry has been coded in ICD-10-CM and ICD-10-PCS for two years. Prior to that, data was coded in ICD-9-CM. You receive requests for data that spans the most recent five years for the following cases. How will you find all applicable cases in the registry for these two requests?

a. Request for cases with an initial acute myocardial infarction of the anterior wall: _____

_____

b. Request for cases with exploration of the common bile duct during an open cholecystectomy: _____

_____

10.28. Code the following operative report using ICD-10-PCS.

Preoperative Diagnosis: Left breast mammographic abnormality.

Postoperative Diagnosis: Same.

Operation: Left breast biopsy with needle localization.

Estimated Blood Loss: Minimal.

Complications: None.

Procedure: The patient was taken to the Operating Room and placed in the supine position and after induction of endotracheal anesthesia, the left breast was prepped using Betadine solution and draped in a sterile fashion.

A transverse incision was made in the left breast medial to the insertion point of the needle. Incision was taken to the subcutaneous layers and the tissue surrounding the guidewire was excised using electrocautery. The amount of tissue excised measured approximately 3 × 2 cm and was submitted for specimen radiography. This was performed and demonstrated a portion of the nodule in question to be in specimen and this was further submitted for a frozen section diagnosis.

With this in mind, the deeper layers of the incision were closed with interrupted 000 Vicryl. The skin was closed with subcuticular 0000 Vicryl and a sterile dressing was applied.

The patient was taken to PACU in good condition after having tolerated this procedure well.

Code(s): _____

10.29. Code the following using ICD-10-PCS.

Preoperative Diagnosis:

Postoperative Diagnosis:

Operation: Transurethral resection of the prostate.

Anesthesia: Spinal.

Procedure: After operative consent, the patient was brought to the operating room and placed on the table in the supine position. With spinal anesthesia induced, the patient was converted to the dorsolithotomy position. The genital area was prepped and draped in the usual and sterile fashion. A 26 French continuous flow resectoscope sheath was inserted per urethra into the bladder with the obturator in place. The obturator was removed and the resectoscope was seated within its sheath. The bladder was visualized. The ureteral orifices were identified. The resectoscope was pulled to the distal portion of the verumontanum and turned to the 12 o'clock position and resection was begun. Resection was carried circumferentially around the glans channeling a large channel. Hemostasis was obtained by means of electrocoagulation. There were no major venous sinuses or capsular perforations encountered. The verumontanum was left intact. After completion of resection, the bladder was evacuated of residual prostatic chips using the Ellik evacuator. The bladder was then visualized. There were no residual chips identified. Ureteral orifices were intact and uninjured. The bladder neck and prostatic fossa were widely patent. Final hemostasis was obtained by means of electrocoagulation and the resectoscope was removed. A 22 French, 3 way, 30 cc Foley catheter was inserted per urethra into the bladder with ease. It was irrigated until clear. It was placed on light traction with continuous bladder irrigation with sterile water and the patient was transported to the recovery room in stable condition.

Code(s): _____

10.30. Code the following operative report using ICD-10-PCS.

Preoperative Diagnosis: Immediately postpartal; desiring sterility.

Postoperative Diagnosis: Same.

Operation: Tubal ligation.

Blood Loss: Negligible.

Blood Replaced: None.

Drains: None.

Procedure: With the patient under an adequate epidural anesthetic, the periumbilical area was prepped with Betadine and sterile drapes were applied.

The abdomen was entered through a small umbilical incision. The fallopian tubes were identified bilaterally and traced to their fimbriated ends. A knuckle of tube was ligated bilaterally with 0 chromic. The tubes were also ligated proximally and distally with 00 Ethibond. A small portion of tube was resected bilaterally. Hemostasis was adequate.

The peritoneum and fascia were closed together with 00 Vicryl. The skin was closed with 000 Vicryl. A sterile dressing was applied.

The patient tolerated the procedure well and was sent to the PACU in good condition.

Code(s): _____

10.31. Code the following using ICD-10-PCS.

Preoperative Diagnosis: Bronchial alveolar cell carcinoma of the left lung.

Postoperative Diagnosis: Same.

Operation: Exploratory left thoracotomy. Left pneumonectomy.

Procedures: This patient was operated on under general endotracheal anesthesia. We had a double lumen tube in where we could selectively ventilate both lungs. He was in the lateral decubitus position. We used a standard posterior lateral left thoracotomy incision and the chest was opened. There was one adhesion to the apical area which was not neoplastic in any manner. I took this down and we were able to easily mobilize the lung. There was a large diffuse lesion in the left upper lobe periphery. I really did not know what to do with this. The lesion had previously been biopsied, and we thought we were dealing with a bronchial alveolar cell. The man did have a past history of non-Hodgkin's lymphoma years ago which was presumably cured. I began dissecting on the pulmonary artery to look at things to see what kind of fissure I had developed, but the inner lobar branches were just too dense, that is, there was no fissure basically and I knew if I did a lobectomy it was really entering the tumor area peripherally. I therefore went ahead and elected to do a left pneumonectomy since his pulmonary function studies were satisfactory pre-op, and this was the best thing I thought. The main pulmonary artery was divided between a vascular staple gun. Dissection was a little tenuous. The artery seemed quite friable but it held nicely. I then reinforced this with a large Chromic tie. We divided the superior and inferior pulmonary vein and prepared for clamping of the bronchus. This completed the pneumonectomy. He lost some blood due to a bleeding adhesion up above which was not recognized until he had about a half a unit of blood in the left upper chest. This was suctioned clean and we transfused him with 2 units of packed cells. He tolerated the procedure well. He had some hypotension but he was hypotensive on induction throughout the entire procedure. Blood gases were satisfactory during clamping of the mainstem bronchus, and he seemed to be reacting well. We closed the chest in layers with Dexon pericostal sutures, approximated clips on the skin.

Code(s): _____

CPT Modifiers

10.32. Dr. Raddy, staff radiologist, interprets a chest x-ray that was obtained in the hospital radiology department. Dr. Raddy is contracted with the hospital to read radiographs. The equipment and staff are owned and/or employed by the hospital. What modifier, if any, should Dr. Raddy report with the chest x-ray code?

   a. No modifier is necessary because Dr. Raddy interpreted the x-ray under contract with the hospital. The hospital will bill the global and pay Dr. Raddy from the reimbursement.
   b. Modifier -26, Professional component
   c. Modifier -TC, Technical component
   d. Modifier -59

10.33. Tiny Patti Sue Smith, 15 days old, currently weighs 1,652 g. She is taken to the operating room for small bowel resection for necrotizing enterocolitis, a frequent complication of prematurity. The remaining portions of the small bowel were anastomosed end-to-end. CPT code 44120 reports a small bowel resection with anastomosis. Is a modifier necessary, and if so, which modifier?

   a. No modifier is needed for the surgery, although the anesthesiologist might need a modifier.
   b. Modifier -63 is reported because the baby weighs less than 4 kg and thus is a higher surgical risk than a larger neonate.
   c. No modifier is needed because code 44120 already applies to neonates who are very low weight.
   d. A modifier is optional and may or may not be assigned depending on the departmental coding guidelines.

10.34. A patient is seen in the emergency department because of hyperkalemia due to an inadvertent overdose of his potassium medication. Over the course of the next six hours he receives infusions and his potassium is measured three times. What is/are the appropriate modifier(s) to report with the second and third potassium determinations?

    a. Modifier -59, to show that these were not duplicate charges but indeed separate incidents.

    b. No modifier is necessary for repeat laboratory tests, only for repeat surgical procedures.

    c. Modifier -91

    d. Modifiers -91 and -59 should be reported for the second and third determinations.

10.35. A patient who was high on PCP stabbed himself in the chest, causing a pneumothorax. He was seen in the emergency department, and Dr. Jones inserted a chest tube. Approximately one hour later, despite soft restraints, the patient managed to free himself and pull out his chest tube. Dr. Jones reinserted the chest tube via a fresh incision. What modifier should be reported on each procedure?

    a. Modifier -76, Repeat procedure by the same physician, should be reported for each chest tube insertion.

    b. Modifier -76 should be reported with the second procedure; no modifier is needed on the first procedure.

    c. Modifier -59 should be reported with the second procedure; no modifier is needed with the first procedure.

    d. Either modifier -59 or -76 may be reported on the first and second procedures.

10.36. A patient underwent gallbladder removal by Dr. Pitts on 4/1 and was discharged home on 4/2. On 4/16, he developed right lower quadrant abdominal pain and evaluation was strongly suggestive of acute appendicitis. Dr. Pitts performed an exploratory laparotomy and appendectomy for an acutely inflamed appendix. What modifier, if any, should be reported with the appendectomy code?

    a. No modifier is needed because the ICD-9-CM diagnosis code and the CPT procedure code clearly identify that this was a procedure not related to the cholecystectomy.

    b. Modifier -79, Unrelated procedure or service by the same physician during the postoperative period, should be reported with the appendectomy code.

    c. Modifier -78, Return to the operating room for a related procedure during the postoperative period, should be reported with the appendectomy code.

    d. Modifier -58, Staged or related procedure or service by the same physician during the postoperative period, should be reported with the appendectomy code.

HCPCS Level II Modifiers

10.37. A patient is brought to the emergency department of Community Hospital following a motor vehicle accident. He appears to have an avulsion of the aortic root and is rushed to the operating room where repair is attempted. The patient expires on the operating room table just as the surgery is being completed and before he can be admitted to the hospital. The CPT code for repair of avulsion of the aortic root is designated as an "inpatient only" code under the outpatient prospective patient system (OPPS). Is there a modifier that the hospital can report to obtain reimbursement for this procedure when performed as an outpatient?

    a. No. If an "inpatient only" procedure is performed on an outpatient basis, the hospital cannot obtain reimbursement under any circumstances.

    b. Modifier -CA, Procedure payable only in the inpatient setting when performed emergently on an outpatient who expires prior to admission, may be appended to the CPT procedure code.

    c. Modifier -ST, Related to trauma or injury, may be appended and a 50 percent reimbursement will be available to the hospital.

    d. Modifier -SC, Medically necessary service or supply, may be appended and a 25 percent reimbursement will be available to the hospital.

10.38. A patient undergoes a bunionectomy on the big toe of the right foot. What modifier is appended to report the location of this procedure?

    a. No modifier. By definition, bunionectomy is performed on the big toe.

    b. Modifier -T5

    c. Modifier -RT

    d. Modifier -TA

10.39. A hospice patient, under hospice care for terminal COPD, falls out of bed and fractures his wrist. He is taken to the emergency department at the local hospital and has a cast applied to the nondisplaced fracture. What modifier is reported to show that these services are not related to the patient's hospice-qualifying condition?

    a. Modifier -GW

    b. Modifier -AT

    c. Modifier -GZ

    d. Modifier -SC

10.40. HCPCS Level II modifiers can be used with which of the following code sets?

    a. CPT codes

    b. HCPCS Level II codes

    c. ICD-9-CM Volume III codes

    d. Both a and b

10.41. Modifiers -G1 through -G5, which report the levels of Urea Reduction Ratio (URR) in the blood, are reported with codes for _____ and measure the efficacy of this modality.

    a. Laboratory tests

    b. Dialysis codes

    c. Coronary artery interventional procedures

    d. Oxygen therapy

10.42. Match the HCPCS Level II modifier in column 2 with its application in column 1.

1. The patient was pronounced dead after the ambulance was called. Ambulance company is entitled to reimbursement.	a. -KA
2. Left hand, fourth digit	b. -SG
3. The beneficiary has been informed of rent/purchase option and has decided to rent the item.	c. -GH
4. Service furnished in an ambulatory surgery center	d. -QY
5. Left circumflex coronary artery	e. -E4
6. Monitored anesthesia care	f. -QL
7. Diagnostic mammogram converted from screening mammogram same day	g. -F3
8. Add-on option or accessory for wheelchair	h. -QS
9. Lower right eyelid	i. -BR
10. Medical supervision of one CRNA by an anesthesiologist	j. -LC

10.43. After a tragic accident where a 75-year-old patient's eye was injured, the patient received a court order for provision of an extended-wear, hydrophilic contact lens. What HCPCS Level II modifier(s) should be appended to code V2523?

_____

Long-term Acute Care (LTAC) Coding

10.44. Patient Julie Jones suffers a massive intracerebral hemorrhage due to right basilar artery bleed. She is admitted to City Acute Hospital where she remains for eight days undergoing acute care and regulation of anticoagulation.

Following her acute hospital stay, she is transferred to City LTAC for continued management. Treatment at City LTAC will focus on continued management and intensive physical, occupational, and speech-language therapy for rehabilitation from the following sequelae of her intracranial bleed:

Left (dominant-sided) hemiplegia involving her upper and lower extremities

Expressive aphasia

Severe dysphagia with impaired swallowing and risk for aspiration

Assign the admission diagnoses that City LTAC will report.

a. 433.00, 438.21, 438.11, 438.82
b. V57.89, 438.21, 438.11, 438.82
c. V58.9, 438.21, 438.11, 438.82
d. V57.2, V57.3, V57.89

10.45. The patient developed buttock and heel decubiti, both stage II, following an extended stay in the acute hospital. He has had resolution of the underlying acute condition that occasioned his admission there and is transferred to the LTAC for treatment of the decubitus ulcers. While in LTAC, he undergoes nonexcisional debridement of the decubiti. He also has underlying diabetes without documented complications and COPD. Assign the appropriate ICD-9-CM diagnoses and procedural codes for this admission.

a. 707.05, 707.07, 707.22, 250.00, 496, 86.28
b. V57.89, 707.05, 707.07, 707.22, 250.00, 496, 86.28
c. 707.05, 707.07, 707.22, 86.28
d. 707.05, 707.07, 707.22, 86.22

10.46. This patient is admitted for pulmonary rehabilitation in a setting of advanced COPD. She also has ASHD and type II diabetes mellitus with peripheral neuropathy. She has been ventilator-dependent at the local acute hospital but was weaned from the ventilator prior to transfer to LTAC. What are the principal diagnosis and secondary diagnoses that the LTAC personnel will report for her stay?

a. 496, 414.00, 250.60, 337.1
b. V57.0, 496
c. V57.89, 496, 414.00, 250.60, 337.1
d. V57.89

10.47. This patient underwent an above-knee amputation of her left leg for severe vascular trauma with transaction of the posterior tibial artery just below the level of the knee and loss of viability of the distal leg, after a motor vehicle accident. She has had continued stump infections and healing has not occurred, now four weeks after amputation. She is transferred to the long-term acute care hospital for management of the stump infection, eventual rehabilitation, and possible prosthetic fitting. What is the principal diagnosis that the LTAC personnel should report for this admission?

a. V57.89
b. V52.1
c. 904.53
d. 997.62

Outpatient Rehabilitation Cases

10.48. Physician Order

Diagnosis: Congenital CP, scoliosis, bilateral congenital dislocated hips

Treatment Goals: Increase in ADLs, strengthening

Therapy Provided

PT: ROM exercises, strengthening, stretching

OT: ADLs, upper extremity strengthening/ROM

What are the correct diagnosis codes for this outpatient therapy visit? (Procedure codes are captured via the chargemaster.) _____

10.49. Physician Order

PT to evaluate and treat IT band syndrome

Therapy Provided

PT: Evaluation and treatment in the weight room

What are the correct diagnosis codes for this outpatient therapy visit? (Procedure codes are captured via the chargemaster.) _____

Inpatient Rehabilitation Cases

10.50. History and Physical for Inpatient Case

Purpose of Consultation: Physical medicine and rehabilitation evaluation at the request of Dr. Brown, status post trochanteric femoral nailing of left IT fracture on 5/19 with touch weight-bearing restrictions.

History of Present Illness: Joe is a 52-year-old male with a history of mental retardation. He resides at home with parents whom I believe are near their 70s. Joe apparently fell in the home setting and sustained a left intertrochanteric femur fracture and was admitted to Regional Hospital on 5/16. He was evaluated by Dr. Smith and then operated on 5/19 with trochanteric femoral nailing, Synthes type, placed by Dr. Brown.

The patient has been followed by Dr. Smith secondary to difficulties with prior arrhythmia and A Fib flutter with him having been on Coumadin chronically until this admission. His INR today is 2.7, his platelets are 283,000, and his hemoglobin preoperative on 5/16 was 15.6 g/dL. His hemoglobin on 5/22 was 13.2 g/dL.

Chemistries of today, 5/25, are sodium 138, potassium 4.3, chloride 99, CO_2 31, BUN 20, creatinine 0.8, glucose 105, magnesium low at 1.4.

He has been working with a physical therapist and has been very slow to progress until significantly improving and tolerating activities and instructions yesterday on

5/24. At that time, he was able with touch to non-weight bearing on the left lower limb with walker ambulate 15 to 20 feet to the doorway and back with contact-guard assistance. He is tall in stature at 6′2″. His admission weight was recorded at 119.3 kg; weight today is 138.5 kg, with a discrepancy likely in his admission weight recording. Pain scores have ranged from a 1 to 2 of 10 today. He has noted some cramping and tightness in his calf, although nontender. He has been working on stretching this out. His medications are as per MAR. He currently remains on telemetry.

Past Medical History:
1. As above, notable for mental retardation and living with parents. He lives in a trilevel home, which he describes as having no stairs to enter the main floor or second level. He lives in the lower level with stair access and frequently is at the upper or higher level. Please refer to the occupational therapy evaluation of tub and difficulties with transfers therein.
2. History of A Fib flutter as above
3. History of gastroesophageal reflux
4. History of chronic Coumadin

Allergies: No known drug allergies

Current Medications: Per MAR, as above

Family History: Noncontributory

Social History: As per above. His care is monitored by his parents. His father has stated that he needs to be more mobile and able to care for himself before returning home. He has been very concerned about his disposition at this time. There is a history of tobacco use approximately 10 years ago. He has a dental bridge prosthesis. He wears glasses for vision and has had a history of night terrors. He is disabled. He is single. His primary care physician is Dr. Allen Smith.

Review of Systems: As per admission H&P of Dr. Brown, as well as ER evaluation of Dr. Canter. See also Dr. Smith evaluation and ongoing care. He has recommended telemetry until discharged from Regional Hospital.

Physical Examination: Admission height: 6′2″

Admission Weight: As above I believe is in error at 119.3 kg

Most Recent Weights: These have been in the 130 to 140 kg range. Today is 138.5.

Vital Signs: BP 133/73, afebrile at 97.6, heart rate in the mid-70s

General: He is alert and conversant. He is sitting up in a chair. He is reading a magazine. He has his lenses in place. He is able to demonstrate functional range of the shoulders and upper extremities and denies any aggravation or irritation with use of the walker for the touch or no weight-bearing on the left. He does have a saline lock. He has significant ecchymotic change about the left posterior elbow and forearm; this is nontender. He is able to demonstrate good strength, and this limits symmetric reflexes.

Lungs: Clear to auscultation

Cardiovascular: Regular rate and rhythm without A Fib at this time

Abdomen: Soft, normoactive bowel sounds

GU: He is voiding spontaneously.

Extremities: Lower limbs demonstrate +1 reflexes, left knee jerk does evoke some left hip discomfort. He is able to ankle plantar flex, somewhat pain-inhibited on the left. There is no distal swelling. He has TED hose in place, knee high. He is able to follow instructions.

Assessment:
1. Status post fall with left intertrochanteric femur fracture on 5/16 in the home setting
2. Status post 5/19 ORIF with trochanteric femoral nailing
3. Touch weight-bearing limitations, left lower extremity
4. History of arrhythmia and A Fib flutter; on chronic Coumadin
5. Gastroesophageal reflux disorder
6. Mild mental retardation; living with parents
7. Pain issues
8. Slow progress but now improving and tolerating therapies per my discussion with his physical therapist

Plan/Comment: I had the pleasure of evaluating Joe today. He appears to be a good candidate for rehab intervention to maximize his functional status so that he can return home with his parents. We will anticipate his admission therein on 5/27 if he continues to progress as well.

Discharge Summary

Date of Discharge: 6/21/20XX

Date of Admission: 5/28/20XX

Discharging Diagnoses:
1. Status post fall with left intertrochanteric femur fracture 5/16/XX, in home setting
2. Status post open reduction and internal fixation with intertrochanteric femoral nailing 5/19/XX, by Dr. Brown, with touch weight-bearing restrictions left lower limb
3. History of arrhythmia and atrial fibrillation flutter, on Coumadin chronically
4. Gastroesophageal reflux disorder
5. Postoperative pain issues
6. Mild cognitive issues, chronic
7. Mobility and self-care deficits

History of Present Illness: The patient is a 52-year-old Caucasian male. He has a history of some mild mental retardation and resides with his parents who are in their 70s.

His primary physician is Dr. Smith, and he is being followed by Dr. Brown in current hospitalization since being admitted on 5/16/XX, at Regional Hospital.

The patient was evaluated by myself in consultation on 5/25/XX, for rehabilitation needs with him coming to the Rehabilitation Hospital on 5/28/XX. Please refer to my consultation of 5/25/XX for specifics.

Hospital Course: The patient was brought to Rehabilitation Hospital for comprehensive therapy programming. He and his parents were in agreement with this.

He is a large Caucasian male who is pleasant and cooperative. He has had problems with pain limitations and some swelling in the left leg. He has remained on Coumadin and was on this chronically before. He has been followed by cardiology and is scheduled to see Dr. Smith in follow-up on 6/22/XX, at 11:15 a.m. He remains on Coumadin, which is followed by his primary physician with him to have further pro time/INR on 6/23/XX, Thursday.

His physical mobility has continued to progress. He has been maintaining touch weight bearing much better with contact guard assistance for gait using front-wheeled walker for 50-feet distances × 2. He has been able to perform total hip arthroplasty exercise program and is independent in 10 repetitions of each.

He has been followed for lymphedema of the left lower limb and has been issued Juzo garments, and his parents were instructed by the physical therapist on his day of discharge on how to don and doff these garments.

With self-care skills, his upper extremities remained with 4/5 strength and active range of motion. Sensation was intact. Somewhat slower on the right side than the left side for 9-hole peg coordination: 38 seconds right, 24 seconds left. Sitting balance was good. Endurance was within functional limits. He has some mild problems with cognition in terms of problem solving and judgment. Visual perceptive skills were thought to be good using his lenses. FIM-level scores were improved by 2 levels for all tasks except for toileting, which improved from a 3 to a 4. He is independent in feeding and dressing. Dressing lower extremities FIM level 5, grooming 6, toileting 4, showering 5. Discharge equipment includes commode.

Medications at Discharge:

1. Fentanyl patch 25 mcg per hour with this having been decreased the day prior to discharge from 50 mcg to 25 mcg with him noting no substantial change in pain levels. He is provided with refill for 5 patches or 15 days with these to be changed every 72 hours with it to then be discontinued.
2. He has also been using oral medications for pain relief, using Percocet (oxycodone/acetaminophen) 5/325 with 10.100 provided for 1 to 2 p.o. every 4 to 6 hours p.r.n. No refills.
3. Coumadin 3 mg daily currently with 2-week supply issued on 6/21/XX.
4. Durable medical equipment includes:

    Front-wheeled walker with large fixed wheels

    Bedside commode

    Rental wheelchair, 20 inches wide. This gentleman is 6′2″ or 6′3″ in height and weighs 116 kg secondary to left hip fracture and mobility defects with limited weight bearing.
5. Ferrous sulfate 650 mg p.o. b.i.d. with meals
6. He has been on Prevacid, but will resume his previous proton pump inhibitor at home for which he has a prescription. His home PPI is Aciphex.

7. He is on Betapace 160 mg p.o. b.i.d.
8. Lanoxin 0.25 mg p.o. every evening
9. Cardizem CD 120 mg p.o. daily
10. He may use over-the-counter stool softeners as needed.

Discharge Instructions:
1. He is to wear his Juzo stockings on the left leg, being placed initially in the morning, removed at bedtime.
2. Fall precautions should be in place.
3. Patient and family chose Regional Hospital Home Health Care for ongoing home health PT, OT, visiting nurse, and aid, with his parents involved in all care decisions.

His prognosis is fair for continued compliance and ongoing follow-up care.

a. What are the correct diagnosis codes (admit, principal, and secondary) for reporting on the UB-04? _____
b. What are the correct diagnosis (etiology and comorbidities) codes for the Patient Assessment Instrument (IRF-PAI)? _____

10.51. Neurology Rehabilitation H&P for Inpatient Case

Date of Consultation: 4/10/XX

Introduction: Rehabilitation consultation is requested to evaluate this 30-year-old man who was injured in a motorcycle accident on 4/3. At that time, he was thrown from his bike and apparently sustained a transient loss of consciousness consistent with concussion. He also apparently had quadriparesis at the scene. He was transported to Regional Hospital where he was ultimately found to have, I believe, a significant hyperflexion injury without major fracture dislocation. He did not require emergency stabilization surgery.

He was clinically and radiographically diagnosed with a cervical spinal cord contusion. This was most prominent at the C3–4 level. There was some initial respiratory impairment, and he was transiently placed on a ventilator. He has since been extubated.

The patient's clinical course has been consistent with a central type of spinal cord contusion such that he has had paralysis of his arms and paresis of the legs. The sensory deficits follow similarly. Patient is now being considered for eventual transfer to the Rehab Hospital.

Current Medications

1. Insulin by sliding scale
2. Bacitracin
3. Dulcolax, p.r.n.
4. Decadron, 4 mg q.6 h. and eventually will be tapered according to protocol
5. Lovenox, 90 mg subcutaneously q.12 h.
6. Prevacid, 30 mg p.o. b.i.d.
7. Claritin, 10 mg p.o. daily
8. Senokot, 8.6 mg p.o. b.i.d.
9. Tylenol, p.r.n.

10. Benadryl, 25 mg p.o. q. 6 h. p.r.n.
11. Ativan, 0.5 mg was used 1 time only
12. Percocet, 5/325, 1 to 2 hours p.o. q. 4 to 6 h. p.r.n.
13. Ambien, p.r.n.
14. Zofran, p.r.n.

Allergies: He has no known medication allergies but has a history of intolerance to morphine and to Motrin. These tend to cause significant itching. He is having some mild itching with his Percocet, but this is relieved with Benadryl.

Past Medical History: He has a torn anterior cruciate ligament.

Review of Systems: Prior to admission, the patient has had no fever, chills, sweats, or weight loss. No change in his vision. No ear, nose, or throat complaints. No chest pains or palpitations. No shortness of breath, coughing, or wheezing. No nausea, vomiting, diarrhea, or constipation. No bladder or kidney dysfunction. No bone or joint problems outside of the anterior cruciate tear. No skin lesions such as rash. No mental illness. No other neurologic problems. No diabetes, thyroid disease, blood or bleeding problems, swollen lymph nodes, or allergic or asthmatic problems.

Family History: Parents are in good health. No neurologic problems.

Social History: He is divorced. Lives in Watson. He is a corrections officer for County Jail. Parents live in Plainsville. He has two children; however, they do not reside with him.

General Exam: Appearance: The appearance is that of a well-developed, athletic-appearing young man who is lying on his back. He has a rigid cervical collar in place. The rigid collar is not to be removed.

Vital Signs: His temperature reached a maximum of 100.3°F but is now down to 99°F. Blood pressure 121/68, pulse is at 72. Respirations 18.

General: He appears normocephalic. The left arm is swollen and wrapped with an ACE-type wrap. No obvious head trauma.

Heart: Is beating at a regular rate and rhythm without murmur. Carotid pulsations cannot be examined at this time. Peripheral pulses cannot easily be examined at this time.

Neurological Exam: He is a bit sleepy. He has received some narcotics and Benadryl. He arouses easily to voice. He is oriented to place and person and thought the date was 4/17. His recent and remote memory is grossly intact, although he has some amnesia for the accident when he was rendered unconscious. His attention span and concentration is grossly normal. Receptive expressive language normal. Fund of knowledge appropriate. His pupils are equal, round, and reactive to light. Funduscopic exam is benign. Visual fields are intact. Visual acuity is grossly normal. Eye movements are intact. Facial sensation, corneal responses, muscles of mastication are normal. Facial movement symmetrical and normal. Hearing intact. Tongue and palate move normally. The sternocleidomastoid is not examined at this time due to the rigid collar. Trapezius testing was not attempted because of his immobilized neck.

He has complete plegia of the upper extremities bilaterally. In the legs, he does have some leg extension, hip extension, and thigh adduction with abduction. He has some ability to extend the legs bilaterally. There is a limited ability to lift the heels off the bed. There is virtual absence of foot dorsiflexion bilaterally; however, there is a weak plantar flexion response bilaterally. Muscle tone slightly increased in the legs. Babinski responses were not attempted. The muscle stretch reflexes are absent in the upper extremities and hyperactive at the knees and ankles. Sensation grossly intact to light touch and temperature in the legs bilaterally. There is anesthesia of the arms bilaterally and reduced sensation of the lower abdomen. The chest sensation and upper shoulders have essentially normal light touch sensation.

Coordination cannot be attempted. Patient obviously not ambulatory at this time.

Lab Studies: Most recent lab studies of note: Glucose is 137, BUN is at 23, creatinine 1.1. Sodium is at 136. The other chemistry parameters are normal. White count is elevated at 12,100, hemoglobin normal at 15.

Imaging Studies: Are most pertinent for the MRI scans. The MRI is most noteworthy for the abnormal signal within the spinal cord, primarily at the C3–C4 disk space level. An additional small area of signal abnormality noted at the C5–C6 disk level. The abnormality within the spinal cord is consistent with spinal cord edema and contusion. There is an additional abnormality in the soft tissues with interspinous ligamentous edema at C3–C4 and C5–C6. Patient coincidentally also has a relatively small spinal canal that appears congenital.

Assessment: Thirty-year-old man with spinal cord injury without significant fracture but is associated with severe cervical spinal cord contusion, primarily at the C3–C4 disk level. Clinically patient has a "central cord" syndrome with paralysis of his arms and paresis of the legs.

Plan: 1. Patient should be an excellent candidate for comprehensive rehabilitation.
2. We will follow along and facilitate transfer when needed.

Interim Discharge Summary for Inpatient Rehab Case

Discharge Diagnosis

1. Cervical instability with plans for cervical fusion and stabilization procedure by Dr. Johnson, neurosurgery
2. Status post motor vehicle accident with cervical trauma and cord myelopathy
3. Quadriparesis and central cord syndrome
4. Neurogenic bowel and neurogenic bladder
5. Dysesthetic pain and numbness
6. Mobility and self-care deficits

John is a 30-year-old Caucasian male who was involved in motor vehicle trauma with subsequent spinal injury and quadriparesis. Please refer to admission H&P for details. He was admitted in transfer from Regional Hospital for comprehensive rehabilitation programming given his quadriparesis. He has been undergoing spinal recovery program with comprehensive therapies and intervention to include neuropsychology.

He has remained somewhat unrealistic and has deferred many of the spinal education efforts that have been offered to him. He is returning on 5/13/XX to Regional

Hospital for cervical stabilization procedure, with Dr. Johnson planning a C3 through C6 anterior cervical diskectomy and fusion.

He has had significant motor recovery from his initial presentation, with his lower extremity strength now +3/5 at the hip extensors and knee extensors. Quadriceps +3/5 bilaterally. Knee flexors, hamstrings were 2/5. Ankle dorsiflexion +1/5. Plantar flexion 3/5. Spasticity and tone does interfere with gait patterning and does limit his ability to progress, with him needing assistance. Bed mobility is rolling with minimal assistance to his stronger right side. Sliding board transfers to bed and chair were with moderate assistance of 1. Supine to sit was with moderate to maximum assist of 1. Gait with ARJO Walker with heavy truncal support is 75 feet with moderate assistance of 1, knee brace on the right, and AFO on the right. Steps and stairs have not yet been attempted.

In terms of self-care skills, the patient remains essentially dependent although he is beginning to show almost antigravity strength being –2 to +2 in the upper limbs with some flicker of hand movement. Palmer grasp on the right 3 lb and left 1 lb. He continues to have a greater degree of sensation proximally than distally, although deep pressure is intact. Light touch is impaired. He is unable to complete a 9-Hole Peg Test and is unable to functionally use the hands bilaterally. Visual perceptive skills are intact.

Medications as per MARS

Plans are for return within 72 hours to the Rehabilitation Hospital if medically stable to resume acute rehabilitation program.

Plan: Disposition is home with support of family and possible spinal cord attendant program via state services. Equipment needs are still to be determined. The patient remains optimistic.

a. What are the correct diagnosis codes (admit, principal, and secondary) for reporting on the UB-04? _____

b. What are the correct diagnosis (etiology and comorbidities) codes for the Patient Assessment Instrument (IRF-PAI)? _____

10.52. Interim History and Physical for Inpatient Case

Subjective: This is an interim history and physical for a 73-year-old woman who sustained an acute right hemisphere ischemic stroke on 03/30/XX. The patient was actually in preadmission at Regional Hospital where she was planning to undergo an orthopedic procedure when she developed acute left hemiparesis. She was transported immediately to the emergency department. It was determined that she had an acute ischemic stroke and received TPA. Despite the TPA, however, the patient was left with severe residual deficits in the form of left hemineglect, left facial weakness, left arm plegia, left leg paresis, and inability to walk. In the course of her workup, she was found to have atrial fibrillation but no significant stenosis of the internal carotid arteries. She was determined to be a suitable candidate for chronic Coumadin therapy.

The patient was fairly stable neurologically, although she had chronic debilitation prior to her admission. This debilitation was related to multiple medical problems, but she was ambulatory, I believe, with a walker. Because of her severe deficits, the patient is now being transferred to the Rehabilitation Hospital for a complete rehabilitation program.

The patient has several comorbid medical problems, including atrial fibrillation, diabetes mellitus, morbid obesity, hyperlipidemia, and degenerative arthritis to include a particular problem with her hip, which was being considered for replacement.

At the time of transfer, she has a temperature of 97.8°F, pulse 108, respirations 20, and blood pressure 134/93. She is awake, alert, and oriented. Her speech is fluent. Her eyes tend to gaze to the right. There is left facial droop consistent with central-type facial weakness. There is left upper extremity plegia, left neglect, and left lower extremity paresis. She is unable to walk.

Assessment:
1. Right hemisphere ischemic infarction with severe residual deficits
2. There are several complicating comorbid problems, which are likely to aggravate her stroke deficit. In particular, these include degenerative arthritis, diabetes, heart disease, and chronic mobility problems.

Plan:
1. Transfer to Rehabilitation Hospital
2. Physical therapy, occupational therapy, speech therapy, and therapeutic recreation
3. Primary goals of therapy will be to improve her ability to ambulate and take care of herself with regard to independence of ADLs.
4. It is anticipated the patient will require 3 to 4 weeks of inpatient rehabilitation.
5. It is anticipated disposition would be to home with the care of family, if possible.

Rehab Hospital Discharge Summary for Inpatient Rehab

Date of Admission: 4/7/XX

Date of Discharge: 5/10/XX

Admission Diagnosis: Right hemisphere infarction with severe residual deficits

Secondary or Comorbid Conditions:
1. Degenerative arthritis
2. Diabetes
3. Coronary artery disease
4. Chronic mobility problems

Discharge Diagnoses:
1. Right hemisphere infarction with severe residual deficits
2. Degenerative arthritis
3. Diabetes
4. Coronary artery disease
5. Chronic mobility problems

History of Present Illness: Patient is a 73-year-old female who sustained a right hemisphere infarction on 3/30/XX. Patient apparently was in the process of undergoing preadmittance for orthopedic procedure when she developed acute left hemiparesis. She was transferred to the emergency room. She received TPA. However, she was left with severe left deficits in the form of left hemineglect, left facial weakness, left arm plegia, and left leg paresis, and an inability to walk.

In the course of her workup, she was found to have atrial fibrillation. It was thought that she was a suitable candidate for chronic Coumadin. Patient was stabilized in the Regional Hospital setting, and it was thought that she would be an appropriate rehabilitation candidate. Her examination at the transfer to the Rehabilitation Hospital showed her general medical exam to be stable. Neurologically, she was awake, alert, and oriented on mental status, and her speech was fluent. The cranial nerves showed a right gaze preference with a left facial droop that was central in nature. There was left upper extremity plegia and left neglect and left lower extremity paresis, and the patient was unable to walk.

During the course of her rehab stay, the patient did undergo some laboratory workup. This consisted of a series of PT and INR values. Initial PT/INR from 4/8/XX showed PT of 24.0 with an INR of 2.2. Prior to discharge on 5/01/XX, the PT was 26.7 with an INR of 2.5. The patient did undergo some limited metabolic profiles including one from 4/22/XX, showing elevated glucose of 143 with a sodium low at 123, chloride low at 88. Uric acid was 6.2. The osmolality was 0.273. On repeat metabolic profile from 4/23/XX showed an elevated glucose of 126 with a sodium low at 123, and a low chloride at 88. On 4/26/XX, glucose was 131. Sodium was 127, chloride 92. On 5/5/XX, patient had sodium level checked and it was at 130. It had improved to 134. Patient had a series of Glucometer checks done throughout the course of her rehabilitation stay. These levels appeared to have remained fairly consistently elevated with values at times near 190, but no values were noted below grossly 120.

During the course of her rehabilitation stay, she underwent some radiographic imaging including a swallowing study from 4/8/XX, which showed some delay in oral phase of swallowing, likely the result of sensory issues. She had a right hip x-ray from 4/10/XX, showing relatively severe arthritic involvement of the right hip. Right shoulder x-ray from 4/10/XX showed a degenerative change with history of previous surgery. A CT of the right shoulder from 4/19/XX showed previous surgery with screws in the proximal right humerus. There were arthritic changes with subluxation of the humeral head superiorly, suggesting a chronic degenerative rotator cuff tear.

During the course of her rehabilitation stay, the patient was seen by the various therapy services. This included speech therapy, who felt that she had trouble swallowing; the patient was to undergo dysphagia management techniques and diet texture modification and full supervision with p.o. She had speech trouble and was to undergo oromotor exercises. She had communication and language deficits and was to undergo standard speech therapy protocol assessment. She had memory trouble and was to undergo assessment, and she was to be 79 percent accurate with auditory and visual memory exercises. The occupational therapy team thought she had decreased independence with ADLs, and she was to be seen three to five times per week to be educated in ADL techniques and in AE. She had decreased use of the left lower extremity and was to be seen for education and weight-bearing techniques and self-range of motion. She had decreased independence with functional transfers and was to be educated in safety with functional transfers. She had decreased independence with leisure participation and was to be seen for education in leisure exploration. The therapeutic recreation team thought she had decreased leisure participation due to hospitalization and was to be provided an opportunity for successful leisure involvement in an activity of choice. The physical therapy team thought that the patient was dependent on transfers and was to undergo transfer training. She had decreased lower extremity strength and was to undergo strengthening exercise. She had dependence with standing and gait and was to undergo standing and gait training.

Rehab Hospital Course: Patient was admitted for an aggressive inpatient rehabilitation stay. The patient was able to participate with rehabilitation efforts and did make slow but steady progress throughout the course of her rehabilitation stay. She was followed by internal medicine during her stay, and various medical issues were addressed in that regard. Patient had no major setbacks during the course of her stay. She was seen by Dr. Benson for a chronic rotator cuff tear and physical therapy was recommended. The patient's hyponatremia gradually improved throughout the course of her rehabilitation stay.

By 5/10/XX, it was thought that the patient had optimized her rehabilitation hospital benefits. As of that date, the various therapy services noted as follows. Occupational therapy thought that the patient had met some but not all of her goals due to inconsistency and poor attention to task. Physical therapy felt that the patient had met almost all of her goals except the first goal of bed mobility and also her standing goal because she still needed moderate assistance. Therapeutic recreation felt that she had met her established goals with recommendations to continue with social and leisure interest and community involvement. Speech therapy staff thought her condition had improved.

On 5/10/XX, the patient was discharged home with outpatient physical therapy, occupational therapy, speech therapy, and nursing. She was on a diabetic, pureed food, full-supervision diet and was to be encouraged to eat a consistent diet. Her activity was as tolerated, and she was not allowed to drive. She was to transfer with 2 on a sliding board, and she was to continue with her knee-high T.E.D. hose. She was to get a PT/INR on 5/11/XX. She was to check her blood sugar before breakfast and evening meals. She was to have a drop-arm shower and transport in a commode. She was to get a hospital bed with rails and a slide board.

Discharge Medications
1. Baby aspirin daily
2. Lemon juice b.i.d. to t.i.d.
3. Over-the-counter stool softeners
4. Novolin insulin subcu b.i.d. on a sliding-scale basis
5. Sinemet 25/100 at bedtime for restless legs
6. Coreg 6.25 mg b.i.d.
7. Klonopin 0.5 mg at bedtime
8. Lanoxin 0.125 mg daily
9. Surfak 240 mg b.i.d.

10. Zetia 5 mg b.i.d.

11. Neurontin 600 mg b.i.d. and then 900 mg at 10 p.m.

12. Prevacid 30 mg b.i.d.

13. Levothyroxine 100 mcg at bedtime

14. Cozaar 100 mg at 8 a.m.

15. Magnesium oxide 400 mg at 8 a.m.

16. Glucophage 1000 mg b.i.d., 500 mg at noon

17. Singulair 10 mg at 10 p.m.

18. Actos 45 mg at 8 a.m.

19. Zoloft 50 mg b.i.d.

20. Zocor 80 mg at 6 p.m.

21. Coumadin 1 mg at 4 p.m.

a. What are the correct diagnosis codes (admit, principal, and secondary) for reporting on the UB-04? _____

b. What are the correct diagnosis (etiology and comorbidities) codes for the Patient Assessment Instrument (IRF-PAI)? _____

Skilled Nursing Facility (SNF) Cases

10.53. The patient was admitted to the acute hospital with a pathological fracture of the left femur due to underlying metastatic cancer from the breast (resected years ago). She underwent percutaneous fixation in the hospital. She had been largely nonambulatory prior to the injury, and remains so. She is admitted to the skilled nursing facility for continued healing of the fracture and for general conditioning. Assign the appropriate diagnosis codes for the skilled facility to report.

a. V54.25, 198.5, V10.3
b. 733.14, 198.5, V10.3
c. V57.89, 733.14, 198.5, V10.3
d. V54.15, 821.00

10.54. This patient had been residing at home until an episode of pneumonia resulted in his hospitalization. While there, it was determined that he really was not able to remain in his home on his own due to rapidly advancing Alzheimer's dementia and episodes where he tried to wander away from the hospital. He was transferred to the skilled nursing facility because of this condition, although no specific therapy was ordered. The pneumonia had completely resolved in the acute hospital, and no further treatment was needed in the skilled nursing facility. The patient does have underlying chronic obstructive pulmonary disease, hypertension, and ASHD that require daily medication. Assign the appropriate diagnosis for this long-term admission.

a. 486, 496, 401.9, 414.00
b. 331.0, 294.11
c. 331.0, 294.11, 496, 401.9, 414.00
d. V57.89, 331.0, 294.11, 496, 401.9, 414.00

10.55. This patient underwent a subtotal colectomy in the acute hospital for resection of a carcinoma of the transverse colon. She was left significantly weak and debilitated following her surgery and was admitted to the skilled nursing facility for conditioning. The surgery appears to have been successful in eradicating the malignancy, and she was receiving no chemotherapy or radiation therapy at the time of her transfer. Assign the appropriate codes for the skilled nursing facility to report for this admission.

a. V58.75, 780.79, V10.05
b. V58.75, 997.99, 780.79, V10.05
c. V10.05, 780.79
d. V58.75, 780.79, 153.1

References

American Hospital Association. 1985–2010. *Coding Clinic for ICD-9-CM*. Chicago: American Hospital Association.

American Medical Association. 1992–2010. *CPT Assistant*. Chicago: American Medical Association.

American Medical Association. 2010. *Current Procedural Terminology (CPT)*. Chicago: American Medical Association.

American Medical Association. 2011. Corrections document—CPT 2011. http://www.ama-assn.org/resources/doc/cpt/cpt-2011-corrections.pdf.

Hazelwood, Anita, and Carol Venable. 2011. *ICD-9-CM Diagnostic Coding and Reimbursement for Physician Services*. Chicago: American Health Information Management Association.

ICD-9-CM Professional for Hospitals: Volumes 1, 2, and 3. 2011. Salt Lake City, UT: Ingenix.

ICD-10-CM: The Complete Official Draft Code Set. 2010. Salt Lake City, UT: Ingenix.

ICD-10-PCS: The Complete Official Draft Code Set. 2010. Salt Lake City, UT: Ingenix.

Kuehn, Lynn. 2010. *CPT/HCPCS Coding and Reimbursement for Physician Services*. Chicago: American Health Information Management Association.

National Center for Health Statistics. 2008 (Oct. 1). *ICD-9-CM Official Guidelines for Coding and Reporting and Present on Admission Reporting Guidelines*. Hyatsville, MD: US Department of Health and Human Services.

Schraffenberger, Lou Ann. 2011. *Basic ICD-9-CM Coding*. Chicago: American Health Information Management Association.

Smith, Gail. 2010. *Basic Current Procedural Terminology (CPT) and HCPCS Coding*. Chicago: American Health Information Management Association.

Exercise Answer Key

Part I

Beginning Coding Exercises

Chapter 1. Basic Principles of ICD-9-CM and ICD-10-CM/PCS Coding

Unless otherwise stated, code set answers given in Chapter 1 are ICD-9-CM.

Characteristics and Conventions of the ICD-9-CM Classification System

1.1.   b. Parentheses

Rationale: Square brackets in ICD-9-CM are used to enclose synonyms, alternative wordings, abbreviations, and explanatory phrases. Slanted brackets are found only in the Alphabetic Index and enclose a code that must be used in conjunction with a code that immediately precedes it. Boxes are not a defined convention of ICD-9-CM.

1.2.   a. Manifestation code

Rationale: Manifestation codes are secondary to the code representing the etiology of the condition. A CC exclusion is a term related to the prospective payment system based on diagnosis-related groups (MS-DRGs), which use ICD-9-CM codes. If the code is designated as an exclusion, the reporting of that code will not affect MS-DRG assignment. In the Alphabetic Index to diseases, the first code represents the underlying condition and the second code, enclosed in italicized brackets, is the manifestation.

1.3.   Uniform Hospital Discharge Data Set

1.4.   Inpatient admissions (short-term, acute, long-term care, and psychiatric hospitals)

Rationale: If a condition has not been ruled out at the termination of an inpatient stay, it may be reported to avoid data loss of a condition that consumed work or resources during an inpatient stay and could not be ruled out. For all other settings, diagnoses are reported only to their highest degree of specificity, and this rule is not applied. Rather, known signs or symptoms are assigned codes.

1.5.   b. The appropriate V code

Rationale: This is an official guideline in ICD-9-CM.

1.6.   c. Highest-degree burn

Rationale: This is an ICD-9-CM guideline. Treatment and anatomic location are not factors in the sequencing of burn conditions.

1.7.   b. Hypertension and chronic kidney disease

Rationale: ICD-9-CM presumes a cause-and-effect relationship between hypertension and chronic kidney disease unless documentation in the health record states the hypertension is secondary. This is not the case with other conditions with hypertension, including heart disease.

1.8.   Morphology codes, M codes

1.9.   October 1, 10/1, 10/01, the first of October

1.10.   b. V codes and E codes

Rationale: The ICD-9-CM system includes only two supplementary classifications:

- Supplementary Classification of Factors Influencing Health Status and Contact with Health Services
- Supplemental Classification of External Causes of Injury and Poisoning

The morphology codes are considered an appendix (A) to ICD-9-CM.

1.11.   a. The nature and status (primary, secondary, in situ) for malignancies

Rationale: The neoplasm table included in the Alphabetic Index of ICD-9-CM provides code numbers by anatomic site. It includes benign, malignant, uncertain behavior, and unspecified categories, and for malignancies only, provides a method to reflect primary, secondary, or in situ status. Morphology codes are not found in the neoplasm table. A benign neoplasm is not reported according to stage because metastasis is not a characteristic of that behavior.

1.12.   c. Either principal diagnosis or secondary diagnosis, depending upon the code and the circumstances of the admission

Rationale: Review the explanation of this supplementary classification included in the ICD-9-CM book for details. The rules for reporting depend on the circumstances of the encounter.

1.13.   Main terms

1.14.   d. All of the above

1.15.   b. When the coder lacks sufficient information to assign a more specific code

Rationale: The Not Otherwise Specified (NOS) designation means that the documentation used to select the code does not provide additional specificity to allow a more granular code assignment. This can be contrasted with Not Elsewhere Classified (NEC), which is assigned when specific details of a condition are available, but the classification system does not include a specific category or code that exactly reflects the concept. Codes are not assigned without appropriate source documents reflecting the physician's diagnosis, even in the outpatient setting.

Infectious and Parasitic Diseases

1.16. 047.1

Rationale: The Alphabetic Index term is Meningitis, subterm ECHO virus.

ICD-10-CM Code(s): A87.0

ICD-10-CM Rationale: The Alphabetic Index main term is Meningitis, subterm echovirus.

1.17. 052.9

Rationale: The Alphabetic Index term is Chickenpox, with an instruction to "*see also* Varicella." Unless this is an encounter for a vaccination against the disease (reported with code V05.4), the code to represent that the patient actually has the disease is 052.9.

ICD-10-CM Code(s): B01.9

ICD-10-CM Rationale: The Alphabetic Index main term Chickenpox refers the coders to see Varicella.

1.18. 022.1

Rationale: The main term in the Alphabetic Index is Anthrax and the subterm is pulmonary, which results in code 022.1.

ICD-10-CM Code(s): A22.1

ICD-10-CM Rationale: The Alphabetic Index main term is Anthrax, subterm pulmonary.

1.19. Negative

Rationale: The Alphabetic term is Infection, subterm Aerobacter aerogenes, which is classified to an NEC code, 041.85. When the Tabular List is consulted to verify the code, you will note that it appears in the code for "other Gram-negative organisms."

1.20. 054.10

Rationale: The Alphabetic term is Herpes, subterm genital. If a specific site is included in the documentation that does not have its own code, code 054.19 is reported. The 054.10 code is reported only if the condition is not further described.

ICD-10-CM Code(s): A60.00

ICD-10-CM Rationale: The Alphabetic Index main term is Herpes, subterm genital, genitalis.

1.21. 042

Rationale: There are specific guidelines for reporting human immunodeficiency virus (HIV) infections. Code 042 is assigned to confirmed cases of HIV infection based on a physician's diagnostic statement. Once a patient develops an HIV-related illness, the 042 code is assigned on every subsequent admission for disease management of this condition. Once the 042 code is reported, it is inappropriate to assign codes 795.71 or V08, because the infection is confirmed.

ICD-10-CM Code(s): B20

ICD-10-CM Rationale: The Alphabetic Index main term is Human, subterm immunodeficiency virus (HIV) disease (infection).

1.22. 098.17

Rationale: The Alphabetic Index entries—main term Salpingitis, subterms venereal, acute; main term Salpingitis, subterms gonococcal, acute; or main term Gonorrhea, subterms fallopian tube, acute—are used to assign code 098.17.

ICD-10-CM Code(s): A54.24

ICD-10-CM Rationale: The Alphabetic Index main term is Salpingitis, subterm gonococcal (acute) (chronic).

1.23. a. 042

Rationale: AIDS stands for acquired immunodeficiency syndrome, frequently called human immunodeficiency infection. When a patient is treated for a complication associated with HIV infection, the 042 code is assigned as the principal diagnosis, followed by the code for the complication—in this case, a specific type of pneumonia. The Alphabetic Index main term is Pneumonia, subterm Pneumocystis (carinii). Whenever an HIV-positive patient is admitted with an HIV-related condition, the principal diagnosis should be 042, followed by additional ICD-9-CM codes for all reported HIV-related conditions.

1.24. c. 070.54

Rationale: The Alphabetic Index main term is Hepatitis, subterms viral, type C, chronic. An outpatient would not have hepatic coma, and this was also not mentioned in the diagnostic statement. Reporting for acute disease is different than for chronic disease.

ICD-10-CM Code: B18.2

ICD-10-CM Rationale: The Alphabetic Index main term is Hepatitis, subterm C, chronic.

1.25. 002.1

Rationale: The Alphabetic Index main term is Fever, subterm paratyphoid A.

ICD-10-CM Code(s): A01.1

ICD-10-CM Rationale: The Alphabetic Index main term is Fever, subterm paratyphoid, A.

1.26. 005.0

Rationale: The Alphabetic Index main term is Poisoning, subterms food, Staphylococcus.

ICD-10-CM Code(s): A05.0

ICD-10-CM Rationale: The Alphabetic Index main term is Poisoning, subterm food, due to, Staphylococcus.

1.27. 009.2

Rationale: The Alphabetic Index main term is Diarrhea, subterm infectious. A different code is assigned if the organism responsible is known.

ICD-10-CM Code(s): A09

ICD-10-CM Rationale: The Alphabetic Index main term is Diarrhea, diarrheal, subterm infectious.

1.28. 011.93

Rationale: The Alphabetic Index main term is Tuberculosis, subterm pulmonary. A fifth digit of 3 is required to show that the tubercle bacilli (in sputum) have been identified by microscopic examination.

ICD-10-CM Code(s): A15.0

ICD-10-CM Rationale: The Alphabetic Index main term is Tuberculosis, subterm pulmonary.

1.29. 034.1

Rationale: The Alphabetic Index main term is Scarlatina. The code 034.1 is assigned alone because there are no further qualifications documented as manifestations.

ICD-10-CM Code(s): A38.9

ICD-10-CM Rationale: The Alphabetic Index main term is Scarlatina.

1.30. 038.2

Rationale: Official coding guidelines state that if the documentation states septicemia, only code 038.2 should be assigned; however, the provider should be queried whether the patient has sepsis, an infection with SIRS.

ICD-10-CM Code(s): A40.3

ICD-10-CM Rationale: The Alphabetic Index main term is Septicemia. A note under Septicemia refers the coder to Sepsis. The main term is now Sepsis, subterm pneumococcal.

1.31. 110.0

Rationale: The Alphabetic Index main term is Dermatophytosis, subterm scalp. Codes are specific to anatomic location.

ICD-10-CM Code(s): B35.0

ICD-10-CM Rationale: The Alphabetic Index main term is Dermatophytosis, subterm scalp.

1.32. 055.1

Rationale: The Alphabetic Index main term is Pneumonia, subterms in, measles.

ICD-10-CM Code(s): B05.2

ICD-10-CM Rationale: The Alphabetic Index main term is Measles, subterm with, pneumonia.

1.33. 072.9

Rationale: The Alphabetic Index main term is the same because mumps without stated complications is assigned to code 072.9. This code is assigned only when the patient has confirmed disease, not for vaccination (V04.6).

ICD-10-CM Code(s): B26.9

ICD-10-CM Rationale: The Alphabetic Index main term is Mumps.

1.34. 078.12

Rationale: The Alphabetic Index main term is Wart, subterm plantar.

ICD-10-CM Code(s): B07.0

ICD-10-CM Rationale: The Alphabetic Index main term is Wart, subterm plantar.

1.35. 075

Rationale: The Alphabetic Index main term is Mononucleosis, infectious. This is an example of a three-digit category.

ICD-10-CM Code(s): B27.90

ICD-10-CM Rationale: The Alphabetic Index main term is Mononucleosis, infectious.

1.36. 078.11

Rationale: The Alphabetic Index main term is Condyloma with subterm acuminatum.

ICD-10-CM Code(s): A63.0

ICD-10-CM Rationale: The Alphabetic Index main term is Condyloma with subterm acuminatum.

1.37. 041.41

Rationale: The Alphabetic Index main term is Infection, subterm *Escherichia coil (E. coli)*, Shiga toxin-producing, with, O157.

ICD-10-CM Code(s): A49.8

ICD-10-CM Rationale: The Alphabetic Index main term is Infection, *Escherichia (E.) coli* NEC.

Neoplasms

1.38. 201.22

Rationale: The Alphabetic Index main term is the eponym Hodgkin's subterm sarcoma, with the fifth digit 2 added to indicate the location of the lymph nodes involved.

ICD-10-CM Code(s): C81.92

ICD-10-CM Rationale: The Alphabetic Index main term is Sarcoma, subterm Hodgkin—there is a note that refers the coder to lymphoma, Hodgkin. The main term now is Lymphoma, subterm Hodgkin. The fifth-digit extension 2 describes the intrathoracic lymph nodes.

1.39. 162.9

Rationale: The neoplasm table in the Alphabetic Index may be used for code selection. In the neoplasm table, the main term is bronchus. Because the character of the disease is stated to be malignant, the first column of the table is used for selection. The code is 162.9.

ICD-10-CM Code(s): C34.90

ICD-10-CM Rationale: The Alphabetic Index main term is Neoplasm, subterm bronchus. The code in the primary neoplasm column should be used. The coder completes the code using the Tabular List. The laterality is not stated, thus code C34.90 is assigned for the unspecified part of bronchus.

1.40. V58.0

Rationale: Encounters for chemotherapy and radiation therapy without other diagnostic workup or disease management are reported with a V code from the supplementary classification in first position. For a hospital inpatient, that is known as the principal diagnosis.

ICD-10-CM Code: Z51.0

ICD-10-CM Rationale: The Alphabetic Index main term is Admission, subterm radiation therapy (antineoplastic).

1.41. d. Either a or b

Rationale: When both treatment methods are used in the same admission, ICD-9-CM allows the reporting of either one as the principal diagnosis, according to guidelines. The disease is not reported in this position when the encounter is specifically for receipt of treatment rather than for diagnosis or disease management.

ICD-10-CM Code: Z51.11

ICD-10-CM Rationale: The Alphabetic Index main term is Chemotherapy, cancer.

1.42. 183.3

Rationale: The Alphabetic Index of ICD-9-CM, under the main term Carcinoma, instructs the coder to "see also neoplasm, by site, malignant." Turning to the neoplasm table, we go to the subterm for broad ligament and choose the code in the first column under the "malignant" heading. Because the cancer has not spread (metastasized), it is considered "primary."

ICD-10-CM Code(s): C57.10

ICD-10-CM Rationale: The Neoplasm Table is the main term, reference the subterm ligament, broad—fifth digit is 0, unspecified.

1.43. 211.7

Rationale: The Alphabetic Index indicates that the main term Adenoma is a benign neoplasm. Note the instructions to the coder to "see also neoplasm, by site, benign." Turning to the neoplasm table, we go to the subterms pancreas, islet cells, and assign code 211.7. Note that this code is different than the codes for benign growths in other parts of the pancreas.

ICD-10-CM Code(s): D13.7

ICD-10-CM Rationale: The Alphabetic Index main term is Adenoma, subterm islet cell, pancreas.

1.44. Benign

Rationale: Knowledge of the disease process is critical for accurate code assignment and correct classification.

1.45. 172.5

Rationale: The Alphabetic Index term is Melanoma, chest wall, resulting in code 172.5.

ICD-10-CM Code(s): C43.59

ICD-10-CM Rationale: The Alphabetic Index main term is Melanoma, subterm skin, chest wall.

1.46. 151.5

Rationale: The Alphabetic Index refers the coder to the neoplasm table and indicates that adenocarcinoma is considered malignant. When not further specified, the lesser curvature is reported with code 151.5.

ICD-10-CM Code(s): C16.5

ICD-10-CM Rationale: The Neoplasm Table is the main term, reference the subterm stomach, lesser curvature. Select the Malignant Primary column because the Alphabetic Index indicated that adenocarcinoma is considered malignant.

1.47. 198.89

Rationale: Malignant neoplasms are the only diseases with "secondary" eligibility in the neoplasm table. In the table, go to salivary gland, subterm submandibular, and choose the code in the secondary column. Note that this code is the same as many others despite the difference in anatomic location. Turn to the Tabular List in ICD-9-CM and review the description of code 198.89, Other specified sites, other, which is very broad.

ICD-10-CM Code(s): C79.89

ICD-10-CM Rationale: The Alphabetic Index main term is Carcinoma, which directs the coder to see also Neoplasm, malignant, by site. Subterm submandibular gland is accessed and the coder chooses the Malignant Secondary column.

1.48. 211.3

Rationale: In the neoplasm table, reference the main term appendix, to select the code in the "benign" column.

ICD-10-CM Code(s): D12.1

ICD-10-CM Rationale: The Neoplasm Table is the main term, reference the subterm appendix and select the code in the Benign column.

1.49. 233.0

Rationale: The term "in situ" indicates "in the original position." In other words, the cancer has not spread from the immediate area. ICD-9-CM has a specific location in the neoplasm table under malignancy. Because the exact location is not provided, the main term is breast, with no subterms. Note that regardless of the anatomic site within the breast, the code for "in situ" disease is the same in ICD-9-CM: 233.0.

ICD-10-CM Code(s): D05.91

ICD-10-CM Rationale: The Alphabetic Index main term is Carcinoma-in-situ, subterm breast Not Otherwise Specified (NOS). The coder completes the code using the Tabular List to report right breast.

1.50. b. Malignant

Rationale: In the Alphabetic Index the main term is Sympathicoblastoma with a note which refers the coder to see neoplasm, malignant, by site.

1.51. Connective tissue

Rationale: The ICD-9-CM classification system often provides clues in the Alphabetic Index concerning the nature of a neoplasm. In this case, it is clear that this is a malignant neoplasm of the connective tissue.

1.52. Primary

Rationale: When the origin of the neoplasm is not known (that is, the physician has stated that there is an unknown [primary] location), there is a specific code for reporting-199.1. Metastatic spread of a primary malignancy is reported as a secondary neoplasm, with the appropriate code according to the location. Code 155.2 is an example of an ICD-9-CM code that is not specified as primary or secondary that allows reporting of malignancy in the liver.

1.53. 162.9

Rationale: The Alphabetic Index refers the coder to the neoplasm table. The main term is bronchus, resulting in code 162.9. It would be important to carefully review the documentation to determine if a more specific code could be reported because this code is unspecified and could refer to either the bronchus or the lung. The term "bronchogenic" suggests that the cancer originated at this location, so the choice of primary malignancy is appropriate.

ICD-10-CM Code(s): C34.90

ICD-10-CM Rationale: The Alphabetic Index main term is Carcinoma, subterm bronchial or bronchogenic. The Index notes to see Neoplasm, lung, malignant which results in code C34.9x. The Tabular List is referenced to assign the 5th digit.

1.54. 233.1

Rationale: The Alphabetic Index refers the coder to the neoplasm table. The main term is uterine cervix, and the "in situ" column is selected for code 233.1.

ICD-10-CM Code(s): D06.9

ICD-10-CM Rationale: The Neoplasm Table is referenced with cervix (uteri) being the main term. The In Situ column is chosen.

1.55. a. Lymph nodes of inguinal region and lower limb

Rationale: The ICD-9-CM codes for malignancies of the lymphatic systems use fifth digits to indicate the location of lymph node involvement. In this case, the digit 5 indicates the lymph nodes of the inguinal region and lower limb. The lymph nodes of the Lymph nodes of axilla and upper limb are reflected in fifth digit 4, the intrapelvic 6, and the head, face, and neck 1.

1.56. 209.32

Rationale: The Alphabetic Index main term is Carcinoma, and subterms Merkel Cell, neck result in code 209.32.

ICD-10-CM Code(s): C4a.4

ICD-10-CM Rationale: The Alphabetic Index main term is Carcinoma, subterm Merkel cell, neck.

1.57. 205.02

Rationale: The Alphabetic Index main term is Leukemia, with subterms myelogenous, acute. Assign the fifth digit of 2 for the patient being in relapse.

ICD-10-CM Code(s): C92.02

ICD-10-CM Rationale: The Alphabetic Index main term is Leukemia, leukemic, subterm myelogenous. The coder is directed to see category C92. The correct code is C92.02.

1.58. 188.0

Rationale: Neoplasm Table with main term Bladder, trigone using the malignant, primary column.

ICD-10-CM Code(s): C67.0

ICD-10-CM Rationale: Neoplasm with main term Bladder, subterm trigone, Malignant, Primary column.

1.59. 173.22

Rationale: The Alphabetic Index main term is Neoplasm, ear, skin, squamous cell carcinoma, malignant.

ICD-10-CM Code(s): C44.22

ICD-10-CM Rationale: The Alphabetic Index main term is Neoplasm, Skin, ear (external), Malignant Primary. The coder completes the code using the Tabular List.

Endocrine, Nutritional, and Metabolic Diseases and Immunity Disorders

1.60. 275.01

Rationale: The Alphabetic Index main term is Hemochromatosis, subterm hereditary, which results in code 275.01.

ICD-10-CM Code(s): E83.110

ICD-10-CM Rationale: The Alphabetic Index main term is Hemochromatosis, subterm hereditary (primary).

1.61. 276.1

Rationale: The Alphabetic Index main term is the same.

ICD-10-CM Code(s): E87.1

ICD-10-CM Rationale: The Alphabetic Index main term is Hyponatremia.

1.62. 272.0

Rationale: The Alphabetic Index main term is the same, subterm primary, which results in the same code assignment.

ICD-10-CM Code(s): E78.0

ICD-10-CM Rationale: The Alphabetic Index main term is Hypercholesterolemia. The term primary is listed in parentheses.

1.63.   b. Hyperaldosteronism

Rationale: The ICD-9-CM index also includes eponyms and provides clues to the nature of the disease. In this case, a description of the disease is also listed as secondary hyperaldosteronism. There are also listings under the main term Syndrome that are useful, in some cases, for locating a specific code. Code 255.13 is listed under Syndromes, Bartter's.

1.64.   250.43, 581.81

Rationale: Coding of diabetes will often involve recognition of diabetes-related complications. The fourth digit indicates the type of diabetes involved and the fifth whether or not the physician has indicated that the diabetes is out of control. Comments such as "under poor control" should not be considered synonymous with uncontrolled. Physician query would be indicated.

ICD-10-CM Code(s): E10.21

ICD-10-CM Rationale: The Alphabetic Index main term is Diabetes, subterms Type I, with, nephropathy.

1.65.   249.00

Rationale: The Alphabetic Index main term is Diabetes, subterm secondary. The fourth digit of 0 is assigned to report without mention of complication. The fifth digit of 0 is assigned to report not stated as uncontrolled, or unspecified.

ICD-10-CM Code(s): E13.9

ICD-10-CM Rationale: The Alphabetic Index main term is Diabetes, subterm secondary. The coder is directed to see Diabetes, specified type.

1.66.   250.51, 362.02

Rationale: The Alphabetic Index main term is Diabetes, subterm retinopathy. The fifth digit of 1 is assigned because the patient is described as a type I (also referred to as juvenile onset). The ophthalmic manifestation is mentioned, which is reflected in the fourth digit, and the additional code, 362.02, is reported to specify what the complication is.

ICD-10-CM Code(s): E10.359

ICD-10-CM Rationale: The Alphabetic Index main term is Diabetes, subterms Type I, with, retinopathy, proliferative.

1.67.   250.13

Rationale: The Alphabetic Index term is Diabetes, subterms with and ketosis, ketoacidosis. The fourth digit of 1 is assigned because the patient is listed as type I and ketoacidosis by definition is uncontrolled.

ICD-10-CM Code(s): E10.10

ICD-10-CM Rationale: The Alphabetic Index main term is Diabetes, diabetic, subterm Type I, with, ketoacidosis.

1.68. 250.51

Rationale: Code 250.51 is assigned for this condition, although it would be very unusual not to also report the manifestation code that describes the complication. Coding professionals are expected to research the documentation for additional conditions that allow more granular data capture.

ICD-10-CM Code(s): E10.39

ICD-10-CM Rationale: The Alphabetic Index main term is Diabetes, subterms Type I, with, ophthalmic complications Not Elsewhere Classified (NEC).

1.69. 251.3

Rationale: The Alphabetic Index term is Hypoinsulinemia, postsurgical, because the patient has had the pancreas removed.

ICD-10-CM Code(s): E89.1, Z90.410

ICD-10-CM Rationale: The Alphabetic Index main term is Hypoinsulinemia, postprocedural. The Tabular List reminds the coder to use an additional code (Z90.41-) to show acquired absence of the pancreas. The coder uses the Tabular List to complete the code.

1.70. d. All of the above

Rationale: Each condition mentioned is indexed and classified in ICD-9-CM to code 255.2, so the answer is all of the above.

1.71. 253.3

Rationale: The Alphabetic Index term is Dwarfism, subterm hypophyseal, or main term Hypophyseal and subterm dwarfism.

ICD-10-CM Code(s): E23.0

ICD-10-CM Rationale: The Alphabetic Index main term is Dwarfism, subterm hypophyseal.

1.72. 276.8

Rationale: The Alphabetic Index main term is the same. Caution is required in assignment of codes based on abnormal findings without physician validation. If the condition is not listed in a diagnostic statement, the best practice is to ask the physician if the condition should be reported with a diagnosis code. Conditions that are integral to the disease process are not separately reported in ICD-9-CM, per coding guidelines.

ICD-10-CM Code(s): E87.6

ICD-10-CM Rationale: The Alphabetic Index main term is Hypopotassemia. There are no subterms.

1.73. 277.02

Rationale: The Alphabetic Index main term is Cystic, subterms fibrosis, with, manifestations, pulmonary.

ICD-10-CM Code(s): E84.0

ICD-10-CM Rationale: The Alphabetic Index main term is Fibrosis, fibrotic, subterm cystic, with, pulmonary manifestations.

1.74. Mucopolysaccharidosis

Rationale: The main term in ICD-9-CM is Syndrome, subterms Hurler's (Hunter) or Sanfilippo's, or an alternative main term is Gargoylism. All are classified to code 277.5 along with other syndromes.

ICD-10-CM Rationale: This main term in the Alphabetic Index lists subterms of Hurler's syndrome and Sanfilippo syndrome. Another main term in the Alphabetic Index may also be referenced—Gargoylism.

1.75. 278.01, V85.41

Rationale: The Alphabetic Index main term is Obesity, subterm morbid. ICD-9-CM defines morbid obesity as increased weight beyond the limits of skeletal and physical requirements (125 percent or more over ideal body weight), as a result of excess fat in subcutaneous connective tissues. Before this code is assigned, the diagnosis should be confirmed with the physician, rather than the coder making a judgment concerning whether the condition is morbid. Unspecified obesity is reported with code 278.00. An additional code should be assigned to identify the Body Mass Index, which is located under the main term Body, bodies, subterms mass index (BMI), adult, 40.0-44.9 V85.41 mass index, 40 and over, to code V85.41.

ICD-10-CM Code(s): E66.01, Z68.41

ICD-10-CM Rationale: The Alphabetic Index main term is Obesity, subterm morbid. The Tabular List E66 category instructs the coder to use an additional code to identify body mass index (BMI), if known (Z68).

1.76. 256.4

Rationale: The Alphabetic Index term is Polycystic, subterm ovary, ovaries, assigned to code 256.4.

ICD-10-CM Code(s): E28.2

ICD-10-CM Rationale: The Alphabetic Index main term is Polycystic, subterm ovary, ovaries.

1.77. 271.4

Rationale: The Alphabetic Index term is Glycosuria, subterm renal. If not designated as renal, this condition is classified as an abnormal finding with code 791.5.

ICD-10-CM Code(s): E74.8

ICD-10-CM Rationale: The Alphabetic Index main term is Glycosuria with subterm renal.

1.78. 242.30

Rationale: The Alphabetic Index main term is Goiter, subterms nodular, with hyperthyroidism. Cross-reference ("see also Goiter, toxic") produces the same code. There is no mention of thyrotoxic crisis or storm, so the correct fifth digit is 0.

ICD-10-CM Code(s): E05.20

ICD-10-CM Rationale: The Alphabetic Index main term Goiter with Hyperthyroidism refers the coder to "See Hyperthyroidism, with, goiter." The main term Hyperthyroidism in the Alphabetic Index is referred with subterms with, goiter, nodular.

1.79. 243

Rationale: The Alphabetic Index main term is Hypothyroidism, subterm congenital. This code is assigned only to patients who were born with this condition.

ICD-10-CM Code(s): E03.1

ICD-10-CM Rationale: The Alphabetic Index main term is Hypothyroidism, (acquired), subterm congenital.

1.80. 279.00

Rationale: Alphabetic Index term Agammaglobulinemia.

ICD-10-CM Code(s): D80.1

ICD-10-CM Rationale: Main term Agammaglobulinemia.

Disorders of the Blood and Blood-Forming Organs

1.81. 280.0

Rationale: The Alphabetic Index main term is Anemia, subterms due to, blood loss (chronic). Note that this condition is classified with iron deficiency anemia. If the coder followed Anemia, deficiency, iron, as subterms, code 280.9 would result and not be as specific. The combination of the Alphabetic Index and the Tabular List is required for accurate code assignment.

ICD-10-CM Code(s): D50.0

ICD-10-CM Rationale: The Alphabetic Index main term is Anemia with subterms deficiency, iron, secondary to blood loss.

1.82. b. Hereditary hemolytic anemias

Rationale: Both conditions are classified to category 282 (codes 282.60 and 282.4X) in the Alphabetic Index in ICD-9-CM. The main terms Sickle-cell and Thalassemia are indexed and are both hereditary hemolytic anemias.

1.83. 282.5

Rationale: Clinical disease is rarely present in patients who carry the sickle-cell trait. To locate this code in the Alphabetic Index, the main term is Sickle-cell, subterm trait, or main term Trait, subterm sickle-cell.

ICD-10-CM Code(s): D57.3

ICD-10-CM Rationale: The Alphabetic Index main term is Trait(s), subterm sickle-cell.

1.84. 285.1

Rationale: The Alphabetic Index main term is Anemia, subterms due to, blood loss, acute. Caution should be used in assignment of this code without confirmation from the physician that this is an appropriate diagnosis for reporting. Transfusions following surgery do not automatically mean the patient has suffered acute blood loss or has acute blood loss anemia. Also, diagnosis codes should not be assigned based on laboratory findings alone without physician confirmation of their significance. Best practice is to ask the physician if this condition is appropriate to add to the diagnostic statement and determine whether a code should be assigned.

ICD-10-CM Code(s): D62

ICD-10-CM Rationale: The Alphabetic Index main term is Anemia, subterm blood loss, acute.

1.85. 285.3

Rationale: The Alphabetic Index main term is Anemia subterms due to, antineoplastic chemotherapy, resulting in code 285.3.

ICD-10-CM Code(s): D64.81

ICD-10-CM Rationale: The Alphabetic Index main term is Anemia with subterms due to, antineoplastic chemotherapy.

1.86. a. Fanconi's anemia

Rationale: The Alphabetic Index directs assignment of code 284.01 for Fanconi's anemia. The main term is Anemia with subterm Fanconi's (congenital pancytopenia).

1.87. 286.4

Rationale: The Alphabetic Index main term is Disease, subterm von Willebrand's (angiohemophilia), or main term von Willebrand's (-Jurgens) (-Minot), subterm disease or syndrome.

ICD-10-CM Code(s): D68.0

ICD-10-CM Rationale: The Alphabetic Index main term is Disease with subterm von Willebrand.

1.88. White

Rationale: The Alphabetic Index main term Agranulocytosis directs the coder to code 288.0. Note that category 288 is for diseases of the white blood cells. This condition is characterized by a reduced number of white cells in the blood.

1.89. 284.9

Rationale: To code aplastic anemia without further qualification, the main term is Anemia, subterm aplastic.

ICD-10-CM Code(s): D61.9

ICD-10-CM Rationale: The Alphabetic Index main term is Anemia with subterm aplastic.

1.90. 281.2

Rationale: The Alphabetic Index main term is Anemia, subterms deficiency, folate. Note that the subterms under folate also are classified to the same code, 281.2, whether dietary or drug-induced. An E code may be used to indicate that the condition is due to a poisoning or adverse reaction to medical treatment. Documentation must reflect the type of cause-and-effect relationship in order to assign the additional E code.

ICD-10-CM Code(s): D52.1

ICD-10-CM Rationale: The Alphabetic Index main term is Anemia, subterm deficiency, folate, drug-induced.

1.91. 281.3

Rationale: The Alphabetic Index main term is Anemia, subterm refractory (primary) megaloblastic, resulting in code 281.3.

ICD-10-CM Code(s): D53.1

ICD-10-CM Rationale: The Alphabetic Index main term is Anemia with subterms megaloblastic, refractory.

1.92. 289.89

Rationale: The Alphabetic Index main term is Anemia, subterm osteosclerotic, or Osteosclerotic anemia, to assign code 289.89. Note that this code is not limited to this type of anemia but includes a variety of other specified diseases of blood and blood-forming organs that is quite broad.

ICD-10-CM Code(s): D64.89

ICD-10-CM Rationale: The Alphabetic Index main term is Anemia, subterm osteosclerotic.

1.93. 287.41

Rationale: The Alphabetic Index main term is Purpura, subterm posttransfusion, which results in code 287.41.

ICD-10-CM Code(s): D69.51

ICD-10-CM Rationale: The Alphabetic Index main term is Purpura with subterm posttransfusion.

1.94. 287.30

Rationale: The Alphabetic Index main term is Purpura, subterm thrombocytopenic, or main term Thrombocytopenia, subterm purpura, to assign code 287.30. Note that this condition is classified as a primary thrombocytopenia and includes other conditions specified using different terms.

ICD-10-CM Code(s): D69.49

ICD-10-CM Rationale: The Alphabetic Index main term is Purpura, subterm thrombocytopenic.

1.95. 287.49

Rationale: The Alphabetic Index main term is Thrombocytopenia, subterms due to, massive blood transfusion, resulting in code 287.49. There are E codes that could also be assigned to reflect the fact that the condition is an adverse reaction to medical treatment. See code category E934.x. Documentation must reflect a cause-and-effect relationship to assign the secondary code and the E code for adverse reaction to substance properly administered.

ICD-10-CM Code(s): D69.59

ICD-10-CM Rationale: The Alphabetic Index main term is Thrombocytopenia with subterms due to, (massive) blood transfusion.

1.96. 285.9

Rationale: This term is indexed as Anemia and is reported with 285.9. Care should be taken to determine if the condition is further specified within the health record for more specific coding than 285.9. Chronic simple anemia is classified to code 281.9 but should not be assigned without clear confirmation of the diagnosis. A fifth digit is required for codes that reflect anemia in chronic diseases but is not required for other specified anemia, 285.8, or the unspecified code in this exercise.

ICD-10-CM Code(s): D64.9

ICD-10-CM Rationale: The Alphabetic Index main term is Anemia.

1.97. 284.01

Rationale: The main terms Anemia or Aplasia can be used in the Alphabetic Index to locate the correct code, 284.01, with the subterms congenital, aplastic, or congenital pure red cell. This condition is also called constitutional anemia.

ICD-10-CM Code(s): D61.09

ICD-10-CM Rationale: The Alphabetic Index main term is Anemia with subterms congenital, aplastic.

1.98. 288.3

Rationale: The Alphabetic Index main term is Leukocytosis, with subterm eosinophilic, to assign code 288.3.

ICD-10-CM Code(s): D72.1

ICD-10-CM Rationale: The Alphabetic Index main term is Leukocytosis, subterm eosinophilic.

1.99. 281.1

Rationale: The Alphabetic Index main term is Anemia, subterms vitamin, and B_{12} deficiency, to assign code 281.1. Using the subterm deficiency, you will note that pernicious anemia has a different fourth digit.

ICD-10-CM Code(s): D51.9

ICD-10-CM Rationale: The Alphabetic Index main term is Anemia with subterms deficiency, vitamin B_{12}.

1.100. 286.0

Rationale: The Alphabetic Index includes this term for assignment of code 286.0. Note that many codes in this category are all congenital factor deficiencies in coagulation. If the coagulation deficiency is acquired and not congenital, code 286.7 applies. This may be due to liver disease or to a deficiency in vitamin K. An E code would be assigned if the cause were drug-induced to reflect the drug involved.

ICD-10-CM Code(s): D66

ICD-10-CM Rationale: The Alphabetic Index main term is Hemophilia (classical).

1.101. 280.9

Rationale: Fe refers to Iron. The Alphabetic Index main term is Anemia with subterm iron (Fe) deficiency.

ICD-10-CM Code(s): D50.9

ICD-10-CM Rationale: The Alphabetic main term is Anemia, with subterms deficiency, iron.

1.102. 284.89

Rationale: The Alphabetic Index main term is Anemia, subterm aplastic, due to, antineoplastic chemotherapy. An additional code would be used to identify the drug.

ICD-10-CM Code(s): T45.1x5A, D61.1

ICD-10-CM Rationale: The Alphabetic Index main term is Anemia, aplastic, due to drugs, resulting in code D61.1. In the Tabular List, code D61.1 indicates to first assign a code from category T36–T50 to identify the drug.

Mental Disorders

1.103. b. Two codes

Rationale: Two ICD-9-CM codes are required. The Alphabetic Index main term Disease, subterm Jakob-Creutzfeldt (code 046.19), with dementia, offers code 294.11 as a manifestation code with behavioral disturbance, code 294.10 without.

1.104. 291.2

Rationale: The Alphabetic Index main term is Syndrome, brain, chronic alcoholic, resulting in code 291.2. When coding a health record, an additional ICD-9-CM code would be assigned for the alcoholism.

ICD-10-CM Code(s): F10.27

ICD-10-CM Rationale: The Alphabetic Index main term is Alcohol, alcoholic, alcohol-induced with subterms brain syndrome, chronic, with dependence.

1.105. 295.34

Rationale: The Alphabetic Index main term is Schizophrenia, subterm paranoid (acute), with the fifth digit of 4 added to reflect an acute exacerbation of a chronic condition, resulting in code 295.34.

ICD-10-CM Code(s): F20.0

ICD-10-CM Rationale: The Alphabetic Index main term is Schizophrenia with subterm paranoid (type).

1.106. 301.11

Rationale: The Alphabetic Index main term is Disorder, subterms personality and hypomanic (chronic), for assignment of code 301.11.

ICD-10-CM Code(s): F60.89

ICD-10-CM Rationale: The Alphabetic Index main term is Disorder, subterm personality. Code F60.9 was found but on review of Tabular List, F60.89 is the correct code.

1.107. 300.01

Rationale: There are two ways to locate this code in the Alphabetic Index. One is under the main term Attack, subterm panic, and the second is found under the main term Panic, to locate code 300.01.

ICD-10-CM Code(s): F41.0

ICD-10-CM Rationale: The Alphabetic Index main term is Attack with subterm panic.

1.108. a. Dissociative identity disorder

Rationale: In the ICD-9-CM Alphabetic Index, look up Multiple, and note the code assignment under the subterm personality, 300.14. Note that ICD-9-CM includes the term "dissociative identity disorder." Looking up disorder, identity results in a different code. The index for Dissociative, subterm identity disorder, also results in code 300.14, so answer "a" is correct.

1.109. 299.00

Rationale: The Alphabetic Index main term is Autism, which results in code 299.00.

ICD-10-CM Code(s): F84.0

ICD-10-CM Rationale: The Alphabetic Index main term is Autism with childhood in parentheses.

1.110. d. All of the above

Rationale: The Alphabetic Index for any of these entries leads to category 302 for sexual deviations and disorders, along with other forms of psychosexual problems/disorders.

1.111. 303.00

Rationale: The Alphabetic Index main term is Intoxication, subterms acute, with alcoholism, to assign code 303.00. Fifth-digit assignments must be based on physician documentation rather than subjective assessment by the coder. Acute intoxication may occur in patients who do not have chronic alcoholism, and the code assignment is then 305.00.

ICD-10-CM Code(s): F10.229

ICD-10-CM Rationale: The Alphabetic Index main term is Alcohol, alcoholic, alcoholic-induced with subterms intoxication (acute), with dependence.

1.112. 304.03

Rationale: Drug addiction is indexed under the main term Dependence in the ICD-9-CM Alphabetic Index. The subterm is morphine. The fifth digit 3 is used to denote that the patient is not currently using the drug and is considered by the physician to be in remission. Coders may not make assumptions about whether or not the patient is in remission from documentation found in the record. This is based on physician specification of the patient's status.

ICD-10-CM Code(s): F11.21

ICD-10-CM Rationale: The Alphabetic Index main term is Dependence, subterm opioid, in remission. An alternate would be Dependence, morphine— see dependence drug, opioid.

1.113. 304.70

Rationale: This combination of recreational drugs and prescription drugs is classified to code 304.70. Morphine or any other opioid-type drug (such as heroin) in combination with any other type of drug is assigned to this category. Because the status of drug use is not known in this statement, the fifth digit 0 is assigned.

ICD-10-CM Code(s): F19.20

ICD-10-CM Rationale: The Alphabetic Index main term is Dependence with subterm polysubstance.

1.114. 306.0

Rationale: The Alphabetic Index main term is Torticollis, which may be a medical condition or psychogenic in origin. The subterm psychogenic results in code assignment of 306.0.

ICD-10-CM Code(s): F45.8

ICD-10-CM Rationale: The Alphabetic Index main term is Torticollis, psychogenic.

1.115. 307.23

Rationale: This mental illness is indexed in ICD-9-CM by the eponym for the disease rather than under Disorder and is assigned to code 307.23.

ICD-10-CM Code(s): F95.2

ICD-10-CM Rationale: The Alphabetic Index main term is Syndrome with subterm Gilles de la Tourette's.

1.116. 296.30

Rationale: The Alphabetic Index main term is Depression, subterm recurrent episode, resulting in code 296.3. The fifth digit of 0 is assigned for unspecified type of depression.

ICD-10-CM Code(s): F33.9

ICD-10-CM Rationale: If you look under Depression, major (recurrent), the Alphabetic Index directs the coder to Disorder, depressive, recurrent.

1.117. 309.21

Rationale: This condition is found in the Alphabetic Index under Disorder, subterms separation, anxiety, and assigned to code 309.21.

ICD-10-CM Code(s): F93.0

ICD-10-CM Rationale: The Alphabetic Index main term is Disorder with subterm separation anxiety of childhood.

1.118. 318.0

Rationale: The Alphabetic Index main term is Disability, disabilities, subterms intellectual, moderate, IQ 35–49.

ICD-10-CM Code(s): F71

ICD-10-CM Rationale: The Alphabetic Index main term is Retardation, subterm mental, moderate (based on IQ).

1.119. 314.01

Rationale: This condition is indexed under the main term Disorder, subterm attention deficit with hyperactivity, resulting in code 314.01.

ICD-10-CM Code(s): F90.9

ICD-10-CM Rationale: The Alphabetic Index main term is Disorder with subterm attention-deficit hyperactivity.

1.120. 291.5

Rationale: The Alphabetic Index main term is Paranoia, subterm alcoholic, for code 291.5. An additional code would be added to reflect alcoholism, according to the documentation provided in the actual health record.

ICD-10-CM Code(s): F10.950

ICD-10-CM Rationale: The Alphabetic Index main term is Alcohol, subterm paranoia, paranoid (type) psychosis.

1.121. 291.0

Rationale: Delirium tremens is a common side effect for a chronic alcoholic who is not drinking. The Alphabetic Index has an entry for the term, with the nonessential modifier (impending) listed, and code 291.0. The appropriate code for alcoholism would be assigned, based on the information available in the record that is not found in this short statement.

ICD-10-CM Code(s): F10.231

ICD-10-CM Rationale: The Alphabetic Index main term is Delirium with subterms due to, alcohol, withdrawal.

1.122. 290.43, 437.0

Rationale: This mental illness that follows cerebral infarctions is indexed under the main term Dementia, multi-infarct, with an instruction to "see also Dementia, arteriosclerotic." Going to this subterm shows additional choices including depressed features and depressed type, both assigned to code 290.43. If this is a late effect of cerebrovascular disease, an additional code should be added from the 438 category, based on the documentation in the health record. Note instructions to also assign 437.0 with this subcategory.

ICD-10-CM Code(s): F01.51, F32.9

ICD-10-CM Rationale: The Alphabetic Index main term is Dementia, subterm multi-infarct. The coder is directed to Dementia, vascular. The depression is considered behavioral disturbance, which results in code F01.51. The Alphabetic Index is Depression.

1.123. 301.84

Rationale: The Alphabetic Index main term is Disorder with subterms personality, passive-aggressive.

ICD-10-CM Code(s): F60.89

ICD-10-CM Rationale: The Alphabetic Index main term is Disorder with subterms personality, passive-aggressive.

1.124. 294.21

Rationale: The Alphabetic Index main term is Dementia, subterm behavioral disturbance.

ICD-10-CM Code(s): F01.51

ICD-10-CM Rationale: The Alphabetic Index main term is Dementia, multi-infarct, with an instruction to "see Dementia, vascular." Going to this subterm shows an additional choice of "with behavioral disturbances" which results in code F01.51.

Nervous System and Sense Organs

1.125. 360.01

Rationale: Index the main term Endophthalmitis, subterm acute, for code 360.01.

ICD-10-CM Code(s): H44.009

ICD-10-CM Rationale: The Alphabetic Index main term is Endophthalmitis with acute in parentheses.

1.126. 359.1

Rationale: This condition is indexed under the main term Dystrophy, with subterms muscular or Duchenne's, resulting in the same code, 359.1.

ICD-10-CM Code(s): G71.0

ICD-10-CM Rationale: The Alphabetic Index main term is Duchenne's, subterm disease, muscular dystrophy.

1.127. c. 250.51, 362.02

Rationale: When retinopathy is due to underlying type 1 diabetes, the diabetes code is sequenced first, followed by a manifestation code for the retinopathy, as in answer "c."

1.128. 362.31

Rationale: This condition is found in the Alphabetic Index under the main term Occlusion, subterms retina and artery, central to result in the selection of code 362.31.

ICD-10-CM Code(s): H34.10

ICD-10-CM Rationale: The Alphabetic Index main term is Occlusion, subterm retinal, central. The code given is incomplete so the coder must reference the Tabular List.

1.129. 370.8, 136.21

Rationale: The Alphabetic Index main term is Keratitis, subterm specified type, which results in code 370.8. The Tabular List instructs to first assign the underlying condition, which is acanthamoeba, 136.21.

ICD-10-CM Code(s): B60.13

ICD-10-CM Rationale: The Alphabetic Index main term is Acanthamebiasis with subterm keratoconjunctivitis.

1.130. 361.81

Rationale: To locate the correct code, use the main term Detachment, then retina, then traction, to assign code 361.81.

ICD-10-CM Code(s): H33.43

ICD-10-CM Rationale: The Alphabetic Index main term is Detachment, subterm retina, traction. The code is completed using the Tabular List.

1.131. 366.14

Rationale: The Alphabetic Index main term is Cataract, subterms senile, posterior subcapsular. Assuming the cataract is "senile" on the basis of the patient's age is inappropriate. A specific diagnosis of senile cataract is required to assign a code from this category. A cataract without further specification as to type is reported with code 366.9.

ICD-10-CM Code(s): H25.049

ICD-10-CM Rationale: The Alphabetic Index main term is Cataract with subterms senile, subcapsular polar, posterior.

1.132. 365.22, 365.71

Rationale: The main term Glaucoma is indexed in the Alphabetic Volume II of ICD-9-CM, and subterms include angle closure, acute, for assignment of code 365.22. When specified as chronic, this code is not appropriate. The Alphabetic Index main term is Glaucoma, subterm stage mild.

ICD-10-CM Code(s): H40.219

ICD-10-CM Rationale: The Alphabetic Index main term is Glaucoma, subterm angle—closure, acute. The coder completes the code using the Tabular List.

1.133. 368.53

Rationale: The main alphabetic term is Defect, subterm tritan to indicate code 368.53.

ICD-10-CM Code(s): H53.55

ICD-10-CM Rationale: The Alphabetic Index main term is Tritanomaly, tritanopia.

1.134. 371.23

Rationale: The main alphabetic term is Keratopathy, subterm bullous, to indicate code 371.23. Note the "see also Keratitis" when this diagnosis is considered for coding.

ICD-10-CM Code(s): H18.13

ICD-10-CM Rationale: The Alphabetic Index main term is Keratopathy, subterm bullous. The coder completes the code using the Tabular List.

1.135. 348.81

Rationale: The main alphabetic term is Sclerosis, subterm temporal for code 348.81.

ICD-10-CM Code(s): G93.81

ICD-10-CM Rationale: The Alphabetic Index main term is Sclerosis with subterm temporal (mesial).

1.136. c. Presbyopia

Rationale: Look up each term in the Alphabetic Index. The term Presbyopia (answer "c") does not result in a code from category 378, but rather code 367.4.

1.137. 381.10

Rationale: When otitis media is specified as chronic serous, code 381.10 results. If the documentation does not further specify this common ear infection in children, the code assignment defaults to 382.9. The main term is Otitis, subterms media, serous, chronic.

ICD-10-CM Code(s): H65.20

ICD-10-CM Rationale: The Alphabetic Index main term is Otitis with subterms media, chronic, serous. Under subterm serous, there is a note to "see Otitis, media, nonsuppurative, chronic, serous."

1.138. 382.01

Rationale: It is important to code this according to ICD-9-CM conventions. The main term is Otitis, subterms media, suppurative, acute with spontaneous rupture of eardrum. This may also be expressed as tympanic perforation. When this occurs postinflammation, the code is 384.20.

ICD-10-CM Code(s): H66.019

ICD-10-CM Rationale: The Alphabetic Index main term is Otitis, subterm media, suppurative, acute with rupture of eardrum. The coder completes the code using the Tabular List.

1.139. 385.33

Rationale: The Alphabetic Index main term is Cholesteatoma, with subterms middle ear, with involvement of mastoid cavity, for code 385.33.

ICD-10-CM Code(s): H71.22

ICD-10-CM Rationale: The Alphabetic Index main term is Cholestatoma (middle) with subterm mastoid. Left ear is H71.22.

1.140. 386.51

Rationale: The Alphabetic Index main term is Hyperactive, labyrinth (unilateral), so the code is 386.51. If present in both ears, code 386.52 is assigned. Take care not to confuse hyper with hypoactivity, which has a different code-386.53.

ICD-10-CM Code(s): H83.2x1

ICD-10-CM Rationale: The Alphabetic Index main term is Labyrinthitis. The coder is directed to see also subcategory H83.

1.141. 379.41

Rationale: Anisocoria is the inequality in the size of the pupils of the eyes. The code assignment depends on whether the condition is congenital or not. Without further qualification, the code is 379.41.

ICD-10-CM Code(s): H57.02

ICD-10-CM Rationale: The Alphabetic Index main term is Anisocoria. The code number H57.09 is listed, but in checking the subcategory H57.0, code H57.02 specifically identifies Anisocoria.

1.142. 380.14

Rationale: The Alphabetic Index main term is Otitis, externa, malignant, resulting in code 380.14. This is a severe necrotic form due to bacteria.

ICD-10-CM Code(s): H60.20

ICD-10-CM Rationale: The Alphabetic Index main term is Otitis, subterm externa, malignant. The coder completes the code using the Tabular List.

1.143. 345.91

Rationale: The Alphabetic Index main term is Epilepsy and the fifth digit, 1, is assigned for poorly controlled, which results in code 345.91.

ICD-10-CM Code(s): G40.919

ICD-10-CM Rationale: The Alphabetic Index main term is Epilepsy with note following the basic code. The note identifies "poorly controlled" as intractable. The subterm intractable is then identified as G40.919.

1.144. 337.21

Rationale: The main term in the Alphabetic Index is Dystrophy, subterm sympathetic (reflex), upper limb, resulting in code 337.21. Even though the condition affects both arms, ICD-9-CM codes are not repeated. This is a convention of a classification system that is different from other coding systems, such as CPT, where a code may have a modifier appended or more than one code assigned when the procedure is performed in more than one location.

ICD-10-CM Code(s): G90.513

ICD-10-CM Rationale: The Alphabetic Index main term is Dystrophy, subterm reflex. The coder is directed to see Syndrome, pain, complex regional 1. The code must be completed using the Tabular List.

1.145. 331.0, 294.11

Rationale: The Alphabetic Index main term is Alzheimer's with subterms dementia, with behavioral disturbance; code 294.11 is for behavioral disturbance.

ICD-10-CM Code(s): G30.0, F02.81

ICD-10-CM Rationale: The Alphabetic Index main term is Alzheimer's disease with subterm with behavioral disturbance. Review of the Tabular List for code G30 includes an instructional note to use an additional code to identify behavioral disturbance—F02.81.

1.146. 348.82

Rationale: In additional to using this code for brain death, any associated injuries would also be coded. The Alphabetic Index main term is Death, subterm brain.

ICD-10-CM Code(s): G93.89

ICD-10-CM Rationale: The Alphabetic Index main term is Brain, death.

Circulatory System

1.147. 417.1

Rationale: The main term in the Alphabetic Index is Aneurysm, subterm pulmonary, resulting in code 417.1.

ICD-10-CM Code(s): I28.1

ICD-10-CM Rationale: The Alphabetic Index main term is Aneurysm with subterm pulmonary.

1.148. d. 402.01, 428.0

Rationale: The Alphabetic Index main term is Hypertension, which takes you to the hypertension table. Note that hypertension with heart involvement has a note to "see also hypertension, heart." There is a specific code for malignant hypertension with heart failure in code 402.01. In the Tabular List there is an instruction to use an additional code to specify the type of heart failure, so code 428.0 is also assigned for that purpose. Answer "b" is incorrect because the code for heart failure is not specific to congestive failure.

ICD-10-CM Code(s): I11.0, I50.9

ICD-10-CM Rationale: The Alphabetic Index main term is Hypertension, hypertensive, heart, with heart failure (congestive), resulting in code I11.0. In the Tabular List, code I11.0 directs the use of an additional code to identify type of heart failure (I50.-).

1.149. 396.1

Rationale: The ICD-9-CM classification system provides a specific category for valve disease that involves both structures and whether or not they are specified as rheumatic. In the Alphabetic Index, the main terms are Stenosis, subterms mitral, with aortic, insufficiency or incompetence, for code 396.1; or Insufficiency, aortic, with mitral valve disease, 396.1.

ICD-10-CM Code(s): I08.0

ICD-10-CM Rationale: The Alphabetic Index main term is Stenosis with subterms mitral, with aortic valve disease.

1.150. 410.21

Rationale: The Alphabetic Index main term is Infarct, subterm myocardium, inferolateral, with code 410.21 resulting. When a myocardial infarct is documented as acute, the initial episode of care fifth digit is assigned to a discharged patient. The use of the fifth-digit 0 should not apply when a health record is available for coding.

ICD-10-CM Code(s): I21.19

ICD-10-CM Rationale: The Alphabetic Index main term is Infarct, infarction, subterm myocardium, ST elevation, inferolateral.

1.151. 8

Rationale: This is an ICD-9-CM convention. The index guides the coder from the main term Infarct, myocardium, with symptoms after 8 weeks, to code 414.8. Turn to the Tabular List for category 410 (acute myocardial infarction). Note the definitions for the use of the fifth-digit 2 and also refer to the notes concerning "stated duration of 8 weeks or less."

ICD-10-CM Rationale: Four weeks or less is the time limit.

1.152. 401.9

Rationale: Hypertension when not otherwise specified by the physician is reported with code 401.9. An assumption cannot be made by a coder that the hypertension is benign or malignant-this must be stated by the physician. The hypertension table in the Alphabetic Index may be referenced to locate this code.

ICD-10-CM Code(s): I10

ICD-10-CM Rationale: The Alphabetic Index main term is Hypertension.

1.153. Stenosis, 425.11

Rationale: The Alphabetic main term is Stenosis with subterms subaortic, hypertrophic (idiopathic).

ICD-10-CM Code(s): I42.1

ICD-10-CM Rationale: The Alphabetic main term is Stenosis, with subterm hypertrophic subaortic (idiopathic).

1.154. 427.32

Rationale: The main term is Flutter, subterm atrial or heart, atrial, resulting in code 427.32.

ICD-10-CM Code(s): I48.1

ICD-10-CM Rationale: The Alphabetic Index main term is Flutter, subterm atrial or auricular.

1.155. 427.41

Rationale: The Alphabetic Index main term is Fibrillation, subterm ventricular, to locate code 427.41.

ICD-10-CM Code(s): I49.01

ICD-10-CM Rationale: The Alphabetic Index main term is fibrillation with subterm ventricular.

1.156. 428.31

Rationale: The main term in the Alphabetic Index is Failure, subterms heart, diastolic, acute, to locate code 428.31.

ICD-10-CM Code(s): I50.31

ICD-10-CM Rationale: The Alphabetic Index main term is Failure, failed, subterm heart, diastolic, acute.

1.157. 411.1

Rationale: The Alphabetic Index main term is Angina, subterm preinfarctional. Angina that evolved into a myocardial infarction in the hospital setting would not be assigned a separate code. Rather, the code for the MI would be assigned because the angina in this circumstance would be considered integral to the disease process.

ICD-10-CM Code(s): I20.0

ICD-10-CM Rationale: The Alphabetic Index main term is Angina with subterm preinfarction—there is a note which directs the coder to angina, unstable.

1.158. 415.19

Rationale: The Alphabetic Index main term is Infarct, subterm pulmonary. A fifth digit is assigned to reflect whether the event was iatrogenic (due to treatment) or not specified as iatrogenic in the "other" category, to result in code 415.19.

ICD-10-CM Code(s): I26.99

ICD-10-CM Rationale: The Alphabetic Index main term is Infarct, infarction, subterm pulmonary. The coder is directed to see Embolism, pulmonary.

1.159. 414.06 (if native artery)

414.07 (if of bypass graft)

Rationale: Patients with a transplanted heart may also get arteriosclerotic heart disease in the new heart, either in the native artery or of a bypass graft. The Alphabetic Index main term is Arteriosclerosis, subterms coronary, of transplanted heart, resulting in code 414.06 or 414.07 depending on the documentation.

ICD-10-CM Code(s): I25.811

ICD-10-CM Rationale: The Alphabetic Index main term is Arteriosclerosis, coronary (artery) with subterm transplanted heart (native).

1.160. 414.04

Rationale: The Alphabetic Index main term is Atherosclerosis, which refers you to arteriosclerosis, subterm bypass graft, coronary artery, autologous artery (internal mammary), to code 414.04. Autologous means that the artery was bypassed with tissue taken from another location in the patient's own body.

ICD-10-CM Code(s): I25.810

ICD-10-CM Rationale: The Alphabetic Index main term is Atherosclerosis, which refers the coder to Arteriosclerosis, subterm coronary (artery), bypass graft, autologous artery.

1.161. 438.13

Rationale: Late effects of a cerebral event that occurred in the past are reported with a code from the 438 category in ICD-9-CM. Using Dysarthria as the main term results in code 784.5 in the Alphabetic Index, which is a symptom code. To locate the appropriate code, go to the index entry Late, subterms effect, cerebrovascular disease, with, dysarthria, resulting in code 438.13.

ICD-10-CM Code(s): I69.922

ICD-10-CM Rationale: The Alphabetic Index main term is Dysarthria with subterms following, cerebrovascular disease.

1.162. 433.21

Rationale: The Alphabetic Index entry is Stenosis, subterm precerebral, which refers you to narrowing, artery, precerebral, which suggests code 433.2, with the fifth digit of 1 added to show the presence of the infarction. If Infarct is used as the main term, subterm cerebral, code 434.91 is suggested; however, the vertebral artery is not considered a cerebral artery, but rather a precerebral artery.

ICD-10-CM Code(s): I63.219

ICD-10-CM Rationale: The Alphabetic Index main term is Infarct, infarction, subterm cerebral, due to, stenosis, precerebral artery. The vertebral artery is a precerebral artery. The code must be completed using the Tabular List.

1.163. 416.2

Rationale: The Alphabetic Index main term is Embolism, subterms pulmonary, chronic, to assign the code 416.2.

ICD-10-CM Code(s): I27.82

ICD-10-CM Rationale: The Alphabetic Index main term is Embolism with subterms pulmonary, chronic.

1.164. 458.0

Rationale: The main term used in the Alphabetic Index is Hypotension.

ICD-10-CM Code(s): I95.1

ICD-10-CM Rationale: The Alphabetic Index main term is Hypotension, subterm orthostatic.

1.165. 454.0

Rationale: The Alphabetic Index main term is Varicose, subterm vein, with, ulcer, resulting in code 454.0.

ICD-10-CM Code(s): I83.029

ICD-10-CM Rationale: The Alphabetic Index main term is Varicose, vein, "see Varix." Main term Varix, subterms, leg, left, with, ulcer.

1.166. 441.3

Rationale: The Alphabetic Index main term is Aneurysm, subterms aorta, abdominal, ruptured, resulting in code 441.3.

ICD-10-CM Code(s): I71.3

ICD-10-CM Rationale: The Alphabetic Index main term is Aneurysm, subterm abdominal, ruptured.

1.167. 428.32

Rationale: The Alphabetic Index main term is Failure with subterms heart, diastolic, chronic.

ICD-10-CM Code(s): I50.32

ICD-10-CM Rationale: The Alphabetic Index main term is Failure with subterms heart, diastolic, chronic.

1.168. 444.01

Rationale: The Alphabetic Index main term is Embolism, subterm saddle, abdominal aorta.

ICD-10-CM Code(s): I74.0

ICD-10-CM Rationale: The Alphabetic Index main term is Embolism aorta, saddle.

Respiratory System

1.169. 466.0

Rationale: The Alphabetic Index main term is Bronchitis, subterm acute, resulting in code 466.0. Note that acute bronchitis with various forms of COPD results in a different code assignment. Bronchitis not specified as acute is classified to code 490.

ICD-10-CM Code(s): J20.9

ICD-10-CM Rationale: The Alphabetic Index main term is Bronchitis with subterm acute or subacute.

1.170. 464.01

Rationale: The Alphabetic Index main term is Laryngitis, subterm with obstruction, resulting in code 464.01.

ICD-10-CM Code(s): J05.0

ICD-10-CM Rationale: The Alphabetic Index main term is Laryngitis, subterm obstructive. Acute is a nonessential modifier.

1.171. 474.10

Rationale: The main term in the Alphabetic Index is Hypertrophy, adenoids and tonsils, or tonsils and adenoids, resulting in code 474.10.

ICD-10-CM Code(s): J35.3

ICD-10-CM Rationale: The Alphabetic Index main term is Hypertrophy with subterms tonsils, with adenoids.

1.172. 471.8

Rationale: The Alphabetic Index main term is Polyp, subterm sinus or maxillary (sinus), resulting in code 471.8.

ICD-10-CM Code(s): J33.8

ICD-10-CM Rationale: The Alphabetic Index main term is Polyp, polypus, subterm sinus. Maxillary is a nonessential modifier.

1.173. b. 480.1

Rationale: RSV is the abbreviation for respiratory syncytial virus. To code this condition, the main term is Pneumonia, subterm respiratory syncytial virus, resulting in code 480.1. Code 079.6 would not be needed to reflect the organism because it is specified in code 480.1. The 466.11 code is for bronchiolitis due to RSV, rather than pneumonia.

ICD-10-CM Code(s): J12.1

ICD-10-CM Rationale: RSV is the abbreviation for respiratory syncytial virus. The Alphabetic Index main term is Pneumonia with subterm respiratory syncytial virus.

1.174. 482.42

Rationale: The Alphabetic Index main term is Pneumonia, subterms Staphylococcus, aureus, methicillin, resistant (MRSA), resulting in code 482.42.

ICD-10-CM Code(s): J15.21, Z16

ICD-10-CM Rationale: The Alphabetic Index main term is Pneumonia, subterm Staphylococcus aureus. The Z16 code identifies the organism as drug resistant. Access Alphabetic Index main term Infection, with, drug resistant organism.

1.175. 491.21

Rationale: The Alphabetic Index main term is Disease, subterms pulmonary, obstructive (chronic), with acute exacerbation, resulting in code 491.21.

ICD-10-CM Code(s): J44.1

ICD-10-CM Rationale: The Alphabetic Index main term is Disease with subterms lung, obstructive (chronic), with, acute, exacerbation.

1.176. 492.8

Rationale: The Alphabetic Index main term is Emphysema. When not otherwise qualified, code 492.8 results. The health record should be evaluated for further specificity as to the type of emphysema when reporting for a healthcare episode or visit.

ICD-10-CM Code(s): J43.9

ICD-10-CM Rationale: The Alphabetic Index main term is Emphysema.

1.177. 486

Rationale: Although this diagnostic statement appears to be very specific, ICD-9-CM does not provide a specific code but rather classifies this condition to pneumonia, not elsewhere classified. The main term is Pneumonia, but it should be noted that bilateral, granulomatous, hemorrhagic, and septic are all nonessential modifiers.

ICD-10-CM Code(s): J18.9

ICD-10-CM Rationale: The Alphabetic Index main term is Pneumonia with bilateral, granulomatous, hemorrhagic, and septic in parentheses.

1.178. 488.81

Rationale: The Alphabetic Index main term is Influenza, influenza, subterms due to identified, novel influenza A virus, with pneumonia.

ICD-10-CM Code(s): J09.110

ICD-10-CM Rationale: The Alphabetic Index main term is Influenza, subterm due to, identified novel H1N1 influenza virus, with, pneumonia, due to identified novel H1N1 influenza virus.

1.179. 493.21

Rationale: The Alphabetic Index main term is Asthma, subterm with chronic obstructive pulmonary disease, resulting in code 493.21. The fifth digit of 1 reflects the status asthmaticus.

ICD-10-CM Code(s): J44.1, J45.902

ICD-10-CM Rationale: The Alphabetic Index main term is Asthma with subterms with, chronic obstructive pulmonary disease, with acute exacerbation. The Tabular List category J44 includes a note to code also the type of asthma, if applicable.

1.180. 512.1

Rationale: The Alphabetic Index main term is Pneumothorax, subterm postoperative, resulting in code 512.1.

ICD-10-CM Code(s): J95.81

ICD-10-CM Rationale: The Alphabetic Index main term is Pneumothorax, subterm postprocedural.

1.181. 518.83

Rationale: The Alphabetic Index main term is Failure, subterms respiration, chronic, resulting in code 518.83.

ICD-10-CM Code(s): J96.10

ICD-10-CM Rationale: The Alphabetic Index main term is Failure, with subterms respiration, chronic.

1.182. 519.02

Rationale: A tracheostomy is an artificial opening created in the trachea to facilitate breathing. The main term in the Alphabetic Index is Stenosis, subterm tracheostomy, resulting in code 519.02.

ICD-10-CM Code(s): J95.03

ICD-10-CM Rationale: The Alphabetic Index main term is Stenosis, subterm tracheostomy.

1.183. 494.0

Rationale: The Alphabetic Index main term is Bronchiectasis. Postinfectious is a nonessential modifier, so code 494.0 is appropriate. If documentation of an acute exacerbation was present, code 494.1 would be assigned.

ICD-10-CM Code(s): J47.9

ICD-10-CM Rationale: The Alphabetic Index main term is Bronchiectasis coded to J47.9.

1.184. c. 493.01

Rationale: The Alphabetic Index main term is Asthma, with subterm extrinsic adding the fourth digit of 0. The fifth digit of 1 reflects the status asthmaticus. The *Official Coding Guidelines* of ICD-9-CM states that it is inappropriate to assign an asthma code with a fifth digit of 2 (with acute exacerbation) together with an asthma code with a fifth digit of 1 (with status asthmaticus). Only the fifth digit of 1 should be assigned to indicate the status asthmaticus.

ICD-10-CM Code(s): J45.902

ICD-10-CM Rationale: The Alphabetic Index main term is Asthma, subterm allergic extrinsic, with status asthmaticus.

1.185. 512.90

Rationale: The Alphabetic Index main term is Pneumothorax, subterm spontaneous.

ICD-10-CM Code(s): J93.1

ICD-10-CM Rationale: The Alphabetic Index main term is Pneumothorax with subterm spontaneous NEC.

1.186. 493.00

Rationale: The main Alphabetic Index term is Asthma, subterm childhood, to assign 493.0x. The fifth digit describes with or without status asthmaticus or acute exacerbation. The appropriate fifth digit in this case is 0 because neither status asthmaticus nor acute exacerbation is mentioned.

ICD-10-CM Code(s): J45.909

ICD-10-CM Rationale: The Alphabetic Index main term is Asthma, asthmatic, subterm childhood.

1.187. 508.0

Rationale: The main term in the Alphabetic Index is Pneumonitis, subterm radiation, resulting in assignment of code 508.0. Depending on the reporting circumstances, an E code from the supplementary classification systems in the ICD-9-CM system might be added to reflect the external cause of this condition.

ICD-10-CM Code(s): J70.0, W88.1xxA

ICD-10-CM Rationale: The Alphabetic Index main term is Pneumonitis with subterm radiation. The Tabular List indicates that the coder should "Use additional code (W88–W90, X39.0-) to identify the external cause. The External Cause Index main term is Radiation (exposure to), radioactive isotope.

1.188. 460

Rationale: The Alphabetic Index main term is Cold, resulting in the three-digit category code 460. Acute upper respiratory illness is often used for patients who seek treatment in the emergency room or physician's office. This condition is classified to code 465.9 in ICD-9-CM, rather than code 460.

ICD-10-CM Code(s): J00

ICD-10-CM Rationale: The Alphabetic Index main term is Cold, subterm common.

1.189. 507.0

Rationale: The Alphabetic Index main term is Pneumonia with subterm aspiration.

ICD-10-CM Code(s): J69.0

ICD-10-CM Rationale: The Alphabetic Index main term is Pneumonia with subterm aspiration.

1.190. 482.41

Rationale: The Alphabetic Index main term is Pneumonia, subterm due to, Staphylococcus, aureus, methicillin, susceptible.

ICD-10-CM Code(s): J15.21, Z16

ICD-10-CM Rationale: The Alphabetic Index main term is Pneumonia, Staphylococcal (broncho) (lobar), aureus. The coder would look up main term Resistance, resistant, organisms to multiple drugs (MDRO) to show that it is MRSA.

1.191. 516.34

Rationale: The Alphabetic Index main term is Disease, subterm lung NEC, interstitial, respiratory bronchiolitis.

ICD-10-CM Code(s): J21.9

ICD-10-CM Rationale: The Alphabetic Index main term is Bronchiolitis (acute) (infective) (subacute).

Digestive System

1.192. 521.00

Rationale: The Alphabetic Index main term is Caries, subterm tooth. Without further qualification, the ICD-9-CM code that results is 521.00.

ICD-10-CM Code(s): K02.9

ICD-10-CM Rationale: The Alphabetic Index main term is Caries with subterm dental.

1.193. 532.00

Rationale: The Alphabetic Index main term is Ulcer, subterms duodenum, acute, with hemorrhage. The fifth digit of 0 reflects the fact that there was no mention of an obstruction in the documentation.

ICD-10-CM Code(s): K26.0

ICD-10-CM Rationale: The Alphabetic Index main term is Ulcer, subterm duodenum, acute, with hemorrhage.

1.194. 531.90

Rationale: The Alphabetic Index main term is Ulcer, subterm stomach, resulting in code 531.90. The fifth digit of 0 indicates there was no mention of obstruction in the source document used for coding.

ICD-10-CM Code(s): K25.9

ICD-10-CM Rationale: The Alphabetic Index main term is Ulcer with subterm gastric—there is a note which refers the coder to stomach.

1.195. 528.6

Rationale: The Alphabetic Index main term is Leukoplakia, subterm tongue, resulting in code 528.6.

ICD-10-CM Code(s): K13.21

ICD-10-CM Rationale: The Alphabetic Index main term is Leukoplakia, subterm tongue.

1.196. b. 530.11

Rationale: The correct answer is "b" with code 530.11. The main term in the Alphabetic Index is Esophagitis, subterm reflux. Code 530.81 is assigned for esophageal reflux, and there is an "Excludes" note in the Tabular List for reflux esophagitis. The other choices are also not as specific as answer "b."

ICD-10-CM Code(s): K21.0

ICD-10-CM Rationale: The Alphabetic Index main term is Esophagitis with subterm reflux.

1.197. d. 531.10

Rationale: The main term in the Alphabetic Index is Ulcer, subterms stomach, with perforation (chronic), and no mention of obstruction, resulting in code 531.10. Category 533 in ICD-9-CM is reserved for a peptic ulcer with the site not specified enough to assign a more concise code. In this case, we know it is the stomach. The term "peptic" can refer to the esophagus, stomach, or duodenum.

ICD-10-CM Code(s): K25.1

ICD-10-CM Rationale: The Alphabetic Index main term is Ulcer, subterm stomach, acute, with, perforation.

1.198. 537.82

Rationale: The main term in the Alphabetic Index is Angiodysplasia, subterm stomach, resulting in code 537.82. When analyzing a health record, the documentation should be searched for evidence of hemorrhage because that would result in a different code assignment.

ICD-10-CM Code(s): K31.819

ICD-10-CM Rationale: The Alphabetic Index main term is Angiodysplasia with subterm stomach.

1.199. 535.31

Rationale: The main term in the Alphabetic Index is Gastritis, subterm alcoholic, with the fifth digit of 1 assigned to indicate hemorrhage, resulting in code 535.31. In reporting services for an encounter, it would be appropriate to report an additional code for the alcoholism, if it could be verified in the documentation.

ICD-10-CM Code(s): K29.21

ICD-10-CM Rationale: The Alphabetic Index main term is Gastritis, subterm alcoholic, with bleeding.

1.200. 540.9

Rationale: The main term in the Alphabetic Index is Appendicitis, subterm acute, resulting in code 540.9. Note that obstructive is a nonessential modifier.

ICD-10-CM Code(s): K35.80

ICD-10-CM Rationale: The main term in the Alphabetic Index is Appendicitis, subterm acute, resulting in code K35.80. Note that obstructive is a nonessential modifier.

1.201. 553.21

Rationale: The Alphabetic Index main term is Hernia, subterm incisional, resulting in code 553.21.

ICD-10-CM Code(s): K43.91

ICD-10-CM Rationale: The Alphabetic Index main term is Hernia, subterm incisional.

1.202. 550.93

Rationale: The main term in the Alphabetic Index is Hernia, subterm inguinal, for code assignment of 550.93. The fifth digit of 3 indicates that both the right and the left sides are involved, and the hernia has recurred.

ICD-10-CM Code(s): K40.21

ICD-10-CM Rationale: The Alphabetic Index main term is Hernia with subterms inguinal, bilateral, recurrent.

1.203. 552.00

Rationale: The main term in the Alphabetic Index is Hernia, subterms femoral, with obstruction. The term "incarcerated" describes an obstruction, so code 552.00 is assigned. The fifth digit of 0 indicates that the source document did not indicate that the hernia involved both sides or was recurrent.

ICD-10-CM Code(s): K41.30

ICD-10-CM Rationale: The Alphabetic Index main term is Hernia, subterm femoral, with obstruction. The term incarcerated is synonymous with obstructed.

1.204. 555.1

Rationale: The main term from the Alphabetic Index is Disease, subterm Crohn's, or Crohn's disease. There is an instructional note to "see Enteritis, regional," so this term is referenced. When specified as located in the large bowel, this condition is reported with code 555.1.

ICD-10-CM Code(s): K50.10

ICD-10-CM Rationale: The Alphabetic Index main term is Disease, Crohn's, which refers the coder to Enteritis, regional, large intestine (colon).

1.205. 556.9

Rationale: The Alphabetic Index main term is Colitis, subterm ulcerative, resulting in code 556.9.

ICD-10-CM Code(s): K51.90

ICD-10-CM Rationale: The Alphabetic Index main term is Colitis, subterm ulcerative.

1.206. 560.31

Rationale: The main term in the Alphabetic Index is Ileus, subterm due to gallstone, resulting in code 560.31.

ICD-10-CM Code(s): K56.3

ICD-10-CM Rationale: The Alphabetic Index main term is Ileus with subterm due to gallstones (in intestine).

1.207. c. 562.10

Rationale: The answer "c" with code 562.10 is correct because the main term Diverticula, subterm colon, is classified there. The other choices involve diverticulitis or hemorrhage (not mentioned) or the small intestine.

ICD-10-CM Code(s): K57.30

ICD-10-CM Rationale: The Alphabetic Index main term is Diverticulosis, subterm large intestine.

1.208. 568.0

Rationale: The Alphabetic Index main term Adhesions, postoperative, results in code 568.0. There is an instructional note to "see also Adhesions, peritoneum," which provides additional choices. In a female patient, the postoperative peritoneal adhesions are reported with code 614.6. It is critical to consider all of the facts available in source documentation before assigning a diagnosis code.

ICD-10-CM Code(s): K66.0

ICD-10-CM Rationale: The Alphabetic Index main term is Adhesions with subterm peritoneum, and postprocedural is enclosed in parentheses.

1.209. 574.00, 574.10

Rationale: The main term in the Alphabetic Index is Cholelithiasis, with subterms cholecystitis, acute, resulting in code 574.00, and chronic, resulting in code 574.10. The fifth digit is 0, because there is no mention in the diagnostic statement of an obstruction. Careful analysis of the health record would be recommended to validate the code choice.

ICD-10-CM Code(s): K80.12

ICD-10-CM Rationale: The Alphabetic Index main term is Cholelithiasis. The coder is directed to Calculus, gallbladder. Under subterm gallbladder, with, cholecystitis, acute, with, chronic cholecystitis.

1.210. 577.1

Rationale: The main Alphabetic Index term is Pancreatitis, subterm chronic.

ICD-10-CM Code(s): K86.1

ICD-10-CM Rationale: The Alphabetic Index main term is Pancreatitis with subterm chronic.

1.211. 569.71

Rationale: Pouchitis is an inflammation of an internal pouch created in patients who have part of their colon removed to treat ulcerative colitis or familial adenomatous polyposis (FAP). This term is indexed in Volume II (Alphabetic Index), and code 569.71 is assigned.

ICD-10-CM Code(s): K91.850

ICD-10-CM Rationale: The Alphabetic Index main term is Pouchitis.

1.212. 530.11

Rationale: The Alphabetic Index main term is Esophagitis with subterm reflux.

ICD-10-CM Code(s): K21.0

ICD-10-CM Rationale: The Alphabetic Index main term is Esophagitis with subterm reflux.

Genitourinary System

1.213. 584.5

Rationale: This condition is indexed under the main term Failure, renal, acute, with tubular necrosis (acute), resulting in code 584.5.

ICD-10-CM Code(s): N17.0

ICD-10-CM Rationale: The Alphabetic Index main term is Failure, with the subterms renal, acute, with, tubular necrosis.

1.214. 592.1

Rationale: The term ureterolithiasis describes a stone or blockage in the ureter. It is indexed in the Alphabetic Index and results in code 592.1. Take care not to confuse it with urethrolithiasis, which is assigned to code 594.2.

ICD-10-CM Code(s): N20.1

ICD-10-CM Rationale: The Alphabetic Index main term Ureterolith, ureterolithiasis directs the coder to see Calculus, ureter. This leads the coder to N20.1.

1.215. 590.10

Rationale: The Alphabetic Index main term is Pyelonephritis, subterm acute.

ICD-10-CM Code(s): N10

ICD-10-CM Rationale: The Alphabetic Index main term is Pyelonephritis with subterm acute.

1.216. 594.2

Rationale: The term urethrolithiasis describes a stone or blockage in the urethra. It is indexed in the Alphabetic Index and results in code 594.2. Take care not to confuse it with ureterolithiasis, which is assigned to code 592.1.

ICD-10-CM Code(s): N21.1

ICD-10-CM Rationale: The Alphabetic Index main term is Urethrolithiasis.

1.217. 591

Rationale: Hydronephrosis occurs when, due to an occlusion or stricture, urine backs up into the kidney. It may result in pyelonephrosis.

ICD-10-CM Code(s): N13.30

ICD-10-CM Rationale: The Alphabetic Index main term is Hydronephrosis. Code N13.30 is listed following this term.

1.218. 599.0

Rationale: Urinary tract infection is located in the Alphabetic Index under Infection as the main term, subterm urinary. Code 599.0 is an NEC code so when specified further, this code should not be assigned, but rather the more specific code. Also, this code must not be assigned based on laboratory results alone, but rather based on a diagnostic statement from the physician. When the organism responsible for the infection has been confirmed by the physician, an additional code may be assigned to reflect the source of the infection.

ICD-10-CM Code(s): N39.0

ICD-10-CM Rationale: The Alphabetic Index main term is Infection, subterm urinary (tract).

1.219. 596.51

Rationale: The main term in the Alphabetic Index is Overactive, subterm bladder, resulting in code 596.51.

ICD-10-CM Code(s): N32.81

ICD-10-CM Rationale: The Alphabetic Index main term is Overactive with subterm bladder.

1.220. 599.71

Rationale: The Alphabetic Index main term is Hematuria, subterm gross, which results in code 599.71.

ICD-10-CM Code(s): R31.0

ICD-10-CM Rationale: The Alphabetic Index main term is Hematuria, subterm gross. The excludes reminds the coder not to use this code with other codes which include hematuria.

1.221. b. 598.9

Rationale: The main term in the Alphabetic Index is Stricture, with the subterm urethral, so answer "b" is correct. Code 598 is further specified. Code 598.00 indicates with infection, which is not stated, and a fourth digit of 8 would require a specified cause to be assigned.

ICD-10-CM Code(s): N35.9

ICD-10-CM Rationale: The Alphabetic Index main term is Stricture with subterm urethra.

1.222. b. The urinary tract infection

Rationale: The UTI is reported first because it is the root cause or etiology. Codes from category 041 are provided to be used as additional codes to identify the bacterial agent in diseases classified elsewhere or for bacterial infections of unspecified nature or sites. Answer "b" is correct.

1.223. c. 600.00

Rationale: The main Alphabetic Index term is Hypertrophy, subterms prostate, benign. Code 222.2 is not appropriate because prostatic hypertrophy is excluded from this category. The fourth digits of 2 or 9 are also not correct because the statement does not indicate localized hyperplasia and specifies the condition enough to assign 0. The fifth digit of "0" is assigned because there is no indication of obstruction.

ICD-10-CM Code(s): N40.0

ICD-10-CM Rationale: In the Alphabetic Index the main term Hypertrophy is referenced with subterm prostate. There is a note to "See Enlargement, enlarged, prostate." The main term Enlargement is then referenced with subterm prostate.

1.224. 602.3

Rationale: The abbreviation PIN II refers to prostatic intraepithelial neoplasia, grade II. The Alphabetic Index main term is PIN II, resulting in code 602.3. Note that this is the appropriate code for grade I and II PIN, but grade III is reported with a code from the neoplasm section, 233.4, Carcinoma in situ of the prostate.

ICD-10-CM Code(s): N42.3

ICD-10-CM Rationale: PIN refers to prostatic intraepithelial neoplasia. There are two grades. The Alphabetic Index main term is Neoplasia, subterm intraepithelial, prostate, grade II.

1.225. a. The tuberculosis

Rationale: In the ICD-9-CM classification system, when indicated in the Alphabetic Index, the etiology of a condition is reported first, followed by any manifestation codes. The correct answer is "a."

1.226. 611.82

Rationale: This term is found in the Alphabetic Index and assigned to code 611.82.

ICD-10-CM Code(s): N64.82

ICD-10-CM Rationale: The Alphabetic Index main term is Micromastia.

1.227. 614.3

Rationale: This abbreviation is for pelvic inflammatory disease. The main term in the Alphabetic Index is Disease, subterms pelvis, inflammatory (female), acute; code 614.3 results. Note that different codes result when the disease is further described as chronic or is due to another condition or complication.

ICD-10-CM Code(s): N73.0

ICD-10-CM Rationale: The Alphabetic Index main term is Disease with subterms pelvis, pelvic, inflammatory, acute.

1.228. 617.3

Rationale: The main Alphabetic Index term is Endometriosis, subterm broad ligament, resulting in code 617.3.

ICD-10-CM Code(s): N80.3

ICD-10-CM Rationale: The Alphabetic Index main term is Endometriosis, subterm broad ligament.

1.229. 620.1

Rationale: The main term in the Alphabetic Index is Cyst, subterms ovary, corpus, luteum, resulting in code 620.1.

ICD-10-CM Code(s): N83.1

ICD-10-CM Rationale: The Alphabetic Index main term is Cyst with subterms corpus, luteum.

1.230. 625.3

Rationale: This term is included in the Alphabetic Index and is assigned to 625.3. Use caution when reporting, because this condition is often integral to other disease processes and may not always warrant separate reporting in ICD-9-CM.

ICD-10-CM Code(s): N94.6

ICD-10-CM Rationale: The Alphabetic Index main term is Dysmenorrhea.

1.231. 627.3

Rationale: The main term in the Alphabetic Index is Vaginitis, subterms postmenopausal, atrophic, resulting in code 627.3.

ICD-10-CM Code(s): N95.2

ICD-10-CM Rationale: The Alphabetic Index main term is Vaginitis with subterm atrophic, postmenopausal.

1.232. 622.12

Rationale: This is an abbreviation for cervical intraepithelial neoplasia II, which is indexed as such in Volume II of ICD-9-CM. Code 622.12 results.

ICD-10-CM Code(s): N87.1

ICD-10-CM Rationale: CIN refers to cervical intraepithelial neoplasia. The Alphabetic Index main term is Neoplasia, subterm cervix, grade II.

1.233. 607.3

Rationale: The Alphabetic Index main term is Priapism (penis).

ICD-10-CM Code(s): N48.31

ICD-10-CM Rationale: The Alphabetic Index main term is Priapism with subterm due to, trauma.

1.234. 596.83

Rationale: The Alphabetic Index main term Stenosis directs the coder to see also stricture. Main term Stricture, cystostomy leads the coder to 596.83.

ICD-10-CM Code(s): N99.518

ICD-10-CM Rationale: The Alphabetic Index main term is Complication, subterm cystostomy, specified type NEC.

Pregnancy, Childbirth, and the Puerperium

1.235. 653.11

Rationale: The Alphabetic Index process for a delivery is indexed under the main term Delivery, with the subterm complicated when there are factors that require treatment. In this case, the subterms contraction, contracted pelvis apply. The fifth digit assignment is 1, for delivered with or without mention of an antepartum condition.

ICD-10-CM Code(s): O33.1

ICD-10-CM Rationale: The Alphabetic Index main term is Pregnancy with subterms complicated by (care of) (management affected by), contracted pelvis.

1.236. 648.83

Rationale: This condition occurs during pregnancy and generally resolves following delivery. The Alphabetic Index main term is Diabetes, with subterm gestational, resulting in code 648.8, with the fifth digit of 3 added to show that this was an antepartum condition in a patient not yet delivered. V58.67, Long-term (current) use of insulin, should also be assigned if the diabetes mellitus is being treated with insulin.

ICD-10-CM Code(s): O24.419

ICD-10-CM Rationale: The Alphabetic Index main term is Diabetes, subterm gestational (in pregnancy).

1.237. 669.22

Rationale: Codes from chapter 11 in ICD-9-CM are organized by antepartum and postpartum conditions. The main term in the Alphabetic Index is Syndrome, maternal hypotension, code 669.2, with the fifth digit of 2 added to show that the condition occurred after the delivery (postpartum).

ICD-10-CM Code(s): O26.53

ICD-10-CM Rationale: The Alphabetic Index main term is Delivery with subterms complicated, by, hypotension. The 5th character "3" specifies the third trimester.

1.238. 6

Rationale: The chapter-specific guidelines general rules item C11, F.1 says, "The postpartum period begins immediately after delivery and continues for six weeks after delivery." The Official Guidelines are maintained by the National Center for Health Statistics and may be found at www.cdc.gov/nchs/data/icd9/icdguide.pdf.

1.239. 35

Rationale: To code this condition, the main term is Pregnancy, subterms management affected by advanced maternal age, primigravida, resulting in code 659.5X. Note the definition of "elderly" in this code and the one for elderly multigravida. Supervision of a pregnancy of either is reported with V23.81 or V23.82.

1.240. 656.61

Rationale: The main term is Pregnancy, subterms management, affected by large-for-dates fetus, resulting in code 656.6 with the fifth digit of 1 added because delivery occurred this admission.

ICD-10-CM Code(s): O36.63x0

ICD-10-CM Rationale: The Alphabetic Index main term is Pregnancy, subterm complicated by, fetal, excessive growth (large for dates). The problem occurred in the third trimester. The seventh character indicates that this is a single gestation. The x is used as a sixth character placeholder.

1.241. 661.01

Rationale: The main term in the Alphabetic Index is Delivery (note that this complication is related to the delivery of the baby rather than to the pregnancy), with subterms inertia, uterine, primary, resulting in code 661.0, with the fifth digit of 1 added to show the patient was delivered during this hospital stay.

ICD-10-CM Code(s): O62.0

ICD-10-CM Rationale: The Alphabetic Index main term is Inertia with subterms uterus, uterine during latent phase of labor.

1.242. 664.21

Rationale: The main term in the Alphabetic Index is Delivery, subterms complicated by, laceration, perineum, third degree, with the fifth digit of 1 assigned for an accomplished delivery during this admission. A corresponding procedure code from Volume III of ICD-9-CM would be expected for the laceration repair.

ICD-10-CM Code(s): O70.2

ICD-10-CM Rationale: The Alphabetic Index main term is Delivery, subterm complicated by, laceration, perineum, third degree.

1.243. 670.24

Rationale: The main term in the Alphabetic Index is Sepsis, subterms puerperal, postpartum, resulting in code 670.2 with the fifth digit of 4 assigned because the postpartum complication is for an episode of care following the admission for delivery.

ICD-10-CM Code(s): O85

ICD-10-CM Rationale: The Alphabetic Index main term is Sepsis with subterm puerperal, postpartum, childbirth.

1.244. 643.13

Rationale: The main term in the Alphabetic Index is Hyperemesis, subterms gravidarum, with dehydration, resulting in code 643.1 with the fifth digit of 3 added to show that the condition occurred before the delivery episode of care.

ICD-10-CM Code(s): O21.1

ICD-10-CM Rationale: The Alphabetic Index main term is Hyperemesis, subterm gravidarum, with, dehydration.

1.245. 644.13

Rationale: The main term in the Alphabetic Index is Pregnancy, subterms complicated by, false labor (pains), resulting in code 644.1 with the fifth digit of 3 added for antepartum status. Note that category 644.1 is limited to a fifth digit of 0 or 3 only.

ICD-10-CM Code(s): O47.1

ICD-10-CM Rationale: The Alphabetic Index main term is False with subterms labor, at or after 37 completed weeks of gestation.

1.246. 654.03

Rationale: The main term in the Alphabetic Index is Bicornuate, subterm in pregnancy or childbirth, resulting in code 654.0, with the fifth digit added to show antepartum status.

ICD-10-CM Code(s): O34.592

ICD-10-CM Rationale: The Alphabetic Index main term is Pregnancy, subterm complicated by, bicornis or bicornuate uterus.

1.247. 674.14

Rationale: The Alphabetic Index main term is Dehiscence, cesarean wound, reported with code 674.1, with fifth digit of 4 added to indicate this is a postpartum condition subsequent to the delivery episode.

ICD-10-CM Code(s): O90.0

ICD-10-CM Rationale: The Alphabetic Index main term is Dehiscence (of) with subterm cesarean wound.

1.248. 673.12

Rationale: The Alphabetic Index main term is Embolism, subterm amniotic fluid (pulmonary), resulting in code 673.1, with the fifth digit of 2 added to reflect the postpartum condition during the delivery episode of care.

ICD-10-CM Code(s): O88.13

ICD-10-CM Rationale: The Alphabetic Index main term is Embolism, subterm obstetric, puerperal, amniotic fluid.

1.249. 2

Rationale: See the fifth-digit categories scattered throughout chapter 11 in Volume I of ICD-9-CM Tabular Lists. The correct answer is 2, delivered with mention of postpartum complication.

1.250. 4

Rationale: See the fifth-digit categories scattered throughout chapter 11 in Volume I of ICD-9-CM Tabular Lists. The fourth-digit description is postpartum condition or complication.

1.251. c. Deficient amount of amniotic fluid

Rationale: The correct answer is "c," deficient amount of amniotic fluid. The other conditions listed would result in different codes.

1.252. 632

Rationale: The Alphabetic Index entry is at the main term Missed, subterm abortion. If the patient has a history of this condition affecting the supervision/management of a current pregnancy, then code V23.1 is reported.

ICD-10-CM Code(s): O02.1

ICD-10-CM Rationale: The Alphabetic Index main term is Missed, subterm abortion.

1.253. 5

Rationale: Look up the main term Abortion, subterms with complications, shock (septic). Code 637.5 results, so the answer is 5.

1.254. d. a and b

Rationale: Any products of conception that are found outside the uterus are considered ectopic pregnancies, so answer "d" is correct because either a tubal (fallopian tube) or an abdominal pregnancy (outside the uterus) is ectopic.

1.255. 630

Rationale: The Alphabetic Index main term is Hydatidiform mole.

ICD-10-CM Code(s): O01.0

ICD-10-CM Rationale: The Alphabetic Index main term is Hydatidiform mole with subterm classical.

1.256. 634.92

Rationale: The Alphabetic Index main term is Abortion, subterm spontaneous. The fifth digit 2 is used as it is described as complete.

ICD-10-CM Code(s): O60.12x0

ICD-10-CM Rationale: The Alphabetic Index main term is Delivery, subterm pre-term. A review of the Tabular List indicates that the correct code for this condition is preterm delivery in the second trimester. In ICD-10-CM a delivery rather than a spontaneous abortion is coded when the gestational age is beyond 20 weeks.

Skin and Subcutaneous Tissue

1.257. 680.4

Rationale: The main term in the Alphabetic Index is Carbuncle, subterm hand, resulting in code 680.4.

ICD-10-CM Code(s): L02.539

ICD-10-CM Rationale: The Alphabetic Index main term is Carbuncle with subterm hand. Sixth character of 9 is assigned for an unspecified hand.

1.258. 681.02

Rationale: The main term in the Alphabetic Index is Paronychia, subterm finger, resulting in code 681.02.

ICD-10-CM Code(s): L03.011

ICD-10-CM Rationale: The Alphabetic Index main term is Paronychia which directs the coder to see also Cellulitis, digit. Main term Cellulitis, digit, refers the coder to Cellulitis, finger. The sixth character is found in the Tabular List.

1.259. 692.71

Rationale: This term is listed in the Alphabetic Index. Code 692.71 results when the burn is first degree or not otherwise specified. For more serious burns (second or third degree), different codes are assigned.

ICD-10-CM Code(s): L55.9

ICD-10-CM Rationale: The Alphabetic Index main term is Sunburn. Since a degree of burn is not specified, fifth character 9 is used.

1.260. 682.0

Rationale: The Alphabetic Index main term is Cellulitis, subterm face (there is no subterm chin, so the more general term of face is referenced), resulting in code 682.0.

ICD-10-CM Code(s): L03.211

ICD-10-CM Rationale: The Alphabetic Index main term is Cellulitis, subterm face. There is no subterm for chin.

1.261. 685.0

Rationale: The Alphabetic Index main term is Cyst, subterms pilonidal, with abscess, resulting in code 685.0.

ICD-10-CM Code(s): L05.01

ICD-10-CM Rationale: The Alphabetic Index main term is Cyst with subterms pilonidal, with abscess.

1.262. 692.6

Rationale: The Alphabetic Index main term is Poison ivy, oak, sumac, or other plant dermatitis, and code 692.6 results for any of them.

ICD-10-CM Code(s): L23.7

ICD-10-CM Rationale: The Alphabetic Index main term is Poison ivy.

1.263. 692.84

Rationale: The Alphabetic Index main term is Dermatitis, subterms due to, animal, dander (cat) (dog), resulting in code 692.84.

ICD-10-CM Code(s): L23.81

ICD-10-CM Rationale: The Alphabetic Index main term is Dermatitis with subterm due to dander (cat).

1.264. 695.4

Rationale: The main Alphabetic Index term is Lupus, subterm erythematosus, resulting in code 695.4.

ICD-10-CM Code(s): L93.0

ICD-10-CM Rationale: The Alphabetic Index main term is Lupus, subterm erythematosus.

1.265. 701.4

Rationale: The main Alphabetic Index term is Keloid (Cheloid), subterm scar, resulting in code 701.4. The main term can also be Scar, but the alternative cheloid is the term that results in the correct coding when you take this route.

ICD-10-CM Code(s): L91.0

ICD-10-CM Rationale: The Alphabetic Index main term is Scar, scarring with subterm keloid.

1.266. 702.0

Rationale: The main Alphabetic Index term is Keratosis, subterm actinic, resulting in code 702.0. Note the various types of keratosis and the need for specificity in getting the correct code assigned. Without further qualification, code 701.1 results.

ICD-10-CM Code(s): L57.0

ICD-10-CM Rationale: The Alphabetic Index main term is Keratosis, subterm actinic.

1.267. 704.01

Rationale: The main Alphabetic Index term is Alopecia, subterm areata, resulting in code 704.01.

ICD-10-CM Code(s): L63.9

ICD-10-CM Rationale: The Alphabetic Index main term Alopecia with subterm areata refers the coder to L63.9.

1.268. 705.83

Rationale: The main Alphabetic Index term is Hidradenitis (suppurativa), resulting in code 705.83.

ICD-10-CM Code(s): L73.2

ICD-10-CM Rationale: The Alphabetic Index main term is Hidradenitis (suppurativa).

1.269. c. 707.07, 707.22

Rationale: The Alphabetic Index main term is Pressure, subterm ulcer, resulting in code 707.07. An additional code is assigned to report the pressure ulcer, stage II.

ICD-10-CM Code(s): L89.602

ICD-10-CM Rationale: The Alphabetic Index main term is Ulcer with subterms pressure, Stage 2, heel. The sixth character "2" specifies stage 2.

1.270. b. The diabetes mellitus

Rationale: Because the foot ulcer is a manifestation of the underlying diabetes, answer "b" is correct. A cause-and-effect relationship must be established for that rule to apply.

1.271. 697.0

Rationale: The Alphabetic Index main term is Lichen, subterm planus, resulting in code 697.0.

ICD-10-CM Code(s): L43.8

ICD-10-CM Rationale: The Alphabetic Index main term is Lichen with subterm planus which refers to code L43.9. Review of the Tabular List indicates code L43.8, other lichen planus, is assigned to report the condition's status of generalized.

1.272. 692.0

Rationale: The Alphabetic Index main term is Dermatitis, subterms due to, detergent, resulting in code 692.0.

ICD-10-CM Code(s): L24.0

ICD-10-CM Rationale: The Alphabetic Index main term is Dermatitis, subterm due (to), detergents (contact) (irritant).

1.273. 682.3

Rationale: The Alphabetic Index main term is Abscess, subterm axilla, resulting in code 682.3.

ICD-10-CM Code(s): L02.411

ICD-10-CM Rationale: The Alphabetic Index main term is Abscess, subterm axilla, resulting in L02.41-. Review of the Tabular List reveals the correct code is L02.411 for the right axilla.

1.274. 691.0

Rationale: The Alphabetic Index main term is Dermatitis, subterm diaper, resulting in code 691.0. Note that due to ammonia refers to household/liquid ammonia that is classified to code 692.4.

ICD-10-CM Code(s): L22

ICD-10-CM Rationale: The Alphabetic Index main term is Dermatitis, with either subterm diaper or ammonia, both resulting in code L22.

1.275. 695.10

Rationale: The Alphabetic Index main term is Erythema, subterm multiforme, resulting in code 695.10.

ICD-10-CM Code(s): L51.9

ICD-10-CM Rationale: The Alphabetic Index main term is Erythema with subterm multiforme.

1.276. 692.76

Rationale: The Alphabetic Index main term is Sunburn, subterm second-degree, resulting in code 692.76.

ICD-10-CM Code(s): L55.1

ICD-10-CM Rationale: The Alphabetic Index main term is Sunburn, subterm second-degree.

1.277. 692.83

Rationale: The Alphabetic Index main term is Dermatitis with subterm jewelry.

ICD-10-CM Code(s): L24.81

ICD-10-CM Rationale: The Alphabetic Index main term is Dermatitis with subterms due to, metals.

1.278. 707.07, 707.22

Rationale: The Alphabetic main term is Ulcer with subterms pressure, heel. The Alphabetic Index main term is Pressure, stage, 2.

ICD-10-CM Code(s): L89.612

ICD-10-CM Rationale: The Alphabetic Index main term is Ulcer, subterms pressure, stage 2, heel resulting in L89.6-. Review of the Tabular List reveals that L89.612 is the correct code. Note that this code is a combination code that specifies the site, including laterality and the stage of the pressure ulcer.

1.279. 704.41

Rationale: The Alphabetic Index main term is Cyst, subterm pilar.

ICD-10-CM Code(s): L72.1

ICD-10-CM Rationale: The Alphabetic Index main term is Cyst, subterm pilar.

1.280. 704.42

Rationale: The Alphabetic Index main term is Cyst, subterm trichilemmal.

ICD-10-CM Code(s): L72.1

ICD-10-CM Rationale: The Alphabetic Index main term is Cyst, trichilemmal.

Musculoskeletal System and Connective Tissue

1.281. 711.05

Rationale: The Alphabetic Index main term is Arthritis, subterm pyogenic or pyemic. The note at the beginning of the index entry for arthritis gives the fifth digits. The fifth digit designating hip (pelvic region and thigh) is 5. The resulting code is 711.05.

ICD-10-CM Code(s): M00.859

ICD-10-CM Rationale: The Alphabetic Index main term is Arthritis with subterm pyogenic with a note to "See Arthritis, pyogenic, bacterial" with subterm hip.

1.282. 714.0

Rationale: The Alphabetic Index main term is Arthritis, subterm rheumatoid, resulting in code 714.0. Subcategory 714.0 does not require a fifth digit to specify anatomic site involved.

ICD-10-CM Code(s): M06.9

ICD-10-CM Rationale: The Alphabetic Index main term is Arthritis, subterm rheumatoid.

1.283. 733.42

Rationale: The Alphabetic Index main term is Necrosis, subterm aseptic, bone, and femur, resulting in code 733.42, with the nonessential modifiers head and neck.

ICD-10-CM Code(s): M87.059

ICD-10-CM Rationale: The Alphabetic Index main term is Necrosis with the subterm bone. There is a note which also refers the coder to the main term Osteonecrosis with subterms idiopathic aseptic, femur. The 6th character "9" refers to unspecified femur.

1.284. 715.36

Rationale: *Coding Clinic* (1995, 2Q:5) and *Coding Clinic* (2003, 4Q:118) state osteoarthrosis, localized, not specified whether primary or secondary, lower leg, is assigned for degenerative joint disease of the knee. The instructional note at the beginning of the index entry for osteoarthritis gives the fifth digit for knees ("lower leg") as 6, resulting in code 715.36.

ICD-10-CM Code(s): M17.0

ICD-10-CM Rationale: The Alphabetic Index main term is Osteoarthritis, subterm knee, bilateral. Although the diagnosis isn't described as primary, the Alphabetic Index directs the coder to category M17.

1.285. 715.09

Rationale: The abbreviation DJD stands for degenerative joint disease. The Alphabetic Index main term is Degeneration, degenerative, subterm joint disease. A cross-reference note refers the coding professional to "see also osteoarthrosis." An entry for "multiple" results in the code 715.09. Review of this code in the Tabular List indicates that generalized DJD is synonymous with DJD of multiple joints.

ICD-10-CM Code(s): M15.9

ICD-10-CM Rationale: The Alphabetic Index main term Disease with subterms joint, degenerative directs the coder to the main term Osteoarthritis with subterm generalized—M15.9.

1.286. 717.41

Rationale: The Alphabetic Index main term is Tear, subterms meniscus, lateral, bucket handle, old, resulting in code 717.41. Note the level of specificity available for injuries to the meniscal structures of the knee.

ICD-10-CM Code(s): M23.201

ICD-10-CM Rationale: The term chronic in this case refers to an old or recurrent condition. The Alphabetic Index main term Tear, torn, subterm meniscus, old, directs the coder to see Derangement, knee, meniscus, due to old tear.

1.287. 717.7

Rationale: The Alphabetic Index main term is Chondromalacia, subterm knee or patella, resulting in code 717.7.

ICD-10-CM Code(s): M22.40

ICD-10-CM Rationale: The Alphabetic Index main term is Chondromalacia with subterm patellae. The 5th character is "0" which refers to unspecified knee.

1.288. 719.12

Rationale: The Alphabetic Index main term is Hemarthrosis, subterm shoulder, resulting in code 719.12. Chronic is a nonessential modifier.

ICD-10-CM Code(s): M25.029

ICD-10-CM Rationale: The Alphabetic Index main term is Hemarthrosis, subterm elbow. A review of the Tabular List determines the sixth character.

1.289. 720.0

Rationale: The Alphabetic Index main term is Spondylitis, subterm ankylosing, resulting in code 720.0. This subcategory does not require a fifth digit to identify anatomic site.

ICD-10-CM Code(s): M45.9

ICD-10-CM Rationale: The Alphabetic Index main term is Spondylitis with subterm ankylosing.

1.290. 721.1

Rationale: The Alphabetic Index main term is Spondylosis. The entry for Osteoarthritis, subterm spine, refers the coding professional to spondylosis, the term for arthritis of the spine. A search under spondylosis leads to subterm cervical, with myelopathy. The documented spinal cord compression constitutes myelopathy. This results in the code 721.1. This subterm does not require a fifth digit.

ICD-10-CM Code(s): M47.12

ICD-10-CM Rationale: The Alphabetic Index main term Osteoarthritis, subterm spine, directs the coder to see Spondylosis. Main term Spondylosis, with, myelopathy, cervical region leads the coder to the correct code.

1.291. 722.10

Rationale: The abbreviation HNP stands for herniated nucleus pulposus. A search for Herniation, nucleus pulposus, in the Alphabetic Index results in a cross-reference note: "see Displacement, intervertebral disc." The main term is Displacement, subterms intervertebral disc, lumbar, lumbosacral. The presence of radicular symptoms does not constitute myelopathy, so the resulting code is 722.10.

ICD-10-CM Code(s): M51.26

ICD-10-CM Rationale: The Alphabetic Index main term Herniation, nucleus pulposus refers the coder to the main term Displacement, intervertebral disc, lumbar region.

1.292. 722.52

Rationale: The Alphabetic Index main term is Degeneration, subterm intervertebral disc. Review of the entry under main term Disease, subterm disc, degenerative, leads the coding professional to the above entry. The subterm lumbar, lumbosacral, results in code 722.52. There is no mention of cord compression in the diagnostic statement, so "with myelopathy" is not the appropriate code.

ICD-10-CM Code(s): M51.36

ICD-10-CM Rationale: The Alphabetic Index main term Disease, diseased, subterm disc, degenerative directs the coder to see Degeneration, intervertebral disc. Under the main term Degeneration, subterm intervertebral, the coder is led to the lumbar region.

1.293. 724.2

Rationale: The Alphabetic Index main term is Pain, subterms back, low, resulting in code 724.2. The term "lumbago" is synonymous with low back pain.

ICD-10-CM Code(s): M54.5

ICD-10-CM Rationale: The Alphabetic Index main term is Pain, back. The Tabular List indicates low back pain to be coded as M54.5.

1.294. 727.40

Rationale: The Alphabetic Index main term is Cyst, subterm synovial, resulting in code 727.40. Review of this code in the Tabular List shows that there is no specific code for the wrist.

ICD-10-CM Code(s): M71.339

ICD-10-CM Rationale: The Alphabetic Index main term Cyst, subterm synovial directs the coder to see also Cyst, bursa. A review of the subterm wrist directs the coder to M71.33 with a review of the Tabular List to complete the code.

1.295. 710.0

Rationale: The abbreviation SLE is for systemic lupus erythematosus. Although localized lupus is a disease of the skin, generalized or systemic lupus is included in the diseases of the musculoskeletal system as it primarily affects the joints. The Alphabetic Index main term is Lupus, subterm erythematosus, disseminated or systemic, resulting in code 710.0. This subcategory does not require a fifth digit.

ICD-10-CM Code(s): M32.9

ICD-10-CM Rationale: The Alphabetic Index main term is Lupus with subterms erythematosus, systemic.

1.296. 730.07

Rationale: The Alphabetic Index main term is Osteomyelitis, subterm acute or subacute. The instructional note at the beginning of the index entry for osteomyelitis indicates that a fifth digit of 7 is appropriate for the bones of the foot, resulting in code 730.07.

ICD-10-CM Code(s): M86.179

ICD-10-CM Rationale: The Alphabetic Index main term Osteomyelitis, subterm acute, metatarsus refers the coder to M86.17 with a review of the Tabular List completing the code.

1.297. 733.01

Rationale: The Alphabetic Index main term is Osteoporosis (with nonessential modifier generalized), subterm postmenopausal, or senile, resulting in code 733.01.

ICD-10-CM Code(s): M81.0

ICD-10-CM Rationale: The Alphabetic Index main term is Osteoporosis with subterm postmenopausal.

1.298. 733.14

Rationale: The Alphabetic Index main term is Fracture, subterm pathologic, femur (neck), resulting in code 733.14. Traumatic fractures are coded to chapter 17, Injury and Poisoning, but pathological fractures, which are due to an underlying bone disease, are categorized to this chapter. Whenever a pathologic fracture code is assigned, the coding professional should also be alert for the presence of a concurrent bone disease, such as osteoporosis, malignancy, bone cyst, and so forth.

ICD-10-CM Code(s): M84.453A

ICD-10-CM Rationale: The Alphabetic Index main term is Fracture, pathological, subterm femur. The coder completes the code using the Tabular List. The seventh character "A" is used for the initial encounter.

1.299. 735.0

Rationale: The Alphabetic Index main term is Hallux, subterm valgus, resulting in code 735.0. Acquired is a nonessential modifier, but congenital is an essential modifier and results in a different code. Because this diagnostic statement does not specify congenital, code 735.0 is appropriate. Note that hallux is not the name of a disease or condition, but merely the term for the big toe.

ICD-10-CM Code(s): M20.10

ICD-10-CM Rationale: The Alphabetic Index main term is Hallux with subterm valgus.

1.300. 737.10

Rationale: The Alphabetic Index main term is Kyphosis, resulting in code 737.10.

ICD-10-CM Code(s): M40.209

ICD-10-CM Rationale: The Alphabetic Index main term is Kyphosis, kyphotic.

Newborn/Congenital Disorders

1.301. 741.03

Rationale: The Alphabetic Index main term is Spina bifida, subterm with hydrocephalus. The fifth digit of 3 is assigned for lumbar region which results in code 741.03.

ICD-10-CM Code(s): Q05.2

ICD-10-CM Rationale: The Alphabetic Index main term is Spina bifida with subterms lumbar, with hydrocephalus.

1.302. 744.42

Rationale: The Alphabetic Index main term is Cyst, subterm branchial, with nonessential modifier cleft, resulting in code 744.42.

ICD-10-CM Code(s): Q18.0

ICD-10-CM Rationale: The Alphabetic Index main term is Cyst, subterm brachial (cleft).

1.303. 745.4

Rationale: The abbreviation VSD stands for ventricular septal defect. The Alphabetic Index main term is Defect, subterm ventricular septal. With no further qualification, the appropriate code is 745.4.

ICD-10-CM Code(s): Q21.0

ICD-10-CM Rationale: The Alphabetic Index main term is Defect with subterms septal, ventricular.

1.304. 747.10

Rationale: The Alphabetic Index main term is Coarctation, subterm aorta, resulting in code 747.10. This code may also be located under main term Anomaly, subterm aorta, coarctation.

ICD-10-CM Code(s): Q25.1

ICD-10-CM Rationale: The Alphabetic Index main term is Coarctation of aorta.

1.305. 749.03

Rationale: The Alphabetic Index main term is Cleft, subterms palate, bilateral, complete. All modifiers here are essential. As there is no mention of cleft lip, code 749.03 is assigned.

ICD-10-CM Code(s): Q35.9

ICD-10-CM Rationale: The Alphabetic Index main term is Cleft with subterm palate.

1.306. 752.61

Rationale: The Alphabetic Index main term is the same. As there is no sex designation in the diagnostic statement, code 752.61 is assigned because male is a nonessential modifier, but female is an essential modifier.

ICD-10-CM Code(s): Q54.9

ICD-10-CM Rationale: The Alphabetic Index main term is Hypospadias.

1.307. 753.12

Rationale: The Alphabetic Index main term is Disease, subterms kidney, polycystic, resulting in code 753.12. None of the essential modifiers that result in other codes are present in this diagnostic statement.

ICD-10-CM Code(s): Q61.3

ICD-10-CM Rationale: The Alphabetic Index main term is Disease with subterms kidney, polycystic.

1.308. 754.35

Rationale: The Alphabetic Index main term is Dislocation, subterms hip, congenital (or congenital, hip), with subluxation of the other hip, resulting in code 754.35.

ICD-10-CM Code(s): Q65.2, Q65.5

ICD-10-CM Rationale: The Alphabetic Index main term is Dislocation, hip, congenital. To find the second code, use main term Dislocation, hip, congenital, partial. Subluxation is a partial dislocation.

1.309. 755.11

Rationale: The Alphabetic Index main term is Syndactylism or syndactyly, subterms fingers, without fusion of bones, resulting in code 755.11.

ICD-10-CM Code(s): Q70.13

ICD-10-CM Rationale: The Alphabetic Index main term is Syndactyly with subterms simple, fingers. Code Q70.13 refers to bilateral.

1.310. 756.12

Rationale: The Alphabetic Index main term is Spondylolisthesis. In the absence of more information, code 756.12 is assigned.

ICD-10-CM Code(s): Q76.2

ICD-10-CM Rationale: The Alphabetic Index main term is Spondylolisthesis, subterm congenital.

1.311. 752.39

Rationale: The Alphabetic Index main term is Fistula, and subterms rectouterine, congenital result in code 752.39.

ICD-10-CM Code(s): Q51.7

ICD-10-CM Rationale: The Alphabetic Index main term is Fistula with subterms rectouterine, congenital.

1.312. 758.7

Rationale: The Alphabetic Index main term is Syndrome, subterm Klinefelter's, resulting in code 758.7.

ICD-10-CM Code(s): Q98.4

ICD-10-CM Rationale: The Alphabetic Index main term is Klinefelter's syndrome.

1.313. 756.51

Rationale: The Alphabetic Index main term is Osteogenesis imperfecta, resulting in code 756.51.

ICD-10-CM Code(s): Q78.0

ICD-10-CM Rationale: The Alphabetic Index main term is Osteogenesis imperfecta.

1.314. 771.1

Rationale: The abbreviation CMV stands for cytomegalovirus. The Alphabetic Index main term is Infection, subterms congenital, cytomegalovirus, resulting in code 771.1.

ICD-10-CM Code(s): P35.1

ICD-10-CM Rationale: The Alphabetic Index main term is Infection, subterm cytomegalovirus, cytomegaloviral, congenital.

1.315. 770.12

Rationale: The Alphabetic Index main term is Syndrome, subterms meconium, aspiration, resulting in code 770.12. This code can also be accessed via main term Syndrome, subterms aspiration, of newborn, massive, or meconium.

ICD-10-CM Code(s): P24.01

ICD-10-CM Rationale: The Alphabetic Index main term is Syndrome with subterms aspiration, meconium.

1.316. 773.0

Rationale: The Alphabetic Index main term is Incompatibility, subterms Rh, fetus, or newborn, resulting in code 773.0. This code can also be accessed via main term Disease, subterms hemolytic, due to or with, incompatibility, Rh-negative mother.

ICD-10-CM Code(s): P55.0

ICD-10-CM Rationale: The Alphabetic Index main term is Disease, subterm hemolytic, due to or with, incompatibility, Rh (blood group) (factor).

1.317. 756.72

Rationale: The Alphabetic Index main term is Omphalocele, resulting in code 756.72.

ICD-10-CM Code(s): Q79.2

ICD-10-CM Rationale: The Alphabetic Index main term is Omphalocele.

1.318. 779.5

Rationale: The Alphabetic Index main term is Syndrome, subterm drug withdrawal, infant, of dependent mother, resulting in code 779.5. This code can also be accessed via main term Withdrawal symptoms or syndrome, subterm newborn, infant of dependent mother.

ICD-10-CM Code(s): P96.1

ICD-10-CM Rationale: The Alphabetic Index main term is Withdrawal state, subterm newborn, infant of dependent mother.

1.319. b. V30.00

Rationale: The Alphabetic Index main term is Newborn, subterm single, born in hospital. Per ICD-9-CM coding guidelines, the code for liveborn infant (V30–V39) is assigned as the principal diagnosis. See Coding Clinic 2002, 4Q. Additional codes would be assigned for all the complications of the newborn period.

1.320. 777.50

Rationale: The Alphabetic Index main term is Enterocolitis, subterms necrotizing, newborn, resulting in code 777.50.

ICD-10-CM Code(s): P77.9

ICD-10-CM Rationale: The Alphabetic Index main term is Enterocolitis, subterm necrotizing, in newborn. The record should be reviewed to determine stage, if possible.

1.321. 756.2

Rationale: The Alphabetic Index main term is Supernumerary with subterms rib, cervical.

ICD-10-CM Code(s): Q76.5

ICD-10-CM Rationale: The Alphabetic Index main term is Supernumerary with subterms rib, cervical.

1.322. Code(s): 747.31

Rationale: The Alphabetic Index main term is Atresia, subterm artery NEC, pulmonary.

ICD-10-CM Code(s): Q25.1, Q25.2

ICD-10-CM Rationale: The Alphabetic Index main term is Coarctation of aorta. The main term is Atresia, subterm aorta.

1.323. 747.32

Rationale: The Alphabetic Index main term is Malformation, subterm arteriovenous, pulmonary.

ICD-10-CM Code(s): Q27.5

ICD-10-CM Rationale: The Alphabetic Index main term is Malformation, subterm pulmonary artery, specified type NEC.

1.324. 773.1

Rationale: The Alphabetic Index main term Hemolysis, subterm fetal directs the coder to see Jaundice, fetus or newborn. The main term is Jaundice, subterm fetus or newborn, due to or associated with incompatibility, maternal, fetal NEC.

ICD-10-CM Code(s): P55.1

ICD-10-CM Rationale: The Alphabetic Index main term is Incompatibility, subterm ABO, newborn. The jaundice is included in code P55.1.

1.325. 760.75

> Rationale: The Alphabetic Index main term is Crack baby.
>
> ICD-10-CM Code(s): P04.41
>
> ICD-10-CM Rationale: The Alphabetic index main term is Crack baby.

Symptoms, Signs, and Ill-Defined Conditions

1.326. 783.0

> Rationale: The Alphabetic Index main term is Anorexia. In the absence of either of the essential modifiers hysterical or nervosa, code 783.0 is assigned.
>
> ICD-10-CM Code(s): R63.0
>
> ICD-10-CM Rationale: The Alphabetic Index main term is Anorexia.

1.327. 783.7

> Rationale: The Alphabetic Index main term is Failure, subterm to thrive, adult, resulting in code 783.7.
>
> ICD-10-CM Code(s): R62.7
>
> ICD-10-CM Rationale: The Alphabetic Index main term is Failure, subterm to thrive, adult.

1.328. 780.91

> Rationale: The Alphabetic Index main term is Fussy infant, resulting in code 780.91. This code can also be accessed via main term Infant, subterm fussy.
>
> ICD-10-CM Code(s): R68.12
>
> ICD-10-CM Rationale: The Alphabetic Index main term is Fussy with subterm infant.

1.329. 780.66

> Rationale: The Alphabetic Index main term is Fever, and the subterm posttransfusion results in code 780.66.
>
> ICD-10-CM Code(s): R50.84
>
> ICD-10-CM Rationale: The Alphabetic Index main term is Fever, subterm posttransfusion.

1.330. 780.2

> Rationale: The Alphabetic Index main term is Syncope. In the absence of any additional information, code 780.2 is assigned.
>
> ICD-10-CM Code(s): R55
>
> ICD-10-CM Rationale: The Alphabetic Index main term is Syncope.

1.331. 780.71

Rationale: The Alphabetic Index main term is Syndrome, subterm fatigue, chronic, resulting in code 780.71. This code can also be accessed via the main term Fatigue, subterms chronic or chronic syndrome, or main term Fatigue, subterm syndrome, chronic.

ICD-10-CM Code(s): R53.82

ICD-10-CM Rationale: The Alphabetic Index main term is Syndrome, subterm fatigue, chronic.

1.332. 786.50

Rationale: The Alphabetic Index main term is Pain, subterm chest. In the absence of any additional information, the code 786.50 is assigned.

ICD-10-CM Code(s): R07.9

ICD-10-CM Rationale: The Alphabetic Index main term is Pain with subterm chest.

1.333. 780.33

Rationale: The Alphabetic Index main term is Seizure, and subterm post-traumatic results in code 780.33.

ICD-10-CM Code(s): R56.1

ICD-10-CM Rationale: The Alphabetic Index main term is Seizure, subterm post-traumatic.

1.334. 799.51

Rationale: The Alphabetic Index main term is Deficit, subterm concentration, which results in code 799.51.

ICD-10-CM Code(s): R41.840

ICD-10-CM Rationale: The Alphabetic Index main term is Deficit with subterm concentration.

1.335. 790.29

Rationale: This code can be accessed via the main term Findings, abnormal, without diagnosis, subterm glucose, 790.29. If there was documentation that the findings were elevated, then code 790.22 (impaired glucose tolerance test) would be assigned.

ICD-10-CM Code(s): R73.09

ICD-10-CM Rationale: The Alphabetic Index main term is Findings, abnormal, inconclusive, without diagnosis, subterm glucose (tolerance test).

1.336. 787.01

Rationale: The Alphabetic Index main term is Nausea, subterm with vomiting, resulting in code 787.01. This code can also be accessed via main term Vomiting, subterm with nausea.

ICD-10-CM Code(s): R11.2

ICD-10-CM Rationale: The Alphabetic Index main term is Nausea with subterm vomiting.

1.337. 789.7

Rationale: The Alphabetic Index main term is Colic, subterm in infant, resulting in code 789.7.

ICD-10-CM Code(s): R10.83

ICD-10-CM Rationale: The Alphabetic Index main term is Colic. Infantile is a nonessential modifier.

1.338. 788.41

Rationale: The Alphabetic Index main term is Frequency (urinary) NEC, resulting in code 788.41. This same code can be accessed via the subterm micturition (synonym for urination).

ICD-10-CM Code(s): R35.0

ICD-10-CM Rationale: The Alphabetic Index main term is Frequency micturition.

1.339. 789.01

Rationale: The abbreviation RUQ stands for right upper quadrant of the abdomen. The Alphabetic Index main term is Pain, abdominal. The Alphabetic Index indicates the need for a fifth digit, and review of subcategory 789.0 reveals that the appropriate fifth digit for the right upper quadrant is 1.

ICD-10-CM Code(s): R10.11

ICD-10-CM Rationale: The Alphabetic Index main term is Pain, subterm abdominal, upper, right quadrant.

1.340. 794.02

Rationale: The abbreviation EEG stands for electroencephalogram. The Alphabetic Index main term is Abnormal, subterm electroencephalogram (EEG), resulting in code 794.02.

ICD-10-CM Code(s): R94.01

ICD-10-CM Rationale: The Alphabetic Index main term is Abnormal with subterm electroencephalogram [EEG].

1.341. 793.3

Rationale: The Alphabetic Index main term is Nonvisualization, subterm gallbladder, resulting in code 793.3. This code can also be accessed via the main term Abnormal, subterms radiologic examination, biliary tract.

ICD-10-CM Code(s): R93.2

ICD-10-CM Rationale: The Alphabetic Index main term is Nonvisualization, gallbladder.

1.342. 793.80

Rationale: The Alphabetic Index main term is Abnormal, subterm mammogram, resulting in code 793.80. This code can also be accessed via the main term Abnormal, subterms radiologic examination, breast, mammogram.

ICD-10-CM Code(s): R92.8

ICD-10-CM Rationale: The Alphabetic Index main term is Abnormal with subterm mammogram.

1.343. 798.0

Rationale: The abbreviation SIDS represents sudden infant death syndrome, considered a sign or symptom rather than a specific diagnosis. The Alphabetic Index main term is Syndrome, subterm sudden infant death, resulting in code 798.0.

ICD-10-CM Code(s): R99

ICD-10-CM Rationale: The Alphabetic Index main term is Death (cause unknown) (of) (unexplained) (unspecified cause). There isn't a more specific code for SIDS.

1.344. 799.4

Rationale: The Alphabetic Index main term is the same, resulting in code 799.4.

ICD-10-CM Code(s): R64

ICD-10-CM Rationale: The Alphabetic Index main term is Cachexia.

1.345. 786.01

Rationale: The Alphabetic Index main term is the same, resulting in code 786.01 in the absence of any additional diagnostic information.

ICD-10-CM Code(s): R06.4

ICD-10-CM Rationale: The Alphabetic Index main term is Hyperventilation.

1.346. 787.23

Rationale: The Alphabetic Index main term is Dysphagia with subterm pharyngeal phase.

ICD-10-CM Code(s): R13.13

ICD-10-CM Rationale: The Alphabetic Index main term is Dysphagia with subterm pharyngeal phase.

1.347. 780.97

Rationale: The Alphabetic Index main term is Alteration (of), altered with subterm mental status.

ICD-10-CM Code(s): R41.82

ICD-10-CM Rationale: The Alphabetic Index main term is Alteration (of), altered with subterm mental status.

1.348. 786.31

Rationale: The Alphabetic Index main term is Hemorrhage, subterm pulmonary, acute idiopathic in infants (AIPHI) (over 28 days old).

ICD-10-CM-Code(s): R04.81

ICD-10-CM Rationale: The Alphabetic Index main term is Hemorrhage, pulmonary, newborn P26.9. However, in the Tabular List, the code P26.9 Excludes 1 note refers to code R04.81 for acute idiopathic hemorrhage in infants over 28 days old.

1.349. 787.60

Rationale: The Alphabetic Index main term is Incontinence, subterm feces, fecal.

ICD-10-CM Code(s): R15.9

ICD-10-CM Rationale; The Alphabetic Index main term is Incontinence, feces.

1.350. 781.2

Rationale:The Alphabetic Index main term is Abnormal, abnormality, abnormalities, subterm gait.

ICD-10-CM Code(s): R26.9

ICD-10-CM Rationale: The Alphabetic Index main term is Abnormal, abnormality, abnormalities, subterm gait. The coder is directed to see Gait. The main term is Gait abnormality.

1.351. 796.2

Rationale: The Alphabetic Index main term is Elevation, subterm blood pressure reading (incidental) (isolated) (nonspecific), no diagnosis of hypertension.

ICD-10-CM Code(s): R03.0

ICD-10-CM Rationale: The Alphabetic Index main term is Elevated, elevation, subterm blood pressure, reading (incidental) (isolated) (nonspecific), no diagnosis of hypertension.

Trauma/Poisoning

1.352. 803.75

Rationale: The Alphabetic Index main term is Fracture, subterms skull, open, with subarachnoid hemorrhage. An instructional note at the beginning of the index entry for fracture defines open vs. closed fractures, and another note at the entry for skull defines the appropriate fifth digits that describe loss of consciousness. The resulting code is 803.75.

ICD-10-CM Code(s): S02.10Xb, S06.6x7A, S06.5x7A

ICD-10-CM Rationale: Open skull fracture: The Alphabetic Index main term is Fracture with subterms skull, base. Subarachnoid hemorrhage: The Alphabetic Index main term is Hemorrhage with subterms intracranial, subarachnoid, traumatic. Subdural hemorrhage: The Alphabetic Index main term is Injury with subterms intracranial, subdural hemorrhage (traumatic). The 7th characters "A" and "B" are used to report the initial encounter.

1.353. 806.01

Rationale: The Alphabetic Index main term is Fracture, vertebra, with spinal cord injury, cervical. A note at the entry for fracture of vertebra defines the fifth-digit subclassifications that describe the extent of spinal cord injury. The appropriate code for a third cervical vertebra fracture, not specified as open, with a complete cord lesion, is 806.01.

ICD-10-CM Code(s): S12.200A, S14.113A

ICD-10-CM Rationale: The Alphabetic Index main term is Fracture, subterm neck, cervical vertebra, third. The Tabular List S12 Category specifies to code also any associated cervical spinal cord injury (S14.0, S14.1-). The 7th character "A" is used for the initial encounter.

1.354. 807.07

Rationale: The Alphabetic Index main term is Fracture, subterm ribs. The instructional table following the entry for Fracture, ribs, indicates that fifth digits are used to describe the number of ribs involved. Fracture, not specified as open, of seven ribs results in code 807.07.

ICD-10-CM Code(s): S22.43xA

ICD-10-CM Rationale: The Alphabetic Index main term is Fracture with subterms ribs, multiple. The 7th character "A" is used for the initial encounter.

1.355. 808.43

Rationale: The Alphabetic Index main term is Fracture, subterms pelvis, multiple, with disruption of pelvic circle, resulting in code 808.43.

ICD-10-CM Code(s): S32.810A

ICD-10-CM Rationale: The Alphabetic Index main term is fracture, subterm pelvis, multiple with disruption of pelvic ring. The coder is directed to see Disruption, pelvic ring. The 7th character "A" is used for the initial encounter.

1.356. 812.01

Rationale: The Alphabetic Index main term is Fracture, subterms humerus, surgical neck, resulting in code 812.01. The instructional note at the beginning of the index entry for fracture indicates that comminuted and impacted fractures are not open.

ICD-10-CM Code(s): S42.211A

ICD-10-CM Rationale: The Alphabetic Index main term is Fracture, traumatic, subterms humerus, surgical neck, "see Fracture, humerus, upper end." Main term is Fracture, traumatic, subterms humerus, upper end, surgical neck, resulting in S42.21-. Review of the Tabular List indicates that S42.211 is the correct code for the right humerus. Additionally, a 7th character of "A" is added to the code to indicate initial encounter for a closed fracture.

1.357. 813.47

Rationale: The Alphabetic Index main term is Fracture, subterms radius, with ulna, torus, resulting in code 813.47. A torus fracture is a type of incomplete break common in children, also known as a buckle fracture.

ICD-10-CM Code(s): S52.622A, S52.522A

ICD-10-CM Rationale: Two separate codes are needed to completely code this diagnosis. The Alphabetic Index main term is Fracture, subterm ulna, lower end, torus (S52.622A) and Fracture, subterm radius, lower end, torus (S52.522A). The 7th character "A" is used for the initial encounter.

1.358. 832.2

Rationale: The Alphabetic Index main term is Nursemaid's, subterm elbow, resulting in code 832.2.

ICD-10-CM Code(s): S53.033A

ICD-10-CM Rationale: The Alphabetic Index main term is Nursemaid's elbow. The seventh character "A" is used for the initial encounter.

1.359. 822.1

Rationale: A missile fracture is a type of open fracture. The Alphabetic Index main term is Fracture, subterms patella, open, resulting in code 822.1. An E code could also be reported to show that the injury was from a bullet.

ICD-10-CM Code(s): S82.002B

ICD-10-CM Rationale: The Alphabetic Index main term is Fracture, traumatic, subterm patella. A missile fracture is a type of open fracture. The 7th character "B" is used for the initial encounter.

1.360. 830.0

Rationale: The Alphabetic Index main term is Dislocation, subterm jaw. There is no indication that the dislocation is open or recurrent, so code 830.0 is appropriate.

ICD-10-CM Code(s): S03.0xxA

ICD-10-CM Rationale: The Alphabetic Index main term is Dislocation with subterm jaw. The 7th character "A" is used for the initial encounter.

1.361. 842.00

Rationale: The Alphabetic Index main term is Sprain, subterm wrist, resulting in code 842.00.

ICD-10-CM Code(s): S63.509A

ICD-10-CM Rationale: The Alphabetic Index main term is Sprain, subterm wrist. The 7th character "A" is used for the initial encounter.

1.362. 860.1

Rationale: The Alphabetic Index main term is Pneumothorax, traumatic, with open wound into thorax, resulting in code 860.1. An E code could be added to report the stabbing with a knife.

ICD-10-CM Code(s): S27.0xxA, S21.319A

ICD-10-CM Rationale: The Alphabetic Index main term is Pneumothorax with subterm traumatic. The 7th character "A" is used for the initial encounter. The coder is instructed to "code also any associated open wound of thorax" (S21.-).

1.363. 911.5

Rationale: The Alphabetic Index main term is Injury, superficial, buttocks. The instructional note at the entry for injury, superficial, indicates that the fourth digit to describe a bite by a nonvenomous insect, infected, is 5, resulting in code 911.5.

ICD-10-CM Code(s): S30.860A, L08.9

ICD-10-CM Rationale: The Alphabetic Index main term is Bite (animal) (human) subterm buttock, superficial insect. A second code is needed to code the infection. The Alphabetic Index main term is Infection, subterm skin. The 7th character "A" is used for the initial encounter.

1.364. 944.35

Rationale: The Alphabetic Index main term is Burn, subterms hand, third-degree. Review of the Tabular List entry for category 944 indicates that the fifth digit to describe burn affecting the palm of the hand is 5, resulting in code 944.35.

ICD-10-CM Code(s): T23.359A

ICD-10-CM Rationale: The Alphabetic Index main term is Burn with subterms palm, third degree. The 7th character "A" is used for the initial encounter.

1.365. 965.1

Rationale: The Alphabetic Index main term is Poisoning. There is no separate entry under poisoning for salicylate, and the coding professional is referred to the Table of Drugs and Chemicals. Review of the table shows that the appropriate code for salicylate poisoning is 965.1. If the circumstances of the poisoning were known, an E code could also be assigned.

ICD-10-CM Code(s): T39.091A

ICD-10-CM Rationale: The Alphabetic Index main term is Poisoning, subterm drug. The coder is directed to the Table of Drugs and Chemicals, by drug, poisoning. The column poisoning accidental is accessed. The 7th character "A" is used for the initial encounter.

1.366. 995.64

Rationale: The Alphabetic Index main term is Anaphylactic shock or reaction, subterms due to, food, nuts, resulting in code 995.64.

ICD-10-CM Code(s): T78.05xA

ICD-10-CM Rationale: The Alphabetic Index main term is Shock with subterm anaphylactic, due to food, nuts. The 7th character "A" is used for the initial encounter.

1.367. 991.0

Rationale: The Alphabetic Index main term is Frostbite, subterm face, resulting in code 991.0. An E code for adverse effect of exposure to cold might also be reported.

ICD-10-CM Code(s): T33.09xA

ICD-10-CM Rationale: The Alphabetic Index main term is Frostbite, subterm face. The 7th character "A" is used for the initial encounter.

1.368. 996.02

Rationale: Search for the entry, Leakage of device or implant, leads to a cross-reference to "see Complications, mechanical." The main term is Complications, subterms mechanical, heart valve prosthesis, resulting in code 996.02.

ICD-10-CM Code(s): T82.03xA

ICD-10-CM Rationale: The Alphabetic Index main term Leakage with subterms device, implant or graft refers the coder to the main term complication with subterm heart, valve, prosthesis, mechanical, leakage. The 7th character "A" is used for the initial encounter.

1.369. 996.82

Rationale: The Alphabetic Index main term is Rejection, subterms transplant, organ, liver, resulting in code 996.82.

ICD-10-CM Code(s): T86.41

ICD-10-CM Rationale: The Alphabetic Index main term is Rejection, subterms transplant, liver.

1.370. 998.2

Rationale: The Alphabetic Index main term is Laceration, accidental, complicating surgery, resulting in code 998.2.

ICD-10-CM Code(s): I97.52

ICD-10-CM Rationale: The Alphabetic Index main term is Laceration with subterm accidental, complicating surgery with a note to "see complications, with subterm intraoperative, circulatory system or organ or structure, during other procedure."

1.371. 995.81

Rationale: The Alphabetic Index main term is Battered, subterm spouse.

ICD-10-CM Code(s): T74.11xA, Y07.01

ICD-10-CM Rationale: The Alphabetic Index main term Battered refers the coder to Maltreatment. Main term Maltreatment, adult, physical abuse, confirmed. The seventh character "A" is used for the initial encounter. Review of the Tabular List for category T74 indicates to report an additional code, if applicable, to identify any associated current injury external cause code to identify perpetrator, if known (Y07.-).

1.372. 997.41

Rationale: The Alphabetic Index main term is Retention, retained, subterm cholelithiasis, following cholecystectomy.

ICD-10-CM Code(s): K91.89, K80.80

ICD-10-CM Rationale: The Alphabetic Index main term is Retention, subterm gallstones. The coder is directed to "Use additional code, if applicable, to further specify disorder." Code K80.80 describes other cholelithiasis, without obstruction.

1.373. 999.42

Rationale: The Alphabetic Index main term is Reaction, subterm anaphylactic—see Anaphylactic reaction. Anaphylactic reaction or shock, due to immunization.

ICD-10-CM Code(s): T80.5xxA

ICD-10-CM Rationale: The Alphabetic Index main term Reaction, anaphylactic directs the coder to see Shock, anaphylactic. Shock, anaphylactic, immunization. The seventh character "A" is used for the initial encounter.

1.374. 997.32

Rationale: The Alphabetic Index main term is Pneumonia, subterm postoperative, aspiration.

ICD-10-CM Code(s): J95.89, J69.0

ICD-10-CM Rationale: The Alphabetic Index main term is Complication, subterm surgical complication, respiratory—see Complication, respiratory system. Complication, respiratory system, postoperative leads the coder to J95.89. The coder is directed to also code J69.0 to report the aspiration pneumonia.

1.375. 808.44

Rationale: The Alphabetic Index main term is Fracture, subterm pelvis, multiple, without, disruption of pelvic circle.

ICD-10-CM Code(s): S32.89xA

ICD-10-CM Rationale: The Alphabetic Index main term is Fracture, pelvis, pelvic (bone), specified site NEC. The seventh character "A" is used for the initial encounter.

ICD-9-CM and ICD-10-CM External Causes of Morbidity

1.376. E886.0, E849.4, E007.0, E000.8

Rationale: The Alphabetic Index main term is Tackle in sport, E886.0; Alphabetic Index main term Accident, subterm occurring football field, E849.4; Alphabetic Index main term Activity, subterm football, tackle, E007.0; Alphabetic Index main term Activity status student, E000.8.

ICD-10-CM Code(s) and Rationale:

W03.xxxA	Index to external cause, Fall, due to, person. The 7th character "A" is used for the initial encounter.
Y92.321	Index to external cause, Place of occurrence, football field.
Y93.61	Index to external cause, Activity, football.
Y99.8	Index to external cause, Status of external cause, specified NEC.

1.377. E881.0, E849.3, E016.2, E000.0

Rationale: The Alphabetic Index main term is Fall, subterms from, ladder, E881.0; Alphabetic Index main term Accident, subterms occurring, construction site, E849.3; Activity, building and construction, E016.2; Alphabetic Index main term Activity status, subterms civilian, work done for pay or income, E000.0.

ICD-10-CM Code(s) and Rationale:

W11.xxxA	Index to external cause, Fall, falling, from, ladder. The 7th character "A" is used for the initial encounter.
Y92.61	Index to external cause, Place of occurrence, building under construction.
Y99.0	Index to external cause, Status of external cause civilian activity done for financial or other compensation.

1.378. E893.1

Rationale: The Alphabetic Index main term is Ignition, subterm clothes, (from controlled fire) in building. This leads to code E893.9. Review of category E893 shows that a more specific code, E893.1, exists for burns from ignition of clothing by controlled fire in a building other than a private dwelling. Thus, code E893.1 is the most appropriate code. It can also be found by accessing Ignition, subterm clothes (from controlled fire) in specified building or structure, except private dwelling, E893.1.

ICD-10-CM Code(s): X02.0xxA

ICD-10-CM Rationale: In the Index to External Cause, the main term Burn with subterm fire refers the coder to main term Exposure, fire with subterms controlled in, building or structure. The 7th character "A" is used for the initial encounter.

1.379. E905.0

Rationale: The Alphabetic Index main term is Bite, subterm rattlesnake, resulting in code E905.0.

ICD-10-CM Code(s): T63.011A

ICD-10-CM Rationale: Index to External Cause, Bite, bitten, snake (nonvenomous) references code W59.11. The Tabular List W59 category excludes 1 note states contact with venomous reptile to see T63.0-, T63.1; a rattlesnake is a venomous snake, which results in code T63.011A. The 7th character "A" is used for the initial encounter.

1.380. E909.2

Rationale: The Alphabetic Index main term is the same, Avalanche, resulting in code E909.2.

ICD-10-CM Code(s): X36.1xxA

ICD-10-CM Rationale: In the Index to External Cause, the main term is Avalanche with a note to see Landslide. The 7th character "A" is used for the initial encounter.

1.381. E917.3, E849.0, E013.9, E000.8

Rationale: The Alphabetic Index main term is Bumping against, into, object, subterm furniture, resulting in code E917.3; Alphabetic Index main term Accident, subterms occurring, home, E849.0; Alphabetic Index main term Activity, subterm household maintenance, E013.9; Activity status, specified NEC, E000.8.

ICD-10-CM Code(s) and Rationale:

W22.03xA	Index to external cause, Striking against, object, furniture. The 7th character "A" is used for the initial encounter.
Y92.010	Index to external cause, Place of occurrence, residence, house single family, kitchen.
Y93e9	Index to external cause, Activity, household (interior) maintenance.
Y99.8	Index to external cause, Status of external cause, specified NEC.

1.382. E910.4

Rationale: A search for the entry Drowning leads the coding professional to a cross-reference to Submersion. Thus, the Alphabetic Index main term is Submersion, subterms in, bathtub, resulting in code E910.4.

ICD-10-CM Code(s): W65.xxxA

ICD-10-CM Rationale: In the Index to External Cause, the main term is Drowning with subterms in, bathtub. The 7th character "A" is used for the initial encounter.

1.383. E923.0

Rationale: The Alphabetic Index main term is the same, Fireworks, resulting in code E923.0.

ICD-10-CM Code(s): W39.xxxA

ICD-10-CM Rationale: In the Index to External Cause, the main term is Fireworks (explosion). The 7th character "A" is used for the initial encounter.

1.384. E004.1

Rationale: The Alphabetic Index main term is Rappelling, resulting in code E004.1.

ICD-10-CM Code(s): Y93.32

ICD-10-CM Rationale: In the Index to External Cause, the main term is Activity. Code Y93.3 refers to activities involving climbing, rappelling, and jumping off.

1.385. 882.0, E966

Rationale: The Alphabetic Index main term is Wound, open, hand. Without documentation of tendon involvement or complication of the wound, the resulting code is 882.0. The E code Alphabetic Index main term is Assault, subterms cut, knife, or stab, resulting in code E966.

ICD-10-CM Code(s): S61.419A

ICD-10-CM Rationale: The Alphabetical Index main term is Laceration, subterm hand, without foreign body.

External Cause: X99.1xxA Assault, cutting or piercing instrument, knife. The 7th character "A" is used for the initial encounter.

1.386. 847.0, E816.0

Rationale: The Alphabetic Index main term is Sprain, subterms cervical or neck, resulting in code 847.0. The E code Alphabetic Index main term is accident, subterm motor vehicle, not involving collision with motor vehicle. A note refers the coding professional to categories E816–E819. Review of these categories and the instructional note preceding category E810, which indicates that the appropriate fourth digit for driver of the motor vehicle is 0, results in code E816.0.

ICD-10-CM Code(s): S16.1xxA, V47.02xA

ICD-10-CM Rationale: The Alphabetic Index main term is Strain, cervical resulting in code S16.1 with a seventh character of "A" for initial encounter. The Alphabetic Index of External Causes main term is Accident, subterms transport, car occupant, driver, collision (with), stationary object, resulting in code V47.52 with a 7th character of "A" for initial encounter.

1.387. 813.82, E818.3

Rationale: The Alphabetic Index main term is Fracture, subterm ulna, resulting in code 813.82, without further information on the specific site of the fracture. The E code Alphabetic Index main term is accident, subterm motor vehicle, not involving collision. A note refers the coding professional to review categories E816–E819. Review of these categories and the instructional note preceding category E810, which indicates that the appropriate fourth digit for passenger on a motorcycle is 3, results in code E818.3.

ICD-10-CM Code(s): S52.201A, V28.1xxA

ICD-10-CM Rationale: The Alphabetic Index main term is Fracture, traumatic, subterm ulna, resulting in code S52.201 with a seventh character of "A." The Alphabetic Index of External Causes main term is Accident, subterms transport, motorcyclist, passenger, noncollision accident, nontraffic, resulting in V28.1 with a 7th character of "A."

1.388. E017.0

Rationale: The Alphabetic Index main term is Activity, subterm riding roller coaster, E017.0.

ICD-10-CM Code(s): Y93.i1

ICD-10-CM Rationale: In the Index to External Cause, the main term is Activity with subterm rollercoaster riding.

1.389. E906.0

Rationale: The Alphabetic Index main term is Bite, subterm dog, resulting in code E906.0.

ICD-10-CM Code(s): W54.0xxA

ICD-10-CM Rationale: The Index to External Cause main term is Bite, bitten by, dog. The 7th character "A" is used for the initial encounter.

1.390. E849.5

Rationale: The Alphabetic Index main term is Accident, subterms occurring at, street, resulting in code E849.5.

ICD-10-CM Code(s): Y92.410

ICD-10-CM Rationale: In the Index to External Cause, the main term is Place of Occurrence with subterm street and highway.

1.391. E871.0

Rationale: The Alphabetic Index main term is Misadventure to patients during surgical or medical care, subterms foreign object left in body during procedure, surgical operation, resulting in code E871.0. A search on the main term Foreign body leads to the cross-reference to Misadventure.

ICD-10-CM Code(s): Y65.4

ICD-10-CM Rationale: External cause of Injury: Y65.4 Failure to, remove tube or instrument.

1.392. E909.0

Rationale: The Alphabetic Index main term is the same, Earthquake (any injury), resulting in code E909.0.

ICD-10-CM Code(s): X34.xxxA

ICD-10-CM Rationale: In the Index to External Cause, the main term is Earthquake. The 7th character "A" is used for the initial encounter.

1.393. E919.3

Rationale: The Alphabetic Index main term is Accident, subterms machine, metal-working, resulting in code E919.3.

ICD-10-CM Code(s): W31.1xxA

ICD-10-CM Rationale: External cause of Injury: W31.1xxA The Index to External Cause indicates Contact, with, machine, machinery, lathe. The 7th character "A" is used for the initial encounter.

1.394. E955.1, E849.3, E000.0

Rationale: The Alphabetic Index main term is Shooting, subterms stated as, intentional purposeful, shotgun, E955.1; Alphabetic Index main term Accident, subterms occurring (at) (in), factory, E849.3; Alphabetic Index main term Activity status, subterms civilian, done for, pay or income, E000.0.

ICD-10-CM Code(s): X94.0xxA, Y92.63, Y99.0

ICD-10-CM Rationale: External cause of injury: In the Index to External Cause, the main term is shooting with subterm inflicted by another person—see Discharge, firearm, by type, homicide. Look up main term Discharge with subterms firearm, shotgun, homicide. The 7th character "A" is used for the initial encounter. Place of occurrence: factory. External cause status: The main term is External cause status with subterm civilian activity done for financial or other compensation.

1.395. 872.11, E928.3

Rationale: The Alphabetic Index main term is Wound, open, ear, external complicated. This leads to subcategory 872.1, where review shows that the appropriate code is 872.11, Auricle of ear. The E code main term is bite, subterm human.

ICD-10-CM Code(s): S01.359x, B99.9

ICD-10-CM Rationale: The Alphabetical Index main term is Bite, ear. External cause of Injury: W50.3xxA Bite, bitten by human being (accidentally), main term Infection. The 7th character "A" is used for the initial encounter.

ICD-9-CM V Codes/ICD-10-CM Z Codes

1.396. V26.1

Rationale: The Alphabetic Index main term is Artificial, subterm insemination, resulting in code V26.1. This code can also be accessed via main term Insemination, artificial.

ICD-10-CM Code(s): Z31.83

ICD-10-CM Rationale: The Alphabetical Index main term is Encounter with subterm assisted reproductive fertility procedure cycle.

1.397. V02.61

Rationale: The Alphabetic Index main term is Carrier of, subterms hepatitis, B, resulting in code V02.61. This code can also be accessed via the main term Hepatitis, subterms viral, type B, carrier status.

ICD-10-CM Code(s): Z22.51

ICD-10-CM Rationale: The Alphabetical Index main term is Carrier, subterm hepatitis, B surface antigen.

1.398. V10.3

Rationale: The Alphabetic Index main term is History of, subterms malignant neoplasm of, breast, resulting in code V10.3.

ICD-10-CM Code(s): Z85.3

ICD-10-CM Rationale: The Alphabetical Index main term is History with subterm personal (of), malignant neoplasm, breast.

1.399. V12.72

Rationale: The Alphabetic Index main term is History of, subterms polyps, colonic, resulting in code V12.72.

ICD-10-CM Code(s): Z86.010

ICD-10-CM Rationale: The Alphabetical Index main term is History, subterm personal, disease or disorder (of), digestive system, colonic polyp.

1.400. V16.41

Rationale: The Alphabetic Index main term is History of, subterms family, malignant neoplasm of, ovary, resulting in code V16.41.

ICD-10-CM Code(s): Z80.41

ICD-10-CM Rationale: The Alphabetical Index main term is History, Family (of), malignant neoplasm, ovary.

1.401. V20.2

Rationale: The Alphabetic Index main term is Admission for, subterm well baby and child care, resulting in code V20.2.

ICD-10-CM Code(s): Z00.129

ICD-10-CM Rationale: The Alphabetical Index main term is Examination, subterm child (over 28 days old).

1.402. V22.2

Rationale: The Alphabetic Index main term is Pregnancy, subterm incidental finding, resulting in code V22.2.

ICD-10-CM Code(s): Z33.1

ICD-10-CM Rationale: The Alphabetical Index main term is Pregnancy, with subterm incidental finding.

1.403. V33.01

Rationale: The Alphabetic Index main term is Newborn, subterms twin, born in hospital, with cesarean delivery or section, resulting in code V33.01.

ICD-10-CM Code(s): Z38.31

ICD-10-CM Rationale: The Alphabetical Index main term is Newborn, subterm twin, born in hospital, by cesarean.

1.404. V28.0

Rationale: The Alphabetic Index main term is Amniocentesis screening, subterm chromosomal anomalies, resulting in code V28.0.

ICD-10-CM Code(s): Z36

ICD-10-CM Rationale: The Alphabetical Index main term is Screening with subterms prenatal, of mother.

1.405. V85.42

Rationale: The Alphabetic Index main term is BMI (body mass index), subterms adult, 45.0–49.9, resulting in code V85.42.

ICD-10-CM Code(s): Z68.42

ICD-10-CM Rationale: The Alphabetical Index main term is Body, bodies, subterm mass index (BMI), 45.0–49.9.

1.406. V45.11

Rationale: The Alphabetic Index main term is Status, subterm renal dialysis, resulting in code V45.11.

ICD-10-CM Code(s): Z99.2

ICD-10-CM Rationale: The Alphabetical Index main term is Status with subterm renal dialysis.

1.407. V45.01

Rationale: The Alphabetic Index main term is Status (post), subterms cardiac, device, pacemaker, resulting in code V45.01. Code V53.31, Fitting or adjustment of cardiac pacemaker, is not appropriate here because there is no mention of such services, only that the pacemaker was present.

ICD-10-CM Code(s): Z95.0

ICD-10-CM Rationale: The Alphabetical Index main term is Status, subterm pacemaker, cardiac.

1.408. V53.32

Rationale: The abbreviation AICD represents an automatic, implantable cardioverter-defibrillator, a device that both detects and corrects cardiac rhythm abnormalities. The Alphabetic Index main term is Reprogramming, subterm cardiac pacemaker, resulting in code V53.31. When reviewing the code choices, code V53.32 is a better choice.

ICD-10-CM Code(s): Z45.02

ICD-10-CM Rationale: The Alphabetical Index main term is Encounter with subterm fitting (of)—see Fitting (and adjustment) (of), automatic implantable cardiac defibrillator (with synchronous cardiac pacemaker).

1.409. V54.27

Rationale: The Alphabetic Index main term is Aftercare, subterms fracture, healing, pathologic, vertebra, resulting in code V54.27. The aftercare codes are appropriate as principal diagnoses for home health agencies, skilled nursing facilities, rehabilitation facilities, and so forth.

ICD-10-CM Code(s): M84.48xD

ICD-10-CM Rationale: The Alphabetical Index main term Aftercare, subterm fracture directs the coder to code to fracture with extension D. The main term Fracture, pathological, subterm vertebra leads the coder to M84.48. The 7th character "D" is used for the initial encounter.

1.410. V55.0

Rationale: The Alphabetic Index main term is Admission for, subterms attention to artificial opening, tracheostomy, resulting in code V55.0.

ICD-10-CM Code(s): Z43.0

ICD-10-CM Rationale: The Alphabetical Index main term is Admission with subterm attention to, tracheostomy.

1.411. V55.3

Rationale: The Alphabetic Index main term is Admission for, subterms attention to artificial opening, colostomy, resulting in code V55.3. This code can also be accessed via the main term Colostomy, subterm attention to.

ICD-10-CM Code(s): Z43.3

ICD-10-CM Rationale: The Alphabetical Index main term is Admission, subterm attention to artificial opening, colostomy.

1.412. V58.11

Rationale: The Alphabetic Index main terms are either Admission for, subterm chemotherapy, or Chemotherapy, subterm encounter for, both resulting in code V58.11. If the purpose of an encounter is the administration of chemotherapy, this is the principal or primary diagnosis, rather than the malignancy, even if the malignancy is still present. An additional code for the malignancy is also used.

ICD-10-CM Code(s): Z51.11

ICD-10-CM Rationale: The Alphabetical Index main term is Encounter with subterm chemotherapy for neoplasm.

1.413. V49.86

Rationale: The Alphabetic Index main term is Status, subterm Do not resuscitate, which results in code V49.86.

ICD-10-CM Code(s): Z66

ICD-10-CM Rationale: The Alphabetical Index main term is DNR.

1.414. V71.4

Rationale: The Alphabetic Index main term is Admission for, subterms observation, following accident, resulting in code V71.4. This code may also be accessed via the main term Observation, subterm accident. The abbreviation MVA stands for motor vehicle accident.

ICD-10-CM Code(s): Z04.1

ICD-10-CM Rationale: The Alphabetical Index main term is Observation (following) with subterms accident, transport.

1.415. V76.12

Rationale: The Alphabetic Index main term is Screening for, subterms malignant neoplasm, breast, mammogram NEC, resulting in code V76.12. This code is appropriate because there is no documentation that this was a patient at high risk for the development of breast cancer.

ICD-10-CM Code(s): Z12.31

ICD-10-CM Rationale: The Alphabetical Index main term is Screening, subterm neoplasm, breast, routine mammogram.

1.416. V12.21

Rationale: The Alphabetic Index main term is History, subterm gestational diabetes.

ICD-10-CM Code(s): Z87.59

ICD-10-CM Rationale: The Alphabetic Index main term is History, subterm personal (of), obstetric complications, pregnancy.

1.417. V87.02

Rationale: The Alphabetic Index main term is Exposure, to, uranium.

ICD-10-CM Code(s): Z77.123

ICD-10-CM Rationale: The Alphabetic Index main term is Contact, subterm radiation, naturally occurring, NEC.

1.418. V62.85

Rationale: The Alphabetic Index main term is Ideation, subterm homicidal.

ICD-10-CM Code(s): R45.80

ICD-10-CM Rationale: The Alphabetic Index main term is Ideation, subterm homicidal.

ICD-9-CM Procedure Coding

1.419. 63.73

Rationale: The Alphabetic Index main term is Vasectomy, resulting in code 63.73. The operative report should be thoroughly reviewed before assigning this code, as surgeons may use the term "vasectomy" synonymously with "ligation of the vas deferens" as a means of male sterilization. The appropriate code for ligation of the vas is 63.71.

1.420. 37.36

Rationale: The Alphabetic Index main term is Stapling, subterm left atrial appendage, resulting in code 37.36.

1.421. 06.2

Rationale: The Alphabetic Index main term is Lobectomy, subterm thyroid (unilateral), resulting in code 06.2.

1.422. 11.62

Rationale: The Alphabetic Index main term is Keratoplasty, subterm lamellar, resulting in code 11.62. Search on the main term Transplant, cornea yields a code, 11.60, that is nonspecific and not appropriate for the degree of information that we have.

1.423. 20.01

Rationale: The Alphabetic Index main term is Myringotomy, subterms with insertion of tube or drainage device, resulting in code 20.01. This code can also be accessed via the main term Tympanotomy, subterm with intubation. The terms "myringotomy" and "tympanotomy" are synonymous, and the physician's choice is usually based on the terminology used at the medical school he or she attended.

1.424. 27.62

Rationale: The Alphabetic Index main term is Repair, subterms cleft, palate, resulting in code 27.62.

1.425. 32.22

Rationale: The Alphabetic Index main term is Reduction, subterm lung volume, resulting in code 32.22.

1.426. 35.51

Rationale: The Alphabetic Index main term is Repair, subterms atrial septal defect, with, prosthesis (open-heart technique), resulting in code 35.51. Mesh is a type of bioinert, manufactured material that is used to patch a hole. Code 35.61, Repair with tissue graft, would not be appropriate as this would involve closure by patching with donor human tissue. Review the documentation in the record to see if 39.61, Cardiopulmonary bypass, is appropriate to use as an additional code.

1.427. 00.66

Rationale: The abbreviation PTCA stands for percutaneous transluminal coronary angioplasty. This is a technique for reducing plaque formation in an artery that is performed through the vessel (percutaneous) rather than via an incision. Search on the abbreviation PTCA leads to a cross-reference. The Alphabetic Index main term is Angioplasty, subterms balloon, coronary artery, resulting in code 00.66. This code can also be accessed via the same main term, subterms percutaneous transluminal, coronary. Only the right coronary artery was treated, so this is the appropriate code.

1.428. 36.16

Rationale: The Alphabetic Index main term is Bypass, subterms internal mammary-coronary artery, double vessel, resulting in code 36.16. The subterm aortocoronary bypass is inappropriate because the internal mammary arteries are sutured directly to the heart without harvesting. In aortocoronary bypass grafting, a segment of vein is sutured to the aorta at one end and to the affected coronary artery at the other end. With an internal mammary graft, the vessel is sutured to the coronary artery but remains attached to its native blood supply on the other end. Because both the left and right internal mammary arteries were used, this is a double-vessel graft, code 36.16. An additional code would be assigned for the use of cardiopulmonary bypass in actual practice. This code may also be accessed via the main term Revascularization, subterms cardiac, internal mammary-coronary artery, double vessel.

1.429. 40.42

Rationale: The Alphabetic Index main term is Dissection, subterms neck, radical, bilateral, resulting in code 40.42. This code may also be accessed via the main term Excision, subterms lymph, node, cervical, radical, bilateral. A search on the term lymphadenectomy, which may be used by the surgeon, leads to this second approach to the code.

1.430. 45.81

Rationale: The Alphabetic Index main term is Colectomy, subterms total, laparoscopic, resulting in code 45.81. This code may also be accessed via the main term Resection, subterms colon, total, laparoscopic.

1.431. 52.7

Rationale: The Alphabetic Index main term is Whipple operation, resulting in code 52.7.

1.432. 53.03

Rationale: The Alphabetic Index main term is Repair, subterms hernia, inguinal, direct unilateral, with prosthesis or graft, resulting in code 53.03.

1.433. 55.53

Rationale: The Alphabetic Index main term is Nephrectomy, subterm removal transplanted kidney, resulting in code 55.53.

1.434. 59.6

Rationale: The Alphabetic Index main term is Pereyra operation, resulting in code 59.6. This code may also be accessed via the main term Suspension, subterm paraurethral.

1.435. 68.8

Rationale: The Alphabetic Index main term is Exenteration, subterms pelvic, female, resulting in code 68.8.

1.436. 75.62

Rationale: Search on the main term Repair, laceration, leads to the cross-reference "see suture, by site." The Alphabetic Index main term is Suture, subterms rectum, obstetric laceration, resulting in code 75.62.

1.437. 81.51

Rationale: The Alphabetic Index main term is Replacement, subterms hip, total, resulting in code 81.51. Surgeons also use the term "total hip arthroplasty," and the code may also be accessed via the main term Arthroplasty, subterms hip, total replacement.

1.438. 84.24

Rationale: The Alphabetic Index main term is Reattachment, subterms arm, upper, resulting in code 84.24.

1.439. 72.21

Rationale: The Alphabetic Index main term is Delivery, subterms forceps, mid, with episiotomy, resulting in code 72.21.

1.440. 60.4

Rationale: The Alphabetic Index main term is Prostatectomy, subterm retropubic, resulting in code 60.4.

1.441. 45.62

Rationale: The Alphabetic Index main term is Jejunectomy, resulting in code 45.62. This code may also be accessed via the main term Resection, subterms intestine, small. An end-to-end anastomosis is not separately coded.

1.442. 36.32

Rationale: The Alphabetic Index main term is Revascularization, subterms cardiac, transmyocardial, percutaneous, resulting in code 36.32.

1.443. 36.07, 00.45

Rationale: The Alphabetic Index main term is Insertion, subterms stent, artery, coronary, drug eluting, resulting in code 36.07, and code 00.45 to indicate the number of stents inserted.

ICD-10-PCS Coding

1.444. ICD-10-PCS Code(s): 0VBQ0ZZ

Rationale: The Alphabetic Index main term is Vasectomy, "see Excision, Male Reproductive System 0VB." Reference the table for 0VB for the remaining characters of the code. For a vasectomy the specific body part is the vas deferens, bilateral (Q), the approach is open (0), and there is no device or qualifier (Z). The definition for the root operation of excision is to cut, out or off, without replacement, a portion of a body part. The code for bilateral vasectomy is 0VBQ0ZZ.

1.445. ICD-10-PCS Code(s): 00160J6

Rationale: During a ventriculoperitoneostomy a shunt is placed leading from skull cavities to the peritoneal cavity to relieve excess cerebrospinal fluid created in the chorioid plexuses of the third and fourth ventricles of the brain. The root operation in ICD-10-PCS for altering the route of passage of the contents of a tubular body part is Bypass. The Alphabetic Index main term is Bypass, Cerebral Ventricle 00160. Reference the table for 001 for the remaining characters of the code. In this instance, the specific body part is the cerebral ventricle (6), the approach is open (0), the device is a synthetic substitute (J), and the qualifier is the peritoneal cavity (6), resulting in code 00160J6.

1.446. ICD-10-PCS Code(s): 0GTH0ZZ

Rationale: The Alphabetic Index main term is Lobectomy, "see Resection, Endocrine System 0GT." The first three characters may also be referenced under the main term Thyroidectomy, "see Resection, Endocrine System 0GT." Reference the table for the remaining characters of the code. For a total right thyroid lobectomy, the body part is the right thyroid gland lobe (H), the approach is open (0), and there is no device or qualifier (Z). The definition for the root operation of resection is cutting out or off, without replacement, all of a body part. The code is 0GTH0ZZ.

1.447. ICD-10-PCS Code(s): 08R93KZ

Rationale: The Alphabetic Index main term is Keratoplasty, "see Replacement 08R." Reference the table for the remaining characters of the code. The body part is the left cornea (9), the approach is percutaneous (3), the device is nonautologous tissue substitute (K), and there is no qualifier (Z), resulting in code 08R93KZ.

1.448. ICD-10-PCS Code(s): 099770Z

Rationale: Myringotomy is a surgical procedure where a small incision is made in the patient's eardrum with a small tube being placed in the eardrum incision to remove fluid. The Alphabetic Index main term is Myringotomy, "see Drainage, Ear, Nose, Sinus, 099." This code can also be accessed via the main term Tympanotomy. The terms "myringotomy" and "tympanotomy" are synonymous and the physician's choice is usually based on the terminology used at the medical school he or she attended. Reference the table for the remaining characters of the code. The body part is right tympanic membrane (7), the approach is via natural or artificial opening (7), the device is drainage device (0), and there is no qualifier (Z), resulting in code 099770Z.

1.449. ICD-10-PCS Code(s): 0Y6J0Z1

Rationale: The Alphabetic Index main term is Amputation, "see Detachment." Following the cross reference, the main term is Detachment, Leg, Lower, Left 0Y6J0Z. Reference the table for the remaining characters of the code. The body part is the left lower leg (J), the approach is open (0), there is no device (Z), and the qualifier is high (1). The qualifier high refers to the portion of the tibia and fibula closest to the knee. The code is 0Y6J0Z1.

1.450. ICD-10-PCS Code(s): 02RG08Z

Rationale: The Alphabetic Index main term is Replacement, Valve, Mitral 02RG. Reference the table for the remaining characters of the code. The approach is open (0), the device is zooplastic tissue (8), and there is no qualifier (Z), resulting in code 02RG08Z.

1.451. ICD-10-PCS Code(s): 02703ZZ

Rationale: The abbreviation PTCA stands for percutaneous transluminal coronary angioplasty. This is a technique for reducing plaque formation in an artery that is performed through the vessel (percutaneous) rather than via an incision. Searching on the abbreviation PTCA, "see Dilation, Heart and Greater Vessels 027." The Alphabetic Index main term is Angioplasty, "see Dilation, Heart and Greater Vessels 027." Reference the table 027 for the remaining characters of the code. The body part value is one coronary artery (0), the approach is percutaneous (3), and there is no device or qualifier (Z), resulting in code 02703ZZ.

1.452. ICD-10-PCS Code(s): 0D5N8ZZ

Rationale: The Alphabetic Index main term is Fulguration, "see Destruction." Following the cross reference, the main term is Destruction, Colon, Sigmoid 0D5N. Reference the table for the remaining characters of the code. The approach is via natural or artificial opening endoscopic (8), and there is no device or qualifier (Z), resulting in code 0D5N8ZZ.

1.453. ICD-10-PCS Code(s): 05CD0ZZ

Rationale: Extirpation is the root operation for taking or cutting out solid material from a body part. For a thrombectomy, the thrombus is the solid material removed. The Alphabetic Index main term is Thrombectomy, "see Extirpation." Following the cross reference, the main term is Extirpation, Vein, Cephalic, Right 05CD. Reference the 05C table for the remaining characters of the code. The body part value is the right cephalic vein (D), the approach is open (0), and there is no device or qualifier (Z), resulting in code 05CD0ZZ.

1.454. ICD-10-PCS Code(s): 0YQA0ZZ

Rationale: The Alphabetic Index main term is Herniorrhaphy, "see Repair, Anatomical Regions, Lower Extremities 0YQ." Reference the 0YQ table for the remaining characters of the code. The body part value is bilateral inguinal region (A), the approach is open (0), and there is no device or qualifier (Z), resulting in code 0YQA0ZZ.

1.455. ICD-10-PCS Code(s): 0TY00Z0

Rationale: The Alphabetic Index main term is Transplantation, Kidney, Right 0TY00Z. Reference the 0TY table for the remaining characters of the code. The body part value is the right kidney (0), the approach is open (0), the device is none (0), and the qualifier is allogenic (0), resulting in code 0TY00Z0.

1.456. ICD-10-PCS Code(s): 01N54ZZ

Rationale: During a carpal tunnel release procedure, the transverse carpal ligament is cut, which releases pressure on the median nerve. The Alphabetic Index main term is Release Nerve, Median 01N5. Reference the 01N table for the remaining characters of the code. The body part is the median nerve (5), the approach is percutaneous endoscopic (4), and there is no device or qualifier (Z), resulting in code 01N54ZZ.

1.457. ICD-10-PCS Code(s): 0QSK04Z

Rationale: The root operation for a fracture reduction is reposition. Reposition is the moving of a body part from an abnormal location to its normal location. The Alphabetic Index main term is Reduction, Fracture, "see Reposition." Following the cross reference, the main term is Reposition, Fibula, Left 0QSK. Reference the 0QS table for the remaining characters of the code. The body part value is left fibula (K), the approach is open (0), the device is internal fixation device (4), and the qualifier is none (Z), resulting in code 0QSK04Z.

1.458. ICD-10-PCS Code(s): 0SR90J7

Rationale: The Alphabetic Index main term is Replacement, Joint, Hip, Right 0SR9. Surgeons also use the term "total hip arthroplasty" and the code may also be accessed via the main term Arthroplasty, "see Replacement, Lower Joints 0SR." Reference the table 0SR for the remaining characters of the code. The body part value is right hip joint (9), the approach is open (0), the device is synthetic substitute (J), and the qualifier is ceramic-on-ceramic (7), resulting in code 0SR90J7.

1.459. ICD-10-PCS Code(s): 0SG1031

Rationale: The Alphabetic Index main term is Fusion, Lumbar Vertebra, 2 or more 0SG1. Reference the table 0SG for the remaining characters of the code. The body part value is lumbar vertebral joints 2 or more (1), the approach is open (0), the device is an interbody fusion device (3), and the qualifier is posterior approach, posterior column (1), resulting in code 0SG1031.

1.460. ICD-10-PCS Code(s): 0SJC4ZZ

Rationale: The Alphabetic Index main term is Arthroscopy, "see Inspection, Lower Joints 0SJ." The main term is Inspection, Joint, Knee, Right 0SJC. Reference the table 0SJ for the remaining characters of the code. The body part value is the right knee joint (C), the approach is percutaneous endoscopic (4), and there is no device or qualifier (Z), resulting in code 0SJC4ZZ.

1.461. ICD-10-PCS Code(s): 0SWD0JZ

Rationale: The Alphabetic Index main term is Revision of device in, Joint, Knee, Left 0SWD. Reference the table 0SW for the remaining characters of the code. The body part value is the left knee (D), the approach is open (0), the device is a synthetic substitute (J), and there is no qualifier (Z), resulting in code 0SWD0JZ.

1.462. ICD-10-PCS Code(s): 0DB98ZX

Rationale: The Alphabetic Index main term is Biopsy, "see Excision." Following the cross reference, the main term is Excision, Duodenum 0DB9. Reference the table 0DB for the remaining characters of the code. The body part value is the duodenum (9), the approach is via natural or artificial opening endoscopic (8), there is no device (Z), and the qualifier is diagnostic (X), resulting in code 0DB98ZX.

1.463. ICD-10-PCS Code(s): 0UT9FZZ, 0UTC4ZZ

Rationale: During a laparoscopic-assisted total vaginal hysterectomy the uterus and cervix are resected. ICD-10-PCS has distinct body part values for both the uterus and cervix; therefore two codes are required to completely code this procedure. The Alphabetic Index main term is Hysterectomy, "see Resection, Uterus 0UT9." Reference the table 0UT for the remaining characters of the first code. The body part value is the uterus (9), the approach is via natural or artificial opening with percutaneous endoscopic assistance (F), and there is no device or qualifier (Z), resulting in code 0UT9FZZ. For resection of the cervix, the main term is Resection, Cervix 0UTC. Reference the table 0UT for the remaining characters of the second code. The body part value is the cervix (C), the approach is percutaneous endoscopic (4) and there is no device or qualifier (Z), resulting in code 0UTC4ZZ.

1.464. ICD-10-PCS Code(s): 0UDB8ZX

Rationale: The root operation of extraction is defined as pulling or stripping out or off all or a portion of a body part. During a D&C a curette is used to scrape the lining of the uterus. The Alphabetic Index main term is Extraction, Endometrium 0UDB. Reference the table 0UD for the remaining characters of the code. The body part value is the endometrium (B), the approach is via natural or artificial opening endoscopic (8), the device is none (Z), and the qualifier is diagnostic (X), resulting in code 0UDB8ZX.

1.465. ICD-10-PCS Code(s): 0TF6XZZ

Rationale: Following the cross reference for Lithotripsy, the main term is Fragmentation, Ureter, Right 0TF6. Reference the table 0TF for the remaining characters of the code. The body part value is the right ureter (6), the approach is external (X), and there is no device of qualifier (Z), resulting in code 0TF6XZZ.

Chapter 2. Basic Principles of CPT Coding

CPT Organization, Structure, and Guidelines

2.1.   a. Patient management

Incorrect answer. This issue is addressed in the Category II codes.

b. New technology

Correct answer. New technology is addressed by the Category III codes.

c. Therapeutic, preventive, or other interventions

Incorrect answer. This issue is addressed in the Category II codes.

d. Patient safety

Incorrect answer. This issue is addressed in the Category II codes.

2.2.   a. Changes in verbiage within code descriptions

Incorrect answer. The symbol ▲ is used to indicate changes in verbiage in code descriptions.

b. A new code

Incorrect answer. The symbol ● is used to indicate a new code.

c. Changes in verbiage other than that in code descriptions, for example, changes in coding guidelines or parenthetical notes

Correct answer.

d. A code for which there is a corresponding HCPCS Level II code

Incorrect answer. There is no such indication in CPT.

2.3.   a. No. All diagnostic procedures are included in therapeutic interventional procedures.

Incorrect answer. This is one of the circumstances when the diagnostic procedure may be reported in addition to the therapeutic intervention.

b. Yes. Per revised coding guidelines, if there is a clinical change during an interventional procedure that requires further diagnostic study, the diagnostic angiogram may be reported in addition to the therapeutic procedure.

Correct answer.

2.4.   a. Kidneys, abdominal aorta, common iliac artery origins, inferior vena cava

Correct answer.

b. Kidneys, abdominal aorta, common iliac artery origins, inferior vena cava, urinary bladder

Incorrect answer. The urinary bladder need be included only if there is a clinical history of urinary system pathology.

c. Liver, gallbladder, common bile duct, pancreas, spleen, kidneys, upper aorta, inferior vena cava

Incorrect answer. These organs are the components of a complete ultrasound of the abdomen.

d. Kidneys, abdominal aorta, common iliac artery origins

Incorrect answer. The inferior vena cava must also be evaluated to complete an examination.

2.5.   a. Appendix E

Incorrect answer. Appendix E contains a list of CPT codes exempt from modifier -51. Appendix G is the correct answer.

b. Appendix F

Incorrect answer. Appendix F contains a list of CPT codes exempt from modifier -63. Appendix G is the correct answer.

c. Appendix G

Correct answer.

d. Appendix H

Incorrect answer. Appendix H contains an alphabetic listing of Category II codes. Appendix G is the correct answer.

2.6.   a. True

Incorrect answer. Category II codes are never used alone. They are supplemental tracking codes and may never be reported first.

b. False

Correct answer.

2.7.   a. Appendix I

Incorrect answer. Appendix I is a detailed listing of genetic code modifiers. Appendix J contains a listing of each of the nerve conduction studies and the nerve that is appropriately reported with that code.

b. Appendix J

Correct answer. Appendix J contains a listing of each of the nerve conduction studies and the nerve that is appropriately reported with that code.

c. Appendix K

Appendix K lists codes assigned in anticipation of FDA approval. Appendix J is a detailed listing of genetic testing code modifiers. Appendix J contains a listing of each of the nerve conduction studies and the nerve that is appropriately reported with that code.

d. Appendix L

Appendix L is a series of diagrams of vascular families. Appendix J contains a listing of each of the nerve conduction studies and the nerve that is appropriately reported with that code.

2.8. d. Both a and b

Rationale: Per CPT guidelines (see Introduction to CPT), in order to be included, a procedure must commonly be performed by many physicians across the country, and it must also be consistent with contemporary medical practice. Answer "c," it must be covered by Medicare, is not correct. Medicare coverage has no bearing upon the creation of CPT codes. Answer "d" is correct.

2.9. a. They are updated only once every two years.

Rationale: All the statements are true except this one. The Category III codes are updated every six months in order to reflect current advances in technology.

2.10. b. Is considered to be an integral part of another, larger service

Rationale: Because a separate procedure is considered a part of, and integral to, another, larger procedure, it is not coded when performed as part of the more extensive procedure. See Surgery Guidelines. It may, however, be coded when it is not performed as part of another, larger service, so answer "c" is not correct.

2.11. a. They are numeric.

Rationale: CPT Category I codes describe primarily physician services and are updated annually by the American Medical Association, so the other statements are all false.

2.12. d. The code has been revised in some way this year.

Rationale: The symbol ▲ is used to designate a code that has been revised this year. See Introduction to CPT for descriptions of the meanings of the various symbols used in the terminology.

2.13. a. The code is new for this year.

Rationale: The symbol ● appears before a code that is new with the current edition of CPT. See Introduction to CPT for descriptions of the meanings of the various symbols used in the terminology.

2.14. b. AMA

Rationale: The AMA developed and maintains CPT. CMS developed and maintains HCPCS Level II codes. The Cooperating Parties and WHO have nothing to do with CPT.

2.15. a. Annually for the main body of codes and every 6 months for Category III codes

2.16. d. All of the above

Rationale: Unlike the Alphabetic Index to Procedures in ICD-9-CM, the Alphabetic Index in CPT includes listings by procedures and services, examinations, and anatomic sites, as well as abbreviations, eponyms, synonyms, and diagnoses.

2.17. b. The procedure can only be reported for that diagnosis.

Rationale: The use of the term "for" followed by a diagnosis means that the code can only be reported with that diagnosis. When a code descriptor contains the term "e.g." followed by one or more diagnoses, the manual is giving examples of the types of diagnoses for which the procedure may be performed.

2.18. b. An unlisted procedure code from the appropriate chapter of CPT

Rationale: There is no "generic" unlisted procedure code in CPT. The unlisted procedure code from the appropriate chapter should be reported. Physicians should never report ICD-9-CM procedure codes. These codes are used only for inpatient hospital coding purposes. The fact that a procedure does not have a code in CPT or HCPCS Level II does not mean that it should not be reported. All services rendered should be reported as specifically as possible. If an unlisted procedure code is reported, the payer will typically request further information, including the operative report.

2.19. Laboratory/Pathology

Rationale: See Introduction to CPT.

2.20. d. All of the above

Rationale: The + sign identifies an add-on code, which can never be reported alone or in the first position. All the statements are true.

2.21. a. Appendix A

2.22. c. Any physician

Rationale: Any physician may use the codes in any section of CPT.

Evaluation and Management (E/M) Services

2.23. a. 99304

Incorrect answer. Code 99304 is for a new patient, which this is not. Assuming that the documentation is supportive, code 99309 would be reported, as it reports subsequent services to a nursing facility patient who requires a detailed interval history, detailed examination, and medical decision making of moderate complexity.

b. 99305

Incorrect answer. Code 99305 is for a new patient and one meeting more extensive criteria. Assuming that the documentation is supportive, code 99309 would be reported, as it reports subsequent services to a nursing facility patient who requires a detailed interval history, detailed examination, and medical decision making of moderate complexity.

c. 99309

Correct answer.

d. 99310

Incorrect answer. Code 99310, which is for an established patient, requires more extensive criteria. Assuming that the documentation is supportive, code 99309 would be reported, as it reports subsequent services to a nursing facility patient who requires a detailed interval history, detailed examination, and medical decision making of moderate complexity.

e. 99318

Incorrect answer. Code 99318 is used to report an annual assessment on an essentially stable patient for administrative reasons. Assuming that the documentation is supportive, code 99309 would be reported, as it reports subsequent services to a nursing facility patient who requires a detailed interval history, detailed examination, and medical decision making of moderate complexity.

2.24. a. Documentation of history, examination, and medical decision making

Rationale: The documentation of history, physical examination, and medical decision making usually determine the level of E/M code because they are the three key components. The final diagnosis may support or justify the level but does not determine it. The amount of time spent with the patient is only a determining factor when more than half the visit is devoted to counseling. See E/M Services Guidelines.

2.25. 99205

Rationale: See E/M Services Guidelines, Instructions for Selecting a Level of E/M Service, in the CPT manual.

2.26. 99202

Rationale: See E/M Services Guidelines, Instructions for Selecting a Level of E/M Service, in the CPT manual.

2.27. 99213

Rationale: See E/M Services Guidelines, Instructions for Selecting a Level of E/M Service, in the CPT manual.

2.28. Time

Rationale: See E/M Services Guidelines, Instructions for Selecting a Level of E/M Service, in the CPT manual.

2.29. d. A patient is placed in designated observation status.

Rationale: See instructional notes preceding code 99217. In order to report these codes, the admission order must designate observation status. Whether or not the patient meets admission criteria or is admitted following surgery does not affect the observation code selection. If the patient is admitted/discharged on the same date, codes 99234–99236 are appropriate.

2.30. d. One code for the inpatient admission only

Rationale: All the E/M services "roll up into" the most intensive service, which is the hospital admission visit. See definitions preceding code 99201. Individual codes should not be assigned for the visits prior to the admission, although the medical decision making that occurred then would be a part of the medical decision making for the hospital admission.

2.31. Key

Rationale: See E/M Services Guidelines, Instructions for Selecting a Level of E/M Service, in the CPT manual.

2.32. d. a and b above

Rationale: Both the occupational history and the marital history are components of the social history. Allergic history is a component of past medical history. See E/M Services Guidelines, Instructions for Selecting a Level of E/M Service, in the CPT manual.

2.33. b. Social history

Rationale: Documentation of history of use of drugs, alcohol, and/or tobacco is considered part of the social history. The review of systems is a part of the history of present illness. See E/M Services Guidelines, Instructions for Selecting a Level of E/M Service, in the CPT manual.

2.34. d. Has a moderate risk of morbidity without treatment, a moderate risk of mortality without treatment, uncertain prognosis, or increased probability of functional impairment

Rationale: See E/M Services Guidelines, Instructions for Selecting a Level of E/M Service, in the CPT manual.

2.35. 99471

Rationale: Index Critical Care Services, pediatric, initial. Note that pediatric critical care is reported in units of days, unlike adult critical care, which is reported in increments of 30 minutes.

2.36. c. Subsequent hospital care codes

Rationale: The subsequent hospital care codes are used. Refer to the E/M Consultations instructional notes.

2.37. 99243

Rationale: See E/M Services Guidelines, Instructions for Selecting a Level of E/M Service, in the CPT manual.

2.38. b. Chief complaint

Rationale: See E/M Services Guidelines, Instructions for Selecting a Level of E/M Service, in the CPT manual.

2.39. d. All of the above

Rationale: See E/M Guidelines, Instructions for Selecting a Level of E/M Service, in the CPT manual.

2.40. c. Domiciliary, rest home, or custodial care services

Rationale: See the instructional note preceding code 99324 for a definition of the care settings for which these codes are reported.

2.41. b. Age of the patient

Rationale: See definitions preceding code 99381.

2.42. b. Office or other outpatient services codes

Rationale: If the department is not open 24 hours, office or other outpatient services codes are used. See instructions preceding code 99281. The services are codable, but the outpatient services codes must be used.

2.43. 30 (thirty)

Rationale: See Guidelines for Critical Care Services in the CPT manual.

Anesthesia Services

2.44. b. When the anesthesiologist is no longer in personal attendance on the patient

Rationale: See Anesthesia Guidelines, Time Reporting.

2.45. b. Has severe systemic disease

Rationale: See Anesthesia Guidelines, Anesthesia Modifiers.

2.46. d. All of the above

Rationale: See Anesthesia Guidelines, Qualifying Circumstances.

2.47. 99140

Rationale: See Anesthesia Guidelines, Qualifying Circumstances.

2.48. 00172

Rationale: Index Anesthesia, cleft palate repair, resulting in code 00172.

2.49. 00326

Rationale: Index Anesthesia, trachea. The codes available are 00320, 00326, and 00542. Index Anesthesia, trachea, reconstruction results in code 00539, which appears to be the most appropriate code. Review of the available codes, however, shows that code 00326 is the correct code for a tracheal reconstruction on a patient under one year of age. A note instructs that code 99100 is not used with 00326.

2.50. 00530

Rationale: Index Anesthesia, pacemaker insertion, resulting in code 00530.

2.51. 00670

Rationale: Index Anesthesia, spine and spinal cord, lumbar, resulting in code range 00630–00670. Review of the available codes shows that code 00670 is appropriate for extensive procedures involving instrumentation.

2.52. 00832, 99100

Rationale: Index Anesthesia, hernia, abdomen, lower, resulting in code range 00830–00836. Review of the available codes indicates that code 00832 is the appropriate code for reporting ventral hernia repair. Because the patient is 76 years old, a qualifying circumstance code may also be assigned.

2.53. 00862

Rationale: Index Anesthesia, nephrectomy, resulting in code 00862. Anesthesia coding does not distinguish between donor nephrectomy and nephrectomy for disease.

2.54. 01400

Rationale: Index Anesthesia, arthroscopic procedures, knee, resulting in code 01382 or 01400. Review of the available codes indicates that code 01382 is used to report anesthesia for diagnostic knee arthroscopies, and 01400 is used for surgical arthroscopic procedures. Thus, code 01400 is the appropriate code.

2.55. 01214

Rationale: Index Anesthesia, hip, resulting in code range 01200–01215. Review of the available codes indicates that code 01214 is the appropriate code for anesthesia for a total hip replacement.

2.56. 00921

Rationale: Index Anesthesia, vasectomy, resulting in code 00921.

2.57. 01967, 01968

Rationale: Index Anesthesia, childbirth, cesarean resulting in codes 01961 or 01963, 01968–01969. Review of the available codes indicates that code 01968 is appropriate for anesthesia for cesarean delivery following neuraxial labor anesthesia. A note following 01968 indicates that this code must be assigned in conjunction with 01967 for the anesthesia administered for the planned vaginal delivery.

2.58. 01232, 99140

Rationale: Index Anesthesia, leg upper, resulting in code range 01200–01274. Review of the available codes indicates that code 01232 is the appropriate code for anesthesia for a femoral amputation. Because the procedure is performed as an emergency, a qualifying circumstance code may also be reported.

2.59. 01480

Rationale: Index Anesthesia, tibia, resulting in code range 01390–01392 or code 01484. Review of the available codes indicates that none of the listed codes are appropriate. In fact, the appropriate code is 01480, Anesthesia for open procedures on bones of the lower leg, ankle, and foot, not otherwise specified. The abbreviation ORIF indicates open reduction, internal fixation, so this was an open procedure.

2.60. 00563

Rationale: Index Anesthesia, heart, resulting in code range 00560–00580. Review of the available codes indicates that code 00563 is the appropriate code for anesthesia for surgery on the heart involving the use of the heart-lung perfusion machinery and systemic hypothermia.

2.61. 00794

Rationale: Index Anesthesia, pancreas, resulting in code 00794. A Whipple procedure is a radical procedure for carcinoma of the pancreas, involving removal of the pancreas and the duodenum.

2.62. 00567

Rationale: Index Anesthesia, heart, coronary artery bypass grafting, resulting in code range 00566–00567. Review of the available codes indicates that code 00567 is the appropriate code for coronary artery bypass grafting with pump oxygenator.

2.63. 00944

Rationale: Index Anesthesia, hysterectomy, vaginal, resulting in code 00944.

Integumentary System

2.64. a. Yes

Incorrect answer. The code for this procedure, 19298, is on the list of procedures that include conscious sedation if administered by the same physician who performed the procedure.

b. No

Correct answer.

2.65. a. Autograft

Incorrect answer. An autograft is tissue transplanted from one part of an individual's body to another part. Tissue transplanted from one individual to another of the same species but different genotype is called an allograft or allogenic graft.

b. Xenograft

Incorrect answer. A xenograft, also called a heterograft, is a graft from another species. Tissue transplanted from one individual to another of the same species but different genotype is called an allograft or allogeneic graft.

c. Allograft or allogeneic graft

Correct answer.

d. Heterograft

Incorrect answer. A heterograft, also called a xenograft, is a graft from another species. Tissue transplanted from one individual to another of the same species but different genotype is called an allograft or allogeneic graft.

2.66.　a. True

Correct answer.

b. False

Incorrect answer. Per the coding guidelines preceding code 15002, "These codes are not intended to be reported for simple graft application alone or application stabilized with dressings (e.g., by simple gauze wrap)." The skin substitute/ graft is anchored using the surgeon's choice of fixation. When services are performed in the office, the supply of the skin substitute/graft should be reported separately. Routine dressing supplies are not reported separately.

2.67.　a. A code for the Z-plasty only

Rationale: Per CPT guidelines, when a lesion is excised and the resultant defect is closed with adjacent tissue transfer, only the tissue transfer is coded. See definitions preceding code 14000. Examples of adjacent tissue transfers include Z-plasty, W-plasty, V–Y-plasty, rotation flap, advancement flap, and double-pedicle flap. It is inappropriate to assign an excision code along with an adjacent tissue transfer code.

2.68.　b. Code each lesion separately.

Rationale: Each lesion is coded separately. Dimensions are only added together when coding repair of wounds. See definitions preceding code 11400. The dimensions that determine the code are now composed of the size of the lesion plus the circumferential margins.

2.69.　a. 19120

Rationale: The fact that the lesion was completely excised makes 19120 the appropriate answer. Code 19125 is for excision of a lesion marked by a radiologic marker. Code 19301 is for a partial mastectomy.

2.70.　b. Measurement of the lesion plus circumferential margins documented by the surgeon preexcision

Rationale: The code is determined by measurement of the lesion plus circumferential margins documented by the surgeon preexcision. See definitions preceding code 11400. This represents a change in the method of measuring excision sizes.

2.71.　Shaving

Rationale: See guidelines preceding code 11300. Note that the surgical code includes the local anesthesia as well as the cautery of the wound. By definition, shavings do not require suturing.

2.72. 11044

Rationale: Index Debridement, skin, subcutaneous tissue, resulting in code range 11042–11044. Review of the available codes indicates that code 11044 is the appropriate code for a debridement involving skin, subcutaneous, muscle, and bone which is 20 sq cm or less.

2.73. 11443

Rationale: Index Excision, skin, lesion, benign, resulting in code range 11400–11471. Review of the available codes indicates that code 11443 is the appropriate code for an excision involving the cheek (face), 2.1 to 3.0 cm. Note that the size of the lesion plus margins as well as the site of the lesion determine the code assignment. A solar keratosis is a type of benign skin lesion.

2.74. 11604

Rationale: Index Excision, skin, lesion, malignant, resulting in code range 11600–11646. Review of the available codes indicates that code 11604 is the appropriate code for a lesion of 3.2 cm (1.2 cm lesion plus 2 cm skin margins). Basal cell carcinoma is a type of malignant skin lesion.

2.75. 11462

Rationale: Index Hidradenitis, excision, resulting in code range 11450–11471. Review of the available codes indicates that code 11462 is the appropriate code for inguinal hidradenitis excision with an intermediate closure. Layered closure is a type of intermediate closure, and inguinal and groin are essentially synonymous.

2.76. 11960

Rationale: Index Tissue, expander, insertion, skin, resulting in code 11960. This code is appropriate for all tissue expander insertions other than the breast and includes the inflation of the tissue expander.

2.77. 12042

Rationale: Index Repair, skin, wound, intermediate, resulting in code range 12031–12057. This code may also be accessed via main term Repair, wound, intermediate, resulting in the same code range. Review of the available codes indicates that code 12042 is the appropriate code for a 5.2-cm laceration of the hand. Refer to the instructional notes preceding code 12001 for a definition of simple, intermediate, and complex repair.

2.78. 12002

Rationale: Index Repair, skin, wound, simple, resulting in code range 12020–12021. Indexing Repair, wound, simple results in code range 12001–12021. Review of the available codes indicates that code 12002 is the appropriate code for this repair. These are both simple closures, and the lacerations are of the same body part (extremity), so they are added together, resulting in a total length of 5.4 cm.

2.79. 12004

Rationale: Index Repair, wound, simple, resulting in code range 12001–12021. In this case, because the repair is simple, and the scalp and extremities are the same body part, the sizes are summed. The total laceration length is thus 11.5 cm. Review of the available codes indicates that code 12004 is the appropriate code in this case (7.6 to 12.5 cm).

2.80. 12015, 13101, 13102, 13102

Rationale: Index Repair, skin, wound, simple; and Repair, skin, wound, complex. Review of the available codes indicates that code 12015 is the appropriate code for the 5.0-cm laceration of the cheek plus the 3.2-cm laceration of the forehead (total 8.2 cm from this body part). Codes 13101 and 13102 × 2 are required for the repair of the complex laceration of the chest wall. Code 13101 reports the first 7.5 cm. Code 13102 is reported for each additional 5 cm or less (13101 = 7.5 cm, 13102 = 5 cm, and 13102 = 3.5 cm, to report a total of 16 cm).

2.81. 10081

Rationale: Index Pilonidal Cyst, incision and drainage, resulting in codes 10080 and 10081. Review of the available codes indicates 10081 is correct.

2.82. Intermediate

Rationale: See definitions of simple, intermediate, and complex repair preceding code 12001.

2.83. 19125

Rationale: Index Breast, excision, lesion, by needle localization, resulting in code range 19125–19126. Review of the available codes indicates that code 19125 is the appropriate code for reporting an excision of a single breast lesion.

2.84. b. Both surgeon and pathologist

Rationale: The physician must act as both surgeon and pathologist. See definitions preceding code 17311.

2.85. 19125

Rationale: Index Excision, breast, lesion, by needle localization, resulting in code range 19125–19126. Review of the available codes indicates that code 19125 is the appropriate code for the first lesion. If the needle was placed during the same session (and at the same site of service), a code for the needle placement (19290–19291) may also be reported. With needle localization excision, there is no discrete lesion identified but, rather, an area of somewhat abnormal appearance on mammography. The tissue at the tip of the needle is excised. If multiple areas are identified by needle placements, additional codes (19126) may be reported for each additional area.

2.86. 14000

Rationale: A V–Y plasty is a type of adjacent tissue transfer. Index Tissue, transfer, adjacent, skin, resulting in code range 14000–14350. Review of the available codes indicates that code 14000 is the appropriate code to report a less than 10-sq-cm excision of the trunk. See the instructional note preceding code 14000 for guidelines on coding lesion excisions with repair by adjacent tissue transfer.

2.87. 19357

Rationale: Index Tissue, expander, breast reconstruction with.

2.88. 11043, 11046

Rationale: Debridement, muscle. Review of the available codes show that code 11043 is used to report the first 20 sq cm and 11046 the additional 2 sq cm. Code 11046 is an add-on code and does not require a modifier.

2.89. a. True

Rationale: Complex repair includes wound repair requiring more than layered closure, viz., scar revision, debridement, extensive undermining, stents, or retention sutures.

2.90. b. False

Rationale: Debridement is considered a separate procedure only when gross contamination requires prolonged cleansing, when appreciable amounts of devitalized or contaminated tissue are removed, or when debridement is carried out separately without immediate primary closure.

2.91. Code(s): 12052

Rationale: Because the simple repair involves extensive cleansing it can be coded as an intermediate repair.

Musculoskeletal System

2.92. a. True

Correct answer.

b. False

Incorrect answer. The type of fracture treatment is based upon the physician's clinical judgment and not the type of fracture.

2.93. a. True

Incorrect answer. A bone biopsy performed in conjunction with a kyphoplasty procedure is not reported separately.

b. False

Correct answer.

2.94. a. CT angiography

Incorrect answer. 3D reconstruction is not to be reported with any of these modalities, nor with nuclear medicine studies or CT (virtual) colonoscopy.

b. MR angiography

Incorrect answer. 3D reconstruction is not to be reported with any of these modalities, nor with nuclear medicine studies or CT (virtual) colonoscopy.

c. PET scans

Incorrect answer. 3D reconstruction is not to be reported with any of these modalities, nor with nuclear medicine studies or CT (virtual) colonoscopy.

d. All of the above

Correct answer.

2.95. b. Comminuted

Rationale: The other terms all describe open fractures.

2.96. d. All of the above

Rationale: All of the scenarios describe open fracture treatment. See Musculoskeletal Guidelines, Definitions. The definitions of open vs. closed treatment of fractures have changed somewhat with CPT 2003, and the guidelines should be carefully reviewed.

2.97. a. A "with manipulation" code

Rationale: The "with manipulation" code is used. The fracture was manipulated, even if the manipulation did not result in clinical anatomic alignment. See Musculoskeletal Guidelines, Definitions.

2.98. 28292

Rationale: Index Bunion Repair, Keller procedure, resulting in code 28292. In a Keller procedure, the base of the proximal phalanx is removed, and the alignment between the phalanx and the first metatarsal is maintained with Kirschner wires. This results in an essentially fused joint, with little motion, so this type of bunionectomy is not usually performed in more active patients.

2.99. 29880

Rationale: Index Arthroscopy, surgical, knee, resulting in code range 29871–29889. Review of the available codes indicates that code 29880 is the most appropriate code for a medial and lateral meniscectomy via the arthroscope. Consistent with guidelines throughout CPT, the diagnostic arthroscopy is not coded separately when performed as a part of a surgical procedure. See the instructional note preceding code 29800.

2.100. 27557

Rationale: Index Dislocation, knee, open treatment, resulting in code range 27556–27558, and individual code 27566 or 27730. Review of all the available codes indicates that the most appropriate code is 27557, Open treatment, with or without internal fixation, with primary ligamentous repair. There is no documentation of ligament augmentation (in which a portion of the lower leg musculature is brought up and sutured to the knee tendon structures) but rather use of a special suture (Anchor suture) to repair the ligament.

2.101. 22520

Rationale: Index Vertebra, osteoplasty, thoracic, resulting in code range 22520–22522. Because only one level was treated, code 22520 is appropriate. In this procedure, methylmethacrylate bone cement is injected into a fractured vertebral body percutaneously under imaging guidance.

2.102. 23031

Rationale: Index Incision and Drainage, shoulder, bursa, resulting in code 23031.

2.103. 23450

Rationale: Index Putti-Platt Procedure, resulting in code 23450. A Putti-Platt procedure is a type of open shoulder repair in which the joint capsule is sutured back to the glenoid labrum of the scapula.

2.104. 24515

Rationale: Index Fracture, humerus, shaft, open treatment, resulting in code 24515. The application of the initial cast is part of the code for the fracture treatment and should not be reported separately. Refer to the instructional note preceding code 29000.

2.105. 25810

Rationale: Index Arthrodesis, wrist, with graft, resulting in code 25810. The term "arthrodesis" is synonymous with fusion. The instructional note with code 25810 indicates that this code includes the harvesting of the graft, so no additional code should be reported for this procedure.

2.106. 25605

Rationale: Index Fracture, radius, with manipulation, resulting in code 25565 or 25605. When a fracture is said to have been reduced, the "with manipulation" code is reported.

2.107. 27130

Rationale: Index Arthroplasty, hip, total replacement, resulting in code 27130. A total hip arthroplasty involves replacement of the femoral neck, femoral head, and acetabulum of the hip bone (ilium). This procedure is typically performed for bone diseases such as arthritis. When a fracture of the femoral neck is the reason for the surgery, a partial hip replacement (partial hip arthroplasty) involving replacement of only the femoral component, not including the acetabulum, is performed.

2.108. d. All of the above

Rationale: Casting is reported in all the listed circumstances. See instructional note for application of casts and strapping preceding code 29000.

2.109. 22864

Rationale: Index Removal, artificial intervertebral disc, cervical interspace, resulting in codes 0095T, 22864. Review of the available codes indicates that code 22864 is the correct code.

2.110. 20240

Rationale: Index Biopsy, bone, resulting in code range 20220–20245. Review of the available codes indicates that code 20240, Biopsy, bone, open, superficial, is the appropriate code because the ilium is listed as an example of a superficial bone structure.

2.111. 29425

Rationale: Index Cast, walking, resulting in code 29355 or 29425. Review of the available codes indicates that code 29425 is the appropriate code. Code 29355 is used to report a long-leg walking cast. Because this cast application was not part of initial fracture treatment, it is appropriate to code. Refer to the instructional note preceding code 29000.

2.112. 29827

Rationale: Index Arthroscopy, surgical, shoulder, resulting in code range 29806–29827. Review of the available codes indicates that code 29827 is the appropriate code for reporting an arthroscopic rotator cuff repair. Code 23412—Repair of ruptured musculotendinous cuff, chronic—is not appropriate because this code is used to report an open procedure.

2.113. 27590

Rationale: Index Amputation, leg, upper, resulting in code range 27590–27592. Review of the available codes indicates that code 27590 is the appropriate code for an amputation through the femur (the thigh bone).

2.114. 21480

Rationale: Index Dislocation, temporomandibular joint, closed treatment, resulting in code range 21480–21485. Review of the available codes indicates that code 21480 is the appropriate code because there is no documentation that this was a complicated reduction.

2.115. a. Manipulation

Correct answer. Manipulation is used throughout the CPT musculoskeletal fracture and dislocation subsections to describe the attempted reduction or restoration of joint dislocation to its normal anatomic alignment through the application of manually applied forces.

b. Traction

Incorrect answer. Manipulation is used throughout the CPT musculoskeletal fracture and dislocation subsections to describe the attempted reduction or restoration of joint dislocation to its normal anatomic alignment through the application of manually applied forces.

c. Percutaneous fixation

Incorrect answer. Manipulation is used throughout the CPT musculoskeletal fracture and dislocation subsections to describe the attempted reduction or restoration of joint dislocation to its normal anatomic alignment through the application of manually applied forces.

d. External fixation

Incorrect answer. Manipulation is used throughout the CPT musculoskeletal fracture and dislocation subsections to describe the attempted reduction or restoration of joint dislocation to its normal anatomic alignment through the application of manually applied forces.

2.116. 29914

Rationale: Index term Arthroscopy, surgical, hip, with femoroplasty.

2.117. 22325, 22328

Rationale: Index term Fracture, vertebra, lumbar, open treatment. Code 22325 is used for the first fracture; add-on code 22328 is used for the second fracture.

2.118. False.

Rationale: Segmental instrumentation is defined as fixation at each end of the construct and at least one additional interposed bony attachment. Refer to the CPT book prior to code 22840 for additional information.

2.119. 20644

Rationale: Index term Application, Halo, Cranial, Thin Skull Osteology 20644.

2.120. Excision of a 2.3-cm soft tissue tumor of the hand

Code(s): 26111

Rationale: Index term Excision, tumor, hand. The range 26111–26118 is given and the correct code, based on size, is 26111.

2.121. Incision and drainage of Infected bursa of the left shoulder.

Code(s): 23031

Rationale: Index term is Incision and Drainage, shoulder, bursa.

2.122. Removal of 19 skin tags.

Code(s): 11200, 11201

Rationale: Index term Removal, skin tags. The coder is directed to range 11200–11201. A review of these codes reveals that both codes are necessary—11200 for the first 15 tags and 11201 for the remaining 4 skin tags.

Respiratory System

2.123. a. Transbronchial lung biopsy

Rationale: If lung tissue is obtained via a puncture through the bronchus, a transbronchial biopsy is the appropriate procedure to report.

2.124. 30140

Rationale: Index Turbinate, submucous resection, nose excision, resulting in code 30140.

2.125. 30901

Rationale: Index Epistaxis, resulting in code range 30901–30906. Review of the available codes indicates that code 30901 is appropriate, even though both cautery and packing were used, because the code description states cautery and/or packing. There is no documentation that this was extensive.

2.126. 31255

Rationale: Index Sinuses, ethmoid, excision, endoscopy, resulting in code range 31254–31255. Review of the available codes indicates that code 31255 is appropriate because this is specified as a total ethmoidectomy, which is defined as anterior and posterior. Note that the FESS (functional endoscopic sinus surgery) codes are unilateral. If this procedure had been performed bilaterally, a modifier -50 would be appended.

2.127. 31365

Rationale: Index Laryngectomy, resulting in code range 31360–31382. Review of the available codes indicates that code 31365 is appropriate for a total laryngectomy with radical neck dissection (removal of regional lymph nodes).

2.128. 31541

Rationale: Index Laryngoscopy, operative, resulting in code range 31530–31561. Review of the available codes indicates that code 31541 is the appropriate code. The instructional note following this code indicates that it is not correct to also report code 69990 (use of operating microscope) with this code.

2.129. 31628

Rationale: Index Bronchoscopy, biopsy, resulting in code range 31625–31629 and code range 31632–31633. Review of the available codes indicates that code 31628 is the appropriate code to report when a transbronchial biopsy is performed. As always, any diagnostic endoscopy is included in the surgical endoscopy and not separately reported.

2.130. 32422

Rationale: Index Thoracentesis, resulting in code range 32421–32422. Review of the available codes indicates that code 32422 is appropriate when a tube is placed.

2.131. 32605

Rationale: Index Thoracoscopy, diagnostics, resulting in code range 32601–32606. Review of the available codes indicates that code 32605 describes the procedure.

2.132. 31030

Rationale: Index Caldwell-Luc Procedure, sinusotomy, resulting in code range 31030–31032. Review of the available codes indicates that code 31030 is appropriate because there is no documentation of removal of polyps.

2.133. 31500

Rationale: Index Insertion, endotracheal tube, resulting in code 31500.

2.134. 31643

Rationale: Index Bronchoscopy, catheter placement, intracavity radioelement, resulting in code 31643.

2.135. 32480

Rationale: Index Lobectomy, lung, resulting in code range 32480–32482. Review of the available codes indicates that code 32480 is appropriate for reporting removal of a single lobe.

2.136. 32853

Rationale: Index Transplantation, lung, double, without cardiopulmonary bypass, resulting in code 32853.

2.137. 31276

Rationale: Index Sinuses, frontal, exploration, with nasal/sinus endoscopy, resulting in code 31276. In the case of the frontal sinus, CPT does not distinguish between procedures with removal of tissue and those without.

2.138. 31238

Rationale: Index Endoscopy, nose, surgical, resulting in code range 31237–31294. Review of the available codes indicates that code 31238 is appropriate when the endoscopy is performed for control of hemorrhage.

2.139. c. The fluoroscopy is included in the bronchoscopy and no code is assigned for it.

Rationale: See instructional note preceding code 31615.

2.140. 32560

Rationale: Index Pleurodesis, chemical, resulting in code 32560.

2.141. 31588

Rationale: Index Laryngoplasty, burns, resulting in code 31588.

2.142. 31380

Rationale: Index Larynx, excision, partial, resulting in code range 31367–31382. Review of the available codes indicates that code 31380 is the appropriate code for this particular approach.

2.143. a. True

Rationale: The correct answer is true.

2.144. Code(s): 31296

Rationale: Index term Sinus/Sinuses, endoscopy with dilation. A range of codes (31295–31297) is given. Code 31296 describes dilation of frontal sinus.

2.145. Code(s): 32151

Rationale: Index term Thoracotomy, removal, foreign body, intrapulmonary.

2.146. Code(s): 32810

Rationale: Index term is Clagett procedure. The coder is directed to see Chest wall, repair, closure. The code 32810 is reported.

Cardiovascular System

2.147. a. Arterial embolization

Correct answer.

b. Angiography of the thoracic aorta

Incorrect answer. Per guidelines in CPT preceding code 33880, angiography of the thoracic aorta, fluoroscopic guidance in delivery of the endovascular components, and preprocedure diagnostic imaging are all included in the repair code. Intravascular ultrasound, if performed, may be separately coded.

c. Fluoroscopic guidance in delivery of the endovascular components

Incorrect answer. Per guidelines in CPT preceding code 33880, angiography of the thoracic aorta, fluoroscopic guidance in delivery of the endovascular components, and preprocedure diagnostic imaging are all included in the repair code. Intravascular ultrasound, if performed, may be separately coded.

d. Preprocedure diagnostic imaging

Incorrect answer. Per guidelines in CPT preceding code 33880, angiography of the thoracic aorta, fluoroscopic guidance in delivery of the endovascular components, and preprocedure diagnostic imaging are all included in the repair code. Intravascular ultrasound, if performed, may be separately coded.

2.148. a. True

Incorrect answer. Separate codes exist for ligation and stripping of the long saphenous vein and ligation and stripping of the short saphenous vein. Code 37718 describes ligation, division, and stripping of the short saphenous vein, and code 37722 describes treatment of the long saphenous vein.

b. False

Correct answer.

2.149. a. Selective catheterization

Rationale: If the tip of the catheter is manipulated, it is a selective catheterization. In the case of a nonselective catheterization, the tip of the catheter remains in either the aorta or the artery that was originally entered.

2.150. 33031

Rationale: Index Pericardiectomy, complete, resulting in code range 33030–33031. Review of the available codes indicates that code 33031 is most appropriate because this procedure is performed under cardiopulmonary bypass.

2.151. 33207

Rationale: Index Insertion, pacemaker, heart, resulting in code ranges 33206–33208 and 33212–33213. Review of all the available codes indicates that code 33207 is most appropriate for placement of this type of pacemaker, in which leads are inserted into only the ventricle. Codes 33212 and 33213 are to report the placement of the pulse generator only, so they are not appropriate in this case.

2.152. c. One code for the final vessel entered

Rationale: The only vessel coded is the final vessel entered. See instructional note preceding code 36000. Intermediate steps along the way are not reported.

2.153. 33430

Rationale: Index Replacement, mitral valve, resulting in code 33430.

2.154. 33510

Rationale: Index Coronary Artery Bypass Graft, venous, resulting in code range 33510–33516. Review of the available codes indicates that code 33510 is appropriate. The harvesting of the vein grafts is included (unless they are obtained from upper extremity veins). Only one artery, the left anterior descending, was grafted, so code 33510 is the correct code. Carefully review the instructional note preceding code 33510 for further discussion of coding of CABGs.

2.155. 33534

Rationale: The abbreviation LIMA stands for left internal mammary artery. Index Coronary Artery Bypass Graft, arterial, resulting in code range 33533–33536. Because two arteries were bypassed (the circumflex and the right), code 33534 is appropriate. Review the instructional note preceding code 33533 regarding coding of arterial conduits for coronary artery bypass grafting.

2.156. 33968

Rationale: Index Balloon Assisted Device, aorta, resulting in code range 33967–33974. Review of the available codes indicates that code 33968 is appropriate for the removal of the device.

2.157. 36200

Rationale: Index Aorta, catheterization, catheter, resulting in code 36200. This procedure, in which a catheter is placed directly into the aorta and stays there, is an example of a nonselective catheterization.

2.158. 36425

Rationale: Index Venipuncture, child/adult, cutdown, resulting in code 36425.

2.159. 36560

Rationale: Index Insertion, Venous Access Device, central, resulting in code range 36560–36566. The coding of a VAD is dependent on the type of insertion (central vs. peripheral), type of catheter (tunneled vs. nontunneled, port vs. pump), and patient age. A VAD is an implanted reservoir attached to a central venous catheter. To determine if the catheter is a VAD, look for an implant sticker in the medical record. Central venous catheters are not considered implants and do not carry implant stickers, while VADs do. Most VADs have the word "port" in their brand name. Some examples are Life-Port, PORT-A-CATH, and Infuse-A-Port. Devices such as pumps and ports always require a tunneled catheter.

2.160. 36821

Rationale: Index Brescia-Cimino Type Procedure, resulting in code 36821. This is a type of AV fistula for dialysis in which an artery and a vein are directly sutured together. The radial artery and cephalic vein are the first choice, followed by the brachial artery and vein.

2.161. 37718, 37722

Rationale: Index Varicose Vein, removal, resulting in code ranges 37718, 37722, and range 37765–37785. Review of all the available codes indicates that codes 37718 and 37722 are the most appropriate because both the long and short saphenous veins were treated.

2.162. 38120

Rationale: Index Splenectomy, laparoscopic, resulting in code 38120. This code may also be accessed via the main term Spleen, excision, laparoscopic.

2.163. 38792

Rationale: Index Sentinel Node, injection procedure, resulting in code 38792.

2.164. 37609

Rationale: Index Biopsy, artery, temporal, resulting in code 37609.

2.165. 36558

Rationale: Index Central Venous Catheter Placement, insertion, central, resulting in code range 36555–36558. It is necessary to know if the catheter is tunneled or nontunneled. It is also necessary to know if the catheter is centrally or peripherally inserted and the age of the patient.

2.166. 36430

Rationale: Index Transfusion, blood, resulting in code 36430. For reporting blood transfusions in the hospital outpatient setting, in order to ensure appropriate reimbursement, this code must be assigned for the actual administration of the blood, along with one or more HCPCS Level II codes from the "C" or "P" codes to describe the product.

2.167. 35646

Rationale: Index Bypass Graft, femoral artery, resulting in codes 35521, 35533, 35540, range 35551–35558, 35566, 35621, range 35646–35647, range 35651–35661, 35666, and 35700. Review of all the available codes indicates that code 35646 is appropriate for a graft from the aorta to both femoral arteries (a Y-type graft).

2.168. 37224

Rationale: Index Revascularization, artery, femoral/popliteal—see range of codes 37224–37227. The correct code is 37224.

2.169. b. Generator

Rationale: According to the CPT Guidelines, when the "battery" of a pacemaker or a cardioverter-defibrillator is changed, it is actually the pulse generator that is changed.

2.170. Code(s): 36584

Rationale: Index term Replacement, venous access device, central. The coder is directed to range of codes 36580–36581, 36584. Note the central venous access procedures table.

2.171. Code(s): 37227

Rationale: Index term Revascularization, artery, femoral. The coder is directed to the range of codes 37224–37227. Code 37227 includes both the stent placement and the atherectomy.

2.172. Code(s): 33620

Rationale: Index term Pulmonary Artery, banding, application.

Digestive System

2.173. 40701

Rationale: Index Repair, cleft lip, resulting in code ranges 40525–40527 and 40700–40761. Review of the available codes indicates that code 40701 is appropriate for a single-stage primary procedure.

2.174. 43282

Rationale: Index Laparoscopy, hernia repair, paraesophageal, resulting in codes 43281 and 43282. Review of the available codes indicate that code 43282 includes implantation of mesh and is the correct code.

2.175. 42145

Rationale: Index Uvula, excision, resulting in code range 42140–42145. Review of the available codes indicates that code 42145 is the appropriate code.

2.176. 42821

Rationale: Index Tonsillectomy, resulting in code range 42820–42826. Indexing the main term Tonsils, excision, with adenoids, results in code range 42820–42821. Review of the available codes indicates that code 42820 is appropriate for a child over 12 years of age.

2.177. 43239

Rationale: Index Endoscopy, gastrointestinal, upper, biopsy, resulting in code 43239. Note that the description states biopsy, single or multiple. This code is assigned once for taking of biopsies, no matter how many are performed. If the same lesion that is biopsied is subsequently excised, only an excision code is assigned. If one lesion is biopsied and another excised, two codes are assigned.

2.178. b. A code for the lesion excision only

Rationale: When a lesion is biopsied and the same lesion is excised, only the excision is coded. If one area is biopsied and a different area excised, codes for both the excision and the biopsy are reported.

2.179. 43215

Rationale: Index Esophagus, endoscopy, removal, foreign body, resulting in code 43215. This code may also be accessed by indexing the main term Endoscopy, esophagus, removal, foreign body.

2.180. 43248

Rationale: The abbreviation EGD stands for esophagogastroduodenoscopy, also called upper gastrointestinal endoscopy. Index Endoscopy, gastrointestinal, upper, dilation, resulting in code 43245 and code range 43248–43249. Review of the available codes indicates that code 43248 is appropriate for reporting dilation over a guidewire as part of an endoscopic procedure. Esophageal dilations can also be performed without an endoscope.

2.181. d. Query the physician as to the method used.

Rationale: It is not appropriate for the coder to assume that the removal was done by either snare or hot biopsy forceps. The ablation code is only assigned when a lesion is completely destroyed and no specimen is retrieved. The coding professional must query the physician to assign the appropriate code.

2.182. 43262

Rationale: The abbreviation ERCP stands for endoscopic retrograde cholangio-pancreatography (examination of the gallbladder, pancreas, and bile ducts). Index Bile Duct, endoscopy, sphincterotomy, resulting in code 43262.

2.183. 43280

Rationale: Index Fundoplasty, esophagogastric, laparoscopic, resulting in code 43280. Indexing the main term Nissen Operation results in this cross-reference. Indexing the main term Nissen procedure, laparoscopic, results in code 43280.

2.184. 43770

Rationale: Index Placement, adjustable gastric restrictive device, resulting in code 43770.

2.185. 43246

Rationale: Index Gastrostomy Tube, placement, percutaneous, endoscopic, resulting in code 43246.

2.186. 46050

Rationale: Index Incision and Drainage, anal, resulting in code range 46045–46050. Review of the available codes indicates 46050 is the correct code.

2.187. 44206

Rationale: Index Colectomy, partial, with colostomy, laparoscopic, resulting in code 44206 or 44208. Review of the available codes indicates that code 44206 is appropriate in this case because an end colostomy is specified.

2.188. 46020

Rationale: Index Placement, seton, anal, resulting in code 46020.

2.189. 44378

Rationale: Index Endoscopy, intestines, small, hemorrhage, resulting in code 44366 or 44378. Review of the available codes indicates that code 44378 is appropriate because the site of the bleeding is specified as being in the ileum. Code 44366 is for a small bowel endoscopy that does not include the ileum, so this cannot be the correct code.

2.190. 45384

Rationale: Index Endoscopy, colon, removal, polyp, resulting in code 44392 and range 45384–45385. Review of the available codes indicates that code 45384 describes polypectomy with hot biopsy forceps.

2.191. 45337

Rationale: Index Endoscopy, colon-sigmoid, volvulus, resulting in code 45337.

2.192. 47563

Rationale: Index Cholecystectomy, any method, with cholangiography, resulting in codes 47563, 47605, and 47620. Review of the available codes indicates that codes 47605 and 47620 are for an open procedure, whereas code 47563 is for a laparoscopic procedure, which is the method described.

2.193. Code(s): 46930

Rationale: Index term Destruction, hemorrhoids, thermal energy. Infrared coagulation is a type of thermal energy.

2.194. Code(s): 45305, 45307

Rationale: Index term Proctosigmoidoscopy, biopsy and then Proctosigmoidoscopy, removal, foreign body.

2.195. Code(s): 43328

Rationale: Index term Fundoplasty, esophagogastric, thoracotomy.

Urinary System

2.196. 50200

Rationale: Index Biopsy, kidney, resulting in code range 50200–50205. Review of the available codes indicates that code 50200 is appropriate for a percutaneous needle biopsy.

2.197. 50320

Rationale: Index Nephrectomy, donor, resulting in code range 50300–50320 or code 50547. Review of the available codes indicates that code 50320 is appropriate in this case involving a living donor and with no mention of laparoscopic assistance.

2.198. 50541

Rationale: Index Kidney, cyst, ablation, resulting in code 50541.

2.199. 50590

Rationale: Index Lithotripsy, kidney, resulting in code 50590 or 52353. Review of the available codes indicates that code 50590 is correct because there is no mention of cystourethroscopy.

2.200. 50688

Rationale: Index Ureterostomy Tube, change, resulting in code 50688.

2.201. 51728

Rationale: Index Cystometrogram, resulting in code range 51725–51729. Review of the available codes indicates code 51728 includes voiding pressure studies and is the correct code.

2.202. 51702

Rationale: Index Bladder, catheterization, resulting in code 51045 and range 51701–51703. Review of the available codes indicates that code 51702 is most appropriate. Indexing the main term Catheterization, bladder, results in codes 51102 and 51045, neither of which is appropriate. Note that codes 51701–51703 should be reported only when performed independently. The insertion of a bladder catheter is an integral part of most genitourinary procedures.

2.203. 52234

Rationale: Index Fulguration, cystourethroscopy with, tumor, resulting in code range 52234–52240. Review of the available codes indicates that code 52234 is appropriate with bladder tumors less than 2 cm in size. Note that the code is assigned once, irrespective of the number of tumors treated. Each tumor should be measured individually to determine the appropriate category (e.g., small, medium, large). CPT code 52234 should be reported once for single or multiple tumors that individually measure 0.5–2.0 cm.

2.204. 52282

Rationale: Index Stent, urethra, insertion, resulting in code 52282. Be careful to distinguish between urethra and ureter.

2.205. 52332

Rationale: Index Cystourethroscopy, insertion, indwelling urethral stent, resulting in code 50947 or 52332. Review of the available codes indicates that code 52332 is appropriate. Code 50947 describes placement of a stent into a ureter via laparoscopy rather than cystoscopy. Indexing the main term Endoscopy, ureter, placement, stent, also results in code 50947, which is not correct for the procedure described.

2.206. 50593

Rationale: Index Ablation, renal tumor, cryotherapy, percutaneous, resulting in code 50593.

2.207. 52601

Rationale: Index Prostate, excision, transurethral, resulting in code 52402, 52601, or 52630. Review of the available codes indicates that code 52601 is correct because there is no mention of this being a staged procedure. The control of postoperative bleeding is included in code 52601, so it is not coded separately.

2.208. 53445

Rationale: Index Prosthesis, urethral sphincter, insertion, resulting in code range 53444–53445. Review of the available codes indicates that code 53445 is appropriate for insertion of a complete inflatable system.

2.209. 53621

Rationale: Index Dilation, urethral, stricture, resulting in code 52281 and range 53600–53621. Review of the available codes indicates that code 52281 is not correct because it describes a cystourethroscopic procedure. Review of codes 53600–53621 shows that code 53621 is correct for a subsequent dilation of a male patient.

2.210. 50945

Rationale: Index Laparoscopy, ureterolithotomy, resulting in code 50945. Note that in this case the procedure is performed laparoscopically, that is, by visualization through the abdomen. Ureterolithotomy can also be performed cystoscopically.

2.211. 53855

Rationale: Index Urethral, stent, insertion, resulting in code 52282. Code 52282 is for a permanent urethral stent. The instructional note beneath code 52282 states to assign code 53855 for placement of a temporary prostatic urethral stent.

2.212. 51840

Rationale: Index Vesicourethropexy, resulting in code range 51840–51841. Review of the available codes indicates that code 51840 is appropriate because there is no documentation that this was a complicated or repeat procedure.

2.213. 52204

Rationale: Index Cystourethroscopy, biopsy, resulting in code choice of 52204 or 52354. Review of the available codes indicates that code 52354 is for a biopsy of the ureter and code 52204 is for biopsy of the bladder or urethra. Code 52204 is therefore the correct code.

2.214. 52352

Rationale: Index Endoscopy, ureter, removal, calculus, resulting in code 50961, 50980, or 52352. Review of the available codes indicates that code 50961 reports a ureteral endoscopy via a ureterostomy, which is not documented here. Code 50980 is for an endoscopy via a ureterotomy, an incision into the ureter, which is also not documented here. Code 52352 describes removal of a ureteral stone via a cystourethroscopy with ureteral catheterization and is the correct code.

2.215. 52630

Rationale: Index Excision, prostate regrowth, resulting in code 52630.

2.216. Code(s): 53860

Rationale: Index term Bladder, reconstruction, and urethra, radiofrequency micro-remodeling.

2.217. 50526

Rationale: Index term Fistula, kidney. The range of codes given is 50520–50526. A review of the codes reveals that 50526 would be used to report the thoracic approach.

2.218. Code(s): 50323

Rationale: Index term Preparation, for transplantation, kidney. Reviewing codes 50323–50329 reveals that 50323 is used for preparation of the cadaval kidney.

Male/Female Genital System and Laparoscopy

2.219. 54057

Rationale: Index Condyloma, destruction, resulting in code range 54050–54065. Review of the available codes indicates that code 54057 is the appropriate code to describe treatment with the laser.

2.220. 54401

Rationale: Index Prosthesis, penile, insertion, resulting in code range 54400–54405. Review of the available codes indicates that code 54401 describes insertion of an inflatable prosthesis. All the other codes describe more complex prostheses.

2.221. 54417

Rationale: Index Prosthesis, penile, removal, resulting in code 54406 or code range 54410–54417. Review of the available codes indicates that code 54417, which describes the infected field and need for debridement of infected tissues, is the most appropriate code.

2.222. 54692

Rationale: Index Laparoscopy, orchiopexy, resulting in code 54692.

2.223. 55250

Rationale: Index Vasectomy, resulting in code 55250.

2.224. 55700

Rationale: Index Biopsy, prostate, resulting in code range 55700–55705. Review of the available codes indicates that code 55700 is appropriate for reporting a needle biopsy. This code may also be accessed via the main term Needle biopsy, prostate, which leads directly to code 55700.

2.225. 55840

Rationale: Index Prostatectomy, retropubic, radical, resulting in code range 55840–55845 or code 55866. Review of the available codes indicates that code 55840 is correct because there is no mention of lymph node dissection and the procedure was not done laparoscopically (55866), according to the limited documentation provided here.

2.226. 56420

Rationale: Index Incision and Drainage, abscess, Bartholin's gland, resulting in code 56420.

2.227. 57456

Rationale: Index Colposcopy, cervix, resulting in code 57421 or code range 57452–57461. Review indicates that code 57456 is most appropriate for a colposcopy of the cervix with curettage. Code 57421 describes colposcopy of the vagina/cervix, and the other cervical colposcopy codes describe procedures other than biopsy with endocervical curettage.

2.228. 58152

Rationale: Index Hysterectomy, abdominal, total, with colpourethropexy, resulting in code 58152. This single code describes the entire procedure, and no separate code should be reported for the Marshall-Marchetti-Krantz procedure.

2.229. 58291

Rationale: Index Hysterectomy, vaginal, resulting in code ranges 58260–58270, 58290–58294, 58550, and 58554. Review of the available codes indicates that code 58291 describes the procedure on a uterus of over 250 grams, with the only secondary procedure being the removal of the tubes and ovaries.

2.230. 58900

Rationale: Index Biopsy, ovary, resulting in code 58900.

2.231. 58546

Rationale: Index Myomectomy, uterus, resulting in code range 58140–58146 or 58545–58546. Review of the available codes indicates that codes 58140–58146 describe open myomectomy, and this procedure was performed laparoscopically. Because eight myomas were removed laparoscopically, code 58546 is correct.

2.232. 58600

Rationale: Index Ligation, fallopian tube, oviduct, resulting in code range 58600–58611 or code 58670. Review of the available codes indicates that code 58600 is the appropriate code because there is no documentation that this procedure was performed postpartum, nor was it performed laparoscopically (58670), based upon the available information.

2.233. 58671

Rationale: Index Laparoscopy, oviduct surgery, resulting in code range 58670–58671 or code 58679. Review of the available codes indicates that code 58671 describes occlusion of the fallopian tubes by a device, procedure performed laparoscopically.

2.234. 58943

Rationale: Index Ovary, excision, total, resulting in code range 58940–58943. Review of the available codes indicates that code 58943 describes the salpingo-oophorectomy and the biopsies.

2.235. 58340

Rationale: Index Hysterosalpingography, injection procedure, resulting in code 58340. In order to fully report this procedure, a radiological supervision and interpretation code would also be reported.

2.236. 54160

Rationale: Index Circumcision, surgical excision, newborn, resulting in codes 54150 and 54160. Review of the available codes indicates that 54160 is the correct code when the circumcision is performed via a surgical excision.

2.237. 54600

Rationale: Index Testis, repair, torsion, resulting in code 54600.

2.238. 58662

Rationale: Index Laparoscopy, destruction, lesion, resulting in code 58662.

2.239. a. 58559

Rationale: Index term is Hysteroscopy, lysis, adhesions. Code 58740 is not needed as the lysis is included in 58559.

2.240. Code(s): 57156

Rationale: Index term is Brachytherapy, vagina, insertion of afterloading apparatus.

2.241. Code(s): 54163

Rationale: Index term is Circumcision, repair.

2.242. Code(s): 54324

Rationale: Index term is Hypospadias, repair, urethroplasty, local skin flaps.

2.243. Code(s): 55041

Rationale: Index term is Hydrocele, excision, bilateral, tunica vaginalis.

2.244. Code(s): 56405

Rationale: Index term is Incision and Drainage, abscess, vulva.

2.245. Code(s): 58558

Rationale: Index term Hysteroscopy, surgical with biopsy.

Endocrine System

2.246. 60000

Rationale: Index Incision and Drainage, cyst, thyroid gland, resulting in code 60000.

2.247. 60100

Rationale: Index Needle Biopsy, thyroid gland, resulting in code 60100.

2.248. 60200

Rationale: Index Thyroid Gland, tumor, excision, resulting in code 60200. An adenoma is a benign tumor, so searching on the main term Thyroid gland, excision, will not lead to the appropriate code.

2.249. 60210

Rationale: Index Thyroidectomy, partial, resulting in code range 60210–60225. Review of the available codes indicates that code 60210 is appropriate for this simple procedure.

2.250. 60212

Rationale: Index Thyroidectomy, partial, resulting in code range 60210–60225. Review of the available codes indicates that code 60212 is correct because there is documentation of isthmusectomy and subtotal resection on the opposite (contralateral) side.

2.251. 60220

Rationale: Index Thyroidectomy, partial, resulting in code range 60210–60225. Review of the available codes indicates that code 60220 is correct because it describes a unilateral complete lobectomy.

2.252. 60225

Rationale: Index Thyroidectomy, partial, resulting in code range 60210–60225. Review of the available codes indicates that code 60225 is correct because it describes a unilateral complete lobectomy and isthmusectomy with subtotal resection on the opposite (contralateral) side.

2.253. 60240

Rationale: Index Thyroidectomy, total, resulting in code 60240 or 60271. Review of the available codes indicates that code 60240 is correct, based upon the available information.

2.254. 60252

Rationale: Index Thyroidectomy, total, for malignancy, limited neck dissection, resulting in code 60252.

2.255. 60254

Rationale: Index Thyroidectomy, total, for malignancy, radical neck dissection, resulting in code 60254.

2.256. 60500

Rationale: Index Parathyroidectomy, resulting in code range 60500–60505. Review of the available codes indicates that code 60500 is appropriate, based upon the available documentation. The parathyroids are routinely removed along with the thyroid due to their proximity, and a separate code should not be reported for the parathyroidectomy in that circumstance.

2.257. 60271

Rationale: Index Thyroidectomy, total, cervical approach, resulting in code 60271.

2.258. 60281

Rationale: Index Thyroglossal Duct, cyst, excision, resulting in code range 60280–60281. Review of the available codes indicates that code 60281 is appropriate when the cyst is documented as recurrent.

2.259. 60505

Rationale: Index Parathyroid Gland, exploration, resulting in code range 60500–60505. Review of the available codes indicates that code 60505 is correct when a mediastinal exploration is documented.

2.260. 60521

Rationale: Index Thymus Gland, excision, resulting in code range 60520–60521. This code range can also be accessed via the main term Thymectomy. Review of the available codes indicates that code 60521 is appropriate when the approach is documented as transthoracic and there is no mention of mediastinal lymph node dissection.

2.261. 60540

Rationale: Index Biopsy, adrenal gland, resulting in code range 60540–60545. Review of the available codes indicates that code 60540 is appropriate when there is no documentation of excision of tumor. Note that adrenalectomy is a separate procedure. The adrenals are routinely removed with the kidneys and a separate code should not be reported for this.

2.262. 60650

Rationale: Index Laparoscopy, adrenal gland, excision, resulting in code 60650. Note that indexing Laparoscopy, adrenalectomy, results in code 50545. Review of the descriptor for this code, however, indicates that it describes a considerably more invasive procedure than a simple adrenalectomy. Code 50545 includes a radical nephrectomy (kidney and ureter), excision of fascia, lymph nodes, and adrenal glands. This illustrates how important it is to reference the Tabular List, even when the index directs the coder to one specific code.

2.263. 60605

Rationale: Index Carotid Body, lesion, carotid artery, resulting in code 60605.

2.264. 60522

Rationale: Index Thymectomy, resulting in code range 60520–60521. Review of the available codes indicates the code that actually best describes the procedure is 60522. This code may be accessed via the main term Thymectomy, sternal split/transthoracic approach, resulting in code range 60521–60522.

2.265. 60300

Rationale: Index Aspiration, cyst, thyroid, resulting in code 60300.

2.266. Code(s): 61690

Rationale: Index term Arteriovenous malformation, cranial, repair. A wide range of codes is given—61680–61692, 61705–61708. The most appropriate code is 61690.

2.267. Code(s): 62310

Rationale: Index term is Injection, anesthetic agent. Several codes are given including 0228T, 0229T, 62310, 62318. The same series of codes are given for the steroid injection. In reviewing these codes 62310 is appropriate to use for a single injection.

Nervous System

2.268. 61154

Rationale: Index Drainage, hematoma, brain, resulting in code range 61154–61156. Review of the available codes indicates that code 61154 describes the procedure for drainage of hematoma.

2.269. 61322

Rationale: Index Craniectomy, decompression, resulting in code range 61322–61323, or code range 61340–61343. Review of all the available codes indicates that code 61322 is appropriate when the procedure is performed for intracranial hypertension and there is no documentation of lobectomy. Note the use of the term "for treatment of intracranial hypertension" in the descriptors for 61322 and 61323. This means that these codes can only be used with that diagnosis.

2.270. 61519

Rationale: Index Brain, meningioma, excision, resulting in codes 61512 and 61519. Review of the available codes indicates that code 61519 is the appropriate code to report excision of a posterior fossa meningioma.

2.271. 61624

Rationale: Index Transcatheter, embolization, percutaneous, cranial, resulting in code range 61624–61626. Code 61624 lists the spinal cord among the treatment areas and is the appropriate code.

2.272. 61798

Rationale: Index Brain, stereotactic, radiosurgery, resulting in code range 61796–61800 in the surgery section. Review of the available codes indicates that code 61798 is correct because the note prior to code 61796 states that a pituitary tumor is always considered complex, regardless of the size of the tumor.

2.273. 62223

Rationale: Index Shunt, brain, creation, resulting in code range 62180–62223. Review of the available codes indicates that code 62223 describes creation of a shunt from the ventricle of the brain to the peritoneal cavity.

2.274. 62270

Rationale: Index Puncture, spinal cord, diagnostic, resulting in code 62270.

2.275. 61885

Rationale: Index Implantation, neurostimulator, pulse generator, resulting in code 61885.

2.276. 64776-F8

Rationale: Index Excision, lesion, nerve, resulting in code range 64774–64792. Review of the available codes indicates that code 64776 describes excision of a neuroma of a digital nerve. The modifiers for the fingers begin with FA for the left thumb and progress to F9 for the right little finger. The appropriate modifier for the right fourth (ring) finger is F8.

2.277. 61340

Rationale: Index Decompression, skull, resulting in code range 61322–61323 or 61340–61345. Review of the available codes indicates that codes 61322–61323 can only be used for a diagnosis of intracranial hypertension, which is not documented here. Code 61340 is the appropriate code. Code 61345 includes a laminectomy of the upper cervical vertebra, which is not documented in the available information.

2.278. 61698

Rationale: Index Aneurysm Repair, vertebral artery, resulting in code 61698 or 61702. Review of both codes shows that code 61698 is the more appropriate code. The instructional note following code 61698 indicates that resection of an aneurysm larger than 15 mm constitutes a complex surgery. The aneurysm in this case is documented at 20 mm.

2.279. 61751

Rationale: Index Biopsy, brain, stereotactic, resulting in code range 61750–61751. Review of the available codes indicates that code 61751 is correct because there is documentation of magnetic resonance imaging guidance.

2.280. 62165

Rationale: Index Neuroendoscopy, intracranial, resulting in code range 62160–62165. Review of the available codes indicates that code 62165 is the correct code for excision of a pituitary tumor via intracranial neuroendoscopy.

2.281. 62252

Rationale: Index Reprogramming, shunt, brain, resulting in code 62252.

2.282. 63077

Rationale: Index Diskectomy, resulting in code range 63075–63078. Review of the available codes indicates that code 63077 is the appropriate code for an anterior diskectomy. Note that indexing Diskectomy, thoracic leads to code 22222. Review of this code indicates that it includes an osteotomy, which is not documented in this case.

2.283. 64415

Rationale: Index Injection, nerve, anesthetic, resulting in code range 01991–01992 or 64400–64530. Review of the codes indicates that code 64415 is appropriate for the brachial plexus.

2.284. 64831-F2, 64832-F3

Rationale: Index Suture, nerve, resulting in code range 64831–64876. Review of the available codes indicates that code 64831 is appropriate for reporting the suture of the first digital nerve, and add-on code 64832 is reported once for the second digital nerve repair. The modifiers for the fingers begin with FA for the left thumb and progress to F9 for the right little finger. The appropriate modifier for the left third (long) finger is F2, and for the left fourth (ring) finger, F3.

2.285. 64600

Rationale: Index Destruction, nerve, resulting in code range 64600–64681. Review of the available codes indicates that code 64600 is appropriate to report the destruction of this branch of the trigeminal nerve.

Eye/Ocular Adnexa

2.286. 65222

Rationale: Index Removal, foreign bodies, cornea, with slit lamp, resulting in code 65222.

2.287. 65750

Rationale: Index Keratoplasty, penetrating, in aphakia, resulting in code 65750.

2.288. 65175

Rationale: Index Removal, ocular implant, resulting in code 65175 or 65920. Review of the available codes indicates code 65175 is the correct code.

2.289. 66984

Rationale: Index Cataract, removal/extraction, extracapsular, resulting in code 66982 or 66984. Review of both codes shows that code 66984 is appropriate because there is no documentation of special equipment being used or that this procedure was more complex than usual.

2.290. 67107

Rationale: Index Retina, repair, detachment, by scleral buckling, resulting in code 67112. Review of this code, however, indicates that it is to be used for a repeat procedure, which is not documented to be the case here. Review of the other codes in the Repair of Retinal Detachment section reveals that code 67107 is most appropriate in this case.

2.291. 67228

Rationale: Index Retina, retinopathy, treatment, photocoagulation, resulting in code 67228.

2.292. 67312

Rationale: Index Strabismus, repair, two horizontal muscles, resulting in code 67312. The horizontal muscles of the eyeball are the lateral and medial recti. The vertical muscles are the superior and inferior recti. The superior and inferior oblique muscles are located on the back portion of the eyeball.

2.293. 67318

Rationale: Index Strabismus, repair, superior oblique muscle, resulting in code 67318.

2.294. 67316, 67335

Rationale: Index Strabismus, repair, two vertical muscles, and Strabismus, repair, adjustable sutures, resulting in code 67316 for the primary procedure and add-on code 67335 to report that adjustable sutures were used. This allows for fine-tuning the alignment when the patient has awakened from anesthesia and is moving the eyeball. Because code 67335 is an add-on code, no modifier such as -51 or -59 is needed.

2.295. 67902

Rationale: Index Blepharoptosis, repair, frontalis muscle technique with fascial sling, resulting in code 67902. Although this is the appropriate code to describe this type of procedure to correct blepharoptosis (droopy eyelids), note that Medicare and some insurance companies may not cover it if performed for purely cosmetic purposes. Documentation of loss of visual fields is usually required to obtain insurance coverage. This does not affect the code assignment, however.

2.296. 67922

Rationale: Index Entropion, repair, thermocauterization, resulting in code 67922.

2.297. 68720

Rationale: Index Dacryocystorhinostomy, resulting in code 68720. Note that some physicians use the term "dacryorhinocystostomy," which means the same thing.

2.298. 68815

Rationale: Index Nasolacrimal Duct, insertion, stent, resulting in code 68815.

2.299. 67805

Rationale: Index Chalazion, excision, multiple, different lids, resulting in code 67805.

2.300. 67145

Rationale: Index Retina, repair, prophylaxis, detachment, resulting in code range 67141–67145. Review of the available codes indicates that code 67145 is the appropriate code when the laser is used for the procedure.

2.301. 66170

Rationale: Index Trabeculectomy ab Externo, in absence of previous surgery, resulting in code 66170. If you arrived at code 65850, you have indexed the term "trabeculotomy ab externo," rather than trabeculectomy.

2.302. 65105

Rationale: Index Enucleation, eye, with implant, muscles attached, resulting in code 65105. There are three terms used for removal of the eyeball: evisceration, enucleation, and exenteration. Evisceration is removal of the contents of the eyeball, leaving the sclera and sometimes the cornea. Enucleation is removal of an entire eyeball, without rupture, leaving the muscles intact to attach to an implant. Exenteration is removal of the entire contents of the orbit, usually including the muscles.

2.303. 65260

Rationale: Index Removal, foreign bodies, posterior segment, magnet extraction, resulting in code 65260.

2.304. 65426

Rationale: Index Pterygium, excision, with graft, resulting in code 65426. The graft is typically obtained from the conjunctiva, and no additional code is assigned for its harvesting.

2.305. 67040

Rationale: Index Vitrectomy, subtotal, with endolaser panretinal photocoagulation, resulting in code 67040.

2.306. Code(s): 65779

Rationale: Index term is Amniotic membrane. The coder is directed to main term Amnion, membrane placement, for wound healing.

2.307. Code(s): 68115

Rationale: Index term is Excision, lesion, conjunctiva, over 1 cm.

2.308. Code(s): 66762

Rationale: Index term is Photocoagulation, iridoplasty. This code is used only once even though there were 3 sessions.

Auditory System

2.309. 69140

Rationale: Index Exostosis, excision, resulting in code 69140. Although exostosis can occur in any part of the body, this code is, in fact, correct for the external auditory canal.

2.310. 69421

Rationale: Index Myringotomy, resulting in code range 69420–69421. Review of the available codes indicates that code 69421 is appropriate when general anesthesia is used. Note that some physicians use the term "tympanotomy," which is synonymous with myringotomy. ("Myrinx" is the Greek root for eardrum; "tympanum" is the Latin root for eardrum.)

2.311. 69433

Rationale: Index Tympanic Membrane, create stoma, resulting in code range 69433–69436. Review of the available codes indicates that code 69433 is appropriate because the use of general anesthesia is not documented.

2.312. 69642

Rationale: Index Tympanoplasty, with mastoidectomy, with ossicular chain reconstruction, resulting in code 69642.

2.313. 69960

Rationale: Index Decompression, auditory canal, internal, resulting in code 69960.

2.314. 69020

Rationale: Index Auditory Canal, external, abscess, incision and drainage, resulting in code 69020.

2.315. 69200

Rationale: Index Removal, foreign bodies, auditory canal, external, resulting in code 69200, which is appropriate because there is no documentation of use of general anesthesia (code 69205).

2.316. 69100

Rationale: Index Biopsy, ear, external, resulting in code 69100.

2.317. 69210

Rationale: Index Cerumen, removal, resulting in code 69210. Review of the descriptor for this code shows that it is bilateral or unilateral in nature, and no modifier is added if the procedure is done bilaterally.

2.318. 69633

Rationale: The abbreviation PORP stands for partial ossicular replacement prosthesis. PORPs are ossicular chain replacements that do not include the stapes. If the prosthesis includes a stapes reconstruction, it is referred to as a total ossicular replacement prosthesis, or TORP. Index Tympanoplasty, without mastoidectomy, with synthetic prosthesis, resulting in code 69633.

2.319. 69436

Rationale: Index Tympanostomy, resulting in code range 69433–69436. Note that the terms "tympanostomy" and "myringotomy" are synonymous. Review of the available codes indicates that code 69436 is appropriate when general anesthesia is used.

2.320. 69552

Rationale: Index Excision, tumor, ear, middle, transmastoid, resulting in code 69552.

2.321. 69610

Rationale: Index Tympanic Membrane, repair, resulting in code 69450 or 69610. Review of both codes reveals that 69450 actually refers to a tympanolysis (freeing of the membrane), and code 69610 is the correct code.

2.322. 69661

Rationale: Index Stapedotomy, with footplate drillout, resulting in code 69661. This procedure is frequently performed with the use of the operating microscope, which may be coded in addition if it is used.

2.323. 69930

Rationale: Index Cochlear Device, insertion, resulting in code 69930.

2.324. 69666

Rationale: Index Oval window, repair fistula, resulting in code 69666.

2.325. 69910

Rationale: Index Labyrinthectomy, with mastoidectomy, resulting in code 69910.

2.326. 69710

Rationale: Index Temporal Bone, electromagnetic bone conducting hearing device, implantation/replacement, resulting in code 69710.

2.327. 69222

Rationale: Index Debridement, mastoid cavity, complex, resulting in code 69222. Review of the descriptor for the code verifies that the need for general anesthesia constitutes a "complex" debridement.

2.328. 69424

Rationale: Index Removal, ventilating tube, ear, middle, resulting in code 69424.

Radiology Services

2.329. a. True

Correct answer.

b. False

Incorrect answer. When applied to the male pelvis, this examination includes the urinary bladder, prostate, seminal vesicles, and any identified pelvic pathology.

2.330. 70100

Rationale: Index Mandible, x-ray, resulting in code range 70100–70110. Review of the available codes indicates that code 70100 is the appropriate code when fewer than four views are obtained.

2.331. 70370

Rationale: Index Pharynx, x-ray, resulting in codes 70370 and 74210. Review of the available codes indicates that code 70370 is the appropriate code since fluoroscopy was utilized.

2.332. 70470

Rationale: Index CT Scan, without and with contrast, brain, resulting in code 70470 or 70496. Review of both codes shows that code 70496 is actually the code for CT angiography. Code 70470 is the correct code.

2.333. 71020

Rationale: Index Chest, x-ray, resulting in code range 71010–71035. Review of the available codes indicates that code 71020 is appropriate for reporting a front-to-back (AP, anteroposterior) and side-to-side (lateral) two-view x-ray.

2.334. 78813

Rationale: Index Nuclear Medicine, tumor imaging, positron emission tomography, resulting in code range 78811–78816. Review of the available codes indicates that 78813 is the correct code.

2.335. 72052

Rationale: Index Spine, x-ray, cervical, resulting in code range 72040–72052. Review of the available codes indicates that code 72052 is appropriate when a complete study, including oblique and flexion views, is done.

2.336. 72240

Rationale: Index Myelography, spine, cervical, resulting in code 72240. Note that to fully report the procedure, a code for the injection of the contrast material must also be reported per the instructional note following code 72240.

2.337. 73040

Rationale: Index Arthrography, shoulder, resulting in code 73040.

2.338. 73530

Rationale: Index Hip, x-ray, intraoperative, resulting in code 73530.

2.339. 74270

Rationale: Index Barium Enema, resulting in code range 74270–74280. Review of the available codes indicates that code 74270 is appropriate. Note that abbreviation KUB stands for kidneys, ureters, and bladder, which may or may not be visualized as part of a barium enema.

2.340. 74320

Rationale: Index Cholangiography, percutaneous, resulting in code 74320. Note that to fully describe the procedure, an injection code must be reported as well.

2.341. 74400

Rationale: Index Urography, intravenous, resulting in code range 74400–74415. Review of the available codes indicates that code 74400 is appropriate for an IVP (intravenous pyelogram) whether or not tomograms are performed.

2.342. 75660

Rationale: Index Angiography, carotid artery, resulting in code range 75660–75671. Review of the available codes indicates that code 75660 is the most appropriate code to describe this procedure.

2.343. 76805

Rationale: Index Ultrasound, pregnant uterus, resulting in code range 76801–76817. Review of the available codes indicates that code 76805 is the appropriate code.

2.344. 75746

Rationale: Index Angiography, pulmonary, resulting in code range 75741–75746. Review of the available codes indicates that code 75746 is the appropriate code when the catheterization is documented to be nonselective. Per the instructional note following code 75746, an injection code is needed to completely report the procedure.

2.345. 78320

Rationale: Index Bone, nuclear medicine, SPECT, resulting in code 78320. The acronym SPECT stands for single photon emission computed tomography, which is a more sophisticated form of CT scanning. Unlike basic x-ray CT scanning, SPECT involves injected radionuclides and is considered a form of nuclear medicine. It is being supplanted to some extent now by PET (positron emission tomography) scanning, which is capable of better resolution and sensitivity.

2.346. 77032

Rationale: Index Mammogram, breast, localization nodule, resulting in code 77032.

2.347. 76770

Rationale: Index Ultrasound, retroperitoneal, resulting in code range 76770–76775. Review of the available codes indicates that code 76770 is correct. Code 76775 reports a limited retroperitoneal ultrasound, such as of one organ, but that is not documented here.

2.348. 78278

Rationale: Index Nuclear Medicine, gastrointestinal, blood loss study, resulting in code 78278.

2.349. c. 74176

Rationale: CPT codes are available for combination abdomen and pelvis codes—the combination code must be used in place of two separate codes. Index term is CT scan, without contrast, abdomen (74150, 74176, 74178) or without contrast, pelvis (72192, 74176, 74178). Code 74176 is assigned to specify CT scan of abdomen and pelvis without contrast material.

2.350. Code(s): 51610, 74450

Rationale: Index term is Urethrocystography, for both the injection code and the supervision and interpretation.

2.351. Code(s): 76946

Rationale: Index term Ultrasound, guidance, amniocentesis.

Pathology/Laboratory Services

2.352. a. This is an add-on laboratory code.

Incorrect answer. The symbol ⊮ designates a laboratory test that has been assigned a Category I code in anticipation of receipt of FDA approval. Ordinarily, AMA does not assign Category I codes to procedures that have not actually received FDA approval.

b. The code is sex specific.

Incorrect answer. The symbol ⊮ designates a laboratory test that has been assigned a Category I code in anticipation of receipt of FDA approval. Ordinarily, AMA does not assign Category I codes to procedures that have not actually received FDA approval.

c. This code should only be reported for Medicare patients.

Incorrect answer. The symbol ⊮ designates a laboratory test that has been assigned a Category I code in anticipation of receipt of FDA approval. Ordinarily, AMA does not assign Category I codes to procedures that have not actually received FDA approval.

d. FDA approval of the vaccine is pending.

Correct answer.

2.353. a. 82270

Correct answer.

b. 82271

Incorrect answer. Code 82271 is occult blood sampling from a site other than fecal. Occult blood assay using multiple samples to screen for colorectal cancer is reported with code 82270.

c. 82272

Incorrect answer. Code 82272 reports fecal occult blood sampling by one to three simultaneous determinations for screening of a condition other than colorectal cancer. Occult blood assay using multiple samples to screen for colorectal cancer is reported with code 82270.

d. 82274

Incorrect answer. Code 82274 is for one to three simultaneous determinations by immunoassay, not three consecutive collected specimens. Occult blood assay using multiple samples to screen for colorectal cancer is reported with code 82270.

2.354. a. True

Incorrect answer. Organ and disease-oriented panel codes, 80047–80076, can only be assigned if all of the tests included in the panel are performed. If one or more of the tests were not performed, each individual test must be coded separately.

b. False

Correct answer.

2.355. a. Cancer patients on toxic chemotherapy agents

Incorrect answer. 87900, Infectious agent drug susceptibility phenotype prediction using regularly updated genotypic bioinformatics, is used in the management of HIV patients on antiretroviral therapy.

b. HIV patients on antiretroviral therapy

Correct answer.

c. Tuberculosis patients on rifampin therapy

Incorrect answer. 87900, Infectious agent drug susceptibility phenotype prediction using regularly updated genotypic bioinformatics, is used in the management of HIV patients on antiretroviral therapy.

d. Organ transplant patients on immunosuppressive therapy

Incorrect answer. 87900, Infectious agent drug susceptibility phenotype prediction using regularly updated genotypic bioinformatics, is used in the management of HIV patients on antiretroviral therapy.

2.356. 82552

Rationale: Index CPK, blood, resulting in code range 82550–82552. Review of the available codes indicates that code 82552 is the appropriate code for reporting complete fractionation into isoenzymes.

2.357. 83090

Rationale: Index Homocysteine, resulting in code 83090.

2.358. 84154

Rationale: Index Prostate specific antigen, resulting in code range 84152–84154. Review of the available codes indicates that code 84154 is the correct code for a free PSA test.

2.359. 83986

Rationale: Index pH, other fluid, resulting in code 83986.

2.360. 80076

Rationale: Index Blood Tests, panels, hepatic function, resulting in code 80076.

2.361. 84300

Rationale: Index Sodium, urine, resulting in code 84300.

2.362. 85025

Rationale: Index Blood Cell Count, hemogram, added indices, resulting in code range 85025–85027. The codes for reporting CBCs (complete blood counts) are very specific and should be carefully reviewed. The appropriate code for a CBC with automated white blood cell differential is 85025.

2.363. 81025

Rationale: Index Urine, pregnancy test, resulting in code 81025.

2.364. 85610

Rationale: Index Prothrombin Time, resulting in code range 85610–85611. Review of the available codes indicates that code 85610 is the appropriate code. There is no documentation of plasma fractionation here.

2.365. 86039

Rationale: Index Antinuclear Antibodies, resulting in code range 86038–86039. Review of the available codes indicates that code 86039 is specified as the titer.

2.366. 86592

Rationale: Index VDRL, resulting in code range 86592–86593. The abbreviation VDRL stands for Venereal Disease Research Laboratory slide test, which is specified as one of the qualitative syphilis tests. Thus, code 86592 is correct.

2.367. 86706

Rationale: In this abbreviation, H stands for hepatitis, b for type B, s for surface, and Ab for antibody. Index Hepatitis Antibody, B surface, resulting in code 86706.

2.368. 86632

Rationale: Index Chlamydia, antibody, resulting in code range 86631–86632. Review of the available codes indicates that code 86632 is appropriate when the IgM antibody is studied. The abbreviation IgM means the "M" immunoglobulin (Ig). Immunoglobulins are protein groups that react in different ways with infectious agents.

2.369. 85652

Rationale: Index Sedimentation Rate, automated, resulting in code 85652.

2.370. 88305

Rationale: Index Pathology, surgical, gross and micro exam, level IV, resulting in code 88305. In practice, each entry in the Surgical Pathology section should be reviewed to determine the appropriate level. An arterial biopsy is categorized to a level IV. Review the instructional note preceding code 88300. Note that the unit of service is the specimen, not the number of slides or cell blocks.

2.371. 88309

Rationale: Index Pathology, surgical, gross and micro exam, level VI, resulting in code 88309. In practice, each entry in the Surgical Pathology section should be reviewed to determine the appropriate level. A specimen consisting of breast and regional lymph nodes is categorized to a level VI. Review the instructional note preceding code 88300. Note that the unit of service is the specimen, not the number of slides or cell blocks.

2.372. 86618

Rationale: Index Antibody, Lyme disease, resulting in code 86617. Review of this code, however, shows that this is a confirmatory test, which is not specified here. The next listed code, 86618, is, in fact, the appropriate code.

2.373. 81001

Rationale: Index Urinalysis, automated, resulting in codes 81001 and 81003. Review of the available codes indicates that 81001 is the appropriate code.

2.374. 88164

Rationale: Index Pap smears, resulting in code ranges 88141–88155, 88164–88167, and 88174–88175. Review of the available codes indicates that code 88164 is for manual screening under physician supervision utilizing the Bethesda System and is therefore the correct code.

2.375. 87040

Rationale: Index Culture, bacteria blood, resulting in code 87040.

2.376. Code(s): 86902

Rationale: Index term is Blood Typing, antigen testing, donor blood.

2.377. Code(s): 87906

Rationale: Index term Genotype Analysis, by nucleic acid, HIV-1.

Medicine

2.378. a. Intravenous infusion

Incorrect answer. An infusion that lasts for less than 15 minutes should be reported with an IV push code per CPT coding guidelines.

b. Intravenous piggyback

Incorrect answer. An infusion that lasts for less than 15 minutes should be reported with an IV push code per CPT coding guidelines.

c. Intravenous or intra-arterial push

Correct answer.

d. Intravenous hydration

Incorrect answer. An infusion that lasts for less than 15 minutes should be reported with an IV push code per CPT coding guidelines.

2.379. a. Chemotherapeutic agents

Incorrect answer. Codes 96360 and 96361 are used to report intravenous infusions for hydration, consisting of prepackaged fluids and/or electrolytes. These codes are not used for infusion of any other types of medications.

b. Sequential drugs of the same drug family

Incorrect answer. Codes 96360 and 96361 are used to report intravenous infusions for hydration, consisting of prepackaged fluids and/or electrolytes. These codes are not used for infusion of any other types of medications.

c. Hormonal antineoplastics

Incorrect answer. Codes 96360 and 96361 are used to report intravenous infusions for hydration, consisting of prepackaged fluids and/or electrolytes. These codes are not used for infusion of any other types of medications.

d. Prepackaged fluids and/or electrolytes

Correct answer.

2.380. a. 99143

Incorrect answer. Code 99149 is assigned for patients five years or older, first 30 minutes, performed by a physician other than the physician providing the service. This code is assigned for patients younger than five years of age and the sedation is performed by the same physician providing the service.

b. 99144

Incorrect answer. Code 99149 is assigned for patients five years or older, first 30 minutes, performed by a physician other than the physician providing the service. This code is assigned for patients five years or older and the sedation is performed by the same physician providing the service.

c. 99149

Correct answer.

d. 99149, 99150

Incorrect answer. Code 99149 is assigned for patients five years or older, first 30 minutes, performed by a physician other than the physician providing the service. Code 99150 is for each additional 15 minutes of intra-service time. Since there were only 10 additional minutes, it would not be appropriate to also assign this code.

2.381. a. 96401

Incorrect answer. 96401 reports nonhormonal antineoplastic. This is a hormonal antineoplastic, as its name suggests, so code 96402 is appropriate.

b. 96402

Correct answer.

c. 96413

Incorrect answer. Code 96402 is specific for hormonal antineoplastic, given subcutaneous tissue. This code reports an intravenous infusion.

d. 96405

Incorrect answer. This code reports intralesional injections of antineoplastics. Code 96402 is specific for hormonal antineoplastic, given subcutaneous tissue.

2.382. a. True

Incorrect answer. It is based upon the primary reason for the encounter.

b. False

Correct answer.

2.383. c. 90375, 96372

Rationale: In order to appropriately report administration of vaccines, both the product administered and the method of administration must be reported. See the instructional note preceding code 90281.

2.384. Interactive

Rationale: See instructions, Psychiatric Diagnostic or Evaluative Interview Procedures, in CPT.

2.385. 90818

Rationale: Index Psychiatric Treatment, individual, insight-oriented, hospital or residential care, resulting in code range 90816–90822. Review of the available codes indicates that code 90818 is appropriate for a 45- to 50-minute session.

2.386. 91020

Rationale: Index Gastric Tests, manometry, resulting in code 91020.

2.387. 92235

Rationale: Index Angiography, Fluorescein, resulting in code 92235.

2.388. 92604

Rationale: Index Cochlear Device, programming, resulting in code range 92601–92604. Review of the available codes indicates that code 92604 is reported for a subsequent reprogramming of such a device in a child older than seven years of age.

2.389. 92980

Rationale: Index Coronary Artery, insertion, stent, resulting in code range 92980–92981. Review of the available codes indicates that code 92980 is appropriate for the first artery treated. It would be appropriate to add modifier -RC to this code to show that the right coronary artery was the one treated in this manner. In addition, radiological supervision and interpretation codes would be reported, as well as catheter placement codes from the cardiovascular chapter.

2.390. 93010

Rationale: Index Electrocardiography, evaluation, resulting in code 93000, 93010, or 93014. Review of the available codes indicates that code 93010 is appropriate. Note that EKG has separate codes for reporting by the physician and the hospital, when a physician reads EKGs performed on hospital equipment.

2.391. 93453

Rationale: Index Cardiac, combined left and right heart, with left ventriculography results in codes 93453, 93460–93461. Review of the available codes indicates that code 93453 is appropriate for the performed procedure.

2.392. 93283

Rationale: Index Analysis, electronic, pacing cardioverter-defibrillator, evaluation of programming, resulting in codes 93282–93284, 93287, 93641–93642. Review of the available codes indicates that based upon the fact that this is a dual-chamber device and reprogramming was required, code 93283 is correct.

2.393. 93926

Rationale: Index Duplex Scan, arterial studies, lower extremity, resulting in code range 93925–93926. Review of the available codes indicates that code 93926 is correct for reporting a unilateral study.

2.394. 94621

Rationale: Index Pulmonology, diagnostic, stress test, resulting in code 94621. Review of this code and surrounding codes shows another code, 94620, for reporting simple pulmonary stress testing, but this is considered a complex test due to the measurements of CO_2 production, O_2 uptake, and electrocardiographic recordings.

2.395. 95819

Rationale: Index Electroencephalography, standard, resulting in code 95819. Review of this code descriptor confirms that standard EEG is awake and asleep.

2.396. 97110 $\times$ 2 or 97110 + 97110

Rationale: Index Physical Medicine/Therapy/Occupational Therapy, procedures, therapeutic exercises, resulting in code 97110. Review of the code indicates that it is reported in 15-minute increments. Thus, a 35-minute session would be reported with code 97110 twice.

2.397. 98941

Rationale: Index Manipulation, chiropractic, resulting in code range 98940–98943. Review of the available codes indicates that code 98941 is appropriate in this case, where four areas of the spine were manipulated.

2.398. 95861

Rationale: Index Electromyography, needle, extremities, resulting in code range 95861–95864. Review of the available codes indicates that code 95861 is appropriate to report an EMG of two extremities with the related paraspinous muscles.

2.399. 94070

Rationale: Index Pulmonology, diagnostic, spirometry, resulting in code range 94010–94070. Review of the available codes indicates that code 94070 is the appropriate code for a bronchospasm provocation evaluation. There is a note to report the bronchodilator antigen administration separately with 99070 or appropriate supply code.

2.400. 97140

Rationale: Index Physical Medicine/Therapy/Occupational Therapy, procedures, traction therapy, resulting in code 97140.

2.401. 96409

Rationale: Index Chemotherapy, intravenous, resulting in code range 96409–96417. Review of the available codes indicates that code 96409 is appropriate when intravenous push technique is used.

2.402. 93620

Rationale: Index Electrophysiology Procedure, resulting in code range 93600–93660. The electrophysiology (EP) studies are complex. The induction of arrhythmia determines the code in this case, which is 93620.

2.403. Code(s): 90668, 90471

Rationale: Index term Vaccines, influenza, pandemic. There are several codes suggested, including 90663, 90664, 90666–90668. A review of these codes indicates that 90668 is the correct code for the product itself. The administration of the vaccine is reported with code 90471 (because of the patient's age).

2.404. Code(s): 92134

Rationale: Index term Ophthalmology, Diagnostic, computerized scanning, posterior. Codes 92133 and 92134 are presented. The correct code for the retina is 92134.

2.405. d. 93451

Rationale: The correct code for this scenario is 93451 which is for a right heart catheterization which also includes oxygen saturation and cardiac output measures. Index term is Cardiac Catheterization, for measurement of O_2, cardiac output.

2.406. Code(s): 93458

Rationale: Index term Angiography, coronary artery with the range of codes 93454–93461, 93563. The coder shall also review main term Catheterization, left heart, with ventriculography. A similar range of codes is presented. After review of all codes, code 93458 is found to include all aspects of the procedure. CPT provides two code families for cardiac catheterization: one for congenital heart disease and one for all other conditions.

2.407. Code(s): 96446

Rationale: Index term is Chemotherapy, peritoneal cavity.

Modifiers

2.408. 51 or -51

2.409. RC or -RC

2.410. d. All of the above.

Rationale: All of the answers reflect circumstances that can be described with the use of a modifier.

2.411. 26 or -26

2.412. 67916E1 or 67916-E1

Rationale: Index Ectropion, repair.

2.413. 54 or -54

2.414. 26045RT or 26045-RT

Rationale: Index Fasciotomy, palm.

2.415. a. Assign the code for a colonoscopy with modifier -74.

Rationale: Per CPT coding guidelines, when a planned procedure is terminated prior to completion for cause, the intended procedure is coded with a modifier. Because general anesthesia was used, modifier -74 is appropriate in this case. See Medicare billing guidelines, which have specific requirements for canceled endoscopic procedures.

2.416. 91 or -91

2.417. c. Assign a code for the procedure and one for the E/M service, with modifier -25 appended to the E/M code.

Rationale: Per coding guidelines, both the procedure and the E/M service should be coded, with modifier -25 appended to the E/M code.

2.418. 50 or -50

2.419. 45307-53

Rationale: Index Proctosigmoidoscopy, removal, foreign body.

2.420. 25 or -25

2.421. 32 or -32

2.422. 27 or -27

2.423. QM or -QM

2.424. 59 or -59

2.425. 80 or -80

2.426. 62 or -62

2.427. 58 or -58

Category III Codes

2.428. d. All of the above

Rationale: All the statements are true. See Introduction to Category III codes.

2.429. b. Report the Category III code.

Rationale: See Introduction to Category III codes. The Category III code should be assigned without a modifier.

2.430. a. Will be archived unless there is evidence that a temporary code is still needed

Rationale: They will be archived unless there is evidence that a temporary code is still needed. See Introduction to Category III codes.

2.431. 0123T

Rationale: Index Fistulization, sclera, for glaucoma.

2.432. 0103T

Rationale: Index Holotranscobalamin, resulting in code 0103T.

2.433. 0184T

Rationale: Index Rectum, tumor, excision, transanal endoscopic, resulting in code 0184T. TEMS stands for transanal endoscopic microsurgical approach.

2.434. 0195T

Rationale: Index Arthrodesis, vertebra, lumbar, pre-sacral interbody, resulting in codes 0195T, 0196T. Review of the codes indicates that code 0195T is correct for one arthrodesis of a single interspace.

2.435. b. Semiannually

Rationale: See Introduction to Category III codes. They are updated more frequently than the main body of CPT in order to better reflect advances in technology.

2.436. 0030T

Rationale: Index Antiprothrombin Antibody, resulting in code 0030T.

2.437. 0188T

Rationale: Index Critical Care Services, remote, video-conferenced evaluation and management, resulting in codes 0188T, 0189T. Review of the codes indicates that code 0188T is the correct code for 60 minutes.

2.438. 0186T

Rationale: Index Eye, injection, medication, suprachoroidal delivery, resulting in code 0186T.

2.439. 22856, 0092T

Rationale: Index Arthroplasty, intervertebral disk, total replacement, resulting in codes 0163T, 22856–22857. Review of these codes reveals that the correct codes are 22856, 0092T.

2.440. c. Hospitals, physicians, insurers, health services researchers

Rationale: Hospitals, physicians, insurers, and health services researchers may use the codes. See Introduction to Category III Codes.

2.441. 0179T

Rationale: Index Cardiology, electrocardiogram, evaluation, resulting in codes 93000, 93010, 93014, 93660, 0178T–0180T. Review of the codes indicates that code 0179T is the most appropriate code for this scenario.

2.442. 0030T

Rationale: Index Antiprothrombin antibody.

2.443. 0156T

Rationale: Index Laparoscopy, electrode removal gastric, resulting in codes 43648, 0156T. Review of the codes indicates that code 0156T is the correct code for removal of electrodes from the lesser curvature of the stomach for laparoscopic approach.

2.444. 0210T

Rationale: Index Audiometry speech gives range 0210T–0211T. The correct code is 0210T.

2.445. 0042T

Rationale: Index Cerebral Perfusion Analysis, resulting in code 0042T.

2.446. 0246T

Rationale: Index term Fracture, rib, internal fixation leads coder to 0245T–0248T. To report 3 ribs the correct code is 0246T.

2.447. 0212T

Rationale: Index term Audiometry, comprehensive offers two choices; code 0212T is for the automated evaluation.

Chapter 3. HCPCS Level II Coding

Drugs

3.1.   d. All of the above

Rationale: HCPCS contains codes for drugs that can be administered by all of these routes. See introduction to J codes.

3.2.   J0295

Rationale: Index Unasyn.

3.3.   J0476

Rationale: Index Balcofen for intrathecal trial.

3.4.   J0585, J0585, J0585, or J0585 × 3

Rationale: Index Botulinum Toxin. Code J0585 reports Botox per unit. To report three units, the code should be reported three times, or once with a unit of "3" in FL 46 (Serv Units) of the UB-04 claim form.

3.5.   J1170

Rationale: Index Dilaudid.

3.6.   J2790

Rationale: Index RhoGAM.

3.7.   J9100

Rationale: Index Cytosar-U.

3.8.   J9280

Rationale: Index Mitomycin, resulting in code J9280.

3.9.   J1160

Rationale: Index digoxin, dosage up to 0.5 mg.

3.10.   J7325

Rationale: Index Synvisc. Code J7325 reports Synvisc per 1 mg. To report 16 mg, the code should be reported once with a quantity of "16" in the FL 46 (Serv Units) of the UB-04 claim form.

3.11.   J0171

Rationale: Using Table of Drugs, Adrenalin, 0.1 mg.

3.12.   J0558

Rationale: Using Table of Drugs, Bicillin CR per 100,000 units. The code should be reported as 2 units.

3.13. J9302

Rationale: Using Table of Drugs, ARZERRA, 10 mg.

Supplies

3.14. E0601

Rationale: Index Continuous positive airway pressure (CPAP) device, resulting in code E0601.

3.15. A4750

Rationale: Index Blood, tubing, resulting in code A4750 or A4755. Review of the available codes indicates that code A4755 is used to report blood tubing for both the arterial and venous limbs of a hemodialysis access. The order specifies venous tubing only, so code A4750, Blood tubing, arterial or venous, is appropriate.

3.16. A5071

Rationale: Index Pouch, urinary, resulting in code range A4379–A4383, A5071–A5073. Review of the available codes indicates that codes A4379–A4383 refer to ostomy pouches with face plates attached, and A4391 is for a pouch with extended-wear barrier, which is not specified here. Code A5071 is appropriate for a urinary ostomy pouch with unspecified barrier attached.

3.17. A6197

Rationale: Index Alginate dressing, resulting in code range A6196–A6199. Review of the available codes indicates that code A6197 is the appropriate code for a dressing of 16–48 sq in. Examples of alginate dressings include AlgiSite, Kalginate, and Tegagen. Alginate dressings are more absorbent than standard dressings and are used for wounds with heavy exudates to decrease the need for frequent dressing changes and to speed healing.

3.18. A9503

Rationale: Index Technetium-99 medronate (Tc-99m). There are multiple analogs of technetium-99m, many of which have their own codes. Care must be taken in assigning these codes. More information may be needed to assign the appropriate code, and input of the nuclear medicine technician and/or the manufacturer may be needed.

3.19. A4346

Rationale: Index Catheter, indwelling, resulting in code range A4338–A4346. Review of the available codes indicates that code A4346 is the appropriate code for a three-way Foley catheter.

3.20. A4605

Rationale: Index Tracheal suction catheter, resulting in code A4624. Code A4624 refers to a tracheal suction catheter, any type other than closed system; therefore, another code (A4605) was referenced for the closed system.

3.21. A4253

Rationale: Index Blood, glucose test strips.

3.22. A7018

Rationale: Index Nebulizer, water.

3.23. A4550

Rationale: Index Surgical, tray.

Ambulance

3.24. A0394

Rationale: Index Ambulance, resulting in code range A0021–A0999. Review of the descriptions of the available codes indicates that code A0394 is the appropriate code for ALS disposable supplies for IV drug therapy.

3.25. -HN

Rationale: See instructional notes regarding ambulance coding preceding code A0021.

3.26. A0380

Rationale: Index Ambulance, resulting in code range A0021–A0999. Review of the descriptions of the available codes indicates that code A0380 is the appropriate code for BLS (basic life support) transport.

3.27. b. Per mile

Rationale: Ambulance services are reported per mile.

3.28. A0436

Rationale: Index Ambulance, air.

3.29. A0424

Rationale: Index Ambulance, resulting in code range A0021–A0999. Review of the descriptions of the available codes indicates that code A0424 is the appropriate code for reporting the circumstance where an extra attendant is required based upon the patient's medical condition.

3.30. c. Half hours

Rationale: Waiting time is measured in half-hour increments. See instructional note preceding code A0420.

3.31. A0382

Rationale: Index Ambulance, disposable supplies, resulting in code range A0382–A0398. Review of the available codes indicates that code A0382 is the appropriate code to report routine disposable supplies, lacking further information.

3.32. A0225

Rationale: Index Ambulance, resulting in code range A0021–A0999. Review of the descriptions of the available codes indicates that code A0225 is the appropriate code for reporting neonatal transport.

3.33. A0422

Rationale: Index Ambulance, oxygen.

3.34. A0392

Rationale: Main Index term Ambulance, disposable supplies, A0382–A0398. A review of these codes finds that A0392 is the correct code.

Durable Medical Equipment

3.35. E0434

Rationale: Index Oxygen, supplies and equipment, resulting in a number of code ranges. Review of the available codes indicates that code E0434 describes rental of a complete liquid oxygen system.

3.36. E0297, E0277

Rationale: Index Bed, hospital, full electric, home care, without mattress, and Mattress, alternating pressure.

3.37. E1594

Rationale: Index Dialysis, peritoneal, resulting in several individual codes and code ranges. Review of all the available codes indicates that code E1594 is the only code that correctly describes the equipment specified here.

3.38. E1300

Rationale: Index Whirlpool equipment, resulting in code range E1300–E1310. Review of the available codes indicates that code E1300 is appropriate to describe a portable unit.

3.39. E1180

Rationale: Index Wheelchair, amputee, resulting in code range E1170–E1200. Review of the available codes indicates that code E1180 describes a chair with the particular combination of accessories detailed.

3.40. E1038

Rationale: Index Transport chair, resulting in code E1037 or E1038. Review of both the available codes indicates that code E1037 reports a pediatric chair, and code E1038 is appropriate for an adult chair.

3.41. E0445

Rationale: Respiratory, equipment, resulting in code range E0424–E0601. Review of the available codes indicates that code E0445 is the appropriate code for an oximeter device.

3.42. E0199

Rationale: Index Eggcrate dry pressure pad/mattress, resulting in code E0184 or E0199. Review of both the available codes indicates that the appropriate code is E0199.

3.43. E0730

Rationale: Index TENS, resulting in code A4595 or code range E0720–E0749. Review of the available codes indicates that code A4595 is used to report the leads, not the unit. Review of the E codes indicates that code E0730 is appropriate to report a four-lead TENS unit.

3.44. E0619

Rationale: Index Monitor, apnea, resulting in code E0618. Review of the description of this code, however, shows that E0618 reports a nonrecording apnea monitor. Review of other codes in this section leads to code E0619 for a recording apnea monitor, which is the correct code. This code may also be accessed by indexing Apnea monitor, which results in code E0618 or E0619.

3.45. E2623

Rationale: Index term Wheelchair, cushion, seat, skin protection. Range of codes given is E2603, E2604, E2607, E2622–E2625.

3.46. E0603

Rationale: Index term Breast, pump, E0602–E0604. Code E0603 is used for an electric breast pump.

Procedures/Services

3.47. a. True

Correct Answer.

b. False

Incorrect answer. Code G0117 should be assigned for glaucoma screenings for high-risk patients furnished by an optometrist or ophthalmologist.

3.48. G0122

Rationale: Index Screening Examination, colorectal cancer, resulting in a series of code listings. Review of the available codes indicates that code G0122 is the appropriate code for reporting barium enema as a means of screening for colorectal cancer.

3.49. G0206

Rationale: Index Mammography, resulting in code range G0202–G0206. Review of the available codes indicates that code G0206 is appropriate to describe a unilateral diagnostic mammography.

3.50. G0219

Rationale: Index PET imaging, whole body, resulting in code G0219.

3.51. G0379

Rationale: Index Hospital, observation, direct referral. G0379 should be reported when observation services are the result of a direct referral for observation care without an associated emergency room visit, hospital outpatient clinic visit, or critical care service on the day of initiation of observation services.

3.52. G0290

Rationale: Index Stent placement, transcatheter, intracoronary, resulting in code G0290 or G0291. Review of the available codes indicates that code G0290 is the appropriate code for the first stent placement, and G0291 for each additional stent.

3.53. G0259

Rationale: Index Injection, arthrography, sacroiliac, joint, resulting in code G0259 or G0260. Review of the available codes indicates that code G0259 is appropriate to describe the injection procedure for the sacroliliac joint for arthrography.

3.54. G0109

Rationale: Index Training, diabetes, resulting in code G0108 or G0109. Review of the available codes indicates that the code for group training is G0109.

3.55. G0127

Rationale: Index Trim nails.

3.56. G0008

Rationale: Index Vaccination, administration, influenza virus, resulting in code G0008.

3.57. L8600

Rationale: Index term Prosthesis, breast. Codes given are reviewed and L8600 is the appropriate selection.

3.58. L8693

Rationale: Index term Auditory osseointegrated device, L8690, L8691, L8692, L8693. A review of codes reveals that L8693 is the correct code.

3.59. G0102

Rationale: Index term Screening, prostate, digital, rectal.

Part II

Intermediate Coding Exercises

Chapter 4. Case Studies from Inpatient Health Records

Unless otherwise stated, code set answers given in Chapter 4 are ICD-9-CM.

Disorders of the Blood and Blood-Forming Organs

4.1.   a. 285.1

Incorrect answer. The anemia may be acute blood loss or a complication due to the surgery, but it is not stated by the physician. Due to incomplete physician documentation, query the physician. *Coding Clinic* (2004, 3Q:4; 2000, 3Q:6; and 1992, 2Q:15–16).

b. 998.11

Incorrect answer. The anemia may be acute blood loss or a complication due to the surgery, but it is not stated by the physician. Due to incomplete physician documentation, query the physician. *Coding Clinic* (2004, 3Q:4; 2000, 3Q:6, and 1992, 2Q:16).

c. 998.11, 285.1

Incorrect answer. The anemia is not documented as a complication of the surgery, nor is the anemia documented as acute blood loss. Due to incomplete physician documentation, query the physician. *Coding Clinic* (2004, 3Q:4; 2000, 3Q:6; and 1992, 2Q:16).

d. Query the physician because opportunity exists to improve documentation of etiology of anemia.

Correct answer.

ICD-10-CM Code(s): D64.9

ICD-10-CM Rationale: Although D64.9 is the correct code, an opportunity exists to improve documentation of etiology of anemia resulting in a more specific diagnosis code.

4.2.   a. 491.21, 284.19, 99.04

Correct answer.

b. 491.21, 284.19, 285.9, 99.04

Incorrect answer. Pancytopenia is a deficiency of all three blood components: white blood cells (neutropenia), red blood cells (anemia), and platelets (thrombocytopenia). Therefore, only the code for pancytopenia (284.19) is assigned.

c. 496, 284.19, 99.04

Incorrect answer. The correct code for an acute exacerbation of COPD is 491.21.

d. 491.21, 284.19, 285.9, 99.02

Incorrect answer. Pancytopenia is a deficiency of all three blood components: white blood cells (neutropenia), red blood cells (anemia), and platelets (thrombocytopenia). Therefore, only the code for pancytopenia (284.19) is assigned. The transfusion was not with previously collected autologous blood.

ICD-10-CM Code(s): J44.1, D61.81

ICD-10-PCS Code(s): 30233N1

ICD-10-CM Rationale: For code J44.1, the Alphabetic Index main term is Disease with subterms lung, obstructive (chronic), with, acute, exacerbation NEC. For code D61.81, the Alphabetic Index main term is Pancytopenia.

ICD-10-PCS Rationale: The Alphabetic Index main term is Transfusion with subterms Vein, Peripheral, Blood, Red Cells.

4.3.   174.4-Y, 85.21, 40.23

Rationale: When a sentinel lymph node biopsy is performed, an excision of the sentinel node is examined to determine the presence of malignancy. *Coding Clinic* (2002, 2Q:7).

ICD-10-CM Code(s): C50.412

ICD-10-PCS Code(s): 0HBU0ZZ, 07B60ZX

ICD-10-CM Rationale: The Alphabetic Index main term is Carcinoma (malignant)—see also Neoplasm, by site, malignant; Neoplasm, breast, upper-outer quadrant.

ICD-10-PCS Rationale: For code 0HBU0ZZ, the Alphabetic Index main term is Excision, Breast, Left. For code 07B60ZX, the Alphabetic Index main term is Excision, Lymphatic, Axillary, Left.

4.4.   a. 286.0, 99.06, 99.04

Incorrect answer. The anemia code of 285.1 would be coded as the principal diagnosis.

b. 285.1, 286.0, 99.04, 99.06

Correct answer.

c. 286.0, 285.1, 99.06, 99.04

Incorrect answer. In accordance with the UHDDS definition for principal diagnosis, the anemia (not the hemophilia) is the reason for admission and sequenced as the principal diagnosis (*ICD-9-CM Official Guidelines for Coding and Reporting*).

d. 285.1, 99.06, 99.04

Incorrect answer. There is a hemophilia code of 286.0 that is needed as a secondary diagnosis code.

ICD-10-CM Code(s): D62, D66

ICD-10-PCS Code(s): 30233N1, 30233V1

ICD-10-CM Rationale: For code D62, the Alphabetic Index main term is Anemia, subterms blood loss, acute. For code D66, the Alphabetic Index main term is Hemophilia.

ICD-10-PCS Rationale: The Alphabetic Index main term is Transfusion with subterms Vein, Peripheral, Blood.

4.5. 284.89-Y, 714.0-Y, 357.1-Y, E933.1-Y, MS-DRG: 810

Rationale: When coding anemia due to drugs, assign two codes, one for the specific type of anemia documented and the appropriate E code. Certain conditions have both an underlying etiology and multiple body system manifestations due to the underlying etiology. In the index both conditions are listed together with the etiology code first followed by the manifestation codes in brackets. The code in brackets is always to be sequenced second (*ICD-9-CM Official Guidelines for Coding and Reporting*).

ICD-10-CM Code(s): T45.1x5A, D61.1, M05.59

ICD-10-CM Rationale: For code T45.1x5A, the Alphabetic Index main term is Azathioprine, subterm adverse effect. For code D61.1, the Alphabetic Index main term is Anemia, subterms aplastic, due to, drugs. For code M05.59, the Alphabetic Index main term is Neuropathy, subterm peripheral (nerve) (see also Polyneuropathy); Polyneuropathy, in (due to), rheumatoid arthritis—see Rheumatoid, polyneuropathy; Rheumatoid, polyneuropathy, multiple sites.

Disorders of the Cardiovascular System

4.6. a. The conditions are reported with two separate codes unless the physician specifically states that there is a cause-and-effect relationship.

Incorrect answer. A cause-and-effect relationship is assumed unless the physician states otherwise.

b. Code 403.9X is assigned, with an additional code for chronic kidney disease.

Correct answer.

c. A cause-and-effect relationship is never assumed.

Incorrect answer. A cause-and-effect relationship is assumed unless the physician states otherwise.

d. Code 403.9X is assigned, with an additional code to specify the type of hypertension.

Incorrect answer. Code 403.9X is assigned with an additional code to specify the stage of the chronic kidney disease.

ICD-10-CM: Correct answer is b.

ICD-10-CM Rationale: A code from category I12.9 is assigned, with an additional code from category N18 to identify the stage of chronic kidney disease.

4.7. 410.51

Rationale: In accordance with the UHDDS definition for principal diagnosis, the acute ST elevation lateral wall myocardial infarction (not the coronary atherosclerosis) is the reason for admission and sequenced as the principal diagnosis. (*ICD-9-CM Official Guidelines for Coding and Reporting*). Code 410.51 is the principal diagnosis, as the MI had not resolved and was still being treated at Hospital B. *Coding Clinic* (2009, 3Q:8)

ICD-10-CM Code: I21.29

ICD-10-CM Rationale: The Alphabetic Index main term is Infarction, subterms myocardium, ST elevation, lateral.

4.8. a. 428.21, 428.31, 410.12, 599.0, 041.49, 89.54

Incorrect answer. It is incorrect to use systolic and diastolic heart failure codes together. The combined code is used in this case. The MI is specified as non-ST so 410.72 is reported.

b. 428.41, 410.72, 599.0, 041.49, 89.54

Correct answer.

c. 428.0, 412, 599.0, 041.49, 89.54

Incorrect answer. The heart failure is not stated as congestive but, rather, the specific types of failure are documented. The non-ST MI would be coded as acute-subsequent admission because it is within the eight-week time frame.

d. 428.41, 410.11, 599.0, 041.49, 89.54

Incorrect answer. It is not correct to use the initial episode fifth digit for the MI because the initial episode of care was completed. The MI is specified as non-ST so 410.72 is reported. The subsequent episode of care fifth digit of 2 should be used instead.

ICD-10-CM Code(s): I50.41, I21.4, N39.0, B96.2

ICD-10-PCS Code(s): 4A12X4Z

ICD-10-CM Rationale: For code I50.41, the Alphabetic Index main term is Failure, subterms heart, diastolic, combined with systolic, acute. For code I21.4, the Alphabetic Index main term is Infarction, subterms myocardium, non-ST elevation. For code N39.0, the Alphabetic Index main term is Infection, subterm urinary (tract). For code B96.2, the Alphabetic Index main term is Infection, subterms *Escherichia (E.) coli* NEC, as cause of disease classified elsewhere.

ICD-10-PCS Rationale: The Alphabetic Index main term is Telemetry.

4.9. 414.01-Y, 415.19-N, 496-Y, 36.12, 36.15, 39.61, MS-DRG: 235

Rationale: In accordance with the UHDDS guidelines for principal diagnosis assignment, the ASHD is the reason for admission and is sequenced as the principal diagnosis (*ICD-9-CM Official Guidelines for Coding and Reporting*). Not all conditions that occur during or following medical care or surgery are classified as complications. Code assignment is based on the provider's documentation of the relationship between the condition and the care or procedure. There must be a cause-and-effect relationship between the care provided and the condition, and an indication in the documentation that it is a complication. Query the provider for clarification if the complication is not clearly documented (2012 *ICD-9-CM Official Guidelines for Coding and Reporting*).

ICD-10-CM Code(s): I25.10, I26.99, J44.9

ICD-10-PCS Code(s): 021109W, 06BQ4ZZ, 02100Z9, 5A1221Z, 5A1935Z

ICD-10-CM Rationale: For code I25.10, the Alphabetic Index main term is Disease, subterms arteriosclerotic, heart—see Disease, heart, ischemic, atherosclerotic. For code I26.99, the Alphabetic Index main term is Embolism, pulmonary. For code J44.9, the Alphabetic Index main term is Disease, subterms lung, obstructive (chronic).

ICD-10-PCS Rationale: For code 021109W, the Alphabetic Index main term is Bypass, subterms Artery, Coronary, Two Sites. For code 06BQ4ZZ, the Alphabetic Index main term is Excision, subterms Vein, Greater Saphenous, left. For code 02100Z9, the Alphabetic Index main term is Bypass, subterms Artery, One Site. For code 5A1221Z, the Alphabetic Index main term is Performance, Cardiac, Continuous, Output. For code 5A1935Z, the Alphabetic Index main term is Performance, Respiratory, Continuous, Less than 24 Consecutive Hours Ventilation.

4.10.   a. Acute ST myocardial infarction, congestive heart failure, Parkinson's disease, emphysema

Correct answer.

b. Acute ST myocardial infarction, congestive heart failure

Incorrect answer. The Parkinson's disease, congestive heart failure, and emphysema are reported as secondary diagnoses based on the UHDDS additional diagnosis guidelines (*ICD-9-CM Official Guidelines for Coding and Reporting, Coding Clinic 2006, 4Q:234, ICD-10-CM Official Guidelines for Coding and Reporting*).

c. Acute ST myocardial infarction, congestive heart failure, Parkinson's disease, emphysema, pneumonia, bleeding ulcer

Incorrect answer. The pneumonia and bleeding ulcer are not current conditions nor evaluated or treated during the hospitalization and should not be coded as secondary diagnoses.

d. Acute ST myocardial infarction, pneumonia, congestive heart failure, emphysema

Incorrect answer. The pneumonia is not a current condition nor evaluated or treated during this hospitalization and should not be coded as a secondary diagnosis. The Parkinson's disease should be added as a secondary diagnosis as a chronic condition requiring monitoring and nursing resources.

4.11. 414.01-Y, 427.81-Y, 37.83, 37.72, 00.66, 36.07, 00.40, 00.45, MS-DRG: 244

Note: In accordance with the UHDDS definition for principal diagnosis, the reason (after study) the patient is admitted to the hospital is to undergo the PTCA for the CAD; therefore, the 414.01 is the principal diagnosis.

ICD-10-CM Code(s): I25.10, I49.5

ICD-10-PCS Code(s): 027034Z, 0JH60P2, 02H63MA, 02HK3MA

ICD-10-CM Rationale: For code I25.10, the Alphabetic Index main term is Disease, subterms arteriosclerotic, heart—see Disease, heart, ischemic, atherosclerotic. For code I49.5, the Alphabetic Index main term is Syndrome, subterms sick, sinus.

ICD-10-PCS Rationale: For code 027034Z, the Alphabetic Index main term is Dilation, Artery, Coronary, One Site. For code 0JH60P2, the Alphabetic Index main term is Insertion of device in, Subcutaneous Tissue and Fascia, Chest, Pacemaker, Dual Chamber. For code 02H63MA, the Alphabetic Index main term is Pacemaker Lead, Atrium, Right. For code 02HK3MA, the Alphabetic Index main term is Pacemaker Lead, Ventricle, Right.

4.12. a. 411.0, 412

Incorrect answer. The angina was documented as "crescendo" and should be assigned to code 411.1, coding to the highest degree of code specificity.

b. 413.9, 412

Incorrect answer. The angina was documented as "crescendo" and should be assigned to code 411.1, coding to the highest degree of code specificity.

c. 411.1, 412

Correct answer.

d. 413.0, 412

Incorrect answer. The angina was documented as "crescendo" and should be assigned to code 411.1, coding to the highest degree of code specificity.

ICD-10-CM Code(s): I20.0, I25.2

ICD-10-CM Rationale: For code I20.0, the Alphabetic Index main term is Angina, crescendo—see Angina, unstable. For code I25.2, the Alphabetic Index main term is Infarction, subterms myocardium, healed or old.

4.13. 434.91-Y, 438.21, MS-DRG: 065

Rationale: Code 436 would not be assigned if there were documentation of infarction. Code V12.59 would not be assigned because it is only for those instances where there are no residual neurologic deficits from a previous stroke. Residual conditions from a previous stroke may be reported with another acute infarct. Category 438 is exempt from the POA requirement.

ICD-10-CM Code(s): I63.50, I69.352

ICD-10-CM Rationale: For code I63.50, the Alphabetic Index main term is Infarction, subterms cerebral, due to, occlusion NEC, cerebral arteries. For code I69.352, the Alphabetic Index main term is Sequelae, subterms stroke, hemiplegia.

4.14.   a. 428.23, 396.2

Incorrect answer. It is correct to add 428.0 with another specified type of heart failure (chronic systolic) based on *Coding Clinic* (2004, 4Q:140) that states CHF is not an inherent component of diastolic or systolic heart failure. Therefore, two codes are required.

b. 428.23, 428.0, 396.2

Correct answer.

c. 428.0, 394.1, 424.1

Incorrect answer. Acute exacerbation of chronic systolic heart failure should be assigned code 428.23 and listed as the principal diagnosis. Mitral regurgitation not otherwise specified is assigned code 424.0. When mitral regurgitation is mentioned with aortic valve stenosis (424.1), a combination code, 396.2, for the mitral regurgitation and aortic stenosis, is assigned.

d. 391.8, 396.2

Incorrect answer. Congestive heart failure is not to be assumed as being rheumatic in nature. *Coding Clinic* (2009, 1Q:18). Acute exacerbation of chronic systolic heart failure should be assigned code 428.23 and listed as the principal diagnosis. It is correct to add 428.0 with another specified type of heart failure (chronic systolic) based on *Coding Clinic* (2004, 4Q:140), which states CHF is not an inherent component of diastolic or systolic heart failure. Therefore, two codes are required.

ICD-10-CM Code(s): I50.23, I08.0

ICD-10-CM Rationale: For code I50.23, the Alphabetic Index main term is Failure, subterms heart, systolic (congestive), acute, and (on) chronic. For code I08.0, the Alphabetic Index main term is Regurgitation, aortic—see Insufficiency, aortic; Insufficiency, aortic, with mitral (valve) disease.

4.15.   00.66, 36.06, 00.45, 00.41

Note: Code 00.66 has a note with instructions to code also any insertion of coronary artery stent(s) and the number of stents inserted.

ICD-10-PCS Code(s): 02703DZ, 02703ZZ

ICD-10-PCS Rationale: For both codes, the Alphabetic Index main term is Dilation, Artery, Coronary, One Site.

Disorders of the Digestive System

4.16. 569.85-Y, 562.11-Y, 45.23

Rationale: The source of the bleeding is angiodysplasia. Therefore, the code with hemorrhage is assigned based on *Coding Clinic* (2005, 3Q:17–18), GI bleeding with multiple possible causes. The diverticulitis was not the source of bleeding; therefore, code is assigned without bleeding. The 578.1 code is not reported in addition because it is included in the 569.85 code.

ICD-10-CM Code(s): K55.21, K57.32

ICD-10-PCS Code(s): 0DJD8ZZ

ICD-10-CM Rationale: For code K55.21, the Alphabetic Index main term is Angiodysplasia, subterm with bleeding. For code K57.32, the Alphabetic Index main term is Diverticulitis, subterms intestine, large.

ICD-10-PCS Rationale: The Alphabetic Index main term is Colonoscopy.

4.17. 531.20-Y, 44.41

Rationale: The ulcer was an acute gastric ulcer with perforation and hemorrhage. The procedure was suture of gastric ulcer. Documentation indicates a laparotomy was done. Therefore, the open technique is coded.

ICD-10-CM Code(s): K25.2

ICD-10-PCS Code(s): 0DQ60ZZ

ICD-10-CM Rationale: The Alphabetic Index main term is Ulcer, subterms stomach, acute, with, hemorrhage, and perforation.

ICD-10-PCS Rationale: The Alphabetic Index main term is Repair, subterm stomach.

4.18. 578.1-Y, 428.22-Y, 428.0-Y, 45.16, MS-DRG: 378

Rationale: The melena is listed as the principal diagnosis. No documented cause is identified for the bleeding. Therefore, melena is the most specific code available. It is correct to add 428.0 with another specified type of heart failure (chronic systolic) based on *Coding Clinic* (2004, 4Q:140), which states CHF is not an inherent component of diastolic or systolic heart failure; therefore, two codes are required.

ICD-10-CM Code(s): K92.1, I50.22

ICD-10-PCS Code(s): 0DB68ZX, 0DB98ZX

ICD-10-CM Rationale: For code K92.1, the Alphabetic Index main term is Melena. For code I50.22, the Alphabetic Index main term is Failure, subterms heart, systolic (congestive), chronic.

ICD-10-PCS Rationale: For code 0DB68ZX, the Alphabetic Index main term is Excision, subterm stomach. For code 0DB98ZX, the Alphabetic Index main term is Excision, subterm duodenum.

4.19.   a. 003.0, 276.51

Incorrect answer. The patient was admitted for treatment of dehydration. The circumstances of inpatient admission always govern the selection of principal diagnosis (*Coding Clinic* 2008, 1Q:10–11).

b. 558.9, 003.0, 276.51

Incorrect answer. The patient was admitted for treatment of dehydration. The circumstances of inpatient admission always govern the selection of principal diagnosis. *Coding Clinic* 2008 (1Q:10–11). Code 558.9 would not be assigned, as the cause of the gastroenteritis is Salmonella.

c. 003.0, 578.9, 276.51, 787.91

Incorrect answer. Acute symptoms of Salmonella gastroenteritis include the sudden onset of nausea, abdominal cramping, and bloody diarrhea. Signs and symptoms that are integral to the disease process should not be assigned as additional codes (*ICD-9-CM Official Guidelines for Coding and Reporting*). Use of category 578, Gastrointestinal hemorrhage, is limited to cases where a GI bleed is documented but no bleeding site or cause is identified (*Coding Clinic* 1992, 2Q:9–10).

d. 276.51, 003.0

Correct answer.

ICD-10-CM Code(s): E86.0, A02.0

ICD-10-CM Rationale: For code E86.0, the Alphabetic Index main term is Dehydration. For code A02.0, the Alphabetic Index main term is Gastroenteritis, subterm Salmonella.

4.20.   550.92-Y, 250.00-Y, 715.36-Y, 17.21, MS-DRG: 352

Rationale: Code 715.36, Degenerative joint disease affecting only one site not identified as primary or secondary, is assigned to subcategory 715.3, Osteoarthrosis, localized, not specified whether primary or secondary. *Coding Clinic* (2003, 4Q:118). Laparoscopic bilateral repair of direct inguinal hernia with graft or prosthesis is coded 17.21. *Coding Clinic* (2008 4Q:165–169)

ICD-10-CM Code(s): K40.20, E11.9, M17.9

ICD-10-PCS Code(s): 0YUA4JZ

ICD-10-CM Rationale: For code K40.20, the Alphabetic Index main term is Hernia, subterms inguinal (direct), bilateral. For code E11.9, the Alphabetic Index main term is Diabetes. For code M17.9, the Alphabetic Index main term is Osteoarthritis, subterm knee.

ICD-10-PCS Rationale: The Alphabetic Index main term is Supplement, subterms inguinal region, bilateral.

4.21. 574.80-Y, 401.9-Y, 51.22, 51.41

Rationale: It is important to review all of the choices at category 574. One code can be selected to show the cholelithiasis, the choledocholithiasis, and the acute and chronic cholecystitis. Hypertension meets the UHDDS definition for reporting additional diagnoses.

ICD-10-CM Code(s): K80.66, I10

ICD-10-PCS Code(s): 0FT40ZZ, 0FC90ZZ

ICD-10-CM Rationale: For code K80.86, the Alphabetic Index main term is Calculus, gallbladder and bile duct, with cholecystitis, acute, with, chronic cholecystitis. For code I10, the Alphabetic Index main term is Hypertension.

ICD-10-PCS Rationale: For code 0FT40ZZ, the Alphabetic Index main term is Resection, subterm gallbladder. For code 0FC90ZZ, the Alphabetic Index main term is Choledocholithotomy.

4.22. 558.3-Y, 558.41-Y, 558.42-Y

Rationale: Three codes are required to completely describe the patient's condition. Allergic gastroenteritis and colitis, code 558.3, Eosinophilic gastroenteritis, code 558.41, and Eosinophilic colitis, code 558.42. No "excludes note" prohibits assigning codes for both allergic and eosinophilic gastroenteritis and colitis. *Coding Clinic* (2008, 4Q:115–116). The symptoms would not be coded, as they are integral to the patient's conditions. All diagnoses were present on admission.

ICD-10-CM Code(s): K52.2, K52.81, K52.82

ICD-10-CM Rationale: For code K52.2, the Alphabetic Index main term is Gastroenteritis, subterm allergic. For code K52.81, the Alphabetic Index main term is Gastroenteritis, subterm eosinophilic. For code K52.82, the Alphabetic Index main term is Colitis, subterm eosinophilic.

4.23. 562.11-Y, 555.1-Y, 560.89-Y, 45.76, 45.73, 45.74, 46.13, MS-DRG: 330

Note: Intestinal obstruction secondary to Crohn's disease is coded 555.9 and 560.89 (*Coding Clinic* 1997, 2Q:3).

ICD-10-CM Code(s): K57.20, K50.112

ICD-10-PCS Code(s): 0DTN0ZZ, 0DTF0ZZ, 0DBL0ZZ, 0D1M0Z4

ICD-10-CM Rationale: For code K57.20, the Alphabetic Index main term is Diverticulitis, subterms intestine, large, with abscess, perforation or peritonitis. For code K50.112, the Alphabetic Index main term is Crohn's disease—see Enteritis, regional; Enteritis, regional, large intestine, with, complication, intestinal obstruction.

ICD-10-PCS Rationale: For code 0DTN0ZZ, the Alphabetic Index main term is Resection, subterms colon, sigmoid. For code 0DTF0ZZ, the Alphabetic Index main term is Resection, subterms intestine, large, right. For code 0DBL0ZZ, the Alphabetic Index main term is Excision, subterms colon, transverse. For code 0D1M0Z4, the Alphabetic Index main term is Bypass, subterms colon, descending.

Endocrine, Nutritional, and Metabolic Diseases and Immunity Disorders

4.24. 276.51-Y, 787.91-Y, 280.9-Y, 486-Y, 344.40-Y, 053.19-Y, 139.8, 45.25, MS-DRG: 640

Rationale: In accordance with *ICD-9-CM Official Guidelines for Coding and Reporting* and *Coding Clinic* (2008, 4Q:206–211), a late effect is the residual effect after the acute phase has ended. Coding requires two codes: one for the condition(s) produced and the late effect code. The pneumonia was being treated prior to admission and is still present. Code 139.8 is POA exempt. All other diagnoses were present on admission.

ICD-10-CM Code(s): E86.0, R19.7, D50.9, J18.9, G83.21, B02.29, B94.8

ICD-10-PCS Code(s): 0DB88ZX, 0DBN8ZX

ICD-10-CM Rationale: For code E86.0, the Alphabetic Index main term is Dehydration. For code R19.7, the Alphabetic Index main term is Diarrhea. For code D50.9, the Alphabetic Index main term is Anemia, subterm iron deficiency. For code J18.9, the Alphabetic Index main term is Pneumonia. For code G83.21, the Alphabetic Index main term is Monoplegia, subterm upper limb. For code B02.29, the Alphabetic Index main term is Neuralgia, subterm postherpetic NEC. For code B94.8, the Alphabetic Index main term is Sequelae, subterm infectious disease, specified NEC.

ICD-10-PCS Rationale: For code 0DB88ZX, the Alphabetic Index main term is Excision, subterms intestine, small. For code 0DBN8ZX, the Alphabetic Index main term is Excision, subterms colon, sigmoid.

4.25. 249.60-Y, 536.3-Y, E932.0-Y, V58.65, MS-DRG: 74

Rationale: Secondary diabetes, category 249, includes drug-induced or chemically induced secondary diabetes. Additional codes, 536.3, Gastroparesis and E932.0, Adverse effect of therapeutic use of adrenal cortical steroids, are needed to completely describe the patient's condition. *Coding Clinic* (2008, 4Q:91–95). All diagnoses are present on admission.

ICD-10-CM Code(s): T38.0x5A, E09.43

ICD-10-CM Rationale: For code T38.0x5A, Steroid, adverse effect. For code E09.43, the Alphabetic Index main term is Diabetes, subterms due to drug or chemical, with gastroparesis.

4.26. 250.13-Y, 276.51-Y

Rationale: The diabetes is coded as the principal diagnosis, as it meets the definition of UHDDS condition, after study, to be the reason the patient was admitted. The fifth digit is 3 because the DM is type I and it is documented as uncontrolled. A symptom such as polydipsia would not be coded, as this symptom is integral to the diabetes. Dehydration meets reporting guidelines as a secondary diagnosis, as the patient's dehydration was evaluated and treated during the hospitalization. Both conditions were present at the time of admission.

ICD-10-CM Code(s): E10.10, E86.0

ICD-10-CM Rationale: For code E10.10, the Alphabetic Index main term is Diabetes, subterms type 1, with, ketoacidosis. For code E86.0, the Alphabetic Index main term is Dehydration.

4.27. 193-Y, 196.0-Y, 06.4 MS-DRG: 626

Rationale: There was documented metastasis to the cervical lymph node; therefore, this meets reporting as a secondary diagnosis. Initially the left lobe was removed, but because of the carcinoma, a total thyroidectomy was done.

ICD-10-CM Code(s): C73, C77.0

ICD-10-PCS Code(s): 0GTK0ZZ

ICD-10-CM Rationale: For code C73, the Alphabetic Index main term is Neoplasm, subterms thyroid, malignant primary. For code C77.0, the Alphabetic Index main term is Neoplasm, lymph, gland, cervical, malignant secondary.

ICD-10-PCS Rationale: The Alphabetic Index main term is Resection, subterm thyroid gland.

4.28. a. 250.71, 440.23, 250.61, 357.2, 83.45

Incorrect answer. Code 440.24 includes any condition classifiable to 440.23 with ischemic gangrene. Assign an additional code for the foot ulceration.

b. 250.71, 440.24, 250.61, 357.2, 707.15, 83.45

Correct answer.

c. 250.01, 440.20, 785.4, 357.2, 707.15, 86.22

Incorrect answer. The gangrene is included in the fifth digit for subcategory 440.2. The debridement was of the muscle.

d. 250.71, 440.24, 250.61, 707.15, 86.22

Incorrect answer. Assign code 250.6X, Diabetes with neurological manifestations, and code 357.2, Polyneuropathy in diabetes, for diabetic neuropathy. *Coding Clinic* (1991, 3Q:9–11). The debridement was of the muscle.

ICD-10-CM Code(s): E10.52, I70.262, E10.621, L97.523, E10.40

ICD-10-PCS Code(s): 0KBW0ZZ

ICD-10-CM Rationale: For code E10.52, the Alphabetic Index main term is Diabetes, subterms type 1, with, gangrene. For code I70.262, the Alphabetic Index main term is Arteriosclerosis, subterms extremities, leg, left, with, gangrene. For code E10.621, the Alphabetic Index main term is Diabetes, subterms type 1, with, skin ulcer NEC. For code L97.523, the Alphabetic Index main term is Ulcer, subterms lower limb, calf, left, with, muscle necrosis. For code E10.40, the Alphabetic Index main term is Diabetes, subterms type 1, with, neuropathy.

ICD-10-PCS Rationale: The Alphabetic Index main term is Excision, subterms muscle, foot, left.

Disorders of the Genitourinary System

4.29.   a. 614.9, 079.98, 59.02

Incorrect answer. Code 614.9 is not specific, while code 614.6 specifies pelvic adhesions and more closely describes the findings at the time of surgery. INTERCEED is an adhesion barrier that should be coded. *Coding Clinic* (1992, 1Q:14).

b. 614.6, 079.98, 59.02, 99.77

Correct answer.

c. 614.6, 079.88, 54.59, 99.77

Incorrect answer. The chlamydia is unspecified, code 079.98. Code 54.59 is an incorrect choice; an "Excludes" note directs code assignment to "lysis of adhesions kidney 59.02 and ureter 59.02–59.03," as the lysis was performed around the kidney and ureter.

d. 614.3, 079.98, 59.02, 99.77

Incorrect answer. The documentation does not state acute inflammatory process.

ICD-10-CM Code(s): N73.6, A56.11

ICD-10-PCS Code(s): 0TN00ZZ, 0TN10ZZ, 3E0M05Z

ICD-10-CM Rationale: For code N73.6, the Alphabetic Index main term is Adhesions, subterms pelvic, female. For code A56.11, the Alphabetic Index main term is Chlamydia, subterms female, pelvic inflammatory disease.

ICD-10-PCS Rationale: For code 0TN00ZZ, the Alphabetic Index main term is Release, subterms kidney, right. For code 0TN10ZZ, the Alphabetic Index main term is Release, subterms kidney, left. For code 3E0M05Z, the Alphabetic Index main term is Introduction, subterms peritoneal cavity, adhesion barrier.

4.30.   a. 183.0, 68.41, 65.61, 40.3

Incorrect answer. The documentation states a radical abdominal hysterectomy was done, coded 68.69, not a laparoscopic total abdominal hysterectomy.

b. 183.0, 68.69, 65.61, 40.3

Correct answer.

c. 198.6, 68.61, 65.61, 40.3

Incorrect answer. Ovarian cancer is a primary cancer, not a secondary one, so the correct code is 183.0. The documentation states a radical abdominal hysterectomy was done, coded 68.69, not a laparoscopic radical abdominal hysterectomy.

d. 183.0, 68.69, 65.61, 40.59

Incorrect answer. The documentation states regional lymph node dissection was done, which would be coded 40.3.

ICD-10-CM Code(s): C56.1

ICD-10-PCS Code(s): 0UT90ZZ, 0UTC0ZZ, 0UBG0ZZ, 0UT20ZZ, 0UT70ZZ, 07TC0ZZ

ICD-10-CM Rationale: The Alphabetic Index main term is Neoplasm, subterm ovary, malignant primary.

ICD-10-PCS Rationale: For code 0UT90ZZ, the Alphabetic Index main term is Resection, subterm uterus. For code 0UTC0ZZ, the Alphabetic Index main term is Resection, subterm cervix. For code 0UT20ZZ, the Alphabetic Index main term is Resection, subterms ovary, bilateral. For code 0UT70ZZ, the Alphabetic Index main term is Resection, subterms fallopian tubes, bilateral. For code 07TC0ZZ, the Alphabetic Index main term is Resection, subterms lymphatic, pelvis. Only part of the vagina was removed so the root operation is excision.

4.31. 599.0-Y, 041.49-Y, 491.21-N, 414.01-Y, 401.9-Y, MS-DRG: 690

Rationale: The symptoms of the UTI are not coded, as they are integral to the UTI. The additional conditions meet reporting guidelines as secondary diagnoses because they are current conditions evaluated and/or treated during the hospitalization. Assign 414.01 if the patient has coronary artery disease and past history does not show coronary artery bypass grafting (*Coding Clinic* 1997, 3Q:15). All conditions *except* the exacerbation of COPD were present at the time of admission. POA reporting guidelines for combination codes instructs coder to report N (no) if any part of the combination code was not present on admission and assign Y (yes) if all parts of the combination code were present on admission.

ICD-10-CM Code(s): N39.0, B96.2, J44.1, I25.10, I10

ICD-10-CM Rationale: For code N39.0, the Alphabetic Index main term is Infection, subterm urinary. For code B96.2, the Alphabetic Index main term is Infection, subterms *Escherichi (E.) coli*, as cause of disease classified elsewhere. For code J44.1, the Alphabetic Index main term is Disease, subterms lung, obstructive (chronic), with, acute, exacerbation NEC. For code I25.10, the Alphabetic Index main term is Disease, subterms heart, ischemic, atherosclerotic. For code I10, the Alphabetic Index main term is Hypertension.

4.32. 218.0-Y, 617.0-Y, 617.1-Y, 617.3-Y, 614.6-Y, 998.2-N, 285.1-N, E870.0-N, E849.7-N

Note: The leiomyoma (218.0) is documented as the reason for the procedure and is sequenced as the principal diagnosis. The patient experienced an intraoperative complication (998.2 and E870.0). A place of occurrence code provides information and is coded. (*ICD-9-CM Official Guidelines for Coding and Reporting*, 19b) Activity codes are not applicable to poisonings, adverse effects, misadventures, or late effects. (*ICD-9-CM Official Guidelines for Coding and Reporting*, 19j)

ICD-10-CM Code(s): D25.0, N80.0, N80.1, N80.3, N73.6, K91.72, D62, Y76.3, Y92.234

ICD-10-CM Rationale: For code D25.0, the Alphabetic Index main term is Leiomyoma, subterms uterus, submucous. For code N80.0, the Alphabetic Index main term is Endometriosis, subterm uterus. For code N80.1, the Alphabetic Index main term is Endometriosis, subterm ovary. For code

N80.3, the Alphabetic Index main term is Endometriosis, subterm pelvic peritoneum. For code N73.6, the Alphabetic Index main term is Adhesions, subterm pelvic, female. For code K91.72, the Alphabetic Index main term is Complication, subterms intraoperative, puncture or laceration, digestive system, during procedure on other organ. For code D62, the Alphabetic Index main term is Anemia, subterms blood loss, acute. For code Y76.3, the Alphabetic Index main term is Misadventure, subterm cut. For code Y92.234, the Alphabetic Index main term is Place of occurrence, subterms hospital, operating room.

4.33. 610.1-Y, V16.3, 85.42

Rationale: This is one procedure code that has a differentiation in ICD-9-CM for bilateral procedures. There is also distinction between simple and other types of mastectomy. Report secondary diagnosis code V16.3 for family history of breast cancer. V16.3 is exempt from POA reporting per the national guidelines.

ICD-10-CM Code(s): N60.11, N60.12, Z80.3

ICD-10-PCS Code(s): 0HTV0ZZ

ICD-10-CM Rationale: For code N60.11, the Alphabetic Index main term is Disease, subterms breast, cystic—see Mastopathy, cystic. For code N60.12, the Alphabetic Index main term is Disease, subterms breast, cystic—see Mastopathy, cystic. For code Z80.3, the Alphabetic Index main term is History, subterms family, malignant neoplasm, breast.

ICD-10-PCS Rationale: The Alphabetic Index main term is Resection, subterms breast, bilateral.

4.34. 584.9-Y, 276.1-Y, 401.9-Y, MS-DRG: 683

Rationale: The acute renal failure and hypertension are coded individually and not combined. The category for hypertensive renal disease does not include "acute" renal failure. Dehydration "with" hyponatremia coded to the highest degree of code specificity is reported as 276.1 (not 276.51). All conditions were present at the time of admission.

ICD-10-CM Code(s): N17.9, E87.1, I10

ICD-10-CM Rationale: For code N17.9, the Alphabetic Index main term is Failure, subterms renal, acute. For code E87.1, the Alphabetic Index main term is Hyponatremia. For code I10, the Alphabetic Index main term is Hypertension.

4.35. 584.9-Y, 403.90-Y, 585.4-Y, 250.41-Y, MS-DRG: 684

Rationale: Code 403.90 is assigned to report hypertensive chronic kidney disease stage IV, and the stage (585.4) is assigned as an additional code. Code 583.81 is not reported because the nephritis/nephropathy is specified as acute and chronic.

ICD-10-CM Code(s): N17.9, I12.9, N18.4, E10.22

ICD-10-CM Rationale: For code N17.9, the Alphabetic Index main term is Failure, subterms renal, acute. For code I12.9, the Alphabetic Index main term is Hypertension, subterm kidney, with, stage 1 through 4 chronic kidney disease. For code N18.4, the Alphabetic Index main term is Disease, subterms kidney, chronic, stage 4. For code E10.22, the Alphabetic Index main term is Diabetes, subterm type 1, with, chronic kidney disease.

4.36. 999.32-Y, 585.6-Y, V45.11

Rationale: Code 999.32 is assigned to report a bloodstream infection due to renal dialysis central venous catheters. An excludes note is found under code 996.62 indicating code 999.32 should be used for bloodstream infection due to central venous catheter. Codes 585.6, End stage renal disease, and V45.11, Renal dialysis status, should be assigned as additional diagnoses. *Coding Clinic* (2008, 4Q:193). No POA indicator is assigned to V45.11, as this code is on the POA exempt list. All remaining diagnoses are present on admission. Therefore, assign a POA indicator of Y.

ICD-10-CM Code(s): T80.21xA, N18.6, Z99.2

ICD-10-CM Rationale: For code T80.21xA, the Alphabetic Index main term is Infection, subterm catheter-related bloodstream (CRBSI). For code N18.6, the Alphabetic Index main term is Failure, subterms renal, end stage. For code Z99.2, the Alphabetic Index main term is State, subterm dialysis.

Infectious Diseases

4.37. 042-Y, 012.13-Y, 014.83-Y, 017.23-Y, 729.81-N

Rationale: In accordance with *ICD-9-CM Official Guidelines for Coding and Reporting* and *Coding Clinic* (2006, 4Q:152), report code 042 as the principal diagnosis when a patient is admitted for an HIV-related condition. The HIV-related conditions are reported as secondary diagnoses. All locations of the lymph node tuberculosis should be coded. Except for the swelling of the extremities, all conditions are present on admission.

ICD-10-CM Code(s): B20, A15.4, A18.39, A18.2, M79.89

ICD-10-CM Rationale: For code B20, the Alphabetic Index main term is Human, subterm immunodeficiency virus disease. For code A15.4, the Alphabetic Index main term is Tuberculosis, subterms lymph gland or node, mediastinal. For code A18.39, the Alphabetic Index main term is Tuberculosis, subterms lymph gland or node, retroperitoneal. For code A18.2, the Alphabetic Index main term is Tuberculosis, subterm lymph gland or node. For code M79.89, the Alphabetic Index main term is Swelling, subterm limb— see Disorder, soft tissue, specified type NEC.

4.38. 038.0-Y, 995.91-Y, 599.0-Y, 041.02-Y, MS-DRG: 872

Rationale: The term "urosepsis" should be queried to determine if the patient has sepsis. Physician response documented sepsis with streptococcal septicemia and urinary tract infection with streptococcus B. In accordance with *ICD-9-CM Official Guidelines for Coding and Reporting* and *Coding Clinic* (2006, 4Q:154–160), report the streptococcal septicemia as the underlying infection and the 995.91 sepsis as the systemic inflammatory response syndrome due to the infectious process without acute organ dysfunction. Urinary tract infection and the causative organism meet secondary diagnosis reporting. All conditions were present at the time of admission.

ICD-10-CM Code(s): A40.1, N39.0, B95.1

ICD-10-CM Rationale: For code A40.1, the Alphabetic Index main term is Sepsis, subterms Streptococcus, group B. For code N39.0, the Alphabetic Index main term is Infection, urinary (tract). For code B95.1, the Alphabetic Index main term is Streptococcus, subterms group, B, as cause of disease classified elsewhere.

4.39. 647.63-Y, 042-Y, 647.83-Y, 136.3-Y, MS-DRG: 781

Rationale: In accordance with *ICD-9-CM Official Guidelines for Coding and Reporting* and *Coding Clinic* (2006, 4Q:153–154), during pregnancy, a patient admitted because of an HIV-related illness is reported with the principal diagnosis of 647.6x followed by 042. The pregnancy is also complicated by the Pneumocystis carinii pneumonia, which meets reporting guidelines for a secondary diagnosis.

ICD-10-CM Code(s): O98.712, B20, O98.612, B59

ICD-10-CM Rationale: For code O98.712, the Alphabetic Index main term is Pregnancy, subterms complicated by, infection, human immunodeficiency. For code B20, the Alphabetic Index main term is Human, subterm immunodeficiency virus disease. For code O98.612, the Alphabetic Index main term is Pregnancy, complicated by, protozoal disease. For code B59, the Alphabetic Index main term is Pneumocystis carinii pneumonia.

4.40. 042-Y, 078.5-Y, 011.03-Y, 492.8-Y, V42.6, 33.24, MS-DRG: 975

Rationale: In accordance with *ICD-9-CM Official Guidelines for Coding and Reporting* and *Coding Clinic* (2006, 4Q:152), report code 042 as the principal diagnosis when a patient is admitted for an HIV-related condition. The HIV-related conditions are reported as secondary diagnoses. Code 33.24 is correct for bronchoscopy with bronchoalveolar lavage (*Coding Clinic* 2006, 2Q:20). Code V42.6 is POA exempt. All other diagnoses were present on admission.

ICD-10-CM Code(s): B20, B25.9, A15.0, J43.9, Z94.2

ICD-10-PCS Code(s): 3E1F88X

ICD-10-CM Rationale: For code B20, the Alphabetic Index main term is Human, subterm immunodeficiency virus disease. For code B25.9, the Alphabetic Index main term is Infection, subterm cytomegalovirus. For code A15.0, the Alphabetic Index main term is Tuberculosis, subterm pulmonary. For code J43.9, the Alphabetic Index main term is Emphysema. For code Z94.2, the Alphabetic Index main term is Transplant, subterm lung.

ICD-10-PCS Rationale: The BAL was performed by washing out the alveolar tissue in order to obtain alveolar tissue for diagnosis. The Alphabetic Index main term is Irrigation, subterm respiratory tract, irrigating substance.

4.41. 482.31-Y, 054.11-Y

Rationale: There is documentation of the cause of the pneumonia. Therefore, the pneumonia due to group A streptococcus is coded. The underlying cause of the vulvovaginitis is determined to be herpes. Therefore, this is reported as a secondary diagnosis. All conditions are present on admission.

ICD-10-CM Code(s): J15.4, A60.04

ICD-10-CM Rationale: For code J15.4, the Alphabetic Index main term is Pneumonia, subterms streptococcal, group, A. For code A60.04, the Alphabetic Index main term is Vulvovaginitis—see Vaginitis; Vaginitis, in, herpesviral infection.

Disorders of the Skin and Subcutaneous Tissue

4.42. 507.0-Y, 438.82, 707.04-Y, 707.21-Y, MS-DRG: 179

Rationale: The documentation links the aspiration to the pneumonia and meets principal diagnosis reporting guidelines. Secondary diagnosis reporting of the dysphagia due to old stroke and stage one decubitus ulcer were evaluated and utilized nursing resources. Code 438.82 is POA exempt. If the documentation had provided further detail about the dysphagia, an additional code from subcategory 787.2 would be assigned.

ICD-10-CM Code(s): J69.0, I69.391, L89.201

ICD-10-CM Rationale: For code J69.0, the Alphabetic Index main term is Pneumonia, subterm aspiration. For code I69.391, the Alphabetic Index main term is Dysphagia, subterms following, cerebrovascular disease, cerebral infarction. For code L89.201, the Alphabetic Index main term is Ulcer, subterm decubitus—see Ulcer, pressure, by site; Ulcer, pressure, stage 1, hip.

4.43. 998.59-Y, 682.2-Y, 041.11-Y, 250.00-Y

Rationale: In accordance with the UHDDS definition for principal diagnosis, the postoperative wound infection meets reporting as principal diagnosis because the condition, after study, caused the admission. Secondary diagnosis reporting of the cellulitis, infectious organism, and diabetes meet secondary reporting guidelines as conditions that were evaluated or treated or increased nursing care during the hospital stay.

ICD-10-CM Code(s): T81.4xxA, L03.311, B95.6, E11.9, Z79.4

ICD-10-CM Rationale: For code T81.4xxA, the Alphabetic Index main term is Complication, subterms surgical procedure, wound infection. For code L03.311, the Alphabetic Index main term is Cellulitis, subterm abdominal wall. For code B95.6, the Alphabetic Index main term is Staphyloccus, subterm aureus, as cause of disease classified elsewhere. For code E11.9, the Alphabetic Index main term is Diabetes, subterm type 2. For code Z79.4, the Alphabetic Index main term is Long-term drug therapy, subterm insulin.

4.44. 682.6-Y, 707.05-Y, 707.20-Y. 438.20, 041.02-Y, MS-DRG: 603

Rationale: The cellulitis is listed in the first position. The infectious organism should be coded as well as the hemiplegia and the decubitus ulcer. Code 438.20 is POA exempt.

ICD-10-CM Code(s): L03.119, L89.329, I69.351, B95.1

ICD-10-CM Rationale: For code L03.119, the Alphabetic Index main term is Cellulitis, subterm lower limb. For code L89.329, the Alphabetic Index main term is Ulcer, subterm decubitus—see Ulcer, pressure, by site; Ulcer, pressure, buttock. For code I69.351, the Alphabetic Index main term is Hemiplegia, subterms following, cerebrovascular disease, cerebral infarction. For code B95.1, the Alphabetic Index main term is Streptococcus, subterms group, B, as cause of disease classified elsewhere.

4.45. 707.05-Y, 707.22-Y, 707.14-Y, 331.0-Y, 83.45, 86.22, MS-DRG: 574

Rationale: The most extensive procedure went into the muscle, so both procedures should be coded. The decubitus as well as the chronic heel ulcer should be coded.

ICD-10-CM Code(s): L89.312, L97.421, G30.9, F02.80

ICD-10-PCS Code(s): 0KBN0ZZ, 0HBNXZZ

ICD-10-CM Rationale: For code L89.312, the Alphabetic Index main term is Ulcer, subterm decubitus—see Ulcer, pressure, by site; Ulcer, pressure, stage 2, buttock. For code L97.421, the Alphabetic Index main term is Ulcer, subterm lower limb, heel, left, with skin breakdown only. For codes G30.9 and F02.80, the Alphabetic Index main term is Disease, subterm Alzheimer's.

ICD-10-PCS Rationale: For code 0KBN0ZZ, the Alphabetic Index main term is Excision, subterms muscle, hip, right. For code 0HBNXZZ, the Alphabetic Index main term is Excision, subterms skin, foot, left.

4.46. 172.5-Y, 493.92-N, 86.4, 86.63, 93.94

Rationale: The melanoma is listed first. The procedure codes reflect the wide excision and the full-thickness skin graft.

ICD-10-CM Code(s): C43.59, J45.901

ICD-10-PCS Code(s): 0HB6XZZ, 0HR6X73, 0HBJXZZ, 3E0F7GC

ICD-10-CM Rationale: For code C43.59, the Alphabetic Index main term is Melanoma, subterms skin, back. For code J45.901, the Alphabetic Index main term is Asthma, subterms with, exacerbation (acute).

ICD-10-PCS Rationale: For code 0HB6XZZ, the Alphabetic Index main term is Excision, subterms skin, back. For code 0HR6X73, the main term is Replacement, subterms skin, back. For code 0HBJXZZ, the Alphabetic Index main term is Excision, subterms skin, upper leg, left. For code 3E0F7GC, the Alphabetic Index main term is Introduction, subterm respiratory tract.

Behavioral Health Conditions

4.47.   a. 291.81, 303.01, 94.63, 94.39

Incorrect answer. When a patient experiences alcohol withdrawal symptoms, one of three codes will apply (291.0, 291.3, or 291.81). Code 291.0 takes precedence over the other two, and 291.3 takes precedence over 291.81. In this case, the patient experienced delirium tremens (DTs); code 291.0 is assigned. See "Excludes" note for 291.3 and 291.81 (*Coding Clinic* 1991, 2Q:9–13).

b. 291.81, 303.90, 94.62, 94.39

Incorrect answer. When a patient experiences alcohol withdrawal symptoms, one of three codes will apply (291.0, 291.3, or 291.81). Code 291.0 takes precedence over the other two, and 291.3 takes precedence over 291.81. In this case, the patient experienced delirium tremens (DTs) and code 291.0 is assigned. See "Excludes" note for 291.3 and 291.81 (*Coding Clinic* 1991, 2Q:9–13). The documentation supports assignment of code 303.01, which indicates acute alcoholic intoxication, continuous. Code 94.63 is correct, as the patient was admitted for both rehab and detox.

c. 291.0, 303.01, 94.63, 94.39

Correct answer.

d. 291.0, 303.90, 94.62, 94.39

Incorrect answer. The documentation supports assignment of code 303.01, which indicates acute alcoholic intoxication, continuous. Code 94.63 is correct, as the patient was admitted for both rehab and detox.

ICD-10-CM Code(s): F10.221

ICD-10-PCS Code(s): HZ2ZZZZ, HZ37ZZZ

ICD-10-CM Rationale: The Alphabetic Index main term is Alcohol, subterms delirium (withdrawal), with intoxication, in, dependence.

ICD-10-PCS Rationale: For code HZ2ZZZZ, the Alphabetic Index main term is Detoxification Services, for substance abuse. For code HZ37ZZZ, the Alphabetic Index main term is Counseling, subterm motivational enhancement.

4.48.   296.24-Y, 94.27, 94.22, 94.08, MS-DRG: 885

Rationale: The procedures assigned would be according to the hospital policy for assigning ICD-9-CM codes for nonsurgical procedures.

ICD-10-CM Code(s): F32.3

ICD-10-PCS Code(s): GZB0ZZZ, GZ3ZZZZ, GZ11ZZZ, GZ13ZZZ

ICD-10-CM Rationale: The Alphabetic Index main term is Disorder, subterms depressive, major, with psychotic symptoms.

ICD-10-PCS Rationale: For code GZB0ZZZ, the Alphabetic Index main term is Electroconvulsive Therapy, subterm electroconvulsive therapy, unilateral-single seizure. For code GZ3ZZZZ, the Alphabetic Index main term is Medication Management. For code GZ11ZZZ, the Alphabetic Index main term is Psychological Tests, subterm personality and behavioral. For code GZ13ZZZ, the Alphabetic Index main term is Psychological Tests, subterm neuropsychological.

4.49. 331.0-Y, 294.11-Y, 891.0-Y, V40.31, E888.9-Y, E849.4, E000.9, 86.59, MS-DRG: 057

Rationale: Code V40.31 is used to indicate wandering in diseases classified elsewhere.

ICD-10-CM Code(s): G30.9, F02.81, S81.011A, W19.xxxA, Y92.830, Y99.9

ICD-10-PCS Code(s): 0JQN0ZZ

ICD-10-CM Rationale: For codes G30.9 and F02.81, the Alphabetic Index main term is Disease, subterm Alzheimer's, with behavior disturbance. For code S81.011A, the Alphabetic Index main term is Laceration, subterm knee. For code W19.xxxA, the Alphabetic Index main term is Fall. For code Y92.830, the Alphabetic Index main term is Place of occurrence, subterm park (public). For code Y99.9, the Alphabetic Index main term is External cause status.

ICD-10-PCS Rationale: The Alphabetic Index main term is Repair, subterms subcutaneous tissue and fascia, lower leg, right.

4.50. 303.01-Y

Rationale: Only one code is assigned for acute and chronic alcoholism, and it was present at the time of admission. The acute inebriation is included in code 303.01. It would be incorrect to assign a code from the 305 category (*Coding Clinic* 1991, 2Q:9–13).

ICD-10-CM Code(s): F10.229

ICD-10-CM Rationale: The Alphabetic Index main term is Alcohol, subterms intoxication, with, dependence.

4.51. 491.21-Y, 293.84-Y, 244.9-Y, 305.1-Y, MS-DRG: 192

Rationale: Code 293.84 is assigned when the anxiety is due to an organic condition (hypothyroidism) (*Coding Clinic* 1996, 4Q:29). The POA indicator is assigned as Y (yes) according to POA guidelines for combination codes that identify both the chronic condition and the acute exacerbation if all parts of the combination code were present on admission.

ICD-10-CM Code(s): J44.1, F06.4, E03.9, F17.210

ICD-10-CM Rationale: For code J44.1, the Alphabetic Index main term is Disease, subterms lung, obstructive (chronic), with, acute, exacerbation NEC. For code F06.4, the Alphabetic Index main term is Disorder, subterms anxiety, due to, general medical condition. For code E03.9, the Alphabetic Index main term is Hypothyroidism. For code F17.210, the Alphabetic Index main term is Smoker—see Dependence, drug, nicotine; Dependence, drug, nicotine, cigarettes.

Disorders of the Musculoskeletal System and Connective Tissue

4.52. 825.25-Y, 79.37, 78.18

Rationale: Open reduction, internal fixation should be coded. The type of external fixator would be coded if documented in the record.

ICD-10-CM Code(s): S92.322A

ICD-10-PCS Code(s): 0QSP04Z, 0QHP04Z

ICD-10-CM Rationale: The Alphabetic Index main term is Fracture, subterms metatarsal bone, second.

ICD-10-PCS Rationale: For code 0QSP04Z, the Alphabetic Index main term is Reposition, subterms metatarsal, left. For code 0QHP04Z, the Alphabetic Index main term is Insertion of device in, subterms metatarsal, left.

4.53. 996.66-Y, V43.64, 00.70, 00.74, MS-DRG: 468

Rationale: "Any time the joint is replaced or revised after the initial replacement would be considered a revision." (*Coding Clinic* 1996, 2Q:13, 1997 3Q:13)

ICD-10-CM Code(s): T84.51xA

ICD-10-PCS Code(s): 0SRB0J5, 0SR90J5, 0SP90JZ

ICD-10-CM Rationale: For code T84.51xA, the Alphabetic Index main term is Complication, subterms joint prosthesis, infection or inflammation, hip.

ICD-10-PCS Rationale: For code 0SRB0J5, the Alphabetic Index main term is Replacement, subterms joint, hip, left. For code 0SR90J5, the Alphabetic Index main term is Replacement, subterms joint, hip, right. For code 0SP90JZ, the Alphabetic Index main term is Removal of device from, subterms joint, hip, right.

4.54. a. 718.31, 81.82

Correct answer.

b. 718.31, 81.82, 83.5

Incorrect answer. Bursectomy is included in acromioplasty.

c. 831.00, 81.82, 83.5

Incorrect answer. Dislocation is not acute; it is stated as recurrent. Bursectomy is included in acromioplasty.

d. 831.00, 81.82, 83.5, 80.41

Incorrect answer. Dislocation is not acute; it is stated as recurrent. Bursectomy and division of ligament are included in acromioplasty.

ICD-10-CM Code(s): M24.412

ICD-10-PCS Code(s): 0RQK0ZZ

ICD-10-CM Rationale: The Alphabetic Index main term is Dislocation, subterms recurrent, shoulder.

ICD-10-PCS Rationale: The Alphabetic Index main term is Repair, subterm joint, shoulder, left.

4.55. a. 722.52, 721.3, 414.00, 401.9, V45.81, V45.82, 03.92, 99.23, 88.93

Correct answer.

Rationale: It is appropriate to assign both 03.92, Injection of other agent into spinal canal, and 99.23, Injection of steroid, for a single injection of steroid into the spinal canal. This code assignment may be repeated for each injection (*Coding Clinic* 2000, 3Q:15).

b. 722.52, 721.3, 724.02, 724.4, 414.00, 401.9, V45.81, V45.82, 03.92, 99.23, 88.93

Incorrect answer. Codes 724.02 and 724.4 should not be assigned. Symptoms and signs associated with (due to) spondylosis and allied disorders or intervertebral disc disorders are included in the 721–722 code series (*Coding Clinic* 1989, 2Q:14). If the physician had stated the lumbar stenosis was not attributable to the displaced disc it would have been assigned (*Coding Clinic* 1994, 3Q:14).

c. 724.4, 414.00, 401.9, V45.81, V45.82, 03.92, 99.23, 88.93

Incorrect answer. The patient has lumbar degenerative disc disease. Code 722.52 should be assigned as the principal diagnosis. Code 724.4 should not be assigned. Symptoms and signs associated with (due to) intervertebral disc disorders are included in the 721–722 code series (*Coding Clinic* 1989, 2Q:14). The arthritis requires a code assignment also.

d. 722.52, 721.3, 414.00, 401.9, V45.81, V45.82, 03.91, 88.93

Incorrect answer. The procedure performed was steroid injections, code 03.92. Code 03.92 does not identify the specific agent injected. Therefore, it would be appropriate to assign both codes 03.92 and 99.23, Injection of steroid, for a single injection of steroid into the spinal canal. This code assignment may be repeated for each injection (*Coding Clinic* 2000, 3Q:15).

ICD-10-CM Code(s): M51.16, M47.26, I25.10, I10, Z95.1, Z95.5

ICD-10-PCS Code(s): 3E0S33Z, BR39ZZZ

ICD-10-CM Rationale: For code M51.16, the Alphabetic Index main term is Disorder, subterms disc, with, radiculopathy, lumbar region. For code M47.26, the Alphabetic Index main term is Osteoarthritis, subterm spine—see Spondylosis; Spondylosis, with, radiculopathy, lumbar region. For code I25.10, the Alphabetic Index main term is Disease, subterms artery, coronary. For code I10, the Alphabetic Index main term is Hypertension. For code Z95.1, the Alphabetic Index main term is Status, subterm aortocoronary bypass. For code Z98.61, the Alphabetic Index main term is Status, subterms angioplasty, coronary artery, with implant.

ICD-10-PCS Rationale: For code 3E0S33Z, the Alphabetic Index main term is Introduction, subterm epidural space, anti-inflammatory. For code BR39ZZZ, the Alphabetic Index main term is Magnetic Resonance Imaging, subterms spine, lumbar.

4.56. 733.13-Y, 733.01-Y, 03.91

Rationale: This is coded as a pathologic fracture because it is due to disease process rather than trauma. Both conditions were present on admission.

ICD-10-CM Code(s): M80.08xA

ICD-10-PCS Code(s): 3E0R3BZ

ICD-10-CM Rationale: The Alphabetic Index main term is Osteoporosis, subterm senile—see Osteoporosis, age-related; Osteoporosis, age-related, with current pathological fracture, vertebra.

ICD-10-PCS Rationale: The Alphabetic Index main term is Introduction, subterm spinal canal, anesthetic, local.

4.57. a. 80.51

Incorrect answer. The discectomy only includes the removal of the disc, not the insertion of the prosthetic device.

b. 80.51, 84.65

Incorrect answer. The discectomy is included in the spinal disc replacement device codes and is not separately assigned.

c. 84.65, 80.51

Incorrect answer. The discectomy is included in the spinal disc replacement device codes and is not separately assigned.

d. 84.65

Correct answer.

ICD-10-PCS Code(s): 0SR20JZ

ICD-10-PCS Rationale: The Alphabetic Index main term is Replacement, subterms disc, lumbar vertebral.

4.58. 77.34

Note: The capitate and lunate are carpal bones found in the wrist.

ICD-10-PCS Code(s): 0P8M0ZZ, 0P8M0ZZ

ICD-10-PCS Rationale: The Alphabetic Index main term is Division, subterms carpal, right. Note: Coding guideline B3.2.b states when performed during the same operative episode, multiple procedures are coded if the same root operation is repeated at different body sites that are included in the same body part value.

4.59. Principal diagnosis: 820.8-Y

Additional diagnoses: 428.0-Y, 492.8-Y, 714.0-Y, 733.00-Y, V15.82, V58.65, V58.68, E884.5-Y, E849.0, E000.8, E013.4

Procedure: 81.52

MS-DRG: 470

Rationale: It is appropriate to code an acute fracture in this case because the physician did not identify the fracture as pathological or correlate the osteoporosis to the fracture in any way. All conditions were present on admission. Code V15.82 is exempt from POA reporting. Assign a code from subcategory V58.6 if the patient is receiving a medication for an extended period as a prophylactic measure, treatment of a chronic condition, or a disease that requires a lengthy course of treatment. Do not assign for medication being administered for a brief period of time, medications for detoxification or maintenance programs, or to treat an acute illness or injury (*ICD-9-CM Official Guidelines for Coding and Reporting*). Category V58 is exempt from POA reporting. Codes E849.0, E000.8, and E013.4 are exempt from POA reporting.

ICD-10-CM Code(s): S72.001A, I50.9, J43.9, M06.9, M81.0, Z87.891, Z79.52, Z79.899, W08.xxxA, Y92.030, Y99.8, Y93.e9

ICD-10-PCS Code(s): 0SRR0JF

ICD-10-CM Rationale: For code S72.001A, the Alphabetic Index main term is Fracture, subterms femur, upper end, neck. For code I50.9, the Alphabetic Index main term is Failure, subterms heart, congestive. For code J43.9, the Alphabetic Index main term is Emphysema. For code M06.9, the Alphabetic Index main term is Arthritis, subterm rheumatoid. For code M81.0, the Alphabetic Index main term is Osteoporosis. For code Z87.891, the Alphabetic Index main term is History, subterms personal, tobacco dependence. For code Z79.52, the Alphabetic Index main term is Long-term drug therapy, subterms steroids, systemic. For code Z79.899, the Alphabetic Index main term is Long-term drug therapy, subterm drug, specified NEC. For code W08.xxxA, the Alphabetic Index main term is Fall, subterms from, off, out of, furniture NEC. For code Y92.030, the Alphabetic Index main term is Place of occurrence, subterms residence, apartment, kitchen. For code Y99.8, the Alphabetic Index main term is External cause status, subterm specified NEC. For code Y93.e9, the Alphabetic Index main term is Activity, subterm household maintenance NEC.

ICD-10-PCS Rationale: The Alphabetic Index main term is Replacement, subterms joint, hip, right, femoral surface.

Neoplasms

4.60. a. 338.3, 199.1, V10.3, 276.51, 250.02, 428.0
Correct answer.

b. 174.9, 276.51, 250.02, 428.0
Incorrect answer. The breast carcinoma was excised three years ago. Therefore, report history of breast cancer V10.3. The widespread metastatic carcinoma, 199.0, is causing the pain and is sequenced as a secondary diagnosis. The reason for the admission is the neoplasm-related pain. Sequence the 338.3 as the principal diagnosis. See *Coding Clinic* (2008, 4Q:231–235).

c. 199.1, V10.3, 276.51, 250.02, 428.0

Incorrect answer. The widespread metastatic carcinoma, 199.0, is causing the pain and is sequenced as a secondary diagnosis. The reason for the admission is the neoplasm-related pain; sequence the 338.3 as the principal diagnosis. See *Coding Clinic* (2008, 4Q:231–235).

d. 786.59, 199.1, 276.51, 250.02, 428.0

Incorrect answer. Per *ICD-9-CM Official Guidelines for Coding and Reporting,* "General Coding Guidelines" state that signs and symptoms are acceptable for reporting when a related definitive condition has not been established (confirmed) by the provider. The neoplasm-related pain is documented by the physician; therefore, delete the 786.59 symptom code and assign 338.3 as the principal diagnosis. The breast carcinoma was excised three years ago. Therefore, report history of breast cancer V10.3.

ICD-10-CM Code(s): G89.3, C79.9, Z85.3, E86.0, E11.65, I50.9

ICD-10-CM Rationale: For code G89.3, the Alphabetic Index main term is Pain, subterms acute, neoplasm related. For code C79.9 refer to the ICD-10-CM *Official Guidelines for Coding and Reporting.* For code Z85.3, the Alphabetic Index main term is History, subterms personal, malignant neoplasm, breast. For code E86.0, the Alphabetic Index main term is Dehydration. For code E11.65, the Alphabetic Index main term is Diabetes, subterm inadequately controlled—code to Diabetes, by type, with hyperglycemia; Diabetes, type 2, with hyperglycemia. For code I50.9, the Alphabetic Index main term is Failure, subterms heart, congestive.

4.61. 162.9-Y, 492.8-Y, 33.24, 33.27, MS-DRG: 168

Rationale: Code 33.24, closed biopsy of bronchus, is assigned for the bronchoalveolar lavage. Code 33.27, closed endoscopic biopsy of lung, is assigned for the biopsy of the lung. *Coding Clinic* (2009, 4Q:9–10).

ICD-10-CM Code(s): C34.12, J43.9

ICD-10-PCS Code(s): 0B9G8ZX, 0B988ZX

ICD-10-CM Rationale: For code C34.12, the Alphabetic Index main term is Neoplasm, subterms lung, upper lobe, malignant primary. For code J43.9, the Alphabetic Index main term is Emphysema.

ICD-10-PCS Rationale: For code 0B9G8ZX, the Alphabetic Index main term is Drainage, subterms lung, upper lobe, left. For code 0B988ZX, the Alphabetic Index main term is Drainage, subterms bronchus, upper lobe, left.

4.62. 276.51-Y, 174.9-Y, 197.7-Y, 198.3-Y, MS-DRG: 641

Rationale: See *ICD-9-CM Official Guidelines for Coding and Reporting* "Neoplasm" guidelines. Because the focus of the admission and treatment was for the dehydration, it meets principal diagnosis reporting. There is no mention that the breast cancer has been resected; therefore, it is coded as current. All conditions were present on admission with a Y indicator assigned.

ICD-10-CM Code(s): E86.0, C50.919, C78.7, C79.31

ICD-10-CM Rationale: For code E86.0, the Alphabetic Index main term is Dehydration. For code C50.919, the Alphabetic Index main term is Neoplasm, subterm breast, malignant primary. For code C78.7, the Alphabetic Index main term is Neoplasm, subterms liver, malignant secondary. For code C79.31, the Alphabetic Index main term is Neoplasm, subterms brain, malignant secondary.

4.63. 198.3-Y, 196.3-Y, V10.3

Rationale: The reason for admission is the metastatic brain cancer. The breast cancer was excised, so it is coded as history. The mets to the axillary lymph nodes should be coded. Both metastatic conditions were present at the time of admission and a POA indicator of Y is assigned. Category V10 is on the POA exempt list. Therefore, no indicator is assigned to V10.3.

ICD-10-CM Code(s): C79.31, C77.3, Z85.3

ICD-10-CM Rationale: For code C79.31, the Alphabetic Index main term is Neoplasm, subterms brain, malignant secondary. For code C77.3, the Alphabetic Index main term is Neoplasm, subterms lymph, gland, axilla, malignant secondary. For code Z85.3, the Alphabetic Index main term is History, subterms personal, malignant neoplasm, breast.

4.64. a. V58.11, 155.0

Incorrect answer. Code 996.32 should be assigned for complication of liver transplant along with code 199.2 for malignancy associated with organ transplant.

b. V58.11, 155.0, 199.2

Incorrect answer. Code 996.32 should be assigned for complication of liver transplant.

c. V58.11, 996.82, 155.0, 199.2

Correct answer.

d. 996.82, 155.0, 199.2

Incorrect answer. The patient was admitted for chemotherapy. Code V58.11, encounter for antineoplastic chemotherapy, should be assigned as the principal diagnosis.

ICD-10-CM Code(s): Z51.11, T86.49, C80.2, C22.0

ICD-10-CM Rationale: For code Z51.11, the Alphabetic Index main term is Chemotherapy, subterm cancer. For code T86.49, the Alphabetic Index main term is Complication, transplant, liver, specified type NEC. For code C80.2, the Alphabetic Index main term is Neoplasm, subterm associated with transplanted organ, malignant primary. For code C22.0, the Alphabetic Index main term is Hepatocarcinoma.

4.65. 183.0-Y, 197.6-Y, 68.69, 65.61, 54.4, MS-DRG: 734

Rationale: The hysterectomy was a radical one, the "Code Also" note instructs the coder to assign BSO in addition, and the omentectomy meets procedure coding guidelines.

ICD-10-CM Code(s): C56.2, C78.6

ICD-10-PCS Code(s): 0DTS0ZZ, 0DTT0ZZ, 0UT90ZZ, 0UTC0ZZ, 0UBG0ZZ, 0UT20ZZ, 0UT70ZZ

ICD-10-CM Rationale: For code C56.2, the Alphabetic Index main term is Neoplasm, subterms ovary, malignant primary. For code C78.6, the Alphabetic Index main term is Neoplasm, subterms omentum, malignant secondary.

ICD-10-PCS Rationale: For code 0DTS0ZZ, the Alphabetic Index main term is Resection, subterms omentum, greater. For code 0DTT0ZZ, the Alphabetic Index main term is Resection, subterms omentum, lesser. For code 0UT90ZZ, the Alphabetic Index main term is Resection, subterm uterus. For code 0UTC0ZZ, the Alphabetic Index main term is Resection, subterm cervix. For code 0UT20ZZ, the Alphabetic Index main term is Resection, subterms ovary, bilateral. For code 0UT70ZZ, the Alphabetic Index main term is Resection, subterm fallopian tubes, bilateral. Only part of the vagina was removed so the root operation is excision.

4.66. 285.3-Y, 157.0-Y

Note: When the admission/encounter is for management of an anemia associated with chemotherapy, immunotherapy, or radiotherapy and the only treatment is for the anemia, the anemia is sequenced first. The appropriate neoplasm code should be assigned as an additional code. (*ICD-9-CM Official Guidelines for Coding and Reporting*) Code E933.1, Antineoplastic and immunosuppressive drugs, is optional since the information regarding an adverse effect of a chemotherapy drug is included in code 285.3. *Coding Clinic* (2009, 4Q:60)

ICD-10-CM Code(s): T45.1x5A, D64.81, C25.0

ICD-10-CM Rationale: For code T45.1x5A, the Alphabetic Index main term is Antineoplastic NEC, subterm adverse effect. For code D64.81, the Alphabetic Index main term is Anemia, subterms due to, antineoplastic chemotherapy. For code C25.0, the Alphabetic Index main term is Neoplasm, subterms pancreas, head, malignant primary.

Disorders of the Nervous System and Sense Organs

4.67. a. 996.2, 331.4, 326, 02.42, 87.02, 87.03
Correct answer.

b. 331.4, 326, 02.42, 87.02, 87.03

Incorrect answer. The reason for admission was for the shunt malfunction (code 996.2).

c. 996.63, 331.4, 02.42

Incorrect answer. The shunt was not infected. Additional codes should be assigned for the late effect of meningoencephalitis, CT scan, and pneumocisternogram.

d. 996.2, 02.42, 87.03

Incorrect answer. Additional codes should be assigned for the hydrocephalus, late effect of meningoencephalitis, and pneumocisternogram.

ICD-10-CM Code(s): T85.01xA, G91.1, G09

ICD-10-PCS Code(s): 00H602Z, 00P602Z, B0201ZZ

ICD-10-CM Rationale: For code T85.01xA, the Alphabetic Index main term is Malfunction, subterm ventricular. For code G91.1, the Alphabetic Index main term is Hydrocephalus, subterm obstructive. For code G09, the Alphabetic Index main term is Sequelae, subterm encephalitis or encephalomyelitis.

ICD-10-PCS Rationale: For code 00H602Z, the Alphabetic Index main term is Insertion of device in, subterm cerebral ventricle. For code 00P602Z, the Alphabetic Index main term is Removal of device from, subterm cerebral ventricle. For code B0201ZZ, the Alphabetic Index main term is Computerized Tomography, subterm brain. Note: The pneumocisternogram also requires coding but the summary does not include enough detail to assign an ICD-10-PCS code.

4.68. 345.51-Y, 348.81-Y, 01.59, 01.18

Rationale: The epilepsy is documented as intractable, partial. Subcategory 345.4 would not be correct because there was not documentation of impairment of consciousness. The procedure code is 01.59. Code 01.39 is not correct because it is for amygdalohippocampotomy. The POA indicator is Y, as epilepsy was present on admission.

ICD-10-CM Code(s): G40.919, G93.81

ICD-10-PCS Code(s): 00B00ZZ, 00K00ZZ

ICD-10-CM Rationale: For code G40.919, the Alphabetic Index main term is Epilepsy, subterm intractable. For code G93.81, the Alphabetic Index main term is Sclerosis, subterm temporal.

ICD-10-PCS Rationale: For code 00B00ZZ, the Alphabetic Index main term is Excision, subterm brain. For code 00K00ZZ, the Alphabetic Index main term is Map, subterm brain.

4.69. 320.1-Y, 481-Y, 03.31, MS-DRG: 094

Rationale: The patient had both meningitis and pneumonia, so both should be coded. The spinal tap should also be coded. Both conditions were present at the time of admission. Therefore, the POA indicator is Y.

ICD-10-CM Code(s): G00.1, J13

ICD-10-PCS Code(s): 009Y3ZX

ICD-10-CM Rationale: For code G00.1, the Alphabetic Index main term is Meningitis, subterm pneumococcal. For code J13, the Alphabetic Index main term is Pneumonia. subterm pneumococcal.

ICD-10-PCS Rationale: The Alphabetic Index main term is Drainage, subterms spinal cord, lumbar.

4.70. 437.3-Y, 38.41, 88.41

Rationale: If the aneurysm was ruptured, then code 430 would be assigned, but in this case the documentation states that it is nonruptured. The POA indicator is Y, as the condition was present on admission. Subcategory codes 38.3 and 38.4 involve surgical removal of aneurysm with restoration of continuity of blood vessel. The former is used with restoration of continuity by anastomosis of the involved vessel after the aneurysm has been excised and the latter is used where the synthetic or venous graft is used for the arterial replacement (*Coding Clinic* 1984, Nov–Dec:10).

ICD-10-CM Code(s): I67.1

ICD-10-PCS Code(s): 03RG0JZ

ICD-10-CM Rationale: The Alphabetic Index main term is Aneurysm, subterms arteriosclerotic, cerebral.

ICD-10-PCS Rationale: The Alphabetic Index main term is Replacement, subterms artery, intracranial. Note: The cerebral angiogram also requires coding but the summary does not include enough detail to assign an ICD-10-PCS code.

4.71. a. 434.91, 438.21, 438.12, 250.00, 305.1, 88.91, 93.39, 93.72

Incorrect answer. This is an acute event. Therefore, code 342.91 and code 784.59 are assigned as additional diagnoses to identify the current neurologic deficits that resulted from the cerebral infarction. When codes from the 430–437 series are used, additional codes are needed to identify any sequelae present, such as category 342 for any associated hemiplegia (*Coding Clinic* 1998, 4Q:87).

b. 434.91, 342.91, 784.59, 250.00, 305.1, 88.91, 93.39, 93.74

Incorrect answer. The patient was receiving speech therapy for dysphasia.

c. 436, 250.00, 305.1, 88.91, 93.39, 93.74

Incorrect answer. The terms stroke and CVA are often used interchangeably to refer to a cerebral infarction. The terms stroke, CVA, and cerebral infarction NOS are all indexed to the default code 434.91, Cerebral artery occlusion, unspecified, with infarction. Code 436, Acute, but ill-defined, cerebrovascular disease, should not be used when the documentation states stroke or CVA (*ICD-9-CM Official Coding Guidelines*). Code 342.91 and code 784.59 are assigned as additional diagnoses to identify the current neurologic deficits that resulted from the cerebral infarction. When codes from the 430–437 series are used, additional codes are needed to identify any sequelae present, such as category 342 for any associated hemiplegia (*Coding Clinic* 1998, 4Q:87). The patient was receiving speech therapy for dysphasia.

d. 434.91, 342.91, 784.59, 250.00, 305.1, 88.91, 93.39, 93.72

Correct answer.

ICD-10-CM Code(s): I63.512, G81.91, R47.02, E11.9, Z72.0

ICD-10-PCS Code(s): B030Y0Z

ICD-10-CM Rationale: For code I63.512, the Alphabetic Index main term is Infarct, subterms cerebral, due to, occlusion, cerebral arteries. For code G81.91, the Alphabetic Index main term is Hemiplegia. For code R47.02, the Alphabetic Index main term is Dysphasia. For code E11.9, the Alphabetic Index main term is Diabetes, subterm type 2. For code Z72.0, the Alphabetic Index main term is Tobacco, subterm harmful use.

ICD-10-PCS Rationale: The Alphabetic Index main term is Magnetic Resonance Imaging, subterm brain. Note: Physical therapy and speech therapy cannot be assigned a code without further information. The first three characters of the code for speech therapy would be F06 and for physical therapy F07.

Newborn/Congenital Disorders

4.72. a. 749.02, 749.12, 27.62, 27.54

Incorrect answer. There is one diagnosis code that includes both the cleft lip and palate, 749.22.

b. 749.22, 27.54, 27.63

Incorrect answer. The 27.63 code is for revision of a previous cleft palate repair.

c. 749.02, 749.12, 27.69

Incorrect answer. There is one diagnosis code that includes both the cleft lip and palate, 749.22. The procedure code 27.69 is an unspecified code. The more specific procedure codes of 27.62 and 27.54 should be used.

d. 749.22, 27.62, 27.54

Correct answer.

ICD-10-CM Code(s): Q37.3

ICD-10-PCS Code(s): 0CQ3XZZ, 0CQ0XZZ

ICD-10-CM Rationale: The Alphabetic Index main term is Cleft, subterms lip, with cleft palate, soft.

ICD-10-PCS Rationale: For code 0CQ3XZZ, the Alphabetic Index main term is Repair, subterms palate, soft. For code 0CQ0XZZ, the Alphabetic Index main term is Repair, subterms lip, upper.

4.73. 771.4-Y, 041.11-Y, 041.09-Y

Rationale: Category 041 codes are used as an additional code to identify the bacterial agent in diseases classified elsewhere. ICD-9-CM does not have a specific code for Group H Streptococcus. Therefore, code 041.09, other Streptococcus, is correct. All conditions are present on admission.

ICD-10-CM Code(s): P38.9, B95.6, B95.4

ICD-10-CM Rationale: For code P38.9, the Alphabetic Index main term is Omphalitis. For code B95.6, the Alphabetic Index main term is Staphylococcus, subterm aureus, as cause of disease classified elsewhere. For code B95.4, the Alphabetic Index main term is Streptococcus, subterm specified NEC, as cause of disease classified elsewhere.

4.74. a. V30.01, 765.03, 765.24

Incorrect answer. A diagnosis code is needed for the respiratory distress syndrome, 769.

b. 765.03, 769

Incorrect answer. A birth code of V30.01 is reported as the principal diagnosis (*ICD-9-CM Official Guidelines for Coding and Reporting*; *Coding Clinic* 2006, 4Q:190). See instructional note under 765.0x to Use Additional Code for weeks of gestation.

c. V30.01, 765.03, 765.24, 769

Correct answer.

d. V30.01, 769

Incorrect answer. The code for prematurity, 765.03, and code 765.24 for weeks of gestation meet reporting guidelines as additional diagnoses.

ICD-10-CM Code(s): Z38.01, P07.03, P07.23, P22.0

ICD-10-CM Rationale: For code Z38.01, the Alphabetic Index main term is Newborn, subterm born in hospital, by cesarean. For code P07.03, the Alphabetic Index main term is Low, subterms birthweight, extreme, with weight of, 750–999 grams. For code P07.23, the Alphabetic Index main term is Immaturity, subterms extreme, with gestation of, 27 weeks. For code P22.0, the Alphabetic Index main term is Syndrome, subterms respiratory, distress, newborn.

4.75. V30.00, 747.10, 745.4, 755.01, 754.79, 755.58

Note: Assign an appropriate code from categories 740–759, Congenital Anomalies, when a specific abnormality is diagnosed for an infant. Such abnormalities may occur as a set of symptoms or multiple malformations. A code should be assigned for each presenting manifestation of the syndrome if the syndrome is not specifically indexed in ICD-9-CM (*ICD-9-CM Official Guidelines for Coding and Reporting*). All codes are POA exempt.

ICD-10-CM Code(s): Z38.00, Q25.1, Q21.0, Q69.1, Q66.8, Q68.1

ICD-10-CM Rationale: For Z38.00, the Alphabetic Index main term is Newborn, subterm born in hospital. For Q25.1, the Alphabetic Index main term is Coarctation of aorta. For Q21.0, the Alphabetic Index main term is Defect, subterms septal, ventricular. For Q69.1, the Alphabetic Index main term is Accessory, subterm thumb. There is no Index entry for cleft hand or foot. The Index entry of Deformity provides codes for both feet and hands. There is another Index option for the Cleft Deformities that produces different codes than the ones obtained by following Deformity. Cleft—see Imperfect closure, Organ or site not listed—see anomaly by site. Under Anomaly, anomalous, there are choices for hand (Q74.0) and foot (Q74.2). After review of the Tabular List, the Q66.8 and Q68.1 codes seem to provide better specificity.

4.76. V30.00, 760.71-Y

Rationale: Because there is no documentation of drug withdrawal, code 760.71 is the best choice. The physician could be queried when reviewing the actual medical record. No POA indicator is assigned to V30.00, as V30–V39 are listed on the POA exempt list.

ICD-10-CM Code(s): Z38.00, Q86.0

ICD-10-CM Rationale: For Z38.00, the Alphabetic Index main term is Newborn, subterm born in hospital. For Q86.0, the Alphabetic Index main term is Syndrome, subterm fetal, alcohol. Because there is no documentation of drug withdrawal, code Q86.0 is the best choice. The physician could be queried when reviewing the actual medical record to determine if P96.1 should be assigned.

Pediatric Conditions

4.77. 945.34-Y, 942.34-Y, 948.10-Y, MS-DRG: 934

Rationale: The highest-degree burn on the lower leg is reported with code 945.34, and the highest-degree burn on the back should also be coded.

ICD-10-CM Code(s): T24.302A, T21.34xA, T31.10

ICD-10-CM Rationale: For T24.302A, the Alphabetic Index main term is Burn, subterms lower, limb, left, third degree. For T21.34xA, the Alphabetic Index main term is Burn, subterms back (lower), third degree. For T31.10, the Alphabetic Index main term is Burn, subterms extent, 10–19 percent, with 0–9 percent third degree.

4.78. a. 201.21, 40.40, 92.29

Incorrect answer. Lymph node biopsy is coded to 40.11. Megavoltage radiotherapy is assigned to a more specific code of 92.24.

b. 201.91, 40.40, 92.29

Incorrect answer. Hodgkin's sarcoma is assigned to code 201.21. Lymph node biopsy is coded to 40.11. Megavoltage radiotherapy is assigned to a more specific code of 92.24.

c. 201.21, 40.11, 92.24

Correct answer.

d. 201.91, 40.11, 92.24

Incorrect answer. Hodgkin's sarcoma is assigned to code 201.21.

ICD-10-CM Code(s): C81.91

ICD-10-PCS Code(s): 07B20ZX

ICD-10-CM Rationale: The Alphabetic Index main term is Sarcoma, subterm Hodgkin—see Lymphoma, Hodgkin.

ICD-10-PCS Rationale: The Alphabetic Index main term is Excision, subterms lymphatic, neck, left. Note: Megavoltage teletherapy is external beam radiotherapy. The first four characters of the ICD-10-PCS code are D703. To assign the remaining characters requires documentation of the type of radiation used and if electrons, whether the procedure was performed intraoperatively.

4.79. 39.50, 39.90, 00.45, 00.40

Rationale: Four codes should be assigned to completely identify the procedure performed. They are: 39.50, angioplasty of other noncoronary vessel; 39.90, insertion of non-drug-eluting peripheral vessel stent(s); 00.45, insertion of one vascular stent; and 00.40, procedure on single vessel, for the insertion of the pulmonary vein stent. *Coding Clinic* (2009, 3Q:13).

ICD-10-PCS Code(s): 027T3DZ

ICD-10-PCS Rationale: The Alphabetic Index main term is Dilation, subterms vein, pulmonary, left.

4.80. a. 008.61, 276.51

Incorrect answer. The patient was admitted for treatment of dehydration. The circumstances of inpatient admission always govern the selection of the principal diagnosis (*Coding Clinic* 2008, 1Q:10–11).

b. 276.51, 558.9

Incorrect answer. The cause of the gastroenteritis was determined to be Rotavirus.

c. 276.51, 008.61

Correct answer.

d. 008.8

Incorrect answer. The cause of the gastroenteritis was determined to be Rotavirus. The dehydration should also be coded as the principal diagnosis.

ICD-10-CM Code(s): E86.0, A08.0

ICD-10-CM Rationale: For E86.0, the Alphabetic Index main term is Dehydration. For A08.0, the Alphabetic Index main term is Gastroenteritis, subterm viral NEC, rotoviral.

4.81. 995.55-Y, 852.23-Y, 361.05-Y, E968.8-Y, E967.8-Y, MS-DRG: 922

Rationale: The shaken infant syndrome code is reported as the principal diagnosis. Instructional note states Use Additional Code(s) to identify associated injuries and Use Additional E-code to identify both the nature of the abuse and the perpetrator per *Coding Clinic* (1996, 4Q:38–43). *ICD-9-CM Official Coding Guidelines for Coding and Reporting and Coding Clinic (2006, 4Q:228)* state that category E967, Perpetrator, goes after the type of assault.

The unconsciousness is not separately coded because it is included as part of the fifth digit reporting in code 852.23. POA indicators are Y (yes), as all were present on admission and none of the codes are on the POA exempt list.

ICD-10-CM Code(s): T74.4xxA, S06.5x4A, H33.051, Y08.89xA, Y07.59

ICD-10-CM Rationale: For T74.4xxA, the Alphabetic Index main term is Syndrome, subterm shaken infant. For S06.5x4A, the Alphabetic Index main term is Hematoma, subdural—see Injury, intracranial, subdural hemorrhage. For H33.051, the Alphabetic Index main term is Detachment, subterm retina, total. For Y08.89xA, the Alphabetic Index main term is Assault, subterm specified means NEC. For Y07.59, the Alphabetic Index main term is Perpetrator, subeterm nonfamily member, specified NEC.

Conditions of Pregnancy, Childbirth, and the Puerperium

4.82.   a. 633.80, 66.62

Incorrect answer. The ectopic pregnancy was documented as tubal.

b. 633.10, 66.62

Correct answer.

c. 633.10, 66.4

Incorrect answer. The salpingectomy was "with removal of tubal pregnancy."

d. 633.10, 66.02

Incorrect answer. The procedure performed was a salpingectomy, not a salpingostomy.

ICD-10-CM Code(s): O00.1

ICD-10-PCS Code(s): 10T24ZZ, 0UT54ZZ

ICD-10-CM Rationale: The Alphabetic Index main term is Pregnancy, subterm tubal.

ICD-10-PCS Rationale: For code 10T24ZZ, the Alphabetic Index main term is Resection, subterm products of conception, ectopic. For code 0UT54ZZ, the Alphabetic Index main term is Resection, subterms fallopian tube, right.

4.83.   a. 635.91, 69.09

Incorrect answer. This was a spontaneous abortion. The D&C should be assigned to code 69.02.

b. 634.91, 69.09

Incorrect answer. The D&C should be assigned to code 69.02.

c. 634.91, 69.02

Correct answer.

d. 635.91, 69.02

Incorrect answer. This was a spontaneous abortion.

ICD-10-CM Code(s): O03.4

ICD-10-PCS Code(s): 10D17ZZ

ICD-10-CM Rationale: The Alphabetic Index main term is Abortion, subterm incomplete.

ICD-10-PCS Rationale: The Alphabetic Index main term is Extraction, subterms products of conception, retained.

4.84. a. 642.41

Correct answer.

b. 659.11

Incorrect answer. The patient was admitted for induction of labor due to pre-eclampsia. In accordance with the UHDDS definition for principal diagnosis, the pre-eclampsia is the reason for admission and sequenced as the principal diagnosis. The *Official Guidelines for Coding and Reporting*, which pertain to selection of obstetric principal diagnosis, state: "When a delivery occurs, the principal diagnosis should correspond to the main circumstances or complication of the delivery. In cases of cesarean delivery, the selection of the principal diagnosis should be the condition established after study that was responsible for the patient's admission. If the patient was admitted with a condition that resulted in the performance of a cesarean procedure, that condition should be selected as the principal diagnosis. If the reason for the admission/encounter was unrelated to the condition resulting in the cesarean delivery, the condition related to the reason for the admission/encounter should be selected as the principal diagnosis, even if a cesarean was performed." (*ICD-9-CM Official Guidelines for Coding and Reporting*; *Coding Clinic* 2009, 4Q:115).

c. 659.01

Incorrect answer. The patient was admitted for induction of labor due to pre-eclampia. In accordance with the UHDDS definition for principal diagnosis, the pre-eclampia is the reason for admission and sequenced as the principal diagnosis. The *Official Guidelines for Coding and Reporting*, which pertain to selection of obstetric principal diagnosis, state: "When a delivery occurs, the principal diagnosis should correspond to the main circumstances or complication of the delivery. In cases of cesarean delivery, the selection of the principal diagnosis should be the condition established after study that was responsible for the patient's admission. If the patient was admitted with a condition that resulted in the performance of a cesarean procedure, that condition should be selected as the principal diagnosis. If the reason for the admission/encounter was unrelated to the condition resulting in the cesarean delivery, the condition related to the reason for the admission/encounter should be selected as the principal diagnosis, even if a cesarean was performed." (*ICD-9-CM Official Guidelines for Coding and Reporting*; *Coding Clinic* 2009, 4Q:115).

d. 652.51

Incorrect answer. The patient was admitted for induction of labor due to pre-eclampsia. In accordance with the UHDDS definition for principal diagnosis, the pre-eclampsia is the reason for admission and sequenced as the principal diagnosis. The *Official Guidelines for Coding and Reporting*, which pertain to selection of obstetric principal diagnosis, state: "When a delivery occurs, the principal diagnosis should correspond to the main circumstances or complication of the delivery. In cases of cesarean delivery, the selection of the principal diagnosis should be the condition established after study that was responsible for the patient's admission. If the patient was admitted with a condition that resulted in the performance of a cesarean procedure, that condition should be selected as the principal diagnosis. If the reason for the admission/encounter was unrelated to the condition resulting in the cesarean delivery, the condition related to the reason for the admission/encounter should be selected as the principal diagnosis, even if a cesarean was performed." (*ICD-9-CM Official Guidelines for Coding and Reporting*; *Coding Clinic* 2009, 4Q:115).

ICD-10-CM Code(s): O14.03

ICD-10-CM Rationale: The Alphabetic Index main term is Pregnancy, subterms complicated by, pre-eclampsia, mild.

4.85. 654.21-Y, 646.81-N, V27.0, 72.1, MS-DRG: 775

Rationale: The previous cesarean delivery code, which is present on admission, is assigned a POA indicator of Y. The fatigue was not present on admission, so a POA indicator of N is assigned. No POA indicator is assigned to V27.0, as category V27 is on the POA exempt list.

ICD-10-CM Code(s): O75.81, O34.21, Z37.0

ICD-10-PCS Code(s): 10D07Z3, 0W8NXZZ

ICD-10-CM Rationale: For O75.81, the Alphabetic Index main term is Exhaustion, subterm maternal, complicating delivery. For O34.21, the Alphabetic Index main term is Cesarean delivery, previous, affecting management of pregnancy. For Z37.0, the Alphabetic Index main term is Outcome of delivery, subterms single, liveborn.

ICD-10-PCS Rationale: For code 10D07Z3, the Alphabetic Index main term is Extraction, subterms products of conception, low forceps. For code 0W8NXZZ, the Alphabetic Index main term is Division, subterm perineum, female.

4.86. 648.83-Y, 646.83-Y, 728.84-Y

Note: Subcategory 648 contains a "use additional code" note instructing coders to use of an additional secondary code to further specify the complication. *Coding Clinic* (1995, 4Q:59)

ICD-10-CM Code(s): O24.410, O99.89, M62.08

ICD-10-CM Rationale: For O24.410, the Alphabetic Index main term is Diabetes, subterms gestational, diet controlled. For O99.89, the Alphabetic Index main term is Pregnancy, subterms complicated by, connective system disorders. For M62.08, the Alphabetic Index main term is Diastasis, subterms muscle, specified site NEC.

Disorders of the Respiratory System

4.87.   a. 491.21

Correct answer.

b. 491.21, 518.82

Incorrect answer. Acute respiratory insufficiency is an integral part of COPD and is, therefore, not coded.

c. 518.81, 491.21

Incorrect answer. The patient had acute respiratory insufficiency, not acute respiratory failure. Acute respiratory insufficiency is an integral part of COPD and is, therefore, not coded.

d. 518.82, 491.21

Incorrect answer. Acute respiratory insufficiency is an integral part of COPD and is, therefore, not coded.

ICD-10-CM Code(s): J44.1

ICD-10-CM Rationale: The Alphabetic Index main term is Disease, subterms lung, obstructive (chronic), with, acute, exacerbation NEC. Acute respiratory insufficiency is an integral part of COPD and is, therefore, not coded.

4.88.   a. 492.8, 276.51, 96.72

Incorrect answer. The dehydration is the reason for admission and should be listed as the principal diagnosis. The code for ventilator-dependent (V46.11) should be listed.

b. 276.51, 492.8, V46.11, 96.72

Correct answer.

c. 276.51, 496, V46.11, 96.71

Incorrect answer. The COPD emphysema should be coded to 492.8. The mechanical ventilation was for 96 continuous hours or more, code 96.72.

d. 492.8, 276.51, V46.11, 96.72

Incorrect answer. The dehydration is the reason for admission and should be listed as the principal diagnosis.

ICD-10-CM Code(s): E86.0, J43.9, Z99.11

ICD-10-PCS Code(s): 5A1955Z

ICD-10-CM Rationale: For E86.0, the Alphabetic Index main term is Dehydration. For J43.9, the Alphabetic Index main term is Emphysema. For Z99.11, the Alphabetic Index main term is Dependence, subterms on, ventilator.

ICD-10-PCS Rationale: The Alphabetic Index main term is Performance, subterms respiratory, greater than 96 consecutive hours, ventilation.

4.89. 486-Y, 276.51-Y, 344.03-Y or 344.04-Y depending on results of physician query, 907.2, V14.0, E929.0, MS-DRG: 193

Rationale: Query the physician to find out if the spinal cord injury was complete or incomplete in order to select the correct code for the quadriplegia. In accordance with *ICD-9-CM Official Guidelines for Coding and Reporting* and *Coding Clinic* (2008, 4Q:206–211), a late effect is the residual effect after the acute phase has ended. Coding requires two codes: one for the condition(s) produced and the late effect code. A late effect E code should be used with any report of a late effect or sequela resulting from a previous injury (*Coding Clinic* 2005, 1Q:90–91). Do not assign a code for hypokalemia unless the physician has included the condition in the discharge statement. There are many factors that may influence a physician's decision to prescribe a medication. It is inappropriate for the coder to assign a code based on the administration of any medication. Query the physician to determine if the patient has hypokalemia, and if so, have it added as a final diagnosis (*Coding Clinic* 1994, 5Q:11). Codes 907.2, V14.0, and E929.0 are POA exempt. All other diagnoses were present on admission.

ICD-10-CM Code(s): J18.9, E86.0, G82.53 or G82.54 depending on results of physician query, S12.400S, S12.500S, S14.105S, S14.106S, Z88.0, V89.2xxS

ICD-10-CM Rationale: For J18.9, the Alphabetic Index main term is Pneumonia. For E86.0, the Alphabetic Index main term is Dehydration. For G82.53 or G82.54, the Alphabetic Index main term is Quadraplegia, subterms complete, C5–C7 level or subterms incomplete, C5–C7 level. For S12.400S, the Alphabetic Index main term is Fracture, subterms neck, cervical vertebra, fifth. For S12.500S, the Alphabetic Index main term is Fracture, subterms neck, cervical vertebra, sixth. For S14.105S, the Alphabetic Index main term is Injury, subterms spinal, cervical, C5 level. For S14.106S, the Alphabetic Index main term is Injury, subterms spinal, cervical, C6 level. For Z88.0, the Alphabetic Index main term is History, subterms personal, allergy, penicillin. For V89.2xxS, the Alphabetic Index main term is Sequelae, subterm motor vehicle accident.

4.90. 493.21-Y

Note: Do not assign an asthma code with fifth digit 2, with acute exacerbation, together with an asthma code with fifth digit 1, with status asthmaticus. Only the fifth digit 1 should be assigned (*ICD-9-CM Official Guidelines for Coding and Reporting*).

ICD-10-CM Code(s): J45.42, J44.1

ICD-10-CM Rationale: For J45.42, the Alphabetic Index main term is Asthma, subterms moderate persistent, with, status asthmaticus. For J44.1, the Alphabetic Index main term is Disease, subterms lung, obstructive (chronic), with, acute, exacerbation NEC.

4.91. 518.81-Y, 482.31-Y, 492.8-Y, 305.1-Y, 96.71, 96.04, MS-DRG: 208

Rationale: *ICD-9-CM Official Guidelines for Coding and Reporting* and *Coding Clinic* (2006, 4Q:178) state acute respiratory failure may be assigned as the principal diagnosis when it is the condition established, after study, to be chiefly responsible for occasioning the admission to the hospital, and the selection is supported by the alphabetic index and tabular list. All conditions are present on admission and assigned a POA indicator of Y (yes).

ICD-10-CM Code(s): J96.00, J15.4, J43.9, F17.210

ICD-10-PCS Code(s): 5A1945Z, 0BH17EZ

ICD-10-CM Rationale: For J96.00, the Alphabetic Index main term is Failure, subterms respiration, respiratory. For J15.4, the Alphabetic Index main term is Pneumonia, subterms streptococcal NEC, group, A. For J43.9, the Alphabetic Index main term is emphysema. For F17.210, the Alphabetic Index main term is Smoker—see Dependence, drug, nicotine; Dependence, drug, nicotine, cigarettes.

ICD-10-PCS Rationale: For code 5A1945Z, the Alphabetic Index main term is Performance, subterms respiratory, 24–96 consecutive hours, ventilation.

Trauma and Poisoning

4.92. a. 852.23, E886.0, E849.4, E007.0, E000.8, 01.31, 88.91, 88.91

Incorrect answer. The patient was unconscious, but the duration is unspecified, so code 852.26 is correct.

b. 852.26, E886.0, E849.4, E007.0, E000.8, 01.31, 88.91, 88.91

Correct answer.

c. 852.33, E886.0, E849.4, E007.0, E000.8, 01.39, 88.91, 88.91

Incorrect answer. This is specified as a subdural hematoma without mention of an open intracranial wound, so code 852.26 is correct. Evacuation of a subdural hematoma is indexed as incision, subdural space, cerebral. Code 01.31 is correct.

d. 852.26, E886.0, E849.4, E007.0, E000.8, 01.39, 88.91, 88.91

Incorrect answer. Evacuation of a subdural hematoma is indexed as incision, subdural space, cerebral. Code 01.31 is correct.

ICD-10-CM Code(s): S06.5x9A, W03.xxxA, Y92.321, Y93.61, Y99.8

ICD-10-PCS Code(s): 00C40ZZ, B030ZZZ, B030ZZZ

ICD-10-CM Rationale: For S06.5x9A, the Alphabetic Index main term is Hematoma, subdural—see Injury, intracranial, subdural hemorrhage. For W03.xxxA, the Alphabetic Index main term is Tackle in sport. For Y92.321, the Alphabetic Index main term is Place of occurrence, subterms sports area, athletic, field, football. For Y93.61, the Alphabetic Index main term is Activity, subterms football, tackle. For Y99.8, the Alphabetic Index main term is Status of external cause, subterm recreation or sport not for income or while a student.

ICD-10-PCS Rationale: For code 00C40ZZ, the Alphabetic Index main term is Extirpation, subterm subdural space. For code B030ZZZ, the Alphabetic Index main term is Magnetic Resonance Imaging, subterm brain.

4.93. 996.41-Y, 332.0-Y, 402.91-Y, 428.0-Y, 365.9-Y, 412, 794.39-Y, V43.65, E878.1-Y

Note: The mechanical complication (aseptic loosening) of the knee prosthesis is sequenced first since it is the reason for the encounter. Abnormal findings (laboratory, x-ray, pathologic, and other diagnostic results) are not coded and reported unless the provider indicates their clinical significance. If the findings are outside the normal range and the attending provider has ordered other tests to evaluate the condition or prescribed treatment, it is appropriate to ask the provider whether the abnormal finding should be added (*ICD-9-CM Official Guidelines for Coding and Reporting*).

ICD-10-CM Code(s): T84.032A, G20, I11.0, I50.9, H40.143, I25.2, R94.39, Y83.1

ICD-10-CM Rationale: For T84.032A, the Alphabetic Index main term is Complication, subterms joint prosthesis, internal, mechanical, loosening, knee. For G20, the Alphabetic Index main term is Parkinsonism. For I11.0, the Alphabetic Index main term is Hypertension, subterms heart, with, heart failure. For I50.9, the Alphabetic Index main term is Failure, subterms heart, congestive. For H40.143, the Alphabetic Index main term is Glaucoma, subterm capsular—see Glaucoma, open angle, primary, capsular. For I25.2, the Alphabetic Index main term is Infarction, subterms myocardium, healed or old. For R94.39, the Alphabetic Index main term is Findings, abnormal, inconclusive, without diagnosis, subterm stress test. For Y83.1, the Alphabetic Index main term is Complication of or following, subterms implant, artificial, internal device.

4.94. 813.33-Y, 847.0-Y, E812.0, 79.32

Rationale: A compound fracture is an open fracture. The site of the fractures was specified. The procedure is ORIF. The POA status indicator is Y for the diagnosis codes, as both were present on admission. No POA indicator is assigned to E812.0, as E810–E819 are included on the POA exempt list.

ICD-10-CM Code(s): S52.201B, S52.301B, S13.4xxA, V43.52xA

ICD-10-PCS Code(s): 0PSH04Z, 0PSK04Z

ICD-10-CM Rationale: For S52.201B, the Alphabetic Index main term is Fracture, traumatic, subterms ulna, shaft. For S52.301B, the Alphabetic Index main term is Fracture, traumatic, subterms radius, shaft. For S13.4xxA, the Alphabetic Index main term is Whiplash injury. For V43.52xA, the Alphabetic Index main term is Accident, subterms transport, car occupant, driver, collision, car.

ICD-10-PCS Rationale: For code 0PSH04Z, the Alphabetic Index main term is Reposition, subterms radius, right. For code 0PSK04Z, the Alphabetic Index main term is Reposition, subterms ulna, right.

4.95. 942.34-Y, 948.00-Y, E923.2-Y, E849.0, E030, MS-DRG: 934

Rationale: The 948 category is used whenever the percent of body surface is documented. The E code selected is based on the documentation in this scenario that states only that there was an explosion. Be advised that if the documentation, such as the actual medical record, states that there was a resultant fire, then a code from category E890 would be correct. All diagnoses are present at the time of admission and assigned indicator Y (yes). Codes E849.0 and E030 are not assigned an indicator because they are on the POA exempt list.

ICD-10-CM Code(s): T21.33xA, T31.0, W40.1xxA, Y92.00, Y93.9

ICD-10-CM Rationale: For T21.33xA, the Alphabetic Index main term is Burn, subterms back, upper, third degree. For T31.0, the Alphabetic Index main term is Burn, subterm extent, less than 10 percent. For W40.1xxA, the Alphabetic Index main term is Explosion, subterms explosive, gas. For Y92.00, the Alphabetic Index main term is Place of occurrence, residence. For Y93.9, the Alphabetic Index main term is Activity.

4.96. 536.41-Y, 682.2-Y, 041.11-Y, 150.4-Y, MS-DRG: 394

Rationale: The infection of the gastrostomy is sequenced first. See the note under the code: "Use additional code to specify type of infection, such as: abscess or cellulitis of abdomen" (682.2). The organism is also coded. The cancer of the esophagus is coded as current because there is no documentation that it has been excised. All diagnoses are reported with status indicator Y (yes) as they were present at the time of admission.

ICD-10-CM Code(s): K94.22, L03.311, B95.6, C15.4

ICD-10-CM Rationale: For K94.22, the Alphabetic Index main term is Complication, subterms gastrostomy, infection. For L03.311, the Alphabetic Index main term is Cellulitis, subterm abdominal wall. For B95.6, the Alphabetic Index main term is Staphylococcus, subterm aureus, as cause of disease classified elsewhere. For C15.4, the Alphabetic Index main term is Neoplasm, subterm esophagus, middle.

4.97. 897.6-Y, E805.2, E001.0, 84.15, 84.15, MS-DRG: 909

Rationale: The complicated code is used because there was documentation of delayed healing. Code 84.3 is not correct for the procedure because it is used for amputation stumps that are not current. Index: Revision, current traumatic, *see* amputation. The excludes note under code 84.3 shows that revision of current traumatic amputation is coded elsewhere. The procedure code may be repeated because it was bilateral (*Coding Clinic*: 1985, Nov/Dec:11). E805.2 and E001.0 are not assigned a status indicator because they are both on the POA exempt list.

ICD-10-CM Code(s): S88.111A, S88.112A, V05.00xA, Y93.01

ICD-10-PCS Code(s): 0Y6H0Z1, 0Y6J0Z1

ICD-10-CM Rationale: For S88.111A and S88.112A, the Alphabetic Index main term is Amputation, subterms traumatic, leg, between knee and ankle. For V05.00xA, the Alphabetic Index main term is Accident, subterms transport, pedestrian, on foot, collision, railway, nontraffic. For Y93.01, the Alphabetic Index main term is Activity, subterm walking.

ICD-10-PCS Rationale: For code 0Y6H0Z1, the Alphabetic Index main term is Detachment, subterms leg, lower, right. For code 0Y6J0Z1, the Alphabetic Index main term is Detachment, subterms leg, lower, left.

4.98.   996.43-Y, V43.64, E878.1-Y, 81.53, 93.22

Rationale: Because this is a mechanical complication, the index entries are as follows: Complications, mechanical, prosthetic, joint, failure, 996.43. Code V43.64 is not assigned an indicator, as V43.64 is on the POA exempt list.

ICD-10-CM Code(s): T84.010A, Y83.1

ICD-10-PCS Code(s): 0SR90J5, 0SP90JZ

ICD-10-CM Rationale: For code T84.010A, the Alphabetic Index main term is Complication, subterm joint prosthesis, internal, mechanical, breakage, broken. For Y83.1, the Alphabetic Index main term is Complication of or following, subterms implant, artificial, internal device.

ICD-10-PCS Rationale: For code 0SR90J5, the Alphabetic Index main term is Replacement, subterms joint, hip, right. For code 0SP90JZ, the Alphabetic Index main term is Removal, subterms joint, hip, right. Note: The code for the gait training cannot be assigned without information about the equipment. The first five characters would be F07Z9.

4.99.   823.20-Y, 850.0-Y, E885.9, E019.0, E849.5, E000.8, 79.36

Note: A comminuted fracture is considered coded as closed unless specified as open or compound per the note in the Index under Fracture. Four "E" codes are necessary to fully describe the circumstances as instructed by the notes in the Tabular List.

ICD-10-CM Code(s): S82.251A, S06.0x0A, W01.198A, Y92.480, Y93.K1, Y99.8

ICD-10-PCS Code(s): 0QSG04Z

ICD-10-CM Rationale: For S82.251A, the Alphabetic Index main term is Fracture, subterms tibia (shaft), comminuted. For S06.0x0A, the Alphabetic Index main term is Concussion. For W01.198A, the Alphabetic Index main term is subterms Fall, due to, slipping, with subsequent striking against object, specified NEC. For Y92.480, the Alphabetic Index main term is Place of occurrence, subterm street or highway, sidewalk. For Y93.K1, the Alphabetic Index main term is Activity, subterm walking an animal. For Y99.8, the Alphabetic Index main term is External cause status, subterm specified NEC.

ICD-10-PCS Rationale: The Alphabetic Index main term is Reposition, subterms tibia, right.

Chapter 5. Case Studies from Ambulatory Health Records

Unless otherwise stated, code set answers given in Chapter 5 are ICD-9-CM and/or CPT.

Disorders of the Blood and Blood-Forming Organs

5.1.   a. 569.85, 45382, 36430-59

Correct answer.

b. 578.9, 569.84, 45382, 36430, 36430, 36430

Incorrect answer. The 36430 is only reported one time. The angiodysplasia of the colon is listed first, and the only code required is the combined code for the angiodysplasia with hemorrhage.

c. 578.9, 45382, 36430-59

Incorrect answer. The GI bleed would be reported with the angiodysplasia code with hemorrhage.

d. 569.84, 578.9, 45382

Incorrect answer. Code 578.9 is not required with 569.84. Code 36430 also should be reported for the administration of the transfusion.

ICD-10-CM Code(s): K55.21

ICD-10-CM Rationale: The Alphabetic Index main term is Angiodysplasia (colon), subterm with bleeding.

5.2.   a. 285.9, 38220

Incorrect answer. The admitting diagnosis was anemia, but the pathologist gave more clarification by providing the diagnosis of iron deficiency anemia.

b. 280.9, 38220

Correct answer.

c. 285.9, 38220, 38221-59

Incorrect answer. The admitting diagnosis was anemia, but the pathology report states bone marrow aspiration and biopsy; however, the technique reported by the surgeon shows that the procedure performed was a bone marrow aspiration, bone trabecula not seen. Code 38221 would not be reported.

d. 280.8, 38230

Incorrect answer. The iron deficiency anemia has not been specified as to the type, so code 280.8 is not correct. The procedure codes listed here would only be used for bone marrow harvesting for transplantation purposes.

ICD-10-CM Code(s): D50.9

ICD-10-CM Rationale: The Alphabetic Index main term is Anemia with subterm iron deficiency.

5.3. 204.00, 38220

Rationale: Acute lymphocytic leukemia is coded to 204.00. There is no remission because this is a new diagnosis. The procedure described is bone marrow aspiration. The code is only assigned once, even though the needle was repositioned to obtain more than one specimen. This is common in this procedure.

ICD-10-CM Code(s): C91.20

ICD-10-CM Rationale: The Alphabetic Index main term is Leukemia, leukemic, subterm lymphoid, specified NEC.

5.4. 172.6, 196.3, 38525-LT, 38792, 78195

Rationale: CPT codes are assigned for the excision and injection procedure. Assign modifier -LT to show that the left axillary lymph node was biopsied.

ICD-10-CM Code(s): C77.3, C43.62

ICD-10-CM Rationale: The Alphabetic Index main term is Melanoma with subterms skin, arm. Also reference main term Neoplasm Table with subterms lymph, gland, axilla, axillary. Select the Malignant Secondary column.

5.5. ICD-9-CM Reason for Visit Code(s): 786.50, 518.3

ICD-9-CM Code(s): 282.62, 517.3

Rationale: Acute chest syndrome (517.3) is to be assigned as an additional code for sickle-cell codes with crisis per instructional note.

ICD-10-CM Reason for Visit Code(s): R07.1, J82

ICD-10-CM Code(s): D57.01

ICD-10-CM Rationale: The Alphabetic Index main term is Pain, subterm chest, on breathing. The Alphabetic Index main term is Infiltrates, subterm pulmonary. The first listed diagnosis code is found in the Alphabetic Index main term Disease, subterm sickle-cell with crisis, with acute chest syndrome.

Disorders of the Cardiovascular System

5.6. a. 33240

Incorrect answer. This code describes only the insertion of the pacing ICD. To completely code the insertion of the leads and the pacing ICD, the coder should choose code 33249. In addition, the documentation states that defibrillator threshold testing was performed. Code 93641 describes the process of testing both the leads and the pulse generator.

b. 33225, 33240

Incorrect answer. Biventricular pacing is not described in the documentation, and therefore, code 33225 cannot be assigned. Code 33240 describes only the insertion of the pacing ICD. To completely code the insertion of the leads and the pacing ICD, the coder should choose code 33249. In addition, the documentation states that defibrillator threshold testing was performed. Code 93641 describes the process of testing both the leads and the pulse generator.

c. 33249, 93641

Correct answer.

d. 33249, 93640, 93641

Incorrect answer. Code 93640 should not be coded with code 93641.
Code 93641 includes testing of both the leads and the pulse generator.

5.7.   a. 745.4, 93315

Incorrect answer. The diagnosis code is not specific to an AV canal defect.

b. 745.69, 93315

Correct answer. The CPT code may be assigned by the chargemaster.

c. 745.69, 93312

Incorrect answer. Conditions present at birth are considered congenital, so
the CPT code would be 93315.

d. 429.71, 93312

Incorrect answer. Conditions present at birth are considered congenital, so
the CPT code would be 93315. The ICD-9-CM code is for an acquired cardiac
septal defect, which means it is not present at birth.

ICD-10-CM Code(s): Q21.2

ICD-10-CM Rationale: The Alphabetic Index main term is Defect, subterm
atrioventricular canal.

5.8.   155.0, 36563

Rationale: Code 155.0 is assigned because there is documentation that it is
primary. Reporting of the chemotherapy agent 5-FU is reported with an HCPCS
"J" code and usually assigned by the chargemaster.

ICD-10-CM Code(s): C22.8

ICD-10-CM Rationale: The Alphabetic Index main term is Liver, primary in the
Neoplasm Table. This is a primary malignancy so a code is chosen from the
Malignant Primary column.

5.9.   ICD-9-CM Reason for Visit Code(s): 786.50
ICD-9-CM and CPT Code(s): 410.11, 428.22, 401.9, 93458

Rationale: The angina is not coded during the same episode of care as an
acute myocardial infarct because the patient was admitted with symptomatic
angina that evolved into or, after study, is found to have an AMI. In this case,
the AMI is sequenced as the principal diagnosis and no additional code would
be assigned, as the angina is an inherent part of this condition (*Coding Clinic*
1993, 5Q: 17–24).

The chronic systolic heart failure and hypertension meet additional diagnosis
reporting to describe coexisting conditions that require and/or affect patient
care treatment or management. The hypertension is coded separately because
there is no cause-effect documentation provided. The correct code for the heart
catheterization is 93458.

ICD-10-CM Reason for Visit Code(s): R07.9

ICD-10-CM Reason for Visit Rationale: The Alphabetic Index main term is Pain, subterm chest.

ICD-10-CM Code(s): I21.09

ICD-10-CM Rationale: The Alphabetic Index main term is Infection, subterm myocardial, ST Elevation, anterior. I50.22 can be found by revealing Alphabetic Index main term Failure, failed, subterm systolic (congestive), chronic. Hypertension is coded to I10 which is found under main term Hypertension.

5.10. ICD-9-CM Reason for Visit Code(s): 427.5

ICD-9-CM Code(s): 427.5

Rationale: The probable MI may not be coded on an outpatient record per *ICD-9-CM Official Guidelines for Coding and Reporting* of Outpatient Services that states "coding for inconclusive diagnoses (probable, suspected, rule out, etc.) were developed for inpatient reporting and do not apply to outpatients."

ICD-10-CM Reason for Visit Code(s): I46.9

ICD-10-CM Code(s): I46.9

ICD-10-CM Rationale: The Alphabetic Index main term is Arrest, with subterm cardiac.

5.11. a. 36475-RT

Correct answer.

b. 36475-RT, 36000
Incorrect answer. The introduction of the catheter into the vein is included in the procedure code, per the instructional note following code 36476.

c. 36478-RT
Incorrect answer. Code 36478 describes laser ablation of incompetent veins. The scenario for coding specifies radiofrequency ablation, 36475.

d. 36475-RT, 76942
Incorrect answer. Per the description of code 36475, the procedure code is inclusive of all imaging guidance and monitoring.

5.12. 185, 36556

Rationale: There are several factors that must be considered when coding insertion of access devices, including the age of the patient and whether or not it is a tunneled or non-tunneled insertion of the central venous catheter. Another consideration is whether or not a port or reservoir is implanted. CPT provides the "Central Venous Access Procedure Table" which is invaluable in assigning these codes. For this encounter the patient is aged 5 years or older and the device is a non-tunneled centrally located central venous catheter. This procedure meets the definition of central VAD as it terminates in the subclavian artery.

ICD-10-CM Code(s): C61

ICD-10-CM Rationale: The Alphabetic Index main term is Prostate in the Neoplasm Table. Then select the Malignant Primary column code.

Disorders of the Digestive System

5.13. a. 553.3, 43327

Incorrect answer. The diagnosis code is correct, but the procedure code is an open abdominal procedure. Because a laparoscopic approach is described for this Nissen procedure, code 43280 is reported.

b. 553.3, 43280

Correct answer. The procedure describes a Nissen fundoplication performed via a laparoscope.

c. 551.3, 43280

Incorrect answer. Code 551.3 would be assigned only when gangrene was documented. The procedure code is correct.

d. 553.3, 43328

Incorrect answer. The CPT code is for a thoracotomy esophagogastric fundoplasty. When the procedure is performed via a laparoscope, designated in this operative report by the use of insufflation, trocars, ports, and direct visualization, code 43280 is reported.

ICD-10-CM Code(s): K44.9

ICD-10-CM Rationale: The Alphabetic Index main term is Hernia, subterm hiatal.

5.14. ICD-9-CM Reason for Visit Code(s): 578.1

ICD-9-CM and CPT Code(s): 578.1, 43235

Rationale: The duodenal ulcer is not coded because it has not been confirmed. Coding guidelines for outpatients state that rule-outs or possible diagnoses are not coded. Code to the highest degree of certainty.

The patient had an esophagoscopy, but the scope also went into the stomach and duodenum. Code 43235 is correct. Code 43200 is a separate procedure code, and the esophagoscopy is included in code 43235. It would be incorrect to assign the separate procedure code in this case. The documentation only states that the endoscopy was done. It does not specify that any techniques were used to control the bleeding.

ICD-10-CM: Reason for Visit Code(s): K92.1

ICD-10-CM Code(s): K92.1

ICD-10-CM Rationale: The Alphabetic Index main term is Melena.

5.15. 263.0, 438.21, 43246

Rationale: The percutaneous endoscopic gastrostomy (PEG) tube placement is coded 43246. V12.59 is for old stroke without residuals, so it is not appropriate. This patient has hemiparesis.

ICD-10-CM Code(s): E44.0, I69.351

ICD-10-CM Rationale: The Alphabetic Index main term is Malnutrition. The Alphabetic Index main term is Sequelae, subterm hemiparesis. The coder completes the code using the Tabular List.

5.16. 574.20, 47562

Rationale: The adhesions did not prevent the surgeon access to the organ and were not documented to be significant. Per ICD-9-CM guidelines, they would not be coded in this instance. Code 44180 is a separate procedure code and per CPT guidelines would not be added on when part of a more extensive, related procedure.

ICD-10-CM Code(s): K80.20

ICD-10-CM Rationale: The Alphabetic Index main term is Cholethiasis. This term refers the coder to the main term Calculus with subterm gallbladder.

5.17. 569.1, 569.0, 562.10, 558.9, 45380

Rationale: The polyps are stated to be nonadenomatous. *CPT Assistant* (1996, Jan.) states that the correct code for a cold biopsy is 45380 or 45385, depending on the technique used, and in this case it was 45380. The biopsy code is used only once. The entire polyps were not removed. Code the postoperative diagnosis rather than the preoperative diagnosis.

ICD-10-CM Code(s): K62.3, K62.1, K57.30, K52.9

ICD-10-CM Rationale: The Alphabetic Index main term is Prolapse, rectum. Rectal polyps are coded by accessing Alphabetic Index main term Polyps, subterm rectum (nonadenomatous). Code K57.30 is referenced under the Alphabetic Index main term Diverticulosis, subterm large intestine. To find K52.9, nonspecific colitis, access main term Colitis.

5.18. 550.90, 49505-RT

Rationale: In CPT, it is not correct to code the implantation of the mesh except for incisional or ventral hernia repairs. Assign HCPCS Level II modifier -RT to indicate the right inguinal hernia.

ICD-10-CM Code(s): K40.90

ICD-10-CM Rationale: The Alphabetic Index main term is Hernia with subterm inguinal (direct) (indirect).

5.19. 574.00, 47563

Rationale: Subacute is a nonessential modifier to acute and listed in parentheses; therefore, subacute is coded to acute. The cholecystectomy includes cholangiography.

ICD-10-CM Code(s): K80.00

ICD-10-CM Rationale: The Alphabetic Index main term is Calculus, calculi, subterm gallbladder, with cholecystitis, acute.

5.20. a. 45384, 45342

Incorrect answer. Code 45384 describes biopsy using a hot biopsy forceps, not the cold forceps mentioned here. In addition, code 45342 is used to report a sigmoidoscopic ultrasound, not ultrasound with colonoscopy.

b. 45380, 45391

Incorrect answer. Code 45391 does not include the transmural biopsy that was performed via the ultrasonic endoscope. Code 45392 is the correct code.

c. 45384, 45392

Incorrect answer. Code 45384 describes biopsy using a hot biopsy forceps, not the cold forceps mentioned here.

d. 45380, 45392

Correct answer.

5.21. 507.0, 44500

Rationale: The documentation confirms placement of the tube in the patient's jejunum. Therefore, code 44500 describes the placement of the long gastrointestinal tube.

ICD-10-CM Code(s): J69.0

ICD-10-CM Rationale: The Alphabetic Index main term is Aspiration, subterm pneumonitis.

5.22. 935.1, 43215

Rationale: Conscious sedation is included in the CPT code.

ICD-10-CM Code(s): T18.190

ICD-10-CM Rationale: The Alphabetic Index main term is Foreign Body with subterms esophagus, causing, tracheal compression, specified type, NEC.

5.23. 211.3, 45380, 45385, 43239

Rationale: Adenomatous polyps are benign. Some payers may require that modifier -59 be added to code 45380. Modifier -59 is used to show that biopsies were taken from polyps other than the ones that were removed. If the same lesion is biopsied and then removed, only the removal code is used.

ICD-10-CM Code(s): D12.3

ICD-10-CM Rationale: The Alphabetic Index main term is Polyp, polypus, subterm colon, transverse.

5.24. 553.20, 49652

Rationale: The marlex mesh that was implanted is included in code 49652; therefore it is not coded separately.

ICD-10-CM Code(s): K43.90

ICD-10-CM Rationale: The Alphabetic Index main term is Hernia with subterm ventral.

Endocrine, Nutritional, and Metabolic Diseases and Immunity Disorders

5.25. 271.3, 625.3

Note: In this case, lactose intolerance is confirmed. It would be inappropriate to code right lower quadrant abdominal pain or cramping because two sources of pain are documented.

5.26. a. 60200

Incorrect answer. The patient has a thyroglossal duct cyst, not a thyroid cyst. CPT code 60280 is specific to a cyst of this location.

b. 60210

Incorrect answer. The patient has a thyroglossal duct cyst that is excised. The thyroid is not excised in this case. CPT code 60280 is specific to the excision of a cyst of this location.

c. 60280

Correct answer.

d. 60281

Incorrect answer. Documentation does not state that the thyroglossal duct cyst is recurrent. In the absence of this documentation, the coder must assign code 60280 for the excision of the cyst.

5.27. 202.00, 60100

Rationale: The lymphoma is in the thyroid gland, which is an organ, so diagnosis code 202.00 is correct. This is not a fine-needle aspiration. A large hollow-core needle is inserted percutaneously. Code 60100 is correct. If needle placement were guided by ultrasound or by computerized tomography, code 76942 or 76360 would also be reported.

ICD-10-CM Code(s): C82.99

ICD-10-CM Rationale: The Alphabetic Index main term is Lymphoma, subterm follicular. The coder completes the code using the Tabular List. The thyroid is an extranodal organ.

Disorders of the Genitourinary System

5.28. a. 625.6, 618.01, 618.2, 57284, 51840

Incorrect answer. Because the cause of the incontinence is likely the vaginal prolapse/cystocele, the reason for visit should be 618.01 followed by the stress incontinence code. Diagnosis code 618.2 is not needed because code 618.01 represents both the cystocele and vaginal prolapse. See *CPT Assistant* (1997, Jan.) regarding the procedure. Additional codes such as 51840 and 51841 should not be reported separately when performed with a paravaginal defect repair.

b. 625.6, 57284-50

Incorrect answer. The diagnosis code (618.01) should be reported first to reflect the incomplete vaginal prolapse and the resulting cystocele, contributing to the stress incontinence. According to *CPT Assistant*, this procedure is inherently bilateral, so a modifier is inappropriate. Also, codes 51845, 57289, and 57240 may be reported in addition to code 57284 if the paravaginal defect repair is performed in conjunction with an abdomino-vaginal vesical neck suspension, such as Stamy, Raz, or a modified Pereyra (*CPT Assistant*, 1997, Jan.). These more complicated procedures are more likely to be performed on an inpatient basis. Careful review of the operative note is required to see if there is enough justification to assign a code for anterior colporrhaphy.

c. 618.02, 57240

Incorrect answer. Urinary incontinence should be added as an additional code per ICD-9-CM coding conventions, by reporting code 625.6. Paravaginal defect repair is reported with CPT code 57284. More documentation would be required to support reporting of anterior colporrhaphy with code 57240.

d. 618.01, 625.6, 57284

Correct answer.

ICD-10-CM Code(s): N39.3, N81.11

ICD-10-CM Rationale: The Alphabetic Index main term is Incontinence with subterm stress (female). For the second diagnosis, the Alphabetic Index main term Prolapse, prolapsed, with subterm vagina states to see Cystocele. The main term is now Cystocele with subterms female, midline.

5.29.   a. 788.37, 788.32, 53445, 51715

Correct answer.

b. 788.39, 51715

Incorrect answer. The diagnosis code can be more specific by reporting code 788.37. Code 788.32 is also necessary to complete the stress incontinence. Additional procedure code 53445 is required to show the incision of the perineum, with the placement of the artificial sphincter.

c. 788.37, 53440

Incorrect answer. Code 788.32 is also necessary to complete the stress incontinence. Code 53440 describes a sling operation.

d. 788.37, 788.32, 53445

Incorrect answer. Code 51715 is reported.

ICD-10-CM Code(s): N39.45, N39.3

ICD-10-CM Rationale: The Alphabetic Index main term is Incontinence, subterm urine, continuous. The main term Is Incontinence, subterm urine, stress (female) (male).

5.30.   a. 788.20, V13.02, 51701

Incorrect answer. The diagnoses are correct. *Coding Clinic for HCPCS*, 3rd Qtr, 2007 directs the coder that code P9612 is the correct code for collection of a urine specimen using a straight catheter. Code 51701 is to be used for the collection of residual urine.

b. 788.20, 51702, P9612

Incorrect answer. Code 51702 is used to describe the insertion of a temporary indwelling (Foley) catheter. Documentation does not support that an indwelling catheter was placed. In addition, the patient has a known history of urinary tract infections, which should be reported as V13.02.

c. 788.20, V13.02, P9612

Correct answer.

d. 599.0, 51701

Incorrect answer. The patient does not have a confirmed urinary tract infection, so code 599.0 should not be reported. Urinary retention and the history of urinary tract infections should be coded as 788.20 and V13.02. *Coding Clinic for HCPCS,* 3rd Qtr, 2007 directs the coder that code P9612 is the correct code for collection of a urine specimen using a straight catheter. Code 51701 is to be used for the collection of residual urine.

ICD-10-CM Code(s): R33.9, Z87.440

ICD-10-CM Rationale: The Alphabetic Index main term is Retention with subterm urine. Another main term is History with subterms personal (of) infection, urinary (recurrent) (tract).

5.31. a. 600.20, 53852

Correct answer.

b. 600.20, 52601

Incorrect answer. When thermotherapy is used, code 53852 is reported. Code 52601 is reported only for electrosurgical resection.

c. 600.00, 53852

Incorrect answer. Adenoma of the prostate is reported with 600.20.

d. 222.2, 53850

Incorrect answer. Adenoma of the prostate is reported with 600.20. Code 53852 is for microwave thermotherapy. In this procedure radiofrequency was used.

ICD-10-CM Code(s): D29.1

ICD-10-CM Rationale: The Alphabetic Index main term is Adenoma, subterm prostate. The coder is directed to see Neoplasm, benign, prostate.

5.32. ICD-9-CM Reason for Visit Code(s): 608.9, 55899

ICD-9-CM and CPT Code(s): 608.20, 55899

Rationale: There is no specific CPT code describing the process of manual detorsion of a testicle, so code 55899 is assigned.

ICD-10-CM Reason for Visit Code(s): N50.8

ICD-10-CM Reason for Visit Rationale: The Alphabetic Index main term is Pain, testis. The code for scrotal swelling is also N50.8.

ICD-10-CM Code(s): N44.00

ICD-10-CM Rationale: The Alphabetic Index main term is Torsion with subterm testis, testicle.

5.33. ICD-9-CM Reason for Visit Code(s): 780.60, 789.07

ICD-9-CM and CPT Code(s): 780.60, V13.02, 290.3, 81000

Rationale: A urinary tract infection was not established, so it is not coded. It may be useful to also report the history of UTI with code V13.02 to establish medical necessity for the urinalysis. It is appropriate to add all diagnoses that affect current patient management. In this case, the fact that the patient has dementia does impact the care and should be reported with code 290.3 (with delirium).

ICD-10-CM Reason for Visit Code(s): R50.9, R10.84

ICD-10-CM Reason for Visit Rationale: The Alphabetic Index main term is Fever (of unknown origin). The Alphabetic Index main term is Pain, subterm abdominal, generalized.

ICD-10-CM Code(s): R50.9, F05, Z87.440

ICD-10-CM Rationale: The Alphabetic Index main term is Fever, unknown origin. The Alphabetic Index main term is Dementia, subterm senile, with acute confusional state. The Alphabetic Index main term is History, subterm personal, urinary tract infection.

5.34. 250.41, 585.6, 583.81, 36821

Rationale: It is correct to report all codes for diagnoses that impact the care or treatment of this patient: nephropathy manifestation code and end-stage renal disease.

ICD-10-CM Code(s): E10.22, N18.6

ICD-10-CM Rationale: The Alphabetic Index main term is Diabetes, diabetic with subterm type I, with, chronic kidney disease. In the Alphabetic Index, the main term is Disease with subterms renal, end-stage (failure).

5.35. 614.6, 58660

Rationale: The adhesions would be considered pelvic, not abdominal.

ICD-10-CM Code(s): N73.6

ICD-10-CM Rationale: The Alphabetic Index main term is Adhesions, subterm tubo-ovarian.

5.36. 600.01, 596.0, 788.20, 52500

ICD-10-CM Code(s): N40.1, N13.8

ICD-10-CM Rationale: The Alphabetic Index main term is Enlargement, enlarged with subterms prostate, with lower urinary tract symptoms (LUTS). There is a note under code N40.1 which directs the coder to "Use additional code for associated symptoms when specified." Urinary obstruction is listed as an additional code and is therefore also coded.

5.37. 50592-RT

Rationale: Code 50592 describes percutaneous radiofrequency ablation of four tumors. The code description states "ablation, one or more renal tumors . . . " so it is not appropriate to report it more than once for multiple tumor ablations. Code 50250 reports an open procedure and 50542 a laparoscopic with tumor ablation, so neither is correct to report a percutaneous procedure.

Infectious Diseases

5.38. ICD-9-CM Reason for Visit Code(s): 789.01, 780.60, 780.79

Rationale: The coder may select any three admitting symptoms as the reason for visit codes: right upper quadrant pain, fever, profound malaise, and bloody diarrhea.

ICD-9-CM Code(s): 006.0

Rationale: The correct code would be 006.0. Symptoms are not reported separately as they are integral to the Entamoeba histolytica dysentery.

ICD-10-CM Reason for Visit Code(s): R10.11, R50.9, R53.81

ICD-10-CM Reason for Visit Rationale: The Alphabetic Index main term is Pain with subterms abdominal, upper, right quadrant. Another main term is Fever; another main term is Malaise.

ICD-10-CM Code(s): A06.0

ICD-10-CM Rationale: The Alphabetic Index main term is Dysentery, dysenteric with subterms Entamoeba with a note to see Dysentery, amebic. Dysentery amebia is now referenced with subterm acute.

5.39. ICD-9-CM Reason for Visit Code(s): 698.1, 709.8

ICD-9-CM Code(s): 133.0

Rationale: Code 133.0 is reported for scabies of any site.

ICD-10-CM Code(s): B86

ICD-10-CM Rationale: The Alphabetic Index main term is Eruption, subterm vesicular. For the pruritus, the main term is Pruritis, subterm scrotum. The itching on the penis, buttocks, and groin is coded as Pruritis, specified NEC. The final diagnosis is found by reviewing main term Infestation, subterm Sarcoptes scabiei.

5.40. ICD-9-CM Reason for Visit Code(s): R19.7

ICD-9-CM Code(s): 008.02

Rationale: The Alphabetic Index main term is Diarrhea.

ICD-10-CM Code(s): A04.1

ICD-10-CM Rationale: The Alphabetic Index main term is Enteritis (acute) with subterms infectious, due to, *Escherichia coli,* enterotoxigenic.

5.41. ICD-9-CM Reason for Visit Code(s): 795.5

ICD-9-CM Code(s): 795.5, 296.52

Rationale: Latent TB means that the patient has had a positive TB test but has no active disease. INH is given prophylactically to keep the patient from converting to active disease later in life. The only code available is 795.5 for a positive PPD. The bipolar disease is coded because this disease process affects the patient's ability to continue taking medication as prescribed.

ICD-10-CM Reason for Visit Code(s): R76.1

ICD-10-CM Reason for Visit Rationale: The Alphabetic Index main term is Positive, subterm skin test tuberculin.

ICD-10-CM Code(s): R76.1, F31.32

ICD-10-CM Rationale: The Alphabetic Index main term is Positive, subterm skin test tuberculin. The bipolar is found in Alphabetic Index under main term Disorder, subterm bipolar (I), current episode, depressed, without psychotic features, moderate.

Disorders of the Skin and Subcutaneous Tissue

5.42. 173.31, 702.19, 11641, 11441, 15260

The lesion on the right nasal tip was a basal cell carcinoma. New code 173.31 describes this condition. The cheek lesion was a seborrheic keratosis which is benign. After removal of the nasal tip lesion a full thickness skin graft was performed (15260). This code is based on the size of the graft. Codes 11641 and 11441 are used to describe the removal of the malignant and benign lesions, respectively.

ICD-10-CM Code(s): C44.31, L82.1

ICD-10-CM Rationale: The Alphabetic Index main term is Skin with subterm ala nasi. Select the code from the Malignant Primary column. In the Alphabetic Index, the main term Keratosis is referenced with subterm seborrheic.

5.43. 214.1, 11406

Code 214.1 is used to report a lipoma which is a benign tumor.

ICD-10-CM Code(s): D17.24

ICD-10-CM Rationale: The Alphabetic Index main term is Lipoma, subterm legs (skin) (subcutaneous). The coder completes the code using the Tabular List.

5.44. a. 172.5, 11603

Incorrect answer. An additional code is required for reporting the layer closure: 12032 for a 3-cm repair.

b. 709.9, 11603

Incorrect answer. When a malignant lesion has been excised and the patient presents for wide excision, the malignant lesion is coded for each case. An additional code is required for reporting the layer closure: 12032 for a 3-cm repair.

c. 172.5, 11603, 12032

Correct answer.

d. V76.43, 11603, 13121

Incorrect answer. When a malignant lesion has been excised and the patient presents for wide excision, the malignant lesion is coded for each case. The code for the layer closure should be reported with 12032. Intermediate repair is generally what is reported for layer closure, unless the report indicates a complicated wound closure involving the procedures described in the CPT manual as complex.

ICD-10-CM Code(s): C43.59

ICD-10-CM Rationale: The Alphabetic Index main term is Melanoma with subterms skin, back.

5.45.   a. 173.31, 15240, 11646

Incorrect answer. Code 11646 is incorrect because the size of the lesion was only 3.2. The size of graft was 10 sq cm.

b. 173.31, 15240, 15004

Incorrect answer. CPT code 15004 is reported for the surgical preparation or creation of a recipient site by excision of open wounds, burn eschar, or scar; therefore, it is not accurate to report this code for the malignant lesion excision. Report code 11644 for the 3.2-cm malignant lesion.

c. 173.31, 15320, 15004, 11644

Incorrect answer. The CPT code for the graft is for an allograft. This uses a homograft from healthy/cadaver skin from another person. When the patient's own tissue is grafted, code 15240 is reported for this size of graft. CPT code 15004 is reported for the surgical preparation or creation of a recipient site by excision of open wounds, burn eschar, or scar; therefore, it is not accurate to report this code for the malignant lesion excision.

d. 173.3, 15240, 11644

Correct answer.

ICD-10-CM Code(s): C44.39

ICD-10-CM Rationale: Reviewing the Neoplasm Table, under skin, cheek, Malignant Primary, the coder is directed to C44.39.

5.46.   ICD-9-CM Reason for Visit Code(s): 703.0

ICD-9-CM and CPT Code(s): 703.0, 281.0, 334.0, 429.9, 11750

Rationale: The digital block is included in the procedure and therefore not coded separately. Code 11750 is reported because the nail matrix is destroyed to achieve permanent removal, even though the physician describes the procedure as a wedge resection. Code 11765 is not used because the nail and the matrix are both removed, not just the skin of the nail fold.

ICD-10-CM Reason for Visit Code(s): L60.0

ICD-10-CM Code(s): L60.0, D51.0, G11.1, I51.9

ICD-10-CM Rationale: The Alphabetic Index main term is Ingrowing with subterm nail (finger) (toe). Another main term is Anemia with subterm pernicious. A third main term is Ataxia with subterm Friedreich's. The final main term is Disease with subterm heart.

5.47. 078.10, 17110

Rationale: The code 17110 includes cryosurgery and curettement of up to 14 lesions, so no other code is assigned.

ICD-10-CM Code(s): B07.9

ICD-10-CM Rationale: The Alphabetic Index main term is wart (viral).

5.48. ICD-9-CM Reason for Visit Code(s): 881.00, 882.0, 891.0

ICD-9-CM and CPT Code(s): 891.0, 881.00, 882.0, E920.8, E849.0, 12031, 12002

Rationale: The intermediate repair is reported in the first position as the most resource-intensive code. The lacerations repaired with simple repair are added together to total 5 cm as all anatomic sites are listed in code 12002.

ICD-10-CM Reason for Visit Code(s): S61.412A, S51.812A, S81.811A

ICD-10-CM Reason for Visit Rationale: The Alphabetic Index main term is Laceration with subterms hand, forearm, leg (lower).

ICD-10-CM Code(s): S61.412A, S51.812A, S81.811A, W25.xxxA, Y92.018, Y93.h9, Y99.8

ICD-10-CM Rationale: The Alphabetic Index main term is Laceration with subterms hand, forearm, leg (lower). The main term in the Index to External Causes is Contact with subterms with, glass. The main term in the Index to External Causes is Activity with subterms maintenance, exterior building. The main term in the Index to External Causes is Place of occurrence with subterms residence, house, single family, specified NEC. In the Index to External Causes the main term is External Cause Status with subterm specified NEC.

5.49. 906.5, 701.4, 15004, 15005, 15175, 15176

Rationale: The late effect code reflects the fact that the contracture and scars were due to a burn. The hypertrophy of the scar/keloid is coded as 701.4. Integra is an acellular dermal replacement that does not require a concurrent epidermal cover.

ICD-10-CM Code(s): T20.07xs, L91.0

ICD-10-CM Rationale: The Alphabetic Index main term is Burn, neck. The degree is not specifically stated so code T20.07 is used. A review of the Tabular List allows the coder to complete the code. The extension "s" is used to indicate there is a sequelae. The keloid is found under main term Keloid.

5.50.   a. 19297-LT

Incorrect answer. Also assign a code for the lumpectomy (partial mastectomy), 19301. Code 19297 is an add-on code and must be reported with the primary procedure code.

b. 19301-LT, 19297-LT
Correct answer.

c. 19301-RT

Incorrect answer. Modifier is reported as -RT (right) and documentation supports procedure on the -LT (left) breast. Report primary procedure and add-on code for the placement of the radiotherapy afterloading balloon catheter.

d. 19120-LT

Incorrect answer. Code 19120 is used to report an excisional biopsy of the breast. A lumpectomy is considered a form of partial mastectomy and is reported with code 19301.

5.51.   a. 707.03, 707.05

Incorrect answer. Two codes are needed to completely describe a pressure ulcer: a code from subcategory 707.0, Pressure ulcer, to identify the site of the pressure ulcer and a code from subcategory 707.2, Pressure ulcer stages.

b. 707.03, 707.05, 707.22

Incorrect answer. Although there is no documentation regarding the stage of the buttock decubitus ulcer, code 707.20 should be assigned.

c. 707.03, 707.22

Incorrect answer. Both decubitus sites are reported even though only one had a debridement: sacrum 707.03 and buttock 707.05.

d. 707.03, 707.05, 707.22, 707.20
Correct answer.

ICD-10-CM Code(s): L89.152, L89.309

ICD-10-CM Rationale: The Alphabetic Index main term is Ulcer, subterm pressure, stage 2, sacral region. The Alphabetic Index entry for the buttock is Ulcer, pressure, buttock. The coder completes the codes using the Tabular List.

Behavioral Health Conditions

5.52.   a. 301.4, 90853

Incorrect answer. The diagnosis reported is a personality disorder (301.4, obsessive compulsive) and is more accurately reported as a phobic disorder (300.3, obsessive-compulsive disorder).

b. 300.3, 90857

Incorrect answer. The diagnosis code is correct; however, the documentation does not support interactive group psychotherapy.

c. 300.3, 90853
Correct answer.

d. 300.3, 90847

Incorrect answer. The service was for a group, not an individual, and there is no documentation of the patient's family being present.

ICD-10-CM Code(s): F42

ICD-10-CM Rationale: The Alphabetic Index main term is Disorder with subterm obsessive-compulsive.

5.53. 300.21, 90849

Rationale: Code 90853 describes multiple-family group psychotherapy. The length of the session is not defined in the code.

ICD-10-CM Code(s): F40.01

ICD-10-CM Rationale: The Alphabetic Index main term is Agoraphobia, subterm with panic disorder.

5.54. ICD-9-CM Reason for Visit Code(s): 881.02

ICD-9-CM and CPT Code(s): 881.02, 296.23, E956, E849.0, 12002

Rationale: The E956 code identifies that it is a suicide attempt.

ICD-10-CM Reason for Visit Code(s)S61.512A, S61.511A

ICD-10-CM Code(s): S61.512A, S61.511A, F32.2, X78.8xxA, Y92.012, Y99.8

ICD-10-CM Rationale: The Alphabetic Index main term is Laceration with subterms wrist, left. The same main term is referenced for the second diagnosis with subterms wrist, right. The seventh character "A" is added to indicate initial encounter. In the Alphabetic Index, the main term is Depression with subterm severe, single episode. In the Index to External Causes, the main term is Suicide, suicidal (attempted) (by) with subterms cutting or piercing instrument, specified NEC. The fourth character "A" is added to indicate initial encounter. In the Index to External Causes, the main term is Place of occurrence with subterms residence, house, single family, bathroom. In the Index to External Causes, the main term is External Cause Status with subterm specified NEC.

5.55. ICD-9-CM Reason for Visit Code(s): 969.05, 969.4

ICD-9-CM and CPT Code(s): 969.05, 969.4, 980.0, 311, E950.3, E950.9, E849.0, 43753, 92950

Rationale: Both drugs and the alcohol are coded to the poisoning codes, with the respective E codes denoting a suicide attempt. The depression is also reported. Report procedure codes for gastric lavage and CPR.

ICD-10-CM Reason for Visit Code(s): T42.4x2A, T43.012A

ICD-10-CM Code(s): T42.4x2A, T43.012A, T51.0x2A, F32.9

ICD-10-CM Rationale: The Table of Drugs and Chemicals is used to code the two drugs and the alcohol. The column for "Poisoning, Intentional, Self-Harm" is used. The Tabular List is used to complete codes. To code depression, the main term is Depression.

Disorders of the Musculoskeletal System and Connective Tissue

5.56. a. 27500, 99148, 99150

Incorrect answer. Manipulation was required to reduce the fracture. Therefore, CPT code 27502 is the most appropriate to describe the service. Conscious sedation cannot be reported with the fracture code due to a CCI edit.

b. 27502

Correct answer.

c. 27506, 99148 ×4

Incorrect answer. CPT code 27502 is the most appropriate to describe the service. Conscious sedation cannot be reported with the fracture code due to a CCI edit.

d. 27506

Incorrect answer. CPT code 27502 is the most appropriate to describe the service.

5.57. a. 812.52, 24577, 29065

Incorrect answer. The diagnosis code is for an open fracture, which is not described here. The CPT code 24577 describes closed reduction of a humeral fracture, rather than the open reduction and internal fixation procedure documented. CPT 29065 should not be assigned with a fracture care code because casting is included in the initial fracture service per CPT guidelines. The HCPCS Level II modifier -RT (right) is added to show laterality.

b. 812.42, 24579, 29065

Incorrect answer. The diagnosis code and CPT code 24579 are correct. CPT 29065 should not be assigned with a fracture care code because casting is included in the initial fracture service per CPT guidelines. The HCPCS Level II modifier of -RT (right) is added to show laterality.

c. 812.42, 24579-RT

Correct answer. The HCPCS Level II modifier of -RT (right) is added to show laterality.

d. 812.52, 24579-RT

Incorrect answer. The diagnosis code is for an open fracture, which is not described here.

ICD-10-CM Code(s): S42.451A

ICD-10-CM Rationale: The Alphabetic Index main term is Fracture, subterm elbow. The coder completes the code using the Tabular List.

5.58. ICD-9-CM Reason for Visit Code(s): 873.41

ICD-9-CM and CPT Code(s): 873.41, 802.0, E917.0, E007.5, E849.4, E000.8, 21320, 12011

Rationale: The fracture is presumed closed. The ER provided fracture care of stabilization, splinting, and taping. This is frequently the only care needed for a nondisplaced nasal fracture. The physician did repair the superficial laceration of the cheek.

ICD-10-CM Reason for Visit Code(s): S01.411A

ICD-10-CM Reason for Visit Rationale: The Alphabetic Index main term is Laceration with subterm cheek (external).

ICD-10-CM Code(s): S01.411A, S02.2xxA, W21.02A, Y92.322, Y93.66, Y99.8

ICD-10-CM Rationale: The Alphabetic Index main term is Laceration with subterm cheek (external). In the Alphabetic Index, the main term is Fracture with subterm nasal (bone(s)). The fracture is assumed closed since the ER physician only stabilized the fracture with a splint and tape. In the Index to External Causes, the main term is Struck (accidentally) by, with subterms ball (hit) (thrown), soccer. In the Index to External Causes, the main term is Place of occurrence with subterms sports area, athletic, field, soccer. In the Index to External Causes, the main term is Activity with subterm soccer. In the Index to External Causes, the main term is External cause status, leisure activity.

5.59. 816.12, E919.8, E849.3, E000.0, E029.9, 26765-F6

Rationale: The fracture is open, and it is documented as distal phalanx; therefore, a fifth digit of 2 is assigned. The E code for external cause status is assigned for civilian work done for income or pay, and the activity E code is assigned as Other activity. The patient works in the food factory but was not preparing food. The CPT code would be assigned for each finger, and in this case there is no documentation that multiple fingers are involved; therefore, one code is assigned with the HCPCS Level II modifier to show which finger was treated.

ICD-10-CM Code(s): S62.630A, W31.82xA, Y92.63, Y93.89, Y99.0

ICD-10-CM Rationale: The Alphabetic Index main term is Fracture, subterm finger, index, distal phalanx. Using the Index to External Causes, the coder accesses Contact, subterm with, machine, machinery, commercial (W31.82). The place of occurrence code is found under Place of occurrence, subterm factory. The External Status Code (found under External Cause Status) is Y99.0, civilian activity for income or pay. Activity code is Activity, specified NEC.

5.60. V54.01, 20680-LT

Rationale: The fracture is not current, so code V54.01 is assigned as the primary diagnosis for removal of internal fixation device. The removal of the hardware is documented as deep (plate and pins), so CPT code 20680 is correct. Add the HCPCS Level II modifier of -LT (left) to report laterality.

ICD-10-CM Code(s): Z47.2

ICD-10-CM Rationale: The Alphabetic Index main term is Aftercare, with subterms following surgery (for) (on), removal of internal fixation device.

5.61. a. Osteochondral autograft

Incorrect answer. An osteochondral autograft involves harvesting tissue from the patient himself or herself. When the graft comes from a cadaver, it is an osteochondral allograft.

b. Osteochondral allograft

Correct answer.

c. Autologous chondrocyte implantation

Incorrect answer. This procedure involves harvesting cells from the patient, growing them to maturity in a laboratory setting, and reinjecting them. When a full osteochondral graft is obtained from a cadaver, it is an osteochondral allograft.

d. Anterior cruciate ligament repair

Incorrect answer. When an osteochondral graft is obtained from a cadaver, it is an osteochondral allograft. A ligament repair may involve cadaveric ligament, but not osteochondral tissue.

5.62. a. 719.46, 717.7, 29873-RT, 29877-RT-59

Correct answer. In a Medicare OPPS case, HCPCS Level II code G0289 would be used in lieu of CPT code 29877-RT-59, since chondroplasty was performed in separate compartments as per the source document.

b. 719.46, 717.7, 27425-RT

Incorrect answer. Diagnosis codes 717.7 and 719.46 are correct. CPT code 27425 is used to report an open retinacular release, rather than the retinacular release via arthroscopy described in the source document.

c. 717.7, 29877-RT

Incorrect answer. Diagnosis and procedure codes are missing. The source document indicates a lateral retinacular release of the right knee was performed to correct lateral patellar compression syndrome in addition to the chondroplasty performed.

d. 719.46, 717.7, 29999-RT, 29877-RT

Incorrect answer. CPT code 29999 is used only when an unlisted arthroscopic procedure is performed. In this case, CPT code 29873 identifies arthroscopic retinacular release as described in the source document.

ICD-10-CM Code(s): M22.41, M25.561

ICD-10-CM Rationale: The Alphabetic Index main term is Chondromalacia with subterm patella. Another main term is Pain with subterms joint, knee.

5.63. 26123, 26125

Rationale: The index code for Dupuytren's contracture leads the coder to the range 26040–26045. However, a note indicates that if a fasciectomy is performed rather than a fasciotomy, then codes 26121–26125 would be used.

5.64. V54.01, 20680-RT

Rationale: The patient is being seen to remove previously placed internal fixation devices. Therefore V code V54.01, Aftercare involving internal fixation device, removal of internal fixation device, is used to describe the reason for encounter. Fracture codes are not used. The correct CPT code is 20680 which is used to describe the removal of "deep" implants. Code 20670 would be used for superficial implants.

ICD-10-CM Code(s): Z47.2

ICD-10-CM Rationale: The Alphabetic Index main term is Encounter with subterms removal (of), internal fixation device.

Neoplasms

5.65. a. V58.0, 77413

Incorrect answer. The malignancy must be reported (149.0 and 196.0), as well as the V code for the encounter.

b. 149.0, 77408

Incorrect answer. The encounter for radiation therapy, V58.0, should be the first-listed code. In addition to the primary malignancy code, the lymph node metastasis should also be reported because this is also treated by radiation (196.0). The radiation treatment CPT code must be 77413 because three treatment areas are involved and custom blocking was employed.

c. V58.0, 149.0, 196.0, 77413

Correct answer.

d. 149.0, 196.0, 77412

Incorrect answer. Encounters for radiotherapy are always coded V58.0, followed by the neoplastic disease. The CPT code is not appropriate for the 6-MV linear accelerator; code 77413 is assigned.

ICD-10-CM Code(s): Z51.0, C14.0, C77.0

ICD-10-CM Rationale: The Alphabetic Index main term is Admission, subterm radiation therapy (antineoplastic). To find the Neoplasm codes, use the Neoplasm Table under Pharynx, wall (lateral) (posterior), Malignant Primary, and Lymph, gland, cervical, Malignant Secondary.

5.66. a. 162.9, 31629

Correct answer.

b. 162.9, 31629, 77002

Incorrect answer. Fluoroscopic guidance is included in all endoscopic biopsy codes in the range of 31622–31646 and is not assigned as an additional code.

c. 162.9, 31625

Incorrect answer. The procedure code is incorrect for a transbronchial aspiration biopsy of lung tissue. Code 31629 is assigned.

d. 235.7, 31629, 77002

Incorrect answer. The carcinoma was not specified as a neoplasm of uncertain behavior, and Volume II of ICD-9-CM directs the coder to malignant neoplasm of the site or, when the site is unspecified, to 162.9. Fluoroscopic guidance is not reported separately in the endoscopic biopsy code range of 31622–31646. This code is also not specific to an intrathoracic needle biopsy.

ICD-10-CM Code(s): C34.90

ICD-10-CM Rationale: The Alphabetic Index main term is Carcinoma, with subterm oat cell. There is a note directing the coder to refer to the Neoplasm Table, specific site (lung), Malignant Primary column.

5.67.　　a. 174.9, 610.1, 19120-RT, 19125-LT, 19290-LT

Correct answer. HCPCS Level II modifiers are used to show that the lesions were not in the same breast and different techniques with separate incisions were employed.

b. 611.72, 610.1, 19120-50

Incorrect answer. When a definitive diagnosis is known, it is reported, so 174.9 for the primary malignancy would be the first-listed code and the breast lump would not be reported. A bilateral modifier -50 applies only to identical procedures on paired organs. The breasts are paired organs, but the procedures involved here are not the same. HCPCS Level II modifier -RT identifies the 19120 procedure on the right breast, while the -LT modifier is appended to CPT codes 19125 and 19290 to show that procedure occurred on the left breast.

c. 174.9, 610.1, 19120-50, 19125-50, 19290-50

Incorrect answer. Appropriate use of the bilateral modifier has it appended to only one CPT code with identical procedures performed on paired organs. Although the breasts may have bilateral procedures using modifier -50, it is only assigned to one code, which communicates to Medicare that 150 percent of the allowed amount should be provided in reimbursement for the case. The correct way to code the procedures is by use of the -RT and -LT Level II HCPCS codes to show that different breasts were involved. Codes 19120 and 19125 would be mutually exclusive otherwise.

d. 174.9, 610.2, 19120, 19125-59, 19290

Incorrect answer. The fibrocystic disease was not stated to be fibroadenosis, so code 610.1 is as specific as the documentation allows. The use of modifier -59 is not appropriate for this case because HCPCS Level II modifiers -RT and -LT would describe the services more concisely.

ICD-10-CM Code(s): C50.911, N60.12

ICD-10-CM Rationale: Using the Neoplasm Table, the coder goes to breast and completes code using the Tabular List. Using Alphabetic Index main term Fibrocystic, subterm disease, breast, the coder is directed to Mastopathy, cystic.

5.68. 153.3, 235.2, 45384, 45380-59

Rationale: Villous adenoma (polyps) is a neoplasm of uncertain behavior. These codes are only appropriately reported when specified as such by a pathologist. Code 235.2 is assigned. Two separate procedures were performed in two distinct locations, so two codes are required—the excision of the polyps by hot biopsy forceps are coded (with one code), and the biopsy of the sigmoid colon is assigned a code because it is a separate lesion. Modifier -59 designates that the two procedures are not components of one another, but distinct.

ICD-10-CM Code(s): C18.7, D37.5

ICD-10-CM Rationale: In the Neoplasm Table, the main term is Colon. Select a code under the Malignant Primary column. Since the listed code (C18.9) refers to an unspecified part of the colon, always review the category to determine if a more specific code can be found. In this case, there is a code for sigmoid colon which is used instead. The main term is Adenoma with subterm villous. There is a note referring the coder to the Neoplasm Table by site and Uncertain Behavior column.

5.69. ICD-9-CM, CPT, and HCPCS Code(s): V58.11, 204.00, 96409, J9070

Rationale: The leukemia is documented as acute lymphocytic (without remission documented), so code 204.00 is correct. The V58.11 code is listed in the first position. Typically the J code is assigned by the chargemaster. Report J9070 with a "2" in the claim units field to specify 200 mg.

ICD-10-CM Code(s): Z51.11, C91.z0

ICD-10-CM Rationale: The Alphabetic Index main term is Encounter, subterm chemotherapy for neoplasm. The Alphabetic Index main term is Leukemia, leukemic, subterm lymphoid, specified, NEC.

Disorders of the Nervous System and Sense Organs

5.70. 996.2, E878.1, 331.5, 62252

Rationale: Malfunction of the CSF shunt is coded as a complication, mechanical, shunt, ventricular, code as 996.2 and E878,1. Headache is not coded, as this is a symptom of the hydrocephalus. Reprogramming of a programmable shunt is coded as 62252.

ICD-10-CM Code(s): T85.09xA, G91.2

ICD-10-CM Rationale: The Alphabetic Index main term is Hydrocephalus with subterm normal pressure. Another main term is Complication with subterms ventricular shunt, mechanical, obstruction.

5.71. a. 335.20, 92265-50, 95861

Incorrect answer. A bilateral modifier is not appropriate for the eye muscle EMG because the code description states "one or both eyes."

b. 335.24, 95868, 95861

Incorrect answer. The diagnosis code is incorrect because this is the code for primary lateral sclerosis. ALS is coded 335.20. The CPT code for the EMG of the eye muscles is 92265 and for the legs (two extremities) is 95861. No modifier is needed for reporting these procedures together because they are for separate sites.

c. 335.20, 95861, 92265-59

Correct answer.

d. 335.29, 95861

Incorrect answer. The diagnosis code requires a fifth digit of 0 for ALS. The correct CPT codes are 95861 for the extremity testing and 92265 for the eye muscle testing.

ICD-10-CM Code(s): G12.21

ICD-10-CM Rationale: The Alphabetic Index main term is Sclerosis, sclerotic, subterm amyotrophic (lateral).

5.72.   a. 250.51, 362.01, 67040-50

Correct answer.

b. 362.01, 362.81, 67040-50

Incorrect answer. When diabetic complications are involved, the code for the diabetes is always listed first, followed by the manifestation codes. Code 250.51 is the reason for service in this case. Although a separate code is available for retinal hemorrhage, this condition is included in the code for diabetic retinopathy, and no additional code is required.

c. 250.50, 362.02, 67039-LT-RT

Incorrect answer. The diabetic code requires a fifth digit of 1 to reflect type I diabetes. The retinopathy should be assigned to code 362.01. The CPT code is for a procedure limited to a small area, such as one or two areas (focal), rather than the increased amount of laser energy required to treat all four quadrants. Correct modifier assignment when both sides are treated is -50.

d. 250.51, 362.02, 67105, 67145

Incorrect answer. The retinopathy should be assigned to code 362.01. The CPT coding is incorrect in this code set. Code 67040 includes the vitrectomy with panretinal laser treatment. The CPT codes listed in this set are for reporting of retinal detachment repairs and prophylaxis of retinal detachment, which would not occur together.

ICD-10-CM Code(s): E10.319, H35.043

ICD-10-CM Rationale: The Alphabetic Index main term is Diabetes with subterms type I, with, retinopathy. Another main term is Disorder with subterms retina, microaneurysms. The bilateral code is used since it was performed on both eyes.

5.73. 366.9, 66984-LT

Rationale: There is no further documentation about the type of cataract, so code 366.9 is correct. The CPT code 66984 describes an extracapsular cataract removal. The insertion of the intraocular lens is included in the code. There is no documentation that this was a complex procedure.

ICD-10-CM Code(s): H26.9

ICD-10-CM Rationale: The Alphabetic Index main term is Cataracts.

5.74. ICD-9-CM Reason for Visit Code(s): 345.91

ICD-9-CM and CPT Code(s): 345.91, 95819

Rationale: There is physician documentation of refractory seizure disorder to support the fifth digit of 1. The procedure code may be assigned by the chargemaster or may be assigned by the coder.

ICD-10-CM Reason for Visit Code(s): G40.319

ICD-10-CM Reason for Visit Rationale: The Alphabetic Index main term is Epilepsy, epileptic, epilepsia with subterms generalized, idiopathic, intractable.

ICD-10-CM Code(s): G40.311

ICD-10-CM Rationale: The Alphabetic Index main term is Epilepsy, epileptic, epilepsia with subterms generalized, idiopathic, intractable. Select the code outlining the epilepsy with status epilepticus.

5.75. a. 66710-LT

Incorrect answer. This code describes a procedure not involving the use of the ophthalmic endoscope. Code 66711 is the correct code.

b. 66711-LT

Correct answer.

c. 66720-LT

Incorrect answer. This code describes destruction of the ciliary body by cryotherapy. Code 66711 is the correct code.

d. 66700-LT

Incorrect answer. This code describes destruction of the ciliary body by diathermy. Code 66711 is the correct code.

5.76. a. 360.00, 67036-LT, 66030-LT

Correct answer. The patient underwent a pars plana vitrectomy with injection of medications for endophthalmitis.

b. 360.03, 67036-LT, 66030-LT

Incorrect answer. The source documentation does not provide specificity of the type of endophthalmitis the patient had.

c. 360.00, 67036-RT

Incorrect answer. The additional code for the injection is needed to completely identify the procedure performed. The procedure was performed on the left eye; therefore, the correct modifier is LT.

d. 998.59, 360.00, 67036-LT, 66030-LT

Incorrect answer. Diagnosis code 998.59 is coded when a postoperative infection is documented by the physician. The source document indicates the patient is status post a procedure; however, it does not link the current infection as a complication of that procedure.

ICD-10-CM Code(s): H44.002

ICD-10-CM Rationale: The Alphabetic Index main term is Endophthalmitis. When reviewing subcategory H44.00, the code for the left eye is listed as H44.002.

Newborn/Congenital Disorders

5.77.   a. 743.30, 760.2, 66984-50

Incorrect answer. The information provided allows greater specificity in the diagnosis code selection. Code 743.32 is the correct code. Category 760 is used to report maternal conditions that affect the fetus or newborn. This was likely reported during the birth episode but is not a reason for health services at this time (evaluation and management are directed at the congenital cataract). Documentation supports the left eye and not bilateral; therefore, the correct HCPCS Level II modifier is -LT.

b. 366.03, 66984-LT

Incorrect answer. There is a specific ICD-9-CM code for congenital cataracts. Code 743.32 is the correct code.

c. V30.00, 771.0, 743.32

Incorrect answer. This is a subsequent episode of care for a seven-month-old, so the V30 code is inappropriate. Code 771.0 is no longer under evaluation or management. CPT code 66984 should be reported.

d. 743.32, 66984-LT

Correct answer.

ICD-10-CM Code(s): Q12.0

ICD-10-CM Rationale: The Alphabetic Index main term is Cataract, subterm congenital.

5.78.   a. 755.02, 11200

Correct answer.

b. 755.02, 11200-RT, 11200-59

Incorrect answer. The CPT code includes up to 15 lesions, so it is not repeated. This makes the use of modifier -59 inappropriate to represent a separate site. The skin does not have a "right" or "left" to it, so the addition of the modifier LT is inappropriate. CMS guidelines state that -RT and -LT modifiers are not to be used for CPT codes with more than one anatomic location included. Code 11200 is such a code.

c. 755.00, 28899

Incorrect answer. The diagnosis code may be specific to the toes in code 755.02. The unlisted code is required only if the procedure involved more than soft tissue removal. In a two-week-old child, this likely is a very small lesion to remove. Code 11200 is used to report this service.

d. 755.02, 26587

Incorrect answer. The procedure code listed is for procedures involving reconstruction of tissue and bone for extra digits found on the hand. Because there is no bone in this case, code 11200 is adequate to report the service.

ICD-10-CM Code(s): Q69.2

ICD-10-CM Rationale: The Alphabetic Index main term is Polydactylism, polydactyly with subterm toes.

5.79. 752.61, 54304

Rationale: Hypospadias is a congenital condition reported with code 752.61. The CPT code 54304 is the correct procedure to report because it is a first-stage procedure requiring transposition of the prepuce.

ICD-10-CM Code(s): Q54.9

ICD-10-CM Rationale: The Alphabetic Index main term is Hypospadias.

5.80. 778.6, 550.92, 49500-50

Rationale: There is a specific code for congenital hydrocele. The 550.92 code includes hernias that are congenital. Because a combination code exists and the procedure is performed on both sides, CPT code 49500 is correct.

ICD-10-CM Code(s): P83.5, K40.20

ICD-10-CM Rationale: The Alphabetic Index main term is Hydrocele with subterm congenital. Another main term is Hernia with subterms inguinal, bilateral.

Pediatric Conditions

5.81. ICD-9-CM Reason for Visit Code(s): 749.12

ICD-9-CM and CPT Code(s): 749.12, 40720

Rationale: This is a secondary repair.

ICD-10-CM Reason for Visit Code(s): Q36.9

ICD-10-CM Reason for Visit Rationale: The Alphabetic Index main term is Cleft, subterm lip.

ICD-10-CM Code(s): Q36.9

ICD-10-CM Rationale: The Alphabetic Index main term is Cleft, subterm lip.

5.82.   a. 42825, 42830

Incorrect answer. A combination code should be used for the combination of the tonsillectomy and the adenoidectomy.

b. 42820, 42820

Incorrect answer. Code 42820 is used for a bilateral T&A.

c. 42821

Incorrect answer. The codes for T&A are age-dependent. This code would be used if the patient is 12 years of age or older. In this case the patient is 6 years old.

d. 42820
Correct answer.

Emergency Room Service

5.83.   ICD-9-CM, CPT, and HCPCS Level II Codes: 493.02, 94640 ×2, J7611

Rationale: Cough is integral to asthma and therefore not coded. Allergic asthma is coded as 493.0X with a fifth digit of 2 for acute exacerbation. The nebulizer treatments are coded as 94640 (nonpressurized inhalation treatment for acute airway obstruction) with units of 2. Some insurers may require that the nebulizers be reported as 94640 and 94640-76 for repeat procedure by the same physician. J7611 is reported for the 1 mg of Albuterol. Note that the medication may be reported as a pharmacy service.

ICD-10-CM Code(s): J45.901

ICD-10-CM Rationale: The Alphabetic Index main term is Asthma, subterm allergic extrinsic, with, exacerbation (acute).

5.84.   a. 14040, 11971

Incorrect answer. Flaps are used in the closure of the defects, but the adjacent tissue transfer codes are not the most appropriate choice for a code. CPT code 26560 most appropriately describes the work of the separation and closure of a syndactyly repair wound.

b. 26560, 11971
Correct answer.

c. 26561

Incorrect answer. This procedure describes the closure with the use of skin flaps and graft. The documentation does not support the use of this code because no grafting was performed. In addition, CPT code 11971 for the removal of the tissue expander is required.

d. 26562

Incorrect answer. This procedure describes the complex repair when the defect involves bone or nails. The documentation does not support the use of this code because the syndactyly does not involve bone. In addition, CPT code 11971 for the removal of the tissue expander is required.

5.85. ICD-9-CM Reason for Visit Code(s): 780.6, 786.2

ICD-9-CM Code(s): 465.9, 372.00

Rationale: The conjunctivitis is unspecified as to the cause.

ICD-10-CM Reason for Visit Code(s): R05, R50.9

ICD-10-CM Code(s): H10.33, J06.9

ICD-10-CM Rationale: The Alphabetic Index main term is Cough. The Alphabetic Index main term is Fever, unspecified. For the final diagnoses, the Alphabetic Index main term is Conjunctivitis, acute. The coder completes the code using the Tabular List. The Alphabetic Index main term is Infection, subterm respiratory, upper NOS.

Conditions of Pregnancy, Childbirth, and the Puerperium

5.86. a. 790.22, V22.2, 82951

Incorrect answer. Code 790.22 excludes that complicating pregnancy and refers the coder to subcategory 648.8. The V code is not appropriate for this encounter because the pregnancy is not incidental. The correct codes are 648.83 and 82951, but laboratory codes are typically coded by the chargemaster.

b. 648.83, 82951

Correct answer. Laboratory codes are typically coded by the chargemaster.

c. 648.83, 82950

Incorrect answer. CPT code 82951 is the appropriate code for this test, which involves obtaining three separate specimens for testing the glucose levels at one hour, two hours, and three hours after the patient drinks the glucose mixture. Laboratory codes are typically coded by the chargemaster.

d. 648.80, 82951, 82952, 82952

Incorrect answer. The fifth digit of 0 is unspecified. This is an antepartum condition. Code 648.83 is the correct code. Three specimens are included in code 82951. CPT code 82952 would only be reported if additional tests, beyond three, were performed. Laboratory codes are typically coded by the chargemaster.

ICD-10-CM Code(s): O99.810

ICD-10-CM Rationale: The Alphabetic Index main term is Pregnancy with subterms complicated by, abnormal, glucose (tolerance) NEC.

5.87. a. 637.91, 58120

Incorrect answer. The abortion was specified as spontaneous; therefore, the diagnosis code 634.91 is reported. Code 58120 is incorrect because this is the surgical completion of an incomplete abortion. The correct CPT code is 59812.

b. 634.91, 59812

Correct answer.

c. 634.91, 58120

Incorrect answer. The CPT code 58120 is used for a nonobstetric procedure. Because this procedure is done for treatment of an incomplete spontaneous abortion, code 59812 is reported.

d. 634.92, 59812

Incorrect answer. The fifth digit is incorrect for the diagnosis of an incomplete abortion.

ICD-10-CM Code(s): O03.4

ICD-10-CM Rationale: The Alphabetic Index main term is Abortion, subterm incomplete.

5.88. V28.4, 76805

Rationale: Because the purpose of the test is antenatal screening, code V28.4 is reported as the reason for the test. It is incorrect to assign V22.0 in this case.

ICD-10-CM Code(s): Z36

ICD-10-CM Rationale: The Alphabetic Index main term is Encounter (for) with subterm antenatal screening.

5.89. 628.2, 58340, 74740, 77002

Rationale: Code 58340 is reported for the injection. Code 74740 is reported for the interpretation of the hysterosalpingogram. The use of the fluoroscope is reported with code 77002.

ICD-10-CM Code(s): N97.1

ICD-10-CM Rationale: The Alphabetic Index main term is Infertility, subterm female, associated with, fallopian tube disease or anomaly.

Disorders of the Genitourinary System

5.90. a. 52332, 50590

Incorrect answer. The cystourethroscopy with stent insertion was done on a previous admission. Only the ESWL was done at this time.

b. 50590

Correct answer.

c. 52353

Incorrect answer. The lithotripsy was not done via cystourethroscopy.

d. 50590, 52353

Code 52353 is not appropriate—a cystourethroscopy was not done on this admission.

5.91. V25.2, 52250

Rationale: The patient presents for contraceptive surgery. V25.2 is used for admissions that are for sterilization surgery. Code 55250 is used for the vasectomy. This code includes any post-surgery semen analysis.

ICD-10-CM Code(s): Z30.2

ICD-10-CM Rationale: The Alphabetic Index main term is Encounter, subterm sterilization.

5.92. 608.23, 54512

Rationale: An appendix testis is a small solid projection of tissue on the upper outer surface of the testis. It is a remnant of the embryonic Mullerian duct. There is no code that specifically refers to the removal of an appendix testis but code 54512 is used for extraparenchymal tissue removal which an appendix testis is.

ICD-10-CM Code(s): N44.03

ICD-10-CM Rationale: The Alphabetic Index main term is Torsion with subterm appendix testis.

Disorders of the Respiratory System

5.93. a. 493.22

Correct answer.

b. 493.21, 491.21

Incorrect answer. When the two conditions occur together, code 493.22 is the only code to report.

c. 493.20

Incorrect answer. The fifth digit should be 2 to show acute exacerbation.

d. 491.21

Incorrect answer. A note under 493.2 includes chronic asthmatic bronchitis and asthma with chronic obstructive pulmonary disease.

ICD-10-CM Code(s): J44.1

ICD-10-CM Rationale: The Alphabetic Index main term is Asthma, subterm with, chronic obstructive bronchitis, with exacerbation (acute).

5.94. 162.3, 305.1, 31625

Rationale: The site is specified as upper lobe of bronchus. The hemoptysis and cough would be integral to the carcinoma.

ICD-10-CM Code(s): C34.10, Z72.0

ICD-10-CM Rationale: The Alphabetic Index main term is Neoplasm with subterms bronchus, upper lobe. Use a code from the Malignant Primary column. Code Z72.0 is referenced under the main term, Use, with subterm tobacco.

5.95. ICD-9-CM Reason for Visit Code(s): V55.0

ICD-9-CM and CPT Code(s): V55.0, 31820

Rationale: The documentation states that plastic repair was not required for the closure, so code 31820 is assigned.

ICD-10-CM Reason for Visit Code(s): Z43.0

ICD-10-CM Code(s): Z43.0

ICD-10-CM Rationale: The Alphabetic Index main term is Attention (to) tracheostomy.

Trauma and Poisoning

5.96. a. 934.0, E912, E000.8, E849.4, 31577

Correct answer.

b. 934.0, E912, E849.4, 31511

Incorrect answer. Code 31511 is for an indirect laryngoscopy rather than the fiberoptic type of scope indicated. Code 31577 is correct.

c. 784.99, E912, E849.4, E000.8, 31530

Incorrect answer. An operative laryngoscopy requires anesthetic support not available in the ED. CPT code 31577 is the correct code for a fiberoptic scope with local anesthesia used. Also, when choking occurs from a foreign body lodged in the airway, the foreign body should be coded rather than the symptom code for choking sensation.

d. 933.1, 31577

Incorrect answer. Code 934.0 is specific to the trachea, while code 933.1 is for a foreign body in the larynx. An E code should be assigned (E912) to show the cause of the problem and code E849.4 reports the place of occurrence.

ICD-10-CM Code(s): T17.490A, Y93.02, Y92.831, Y93.02, Y99.8

ICD-10-CM Rationale: The Alphabetic Index main term is Foreign body with subterms trachea, causing, asphyxiation, specified type NEC. In the Index to External Causes, the main term is Activity with subterm running. specified NEC. In reviewing the Y93 category, the best code was found to be Y93.9. In the Index to External Causes, the main term is Place of occurrence with subterm amusement park. In the Index to External Causes, the main term is External cause status, leisure activity. In the Index to External Causes, the main term is Activity with subterm running.

5.97. ICD-9-CM, CPT, and HCPCS Level II Code(s): 972.9, E950.4, 43753, 96374-59, 96367, 96366, J1610 × 20, J7060

Rationale: Verapamil is not listed specifically in the Table of Drugs and Chemicals but is a cardiovascular medication and can be accessed in the Table under that term. For a suicide attempt, the code is 972.9 with an E-code of E950.4. The initial IV is a push of Glucagon (96374) with two additional hours of sequential IV (96367 and 96366). The Glucagon HCl is J1610 for 20 units (10 mg push and 5 mg per hour over 2 hours) and D5W is J7060.

ICD-10-CM Code(s): T46.1x2A

ICD-10-CM Rationale: The Drug and Chemical Table is used to locate the drug Verapamil. The column Poisoning, Intentional, self-harm is used.

5.98. V58.30, 16030

Rationale: The specific site of the burns is not documented, so code 943.20 is the most specific code. However, the patient is being seen in aftercare (after the acute phase of the injury was treated) for dressing changes. The correct code to report is V58.3X (attention to dressing and sutures) with a fifth digit of 0 to denote encounter for change or removal of nonsurgical wound dressing; therefore, code 943.20 (second-degree burn of upper extremity) would not be reported. E codes are not assigned for subsequent visits of an accident, only the initial visit, or when a late effect applies. Code 16030 was selected because dressings were applied to more than one extremity.

ICD-10-CM Code(s): Z48.00

ICD-10-CM Rationale: The Alphabetic Index main term is Change(s) (of) with subterm dressing (nonsurgical).

5.99. 162.9, 511.81, 32421, 32421-76

Rationale: The thoracentesis was repeated in the same day by the same physician. The procedure code is reported twice with modifier -76 reported on the second procedure. The malignant pleural effusion is coded as 511.81.

ICD-10-CM Code(s): C34.90, J91.0

ICD-10-CM Rationale: The Alphabetic Index main term is found in the Neoplasm Table under Lung. The Alphabetic Index main term is Effusion, subterm pleura, malignant.

5.100. ICD-9-CM Reason for Visit Code(s): 882.0, 881.0, 890.0

ICD-9-CM and CPT Code(s): 882.0, 881.00, 890.0, E888.0, E920.9, E849.1, E000.8, E001.1, 12042, 12004

Rationale: When the sites of the open wounds are known, do not assign a code for multiple. Code the sites individually. The External cause of injury code E888.0 instructs the coder to use an additional E code to identify the sharp object (E920.9). Place of occurrence is a farm (E849.1). The external cause status of E000.8 is assigned for leisure activity and the activity code is assigned as E001.1 because the patient was running in the field.

The lengths of all three wounds are not added together. Only the lengths of wounds that are in the same repair category and anatomic site are added together. In this case, the forearm and thigh are both simple repairs, while the hand is an intermediate repair, which is separately reported. The intermediate repair is listed as the first procedure since it is the more resource-intensive procedure.

ICD-10-CM Reason for Visit Code(s): S51.811A, S61.411A, S71.112A

ICD-10-CM Code(s): S51.811A, S61.411A, S71.112A, W01.118A, Y92.79, Y93.02, Y99.8

ICD-10-CM Rationale: In the Index to External Causes, the main term is Fall, falling with subterms due to, slipping, with subsequent striking against object, specified NEC. In the Index to External Causes, the main term is Place of occurrence with subterm farm. In the Index to External Causes, the main term is Activity with subterm running. In the Index to External Causes, the main term is External Cause Status with subterm specified NEC.

5.101. a. 961.0, 786.09, 995.1, 693.0, E857, E849.0

Incorrect answer. There is no evidence in the source document of an overdose of the medication; therefore, an ICD-9-CM code for poisoning is inappropriate.

b. 995.20, E931.0, E849.0

Incorrect answer. Code 995.20 is less specific while code 995.1 accurately reflects the documentation.

c. 995.1, 786.09, E931.0, E849.0

Correct answer.

d. 995.1, 786.09, 693.0, E930.9, E849.0

Incorrect answer. The diagnosis codes are correct except the E code. According to the source document, the antibiotic Bactrim (sulfonamide) was the cause of the adverse reaction, requiring assignment of an E code with a higher level of specificity.

ICD-10-CM Code(s): T36.8x5A, R06.00, T78.3xxA

ICD-10-CM Rationale: The code for angioedema is found in the Alphabetic Index under main term Angioedema. The Alphabetic Index main term is Distress, subterm respiratory. The Drug and Chemical Table is used to select the adverse effect code for Bactrim. There is no entry for Bactrim, but the code for sulfamethazole with trimethoprim is used.

5.102. 816.11, E919.4, E849.0, 26418-F1, 26540-F1, 11012-F1

Rationale: The source document reveals the patient had a compound fracture that was debrided down to the bone with extensor tendon and collateral ligament repair. The left hand modifiers are as follows: first digit (thumb) is -FA, second digit (index finger) is -F1, third digit (middle finger) is -F2, fourth digit (ring finger) is -F3, and fifth digit (pinky) is -F4.

ICD-10-CM Code(s): S62.621A, W31.2xxA, Y92.015, Y93.h9, Y99.8

ICD-10-CM Rationale: The Alphabetic Index main term is Fracture with subterms finger, index, medial phalanx (displaced). In the Index to External Causes, the main term is Contact (accidental) with subterms with, circular saw. In the Index to External Causes, the main term is Activity with subterms maintenance, property. In the Index to External Causes, the main term is Place of occurrence with subterms residence, houses, single family, garage. In the Index to External Causes, the main term is External Cause Status with subterm specified NEC.

Chapter 6. Case Studies from Physician-based Health Records

Unless otherwise stated, code set answers given in Chapter 6 are ICD-9-CM and/or CPT.

Anesthesia Services

6.1.   a. 00404

Incorrect answer. Code 00402 specifies reconstructive procedures on the breast.

b. 00406

Incorrect answer. Code 00402 specifies reconstructive procedures on the breast.

c. 00402

Correct answer.

d. 00400

Incorrect answer. Code 00402 specifies reconstructive procedures on the breast.

6.2.   a. 660.11, 653.41, 64493

Incorrect answer. Code 64493 is for injection of the facet joint or facet nerve. The correct answer is 01967 and 01968.

b. 660.11, 653.01, 01961

Incorrect answer. This is for a C-section delivery that does not involve an epidural (that is, general anesthesia). The correct answer is 01967 and 01968. The disproportion was specified as cephalopelvic; thus, the correct ICD-9-CM code is 653.41.

c. 660.11, 653.41, 01967, 01968

Correct answer.

d. 660.11, 653.91, 01996

Incorrect answer. The code 01996 should be used only for each subsequent day if a long-term epidural is used for pain control. The correct answer is 01967 and 01968. The disproportion was specified as cephalopelvic; thus, the correct ICD-9-CM code is 653.41.

ICD-10-CM Code(s): O65.4

ICD-10-CM Rationale: The Alphabetic Index main term is Delivery with subterms complicated by, obstruction, due to, fetopelvic disproportion.

6.3.   a. 521.00, 00170-AA-23

Correct answer.

b. 521.00, 00170-AA

Incorrect answer. The patient was not under one year of age. Modifiers should be attached to the anesthesia code.

c. 520.7, 00170-P1-23-AA

Incorrect answer. The diagnosis code should be 521.00, and the P1 modifier may not be required if it does not add additional unit value.

d. 521.30, 00170

Incorrect answer. The diagnosis code should be 521.00. The patient was not under one year of age. Modifiers should be attached to the anesthesia code.

ICD-10-CM Code(s): K02.9

ICD-10-CM Rationale: The Alphabetic Index main term is Caries, subterm dental.

6.4.   a. 12031, 99143

Incorrect answer. The patient age of five years is reported with code 99144.

b. 12031, 99144

Correct answer.

c. 12031-47

Incorrect answer. Neither regional nor general anesthesia was given to the patient, so modifier -47 is not appropriate. The code for conscious sedation with Versed, 99144, must be reported.

d. 12031-QS

Incorrect answer. The -QS modifier for monitored anesthesia care applies to anesthesia providers who are monitoring the patient. In this case, the staff nurse monitored the patient. The code for conscious sedation with Versed, 99144, must be reported.

6.5.   747.10, 00561-AA-P5

Rationale: The physical status modifier is -P5 because the patient is not expected to survive without the surgery. Code 99100 is not assigned due to an instructional note under 00561 that states "do not report 00561 in conjunction with 99100."

ICD-10-CM Code(s): Q25.1

ICD-10-CM Rationale: The Alphabetic Index main term is Coarctation of aorta.

Disorders of the Blood and Blood-Forming Organs

6.6.   269.0, 286.7

Rationale: Vitamin K deficiency (269.0) is the underlying cause and is therefore sequenced first. The acquired coagulopathy (286.7) is different from a defect in coagulopathy. In the Index under Coagulopathy, the coder is directed to See also Defect, Coagulopathy, where an entry for acquired coagulopathy is found.

ICD-10-CM Code(s): D68.4

ICD-10-CM Rationale: The Alphabetic Index main term is Coagulopathy where there is a note to "See also Defect, coagulation." Under the main term Defect, defective, the subterms are coagulation, due to, Vitamin K deficiency.

6.7. a. 201.21, 38505

Correct answer.

b. 201.91, 38505

Incorrect answer. Hodgkin's sarcoma is assigned to code 201.21.

c. 201.21, 38500

Incorrect answer. The biopsy was performed with a needle, so code 38500 is not correct.

d. 785.6, 38510

Incorrect answer. Because the Hodgkin's sarcoma was confirmed by a pathologist, the definitive diagnosis should be coded. There is no documentation that the lymph node is deep, and it was biopsied with a needle, so code 38510 is not correct.

ICD-10-CM Code(s): C81.91

ICD-10-CM Rationale: The Alphabetic Index main term Hodgkin's directs the coder to Lymphoma, Hodgkin.

6.8. a. 282.61, 789.09, 427.31, 250.00

Incorrect answer. The sickle-cell anemia is in crisis, so 282.61 is not correct. It is not necessary to code the inguinal pain because pain, fever, and so forth are part of a sickle-cell crisis.

b. 282.62, 733.42, 427.31, 250.00

Incorrect answer. The avascular necrosis was not confirmed, but only documented as "rule-out." This would not be coded in the physician setting.

c. 282.62

Incorrect answer. The atrial fib and diabetes should be coded.

d. 282.62, 427.31, 250.00

Correct answer.

ICD-10-CM Code(s): D57.00, I48.0, E11.9

ICD-10-CM Rationale: The Alphabetic Index main term is Crisis with subterm sickle-cell. Another main term is Fibrillation with subterm atrial or auricular. The diabetes code is located at the main term Diabetes with subterm type 2.

6.9. 36415, 82951

Rationale: The correct code assignment would be code 36415 for the venipuncture, all three specimens, and code 82951 for the glucose tolerance test, three specimens.

6.10. a. 280.0

Correct answer. The physician did not document the type of anemia. Without that documentation, code 280.0 is the default for unspecified anemia.

b. 285.1

Incorrect answer. The physician did not document the type of anemia. Without that documentation, code 280.0 is the default for unspecified anemia.

c. 285.8

Incorrect answer. The physician did not document the type of anemia. Without that documentation, code 280.0 is the default for unspecified anemia.

d. 285.9

Incorrect answer. The physician did not document the type of anemia. Without that documentation, code 280.0 is the default for unspecified anemia.

ICD-10-CM Code(s): D50.0

ICD-10-CM Rationale: The Alphabetic Index main term is Anemia with subterm blood loss (chronic).

Disorders of the Cardiovascular System

6.11. 458.9, 427.89, 787.91, 715.36

Symptoms of hypotension and sinus bradycardia are coded because the cause is not established. Diarrhea is coded. GI bleed is stated a "potential" and is not an established diagnosis. Osteoarthrosis is localized to the knee and therefore coded as 715.36.

ICD-10-CM Code(s): I95.9, R00.1, R19.7, M17.9

ICD-10-CM Rationale: The Alphabetic Index main term is Hypotension. The Alphabetic Index main term is Bradycardia (sinoatrial) (sinus) (vagal). The Alphabetic Index main term Diarrhea (disease) is reviewed to get the code R19.7. The Alphabetic Index main term Osteoarthrosis directs the coder to "See Osteoarthritis if appropriate." Main term Osteoarthritis, subterm knee yields code M17.9.

6.12. a. 427.0, 414.01, 92982, 33206

Incorrect answer. Patient had sick sinus syndrome (not paroxysmal supraventricular tachycardia), which should be listed as a secondary diagnosis code. The pacemaker is documented as AV, which means atrial-ventricular or dual chamber. Code 33208 is correct.

b. 414.01, 427.81, 92995, 33208

Incorrect answer. The angioplasty is not documented as with atherectomy. The correct code is 92982.

c. 414.01, 427.81, 92982, 33208

Correct answer.

d. 427.81, 414.01, 92982, 33206

Incorrect answer. The documentation states that the patient was transferred to the hospital specifically to undergo the PTCA for the CAD, so the 414.01 code should be sequenced first. The documentation shows that the pacemaker was inserted percutaneously. The correct code is 33208.

ICD-10-CM Code(s): I25.10, I49.5

ICD-10-CM Rationale: The Alphabetic Index main term is Disease with subterm coronary (artery) along with a note to "See Disease, heart, ischemic, atherosclerotic." Another main term Syndrome is referenced with subterms sick, sinus.

6.13. 404.93, 428.0, 585.5, 250.01

Rationale: The combination code for hypertensive heart and renal disease is used because the hypertension was documented as the cause of the heart disease. The fifth digit of 3 is assigned and code 585.5 is assigned to identify the stage of chronic kidney disease. A separate code is not assigned for the hypertension. The type of heart failure (428.0) should be the second code. The DM should also be coded.

ICD-10-CM Code(s): I13.2, I50.9, N18.5, E10.9

ICD-10-CM Rationale: The Alphabetic Index main term is Hypertension, subterm cardiorenal (disease) with heart failure, with stage 5 or end-stage renal disease. The Tabular List directs the coder to use an additional code to identify the type of heart failure (I50-) as well as a code to identify the stage of CKD (N18.5, N18.6). The Diabetes mellitus is coded by reviewing the Alphabetic Index main term Diabetes, subterm type I.

6.14. ICD-9-CM Code(s): 411.1

Rationale: The patient did not have a myocardial infarction. See Syndrome, preinfarction.

ICD-10-CM Code(s): I20.0

ICD-10-CM Rationale: The Alphabetic Index main term is Syndrome with subterm preinfarction.

6.15. ICD-9-CM and CPT Code(s): V58.81, 153.3, 36589

Rationale: The V code is used because the episode was not directed at the cancer. The cancer is coded as current because it has not been resected. It is appropriate to assign a procedure code for removal of an implantable venous access device. The coding of the removal of a VAD is dependent on a tunneled central venous catheter and whether or not a port or pump was present.

ICD-10-CM Code(s): Z45.2, C18.7

ICD-10-CM Rationale: The Alphabetic Index main term is Removal, subterm vascular access device or catheter. Using the Neoplasm Table, review intestine, large, colon, sigmoid, Malignant Primary.

Disorders of the Digestive System

6.16. a. 278.00, 43842, 43846-51

Incorrect answer. The documentation states that the patient has morbid obesity, so code 278.01 is correct. The contributing risk factors should be coded because they were treated and affect the care of the patient. The CPT code 43846 should not be added because there was no documentation that a bypass was also performed.

b. 278.01, 401.9, 272.0, 43842

Correct answer.

c. 278.01, 401.1, 272.0, 43842, 43843-59

Incorrect answer. The hypertension was not documented as benign; therefore, it should be coded 401.9 without further query to the physician. Code 43842 is the only procedure code that is needed.

d. 278.01, 43848

Incorrect answer. The contributing risk factors should be coded because they were treated and affect the care of the patient. CPT code 43848 is incorrect because this is the original procedure, not a revision.

ICD-10-CM Code(s): E66.01, I10, E78.0

ICD-10-CM Rationale: The Alphabetic Index main term is Obesity with subterms morbid, due to excess calories. Another main term is Hypertension, hypertensive. Another main term is Hypercholesterolemia.

6.17. a. 560.89, 555.0, 44120, 44121-51

Incorrect answer. *Coding Clinic* (1997, 2Q) states that the regional enteritis is sequenced first followed by the bowel obstruction. Code 44121 is an add-on code and therefore the modifier -51 is not appropriate.

b. 555.0, 560.89, 44120, 44121-51

Incorrect answer. Code 44121 is an add-on code and therefore the modifier -51 is not appropriate.

c. 555.0, 560.89, 44120, 44121

Correct answer.

d. 555.2, 560.89, 44020

Incorrect answer. The correct code for Crohn's disease of the small intestine is 555.0. There is no documentation of exploration, biopsy, or removal of foreign body. The correct code for the enterectomy, which is excision, is 44120.

ICD-10-CM Code(s): K50.012

ICD-10-CM Rationale: The Alphabetic Index main term Crohn's disease directs the coder to Enteritis, regional. The code is found at Enteritis, regional, regional, small intestine, with complication, intestinal obstruction.

6.18. 45384, 45380-51

Rationale: Because the biopsy and the polypectomy were done on different sites, they should both be coded. The polypectomy was done by hot biopsy, forceps. Some payers may require a -59 modifier appended to code 45380.

6.19. 789.00, 578.1, 91110

Rationale: The procedure is located in the index under Gastrointestinal tract, Imaging and the Intraluminal. The physician documents a site "suggestive of possible..." and therefore the erosion is not coded.

ICD-10-CM Code(s): R10.9, K92.1

ICD-10-CM Rationale: The Alphabetic Index main term is Pain, abdominal. The Alphabetic Index main term is Blood, subterm in, feces.

6.20. 47610, 44950-52

Rationale: For reporting purposes, some payers require that the appendectomy be identified. In those cases, CPT code 44950-52 would be reported in addition to the major abdominal procedure performed, as per CPT instructions. The correct code for cholecystectomy with common duct exploration is 47610. The appendectomy code 44955 is not correct because there is no documentation that the patient had a condition of the appendix. Documentation states incidental.

6.21. a. 455.4, 455.1, 46255

Correct answer.

b. 455.5, 455.2, 46260

Incorrect answer. The hemorrhoids are thrombosed and in a single column. Therefore, CPT code 46255 describes the hemorrhoidectomy of internal and external hemorrhoids in a single column or group.

c. 455.4, 455.1, 46945, 46320

Incorrect answer. CPT code 46255 is a combination for hemorrhoidectomy of internal and external hemorrhoids in a single column or group. Coding these procedures separately is inappropriate.

d. 455.7, 46083, 46320

Incorrect answer. The hemorrhoids are thrombosed and in a single column. Therefore, CPT code 46255 describes the hemorrhoidectomy of internal and external hemorrhoids in a single column or group. Coding these procedures separately is inappropriate.

ICD-10-CM Code(s): I84.03

ICD-10-CM Rationale: The Alphabetic Index main term is Hemorrhoids, subterm external, with internal, thrombosed. Only one code is needed.

6.22. 574.00, 574.10, 47563

Rationale: Coding guidelines state that when an acute and a chronic condition are both present and there is no combination code, you code both, with the acute condition sequenced first. The procedure was done via laparoscope.

ICD-10-CM Code(s): K80.12

ICD-10-CM Rationale: The Alphabetic Index main term is Calculus with subterms gallbladder, with, cholecystitis, acute, with, chronic cholecystitis.

6.23. a. 43773

Correct answer. Code 43773 describes removal and replacement of an adjustable gastric band.

b. 43771, 43770

Incorrect answer. Reporting both codes 43771 and 43770 for removal of a band and placement of a band could be construed as unbundling, since there is a single code that reports the procedure.

c. 43774, 43770

Incorrect answer. Code 43774 is inappropriate as it describes removal of both the band and subcutaneous port, which was not done here.

d. 43888

Incorrect answer. Code 43888 describes removal and replacement of a gastric band, but this is the code for an open procedure, not the laparoscopic procedure noted here.

6.24.   ICD-9-CM and CPT Code(s): 750.0, 41520

Rationale: The coder should note that 41520 is for a frenoplasty while code 40806 is used when only a frenotomy is done.

ICD-10-CM Code(s): Q38.1

ICD-10-CM Rationale: The Alphabetic Index main term is Ankyloglossia.

6.25.   ICD-9-CM and CPT Code(s): 562.10, 455.0, 211.3, 45384

Rationale: Code 45384 includes the use of conscious sedation so no additional code is needed. It also includes both the colonoscopy and the removal of the tumor.

ICD-10-CM Code(s): K57.30, D12.5, I84.21

ICD-10-CM Rationale: The Alphabetic Index main term is Diverticulosis, large intestine. The Alphabetic Index main term is Polyp, polyps, subterm colon, sigmoid. The Alphabetic Index main term is Hemorrhoids, subterm internal.

Evaluation and Management (E/M) Services

6.26.   a. 99284

Incorrect answer. Note the description for code 99285, "with the constraints imposed by the urgency of the patient's clinical condition and/or mental status."

b. 99285

Correct answer.

c. 99285-52

Incorrect answer. The description for code 99285 allows for the constraints of urgency. Modifier -52 for reduced services is not necessary with the E/M code.

d. 99291

Incorrect answer. No mention was made of critical care services being provided, and time spent performing critical care is not documented.

6.27.   a. 784.99, 783.3, 99335

Incorrect answer. The choking was caused by a foreign body, code 933.1.

b. 933.1, 99334

Incorrect answer. The correct CPT code for the key components listed is 99335 as this is an established patient with two out of the three components being met (expanded problem focus exam and low-complexity MDM).

c. 933.1, 99335

Correct answer.

d. 783.3, 99334

Incorrect answer. The choking was caused by a foreign body, code 933.1. The correct CPT code for the key components listed is 99335, as this is an established patient with two out of the three components being met (expanded problem focus exam and low-complexity MDM).

ICD-10-CM Code(s): T17.328A

ICD-10-CM Rationale: The Alphabetic Index main term is Foreign body, subterm larynx, causing, injury NEC.

6.28. 99396, 99214-25

Rationale: The physician codes 99396 for the preventive medicine visit, and 99214-25 for the additional diagnosis and workup related to the mass.

6.29. 427.5, 99291, 99292 × 2

Rationale: Reference the Critical Care Services section preceding the critical care codes. Codes 99291 and 99292 are used to report the total duration of time spent by the physician providing critical care to the patient, even if the time spent is not continuous for that date. This requires that the physician devote his or her full attention to the patient and therefore cannot provide services to any other patient during the same period of time. Critical care time may or may not be direct bedside care, but also includes nursing unit time for care assessment and planning that contributes directly to the treatment of the patient.

ICD-10-CM Code(s): I46.9

ICD-10-CM Rationale: The Alphabetic Index main term is Arrest, arrested, cardiac.

6.30. a. 381.4, 493.90, 787.03, 758.0, 99214, 96372, J0696

Incorrect answer. The otitis is documented as acute, so code 382.9 is the correct code. The patient is a first-time wheezer who has not been diagnosed with asthma. Code 786.07 correctly describes the wheezing. The documented components support 99214 as the E/M code assignment but a -25 modifier is required. The patient received an IM injection, 96372, with two units of Ceftriaxone sodium, J0696, because each unit is worth 250 mg. The patient and mother are taught how to use the inhaler, which is coded as 94664.

b. 382.9, 758.0, 99214, 94640, 96372, J0696 × 2 units

Incorrect answer. The documented components support 99214 as the E/M code assignment, but a -25 modifier is required. The patient and mother are taught how to use the inhaler, which is coded as 94664. The patient was not provided with a nebulizer treatment (94640).

c. 382.9, 786.07, 787.03, 758.0, 99214-25, 94664, 96372, J0696 × 2 units

Correct answer.

d. 382.9, 786.07, 787.03, 758.0, 99214-25, 96372, J0696

Incorrect answer. The patient received an IM injection, 96372, with two units of Ceftriaxone sodium, J0696, because each unit is worth 250 mg. The patient and mother are taught how to use the inhaler, which is coded as 94664.

ICD-10-CM Code(s): H66.93, R06.2, R11.10, Q90.9

ICD-10-CM Rationale: The Alphabetic Index main term is Otitis with subterms media, acute, subacute. Because the otitis media was bilateral, code H66.93 is used. Another main term is Wheezing. A third main term is Vomiting. The final main term is Syndrome with subterm Down.

6.31. a. 99304

Incorrect answer. This reports initial evaluation and management services to a nursing facility patient. Code 99318 is the appropriate code for an annual physical examination.

b. 99308

Incorrect answer. This reports subsequent evaluation and management services that are performed to assess a change in the patient. Annual examinations performed for administrative reasons are reported with code 99318.

c. 99318

Correct answer.

d. 99306

Incorrect answer. Code 99306 reports an initial new or established nursing facility evaluation meeting comprehensive history, comprehensive exam, and high-complexity MDM.

6.32. 99225

Rationale: New CPT E&M codes have been added for subsequent observation care. These codes are based on history, examination, and medical decision making. Two of the three key elements are required to select the appropriate level. Based on a detailed examination and moderate decision making the correct code to use is 99225.

6.33. a. 99292, 99292, 92950

Incorrect answer. Code 99292 is an add-on code and must be used with 99291.

b. 99291, 99292, 99292, 92950

Correct answer.

c. 99291, 99292, 99292, 99090, 92950, 43752

Incorrect answer. Codes 99090 and 43752 are not appropriate to use. These services are included in the codes for the critical care services provided.

d. 99291, 99292, 92950

Incorrect answer. In order to capture the entire time spent with the patient, code 99292 should be reported two times.

Endocrine, Nutritional, and Metabolic Diseases and Immunity Disorders

6.34. a. 60220-50

Incorrect answer. Code 60220 describes the removal of one lobe of the thyroid. This is correct on the left side, but the right side is more appropriately coded with 60260 because part of the right thyroid was previosuly removed. In addition, a code is needed for sparing the parathyroid glands and the replantation into the local tissue.

b. 60240

Incorrect answer. Code 60240 describes a total thyroidectomy. However, in this case, a portion of the right thyroid gland has already been removed. Codes 60260 and 60220 more appropriately describe this procedure. In addition, a code is needed for sparing the parathyroid glands and the replantation into the local tissue.

c. 60260-50, 60512

Incorrect answer. Code 60260 describes removal of the remaining portion of the thyroid when a portion has been previously removed. This describes the procedure on the right but not on the left. Codes 60260 and 60220 more appropriately describe this procedure. The parathryoid procedure is correct.

d. 60260-RT, 60220-LT, 60512

Correct answer.

6.35. a. 90700

Incorrect answer. Code 90461 is used to report additional vaccinations and must be reported with code 90460. The code for the vaccine is appropriate.

b. 99213, 90460, 90700

Incorrect answer. An evaluation and management code should not be reported unless a separate E&M service was performed.

c. 90460, 90461, 90461, 90700

Correct answer. For vaccines with multiple components, the 2011 CPT code book instructs to assign code 90460 for each vaccine administered in conjunction with 90461 for each additional component in a given vaccine. According to CPT, a component is defined as each antigen within a vaccine that prevents disease(s) caused by one organism. An example of a combination vaccine by this definition is DTaP, a combination of diphtheria, tetanus, and pertussis components (AMA 2011, 6).

d. 90460

Incorrect answer. This code is appropriate for reporting the administration, but an additional code should be reported for the vaccine itself, 90700.

6.36.   a. 253.0, 225.0

Incorrect answer. A pituitary tumor is not confirmed and would not be coded until it was confirmed. If it was confirmed, a pituitary adenoma would be coded to 227.3 rather than 225.0.

b. 253.0

Correct answer.

c. 227.3

Incorrect answer. A pituitary tumor is not confirmed and would not be coded until it was confirmed. Code only the known diagnosis at the time of the visit—in this case, the acromegaly.

d. 253.0, 227.3

Incorrect answer. A pituitary tumor is not confirmed and would not be coded until it was confirmed.

ICD-10-CM Code(s): E22.0

ICD-10-CM Rationale: The Alphabetic Index main term is Acromegaly, acromegalia.

6.37.   a. 627.2, V07.4, 99213

Correct answer. The elements of E/M are an expanded problem-focused history based on one to three elements of HPI, examination not documented, and low medical decision making based on one stable chronic disease and medication management. The E/M code is therefore 99213.

b. V07.4, V49.81, 99212

Incorrect answer. The patient has symptoms that are being controlled with medication. Code 627.2 should be used instead of the asymptomatic menopause code. The elements of E/M are an expanded problem-focused history based on one to three elements of HPI, examination not documented, and low medical decision making based on one stable chronic disease and medication management. The E/M code is therefore 99213.

c. 627.2, 99213

Incorrect answer. Code V07.4 should be assigned to report the use of hormone replacement therapy. The elements of E/M are an expanded problem-focused history based on one to three elements of HPI, examination not documented, and low medical decision making based on one stable chronic disease and medication management. The E/M code is therefore 99213.

d. V07.4, 99212

Incorrect answer. The patient has symptoms that are being controlled with medication. Code 627.2 should be added. The elements of E/M are an expanded problem-focused history based on one to three elements of HPI, examination not documented, and low medical decision making based on one stable chronic disease and medication management. The E/M code is therefore 99213.

ICD-10-CM Code(s): N95.1; Z79.890

ICD-10-CM Rationale: The Alphabetic Index main term is State (of) with subterms menopausal, symptomatic. Another main term is Therapy with subterms drug, hormone replacement (postmenopausal).

6.38. 250.41, 583.81, 250.51, 362.01

Rationale: Both diabetic complication codes are assigned with the fifth digit of 1.

ICD-10-CM Code(s): E10.21, E10.319

ICD-10-CM Rationale: The Alphabetic Index main term is Diabetes, diabetic, subterm type I, with, nephropathy (E10.21) and retinopathy (E10.319).

6.39. 250.11, 276.51

Rationale: The ketoacidosis should be sequenced first and the DM is not specified as uncontrolled, so a fifth digit of 1 is used. The symptoms of increased urination and polydipsia are related to the diabetic condition. The dehydration, however, is treated separately.

ICD-10-CM Code(s): E10.10, E86.0

ICD-10-CM Rationale: The Alphabetic Index main term is Diabetes with subterms type I, ketoacidosis. Another main term is Dehydration.

6.40. a. 250.60, 536.3, V58.67

Correct answer.

b. 250.60, 586.3, 337.1, V58.67

Incorrect answer. *Coding Clinic* (2004, 2Q), published as superseding advice, states that only two codes are needed for this condition. Code 337.1 is no longer assigned.

c. 250.61, 536.3

Incorrect answer. The patient is a type II diabetic who is on insulin. This is not the same as a type I diabetic. The fifth digit of 0 is assigned. The V58.67 code is reported to show the current insulin usage.

d. 250.62, 536.3, V58.67

Incorrect answer. Just because the patient is on insulin, it cannot be presumed that the diabetes is uncontrolled.

ICD-10-CM Code(s): E11.43, Z79.4

ICD-10-CM Rationale: The Alphabetic Index main term is Diabetes, diabetic, subterms type 2, with, gastroparesis. A note under main term E11 directs the coder to "Use additional code to identify insulin use" (Z79.4).

6.41. a. 250.50, 362.07

Incorrect answer. The diabetes needs to be listed first, followed by the code for the proliferative retinopathy (362.02). Per the coding notes, the code for macular edema would be added (362.07), along with a code from 362.01–362.06.

b. 250.50, 362.06, 362.07

Incorrect answer. The diabetes needs to be listed first, followed by the code for the proliferative retinopathy (362.02). Per the coding notes, the code for macular edema would be added (362.07), along with a code from 362.01–362.06.

c. 250.50, 362.02, 362.07

Correct answer.

d. 362.02, 363.07

Incorrect answer. The diabetes needs to be listed first, followed by the code for the proliferative retinopathy (362.02). Per the coding notes, the code for macular edema would be added (362.07), along with a code from 362.01–362.06.

ICD-10-CM Code(s): E11.351

ICD-10-CM Rationale: The Alphabetic Index main term is Diabetes, diabetic with subterms type 2, with, retinopathy, proliferative, with macular edema.

Disorders of the Genitourinary System

6.42. ICD-9-CM and CPT Code(s): 600.10, 600.01, 788.43, 788.64, 55700, 76942

Rationale: Code 600.10 is used to report the nodular prostate. Code 600.01 is used to report the BPH. The code book reminds the coder that an additional code should be used for the nocturia and the hesitancy. Code 76942 is used to reflect the imaging guidance. A note under code 55700 directs the coder to use code 76942.

ICD-10-CM Code(s): N40.1, R35.1, R39.11

ICD-10-CM Rationale: The Alphabetic Index main term Nodule(s), nodular, subterm prostate directs the coder to Enlargement, enlarged prostate. Main term Enlargement, enlarged prostate is reviewed with subterm prostate, with lower urinary tract symptoms. A review of code N40.1 directs the coder to code associated symptoms of nocturia (R35.1) and hesitancy (R39.11).

6.43. a. 585.6, 90970

Incorrect answer. The services are for a month, so 90970 is incorrect.

b. V56.0, 90960

Incorrect answer. The patient is receiving dialysis, but for physician services, the ESRD code would be used, not V56.0. When the facility performed dialysis, they would use the V56.0 code.

c. 585.6, V56.8, 90999

Incorrect answer. The V56.8 code is not needed. The procedure code is incorrect and is more appropriately coded as 90960.

d. 585.6, 90960

Correct answer. Any E/M services that are unrelated to the dialysis care may be reported in addition.

ICD-10-CM Code(s): N18.6, Z99.2

ICD-10-CM Rationale: The Alphabetic Index main term is Failure, failed with subterms renal, end stage (chronic). There is a note in the Tabular List instructing the coder to "Use additional code to identify dialysis status."

6.44. a. V67.6, V10.51, 600.00, 52000

Correct answer.

b. 188.9, 600.00, 52000

Incorrect answer. The cancer has been resected and has not recurred in seven years. This encounter is for follow-up after combined therapy (surgery and chemotherapy). The cancer is expressed as a history code using V10.51. The procedure code is correct.

c. 600.00, V10.51, 52010

Incorrect answer. Code V67.6 is the appropriate code to report because this procedure is for surveillance only following completed treatment. The procedure code is incorrect. Code 52000 is appropriate for this follow-up diagnostic procedure.

d. V67.00, 188.9, 52000

Incorrect answer. It is mentioned that the patient was treated with both surgery and chemotherapy, so the follow-up code V67.6 is a better choice. If the patient still had cancer, the 188.9 would be assigned instead of follow-up. Code V10.51 is assigned because the cancer was resected and there has been no recurrence. The additional code of prostatic hypertrophy should also be reported because it may require future follow-up. The other codes are correct.

ICD-10-CM Code(s): Z08, Z85.51, N40.0

ICD-10-CM Rationale: The Alphabetic Index main term is Examination, follow-up, chemotherapy, malignant neoplasm. The Alphabetic Index main term is History, personal (of), malignant neoplasm (of), bladder. The Alphabetic Index main term is Enlargement, enlarged, prostate.

6.45. 58563

Rationale: This is a combination code that describes the hysteroscopy, the endometrial ablation, and the D&C that were performed.

6.46. ICD-9-CM and CPT Code(s): V25.2, V61.5, 58671

Rationale: The tubal ligation was performed with Falope Rings and was performed laparoscopically. Code V61.5 identifies the multiparity as the reason for desiring the tubal ligation.

ICD-10-CM Code(s): Z30.2, Z64.1

ICD-10-CM Rationale: The Alphabetic Index main term is Encounter, sterilization. The Alphabetic Index main term is multiparity.

6.47.   ICD-9-CM and CPT Code(s): 078.0, 54057, 54056-51

Rationale: It is appropriate to assign both techniques when performed. Some payers may require the use of the -59 modifier to show that the procedures were done independently. Because there is documentation that cryosurgery and laser were used, they both should be coded.

ICD-10-CM Code(s): B08.1

ICD-10-CM Rationale: The Alphabetic Index main term is Molluscum contagiosum.

Infectious Diseases

6.48.   ICD-9-CM, CPT, and HCPCS Code(s): 034.0, 034.1, 99214, 87880, 96372, J0561

Rationale: Long-acting Penicillin G has a HCPCS code, J0561, for the dosage of 1,000,000 units. Code J0561 would be used with a "12" in the units field.

ICD-10-CM Code(s): A38.9

ICD-10-CM Rationale: Code A38.9 includes both scarlet fever and scarlatina. Either scarlatina or scarlet fever in the Alphabetic Index gives code A38.9.

6.49.   ICD-9-CM and CPT Code(s): V05.3, 90471, 90746

Rationale: Code V05.3 is used for this purpose. CPT codes for the injection and for the hepatitis B are assigned.

ICD-10-CM Code(s): Z23

ICD-10-CM Rationale: The Alphabetic Index main term is Vaccination (prophylactic) with subterm encounter for.

6.50.   ICD-9-CM and CPT Code(s): V20.2, 799.51, 90707, 90471, 99393

Rationale: It is correct to assign the immunizations with the preventive medicine visit and V20.2 is the only diagnosis required to establish medical necessity for the immunizations. The patient has not been diagnosed with attention deficit disorder but has the symptom of concentration deficit that is to be evaluated. This patient is stated as "patient of ours," implying an established patient status.

ICD-10-CM Code(s): R41.840, Z00.121

ICD-10-CM Rationale: The Alphabetic Index main term is Deficit, subterm attention and concentration. The Alphabetic Index main term is Examination, subterm child, with abnormal findings.

Disorders of the Skin and Subcutaneous Tissue

6.51.   a. 996.61, 682.2, 33222
   Correct answer.

   b. 682.2, 33222
   Incorrect answer. Devices that cause inflammation or infection are coded to the 996 category in ICD-9-CM. The correct code is 996.61. The procedure code is correct.

c. 996.61, 33233

Incorrect answer. This CPT code is for a revision of the skin pocket for a cardioverter-defibrillator. Code 33222 is the correct code. Code 682.2 is coded per the instructions under code 996.6.

d. 996.72. 682.2, 33999

Incorrect answer. An abscess is an infection, so subcategory 996.6 is more applicable than 996.7. The unlisted code is not appropriate, because there is a specific CPT code available for relocation of a pacemaker pocket. Code 33222 is correct.

ICD-10-CM Code(s): T82.7xxA, L02.213

ICD-10-CM Rationale: The Alphabetic Index main term is Complication with subterms cardiac, device, implant or graft, infection or inflammation. Another main term is Abscess with subterms chest, wall.

6.52. ICD-9-CM and CPT Code(s): 706.1, 10040

Rationale: Pustular acne is classified to ICD-9-CM code 706.1. Acne surgery is reported with code 10040. An evaluation and management service (even the lowest level) is not reported when no separate E/M services are rendered.

ICD-10-CM Code(s): L70.0

ICD-10-CM Rationale: The Alphabetic Index main term is Acne, subterm pustular.

6.53. ICD-9-CM and CPT Code(s): 701.1, 15786, 15787, 15787

Rationale: Keratosis, NOS, is assigned to 701.1. To correctly report the abrasion of the keratoses, code 15786 is reported for the first lesion. Add-on code 15787 is used for each additional four lesions. The 15787 code needs to be repeated one additional time for the sixth lesion. The add-on code is exempt from modifier -51 use.

ICD-10-CM Code(s): L57.0

ICD-10-CM Rationale: The Alphabetic Index main term is Keratosis.

6.54. 15002, 15003, 15400, 15401, 15401, 15401

Rationale: The documentation supports assignment of codes 15002 and 15003, since it states that necrotic eschar was debrided to bleeding subcutaneous tissue. Code 15400 describes application of the first 100 sq cm of Mediskin, which is a type of xenogeneic (porcine) dermis. Code 15401 is reported three times to report sq cm 100–200, 200–300, and >300.

6.55. 15365

Rationale: TranCyte is an example of tissue-cultured allogeneic dermal substitute, most often used to treat diabetic foot ulcers. It is reported with codes in the range 15360–15366. Because this graft involved the foot, code 15365 is correct. There is no documentation of preparation of the recipient site by excision of tissue, so the reporting of code 15004 is not correct.

6.56. ICD-9-CM and CPT Code(s): 078.12, 17110

Rationale: Code 17110 is used to report the destruction of up to 14 separate lesions. Four lesions were destroyed so only 1 code is needed.

ICD-10-CM Code(s): B07.0

ICD-10-CM Rationale: The Alphabetic Index main term is Wart, subterm plantar.

Behavioral Health Conditions

6.57. a. 90805

Correct answer.

b. 90804, 99212

Incorrect answer. The combination code for psychotherapy and E/M service is reported, 90805.

c. 90811

Incorrect answer. The psychotherapy is described as insight-oriented, not interactive type. Code 90805 is correct.

d. 90810, 99212

Incorrect answer. The combination code for insight-oriented type of psychotherapy with E/M service is reported, 90805.

6.58. a. 314.00, 99214

Incorrect answer. A new patient visit code should be reported, 99204.

b. 314.00, 99204

Correct answer.

c. 314.01, 99204

Incorrect answer. The diagnosis does not include hyperactivity. The correct code is 314.00.

d. 314.9, 99214

Incorrect answer. The DSM-IV code for ADD is 314.9; however, the correct code in ICD-9-CM is 314.00. Also, a new patient visit code should be reported, 99204.

ICD-10-CM Code(s): F90.9

ICD-10-CM Rationale: The Alphabetic Index main term is Disorder, subterm attention-deficit without hyperactivity.

6.59. 90880

Rationale: Hypnotherapy is coded as 90880. The length of time is not specified in the code.

6.60. ICD-9-CM Code(s): 331.0, 294.11

Rationale: The dementia is coded as that with behavioral disturbance because of the wandering off. Assign code 294.11. It is very clear in the tabular notes under subcategory 294.1 that the Alzheimer's disease is listed first.

ICD-10-CM Code(s): G30.9, F02.81

ICD-10-CM Rationale: The Alphabetic Index main term is Disease, subterm Alzheimer's, with behavioral disturbance. The format of the entry directs the coder to assign two codes. Wandering off is a behavioral disturbance.

Disorders of the Musculoskeletal System and Connective Tissue

6.61. a. 739.7, 99213-25, 98925

Correct answer. Somatic dysfunction is found in ICD-9-CM under the main term "dysfunction" and subterm "somatic." E/M services on the same day must have documentation that shows they are separate from the procedure and include the key elements of an evaluation and management code (history, exam, and medical decision making).

b. 739.2, 98925

Incorrect answer. The wrong region is described by this ICD-9-CM code. Also, not reporting the E/M service with the procedure is underreporting the physician work for the visit.

c. 786.59, 99212-25, 98925

Incorrect answer. The ICD-9-CM code is too vague and the E/M service level is not as high as the documentation supports.

d. 739.8, 99213

Incorrect answer. The ICD-9-CM code is not as specific as the documentation allows. Failure to report the osteopathic manipulation in addition to the E/M service is underreporting the physician service.

ICD-10-CM Code(s): M99.07

ICD-10-CM Rationale: The Alphabetic Index main term is Dysfunction with subterms somatic, sternoclavicular.

6.62. a. 824.8, E917.0, 27788, Q4046

Correct answer.

b. 824.2, E917.0, 27788, 29515-51

Incorrect answer. The diagnosis code is specific to the lateral malleolus, which is not documented. Code 29515 should not be reported with a fracture care code because casts and strapping are included with initial fracture care.

c. 823.81, E917.0, 27786, L4350

Incorrect answer. Code 823.81 is not the correct classification for distal fibula. The CPT code for fracture care is for closed treatment without manipulation. The HCPCS code is for an air splint, but this splint is molded from fiberglass.

d. 824.4. E917.0, 27810, 29515-51, L4396

Incorrect answer. The diagnosis code is specific to a bimalleolar fracture, which is not documented. CPT code 27810 is for fracture care of a bimalleolar fracture with manipulation, so it is also inappropriate. Code 29515 for the splint should not be reported with a fracture care code, and the supply code L4396 is not appropriate because it is a splint for ankle contracture, not a fracture.

ICD-10-CM Code(s): S82.452A, Y92.39, Y93.43, Y99.8

ICD-10-CM Rationale: The Alphabetic Index main term is Fracture, subterm fibula, comminuted (displaced). The coder completes the code using the Tabular List. The Activity Code is found in the Index to External Causes under Activity, gymnastics (Y93.43). External status is found in the Index to External Causes under main term External cause status, subterm leisure activity (Y99.8). The place of occurrence code is found in the Index to External Causes under the main term Place of occurrence, subterm gymnasium (Y92.39).

6.63. ICD-9-CM and CPT Code(s): V54.16, 29440, 73590

Rationale: It is correct to use the orthopedic aftercare code. The CPT codes would be for conversion to a walking cast and the x-ray. It is incorrect to code fracture care codes in this scenario. Do not report an E code because this is not the first encounter for the injury.

ICD-10-CM Code(s): S82.451D

ICD-10-CM Rationale: The Alphabetic Index main term is Aftercare with subterm fracture. There is a note which directs the coder to "code to fracture with extension D." Main term is now Fracture with subterms fibula, comminuted.

6.64. a. 23140

Incorrect answer. Code 23140 describes the excision of a bone cyst or tumor. In this case, the physician excises a piece of dead bone, not a cyst or tumor.

b. 23172

Correct answer. A sequestrum is a piece of dead bone that has become separated during the process of necrosis from normal/sound bone. It is a complication (sequela) of osteomyelitis. A sequestrectomy is the removal of this dead bone.

c. 23182

Incorrect answer. Code 23182 describes the process of creating a crater or saucer on the body of the scapula. Code 23172 describes the exact procedure performed on the scapula and is therefore a better choice.

d. 23190

Incorrect answer. Code 23190 describes the removal of a portion of the scapula but does not address the specific reason the bone was removed. Code 23172 describes the exact procedure performed on the scapula and is therefore a better choice.

6.65. ICD-9-CM and CPT Code(s): 729.6, V90.81, 26075

Rationale: This foreign body is a retained foreign body because the wound healed around the foreign body. A coding note directs the coder to assign a code from category V90 to identify the type of retained foreign body. V90.81 is assigned to identify a retained glass foreign body.

ICD-10-CM Code(s): M79.5, Z18.81

ICD-10-CM Rationale: The Alphabetic Index main term is Foreign body with subterms retained (old), soft tissue. A second code is assigned to describe the object retained by going to the main term Retained, subterm glass.

6.66. a. 724.5

Incorrect answer. The site of the pain is coded first, followed by the 307.89 code. Because of the instructional note, the site of the pain is sequenced first.

b. 724.5, 307.89

Correct answer. An instructional note under code 307.89 states to code first the type or site of pain.

c. 307.89

Incorrect answer. The site of the pain is coded first, followed by the 307.89 code. Because of the instructional note, the site of the pain is sequenced first.

d. 307.89, 724.5

Incorrect answer. The site of the pain is coded first, followed by the 307.89 code. Because of the instructional note, the site of the pain is sequenced first.

ICD-10-CM Code(s): F45.41

ICD-10-CM Rationale: The Alphabetic Index main term is Pain, subterm psychogenic. There is no note under F45.41 instructing the coder to also use a code for the back pain.

Neoplasms

6.67. a. V58.12, 149.8, 96401, J9213

Correct answer.

b. 149.8, 96372, J9213

Incorrect answer. The patient is coming in for antineoplastic immunotherapy, so the first-listed diagnosis should be V58.12. The patient is receiving an antineoplastic immunotherapy injection, so the correct code would be 96401.

c. 145.9, 140.9, 96372

Incorrect answer. The cancer is reported with one code because the lip and oral cavity are contiguous sites. Code 149.8 is correct. The patient is receiving an antineoplastic immunotherapy injection, so the correct code would be 96401. Also, the J9213 code is required to report the agent administered.

d. V58.11, 96549

Incorrect answer. Interferon is considered an immunotherapy agent, not chemotherapy. Assign a code for the neoplasm. Interferon is an immunotherapy antineoplastic agent, so the correct procedure code is 96401. An HCPCS code (J9213) to describe the agent administered should be reported as well.

ICD-10-CM Code(s): Z51.12, C00.4

ICD-10-CM Rationale: In the Neoplasm Table, the main term is Lip with subterms internal, lower. Use the code from the Malignant Primary column. Another main term is Encounter (for) with subterm immunotherapy for neoplasm.

6.68. ICD-9-CM and CPT Code(s): 233.1, 493.90, 57454

Rationale: Cervical dysplasia is a precursor condition of carcinoma in situ of the cervix and should not be coded. Carcinoma in situ (233.1) should be assigned. The endocervical biopsy was performed endoscopically. Code 57454 is correct, and it includes endocervical curettage. Other pre- and postoperative services are not included and are reported separately.

ICD-10-CM Code(s): D06.9, J45.909

ICD-10-CM Rationale: The Neoplasm Table is used to find the correct code. Under Neoplasm, the coder finds Cervix. The in-situ column is selected. The Alphabetic Index main term is Asthma.

6.69. ICD-9-CM and CPT Code(s): 214.3, V10.05, 50543

Rationale: Lipoma of the kidney is assigned to code 214.3; history of colon cancer is assigned to code V10.05; laparoscopic partial nephrectomy is assigned to code 50543.

ICD-10-CM Code(s): D17.5, Z85.038

ICD-10-CM Rationale: The Alphabetic Index main term is Lipoma with subterms site classification, intra-abdominal. Another main term is History with subterm personal (of), malignant neoplasm (of), colon.

6.70. a. 173.4, 11622

Incorrect answer. The ICD-9-CM index directs the coder to Merkel Cell carcinoma and provides the code of 209.32 for Merkel Cell Ca of the neck. The total excised diameter of this lesion is 2.0 cm plus 0.2 cm for each of the two margin measurements, for a total of 2.4 cm. CPT code 11623 correctly describes this service.

b. 209.32, 11623

Correct answer.

c. 209.36, 11422

Incorrect answer. The documentation states that the Merkel Cell is located on the patient's neck. There is a specific entry for the location of neck, providing the code 209.32. A Merkel Cell tumor is a carcinoma. Therefore, the category for excision of malignant lesion should have been used. The total excised diameter of this lesion is 2.0 cm plus 0.2 cm for each of the two margin measurements, for a total of 2.4 cm. CPT code 11623 correctly describes this service.

d. 216.4, 11423

Incorrect answer. The ICD-9-CM index directs the coder to Merkel Cell carcinoma and provides the code of 209.32 for Merkel Cell Ca of the neck. A Merkel Cell tumor is a carcinoma. Therefore, the category for excision of malignant lesion should have been used.

ICD-10-CM Code(s): C4a.4

ICD-10-CM Rationale: The Alphabetic Index main term is Carcinoma, subterm Merkel cell, neck.

6.71.   ICD-9-CM and CPT Code(s): 183.0, 250.03, 58943

Rationale: Ovarian carcinoma is assigned to code 183.0. The diabetes is insulin-dependent and was out of control. The staging of the ovarian malignancy and excision for malignancy CPT code is 58943.

ICD-10-CM Code(s): C56.1, E10.65

ICD-10-CM Rationale: In the Neoplasm Table, the main term is Ovary. Select a code from the Malignant Primary column. Another main term is Diabetes with subterm out of control. There is a note to "code to Diabetes by type, with hyperglycemia." Therefore, the main term is Diabetes with subterms type I, with, hyperglycemia.

Disorders of the Nervous System and Sense Organs

6.72.   a. 61796, 20660

Incorrect answer. Code 61796 is not reported in conjunction with code 20660. Code 61800 is reported for the stereotactic headframe application.

b. 61796, 61800

Correct answer.

c. 64600

Incorrect answer. The correct CPT codes for this procedure are 61796 and 61800; code 64600 is for destruction by a neurolytic agent, not a gamma knife.

d. 61796

Incorrect answer. Code 61800 is reported for the stereotactic headframe application.

6.73.   a. 63655

Incorrect answer. This CPT code is for reporting laminectomy for implantation of neurostimulator electrodes, plate/paddle, epidural.

b. 63685

Correct answer.

c. 63650

Incorrect answer. This CPT code is for reporting percutaneous insertion of a catheter with electrodes generally performed under fluoroscopic guidance.

d. 63688

Incorrect answer. This CPT code is for a revision or removal of implanted spinal neurostimulator pulse generator or receiver.

6.74. a. 365.9, 250.00, 66172-RT

Incorrect answer. The glaucoma is specified as being open angle, so code 365.10 is correct. The diabetes mellitus is documented as type I, so the correct fifth digit is 1. This is the initial procedure according to the documentation, so code 66170 is correct.

b. 365.11, 250.01, 65850

Incorrect answer. The documentation only specifies the glaucoma as open angle, not primary open angle, so code 365.10 is correct. The section of codes 66150–66172 is for treatment of glaucoma, and code 66170 describes the procedure.

c. 250.51, 365.44, 66170-52

Incorrect answer. The patient has diabetes mellitus, but there is no cause-effect stated as to the cause of the glaucoma. In order to use this diagnosis coding, the physician would need to state "diabetic glaucoma" or "glaucoma due to diabetes." Each disorder needs to be separately coded. The procedure does not need the modifier -52 because these are inherently unilateral procedures.

d. 365.10, 250.01, 66170-RT

Correct answer. If the payer accepts HCPCS Level II modifiers, the -RT gives information about the side operated on.

ICD-10-CM Code(s): H40.10, E10.9

ICD-10-CM Rationale: The Alphabetic Index main term is Glaucoma, subterm open angle. The Alphabetic Index main term is Diabetes, subterm type I.

6.75. a. 374.00, 67921-RT

Correct answer. Entropion is the turning inward of the eyelid edge toward the eyeball. If the payer accepts HCPCS Level II modifiers, modifier -RT gives information about the correct site of the procedure.

b. 374.00, 67921-50

Incorrect answer. It is incorrect to use the modifier -50 with this procedure. It is inherently a unilateral procedure. This patient has bilateral entropion, but only the right side was repaired at this session. If the payer accepts HCPCS Level II modifiers, the -RT modifier gives information about the correct site of the procedure.

c. 374.10, 67921-RT

Incorrect answer. Code 374.10 is the code for ectropion, the turning outward (eversion) of the eyelid edge causing the palpebral conjunctiva to be exposed. Code 374.00 is correct. The CPT code is correct.

d. 374.00, 67923

Incorrect answer. Code 374.00 is correct. The CPT code is incorrect because this would describe an entropion repair with tarsal wedge excision, which is not documented. The correct code is 67921-RT.

ICD-10-CM Code(s): H02.003, H02.006

ICD-10-CM Rationale: In the Alphabetic Index, the main term is Entropion with subterms right, left.

6.76. ICD-9-CM Code(s): 438.20, 438.11, 401.9, 250.00

Rationale: The dominant side is not specified, so code 438.20 is the most specific code for this scenario. The aphasia is coded because it is still current, and the hypertension and DM should be coded.

ICD-10-CM Code(s): I69.320, I69.351, I10, E11.9

ICD-10-CM Rationale: To access the codes for the hemiplegia and aphasia, the Alphabetic Index main term is Sequelae (of), subterm stroke, aphasia (I69.320), and hemiplegia (I69.35-). The Alphabetic Index main term is Hypertension. The Alphabetic Index main term is Diabetes, diabetic, subterm type 2.

6.77. ICD-9-CM and CPT Code(s): 871.5, E914, E849.3, E000.0, 65235

Rationale: The code for external status is used to reflect the fact that the patient was involved in a job for payment. Code 69990 for operating microscope is not used in addition to code 65235 as directed by the note in the CPT book.

ICD-10-CM Code(s): S05.51xA, W31.1xxA, Y92.63, Y93.89, Y99.0

ICD-10-CM Rationale: The Alphabetic Index main term is Puncture with subterms eyeball, with foreign body. In the Index to External Causes, the main term is Contact with subterms with, machine, metalworking. In the Index to External Causes, the main term is Place of occurrence with subterm factory. In the Index to External Causes, the main term is Activity with subterm specified NEC. In the Index to External Causes, the main term is External cause status with subterm civilian activity done for financial or other compensation.

6.78. a. 382.9, 69436-50

Correct answer.

b. 381.00, 69421-50

Incorrect answer: Code 381.00 is used to report acute otitis media not chronic. Code 69421 is not correct because it does not reflect the ventilating tube placement.

c. 382.9, 69433-50

Incorrect answer. Code 69433 is incorrect because general anesthesia was used on this patient—this code is for topical or local.

d. 382.9, 69436

Incorrect answer. The CPT directs the coder to use the modifier -50 for a bilateral procedure.

ICD-10-CM Code(s): H66.93

ICD-10-CM Rationale: The Alphabetic Index main term is Otitis, subterm media, chronic. The code for bilateral is used even though the Alphabetic Index directs the coder to H66.90.

Newborn/Congenital Disorders

6.79.   a. 773.0, 770.84, 99469

Incorrect answer. For a birth episode, code V30.00 is reported in the first position for a spontaneous vaginal delivery. The management of the ventilator is included with the intensive care code, but the exchange transfusion is not included per the CPT manual. Code 36450 is assigned in addition.

b. V30.00, 99468, 36450, 94660

Incorrect answer. Code 99469 is the appropriate choice for the second day of care. Code 99468 is used to report initial services, which in this case would be the date of birth. Code 94660 is not reported with neonatal intensive care because the listed services are considered bundled. The exchange transfusion is not a bundled service, so it is correctly reported as a separate code.

c. V30.00, 773.0, 770.84, 99469, 36450

Correct answer.

d. 773.0, 770.84, 99469

Incorrect answer. The exchange transfusion procedure, code 36450, should also be reported in CPT because it is not bundled with the intensive care services like the CPAP management. ICD-9-CM code V30.00 must be reported in first position when reporting an episode of care where a birth occurred.

ICD-10-CM Code(s): Z38.00, P28.5, P55.0

ICD-10-CM Rationale: The Alphabetic Index main term is Newborn, subterm born in hospital. Another main term is Failure with subterms respiration, respiratory, newborn. A third main term is Erythroblastosis with subterms due to, Rh (antibodies).

6.80.   a. 33813

Incorrect answer. CPT code 33813 is the repair of the aortopulmonary septal defect, or window, that is a communication between the ascending aorta and the main pulmonary artery above the two distinct semilunar valves. A patent ductus arteriosus is a connect between the aorta and the pulmonary artery within the aortic arch, well above the heart. PDA closure is described by 33820–33824, based on the method used for closure. In this case, the physician divides the connection and suturing each of the defects closed. CPT code 33824 describes this service for this 22-year-old patient.

b. 33820

Incorrect answer. This code describes a closure method by ligation, or tying off the connect with several heavy sutures. In this case, the physician divides the connection and suturing each of the defects closed. CPT code 33824 describes this service for this 22-year-old patient.

c. 33822

Incorrect answer. This code describes the correct method of closure, but the patient in this case is 22 years old. CPT code 33824 describes this service for this 22-year-old patient.

d. 33824
Correct answer.

6.81.   a. 569.89, 49580

Incorrect answer. This is a congenital condition, not an acquired condition. Code 756.73 correctly describes the congenital gastroschisis, which is a specific type of abdominal hernia. It is not related to the umbilicus. Code 49605 is the correct code.

b. 756.73, 49605
Correct answer.

c. 569.89, 49600

Incorrect answer. This is a congenital condition, not an acquired condition. Code 756.73 correctly describes the congenital gastroschisis. An omphalocele is a different type of abdominal hernia. CPT code 49600 is specific to an omphalocele and code 49605 describes the repair of the gastroschisis.

d. 756.73, 49600

Incorrect answer. An omphalocele is a different type of abdominal hernia. CPT code 49600 is specific to an omphalocele and code 49605 describes the repair of the gastroschisis.

ICD-10-CM Code(s): Q79.3

ICD-10-CM Rationale: The Alphabetic Index main term is Gastroschisis.

6.82. a. 754.69, 29450

Incorrect answer. The diagnosis code reported is for equinovarus, which is not what the documentation states and which represents a different type of clubfoot. The evaluation and management service should also be reported with a -25 modifier to show that it is distinct from the cast replacement.

b. 736.71, 29405

Incorrect answer. The condition is congenital, not acquired, if the patient is a newborn. Clubfoot manipulation and casting has a specific CPT code to report, which is 29450. In addition, if the evaluation and management service is distinct from the procedure, it may be reported separately with modifier -25.

c. 754.51, 29405

Incorrect answer. Clubfoot manipulation and casting has a specific CPT code to report, which is 29450. In addition, if the evaluation and management service is distinct from the procedure, it may be reported separately with modifier -25.

d. 754.51, 99212-25, 29450

Correct answer. Selected payers may question or refuse to reimburse for an E/M service on the same date as a procedure, but it is correct from a CPT coding standpoint if the E/M service is above and beyond what is provided as part of the routine pre- and postop services connected with the procedure.

ICD-10-CM Code(s): Q66.0

ICD-10-CM Rationale: The Alphabetic Index main term is Talipes (congenital), subterm equinovarus.

6.83. a. V30.2, 99460, 99238

Incorrect answer. When admission and discharge occur on the same date, code 99463 is reported. Code 99238 is not used when admission and discharge occur on the same day.

b. V30.00, 99463

Incorrect answer. A birthing center is not a hospital birth. The correct code is V30.2.

c. V30.2, 99460

Incorrect answer. Code 99460 is used in birthing room deliveries but not when the admission and discharge services occur on the same date. Code 99463 is the correct CPT code for this service.

d. V30.2, 99463

Correct answer. A birthing center is not considered a hospital birth, so the fourth digit is 2 for the liveborn infant type of birth.

ICD-10-CM Code(s): Z38.1

ICD-10-CM Rationale: The Alphabetic Index main term is Newborn with subterm born outside the hospital.

Pediatric Conditions

6.84. a. 99212, 90378, 96372

Incorrect answer. There is nothing in the brief description of this service to substantiate a Level II office visit (99212).

b. 90378, 90471

Incorrect answer. This is not a vaccine. Administration via IM injection of an immune globulin is reported with code 96372.

c. 99212, J1459

Incorrect answer. This J code is for intravenous administration of RSV immune globulin, not an intramuscular injection. There is nothing in the brief description of this service to substantiate a Level II office visit (99212). Administration of the IM injection is reported with code 96372.

d. 90378, 96372

Correct answer.

6.85. ICD-9-CM and CPT Code(s): 382.01, V60.81, 99213

Rationale: The otitis media is documented as acute with perforation of eardrum. The highest level of E/M code that can be assigned is 99213.

ICD-10-CM Code(s): H66.001, H66.012, Z62.21

ICD-10-CM Rationale: The Alphabetic Index main term is Otitis with subterms media, suppurative, acute, with rupture of eardrum. Another main term is Otitis with subterms media, suppurative, acute. Another main term is Upbringing, institutionalized with subterm in foster care.

6.86. ICD-9-CM and CPT Code(s): 382.3, 69436-50

Rationale: The procedure was performed bilaterally, so modifier -50 would apply.

ICD-10-CM Code(s): H66.3x3

ICD-10-CM Rationale: The Alphabetic Index main term is Otitis, subterm media, chronic, suppurative. The Alphabetic Index directs the coder to Otitis, media, suppurative, chronic. The coder is directed to see category H66.3.

6.87. ICD-9-CM and CPT Code(s): 493.01, 99283, 94060

Rationale: The intractable wheezing would be assigned to the fifth digit of 1.

ICD-10-CM Code(s): J45.902

ICD-10-CM Rationale: The Alphabetic Index main term is Asthma with subterms childhood, with, status asthmaticus.

Conditions of Pregnancy, Childbirth, and the Puerperium

6.88.   a. 654.53, 59871

Correct answer.

b. 654.53 (The cerclage removal is part of the global package.)

Incorrect answer. CPT guidelines state that the cerclage removal may be coded if done under anesthesia other than local.

c. 622.5, with appropriate E/M procedure

Incorrect answer. Code 622.5 is used for incompetent cervix when the patient is not pregnant. CPT guidelines state that the cerclage removal may be coded if done under anesthesia other than local.

d. 622.5, 59871

Incorrect answer. Code 622.5 is used for incompetent cervix when the patient is not pregnant.

ICD-10-CM Code(s): O34.33

ICD-10-CM Rationale: The Alphabetic Index main term is Pregnancy, complicated by, incompetent cervix. Because the due date is in 2 weeks it is coded to the third trimester.

6.89.   59510

Rationale: This is a classic primary cesarean section delivery, without complication.

6.90.   a. 637.91, 59812

Incorrect answer. The abortion was specified as spontaneous. It is appropriate to also report the antepartum visits.

b. 634.91, 59812, 59425

Correct answer.

c. 634.91, 58120

Incorrect answer. Code 58120 is incorrect because this is an abortion. The correct code is found under the abortion subheading. It is correct to also report the antepartum visits.

d. 634.92, 58120, 59425

Incorrect answer. The abortion was incomplete, so the fifth digit is incorrect. 58120 is incorrect because this is an abortion. The correct code is found under the abortion subheading.

ICD-10-CM Code(s): O03.4

ICD-10-CM Rationale: The Alphabetic Index main term is Abortion (complete) (spontaneous), subterm incomplete (spontaneous).

6.91. ICD-9-CM Code(s): 643.23

Rationale: Because this started after the 22 completed week of gestation, it is considered to be excessive vomiting of late pregnancy.

ICD-10-CM Code(s): O21.2

ICD-10-CM Rationale: The Alphabetic Index main term is Pregnancy with subterms complicated by, vomiting, late.

6.92. ICD-9-CM Code(s): 647.63, 042, 136.3

Rationale: According to the coding guidelines, when a pregnant patient with AIDS is admitted with a condition related to the AIDS, code 647.6X is assigned, followed by 042 and the condition being treated.

ICD-10-CM Code(s): O98.713, B20, B59

ICD-10-CM Rationale: The Alphabetic Index main term is Pregnancy, subterm complicated by, HIV. Code O98.713 directs the coder to also code the acquired immune deficiency syndrome (AIDS) (B20). A review of code B20 in the Tabular List directs the coder to use an additional code to identify the manifestation of AIDS. The Alphabetic Index main term is Pneumocystitis carinii pneumonia.

6.93. 654.53, 59320

Rationale: The fifth digit "3" is used because the patient did not deliver on this admission.

ICD-10-CM Code(s): O34.32

ICD-10-CM Rationale: The Alphabetic Index main term is Pregnancy with subterms complicated by, incompetent cervix.

6.94. a. 634.91, 59820

Incorrect answer. Code 59820 is used to report the treatment of a missed abortion. This is a case of a spontaneous abortion.

b. 634.92, 59820

Incorrect answer. The fifth digit of '2' indicates a complete abortion—this was an incomplete abortion.

c. 634.81, 59812

Incorrect answer. There were no complications of this spontaneous abortion; therefore the correct fourth digit is "9".

d. 634.91, 59812
Correct answer.

ICD-10-CM Code(s): O03.4

ICD-10-CM Rationale: The Alphabetic Index main term is Abortion (complete) (spontaneous), subterm incomplete (spontaneous).

Disorders of the Respiratory System

6.95. a. 519.00, V46.11, 31614

Incorrect answer. This was not a complication of the tracheostomy, such as an infection or a mechanical breakdown of the tube or tracheal stenosis. Code V55.0 is more appropriate for scar tissue redundancy.

b. V55.0, V46.11, 31614

Correct answer. Because the scar tissue is not a true complication of the stoma, the V code is the correct code to communicate the reason for the service.

c. V55.0, 31610

Incorrect answer. An additional code could be assigned for the respirator dependence because it would affect the evaluation and management of the case. Code 31610 is incorrect because this is a revision of a tracheostomy already established, not a fenestration procedure.

d. 519.00, 31613

Incorrect answer. This was not a complication of the tracheostomy, such as an infection or a mechanical breakdown of the tube or tracheal stenosis. Code V55.0 is more appropriate for scar tissue redundancy. The CPT code is also incorrect. Because flap rotation was documented, code 31614 is warranted. Also, code V46.11 could be added because the respirator dependence is likely to affect evaluation and management of the case.

ICD-10-CM Code(s): Z43.0, Z99.11

ICD-10-CM Rationale: The Alphabetic Index main term is Attention (to) with subterms artificial, opening of, trachea. Another main term is Dependence with subterms on, respirator.

6.96. a. 518.89, 32657

Incorrect answer. The emphysematous nodules are assigned to code 492.8.

b. 492.8, 32657, 32657-51

Incorrect answer. The procedure code is correct, but it should only be reported one time because the description states "single or multiple."

c. 518.89, 32500

Incorrect answer. The emphysematous nodules are assigned to code 492.8. The procedure was done endoscopically with a thoracoscope. The open procedure code is not used. The correct CPT code is 32657.

d. 492.8, 32657

Correct answer.

ICD-10-CM Code(s): J43.9

ICD-10-CM Rationale: The Alphabetic Index main term is Emphysema.

6.97. a. 231.2, 31641

Correct answer. Per individual payer guidelines, review should be done of the postop period because the diagnostic procedure was done. If the criteria are met, then modifier -58 might be appropriate.

b. 162.2, 31641, 31623-59

Incorrect answer. The lesions were not described as a primary neoplasm, so code 162.2 is not accurate. Code 231.2 is assigned. The CPT code for the bronchial washings is incorrect because the lesions were identified by this means in a previous bronchoscopy, and this episode was for the laser treatment through a rigid scope.

c. 231.2, 31641, 31623-59

Incorrect answer. The only CPT code to report for this session is 31641. The CPT code for the bronchial washings is incorrect because the lesions were identified by this means in a previous bronchoscopy, and this episode was for the laser treatment through a rigid scope.

d. 162.2, 31641

Incorrect answer. The lesions were not described as a primary neoplasm, so code 162.2 is not accurate. Code 231.2 is assigned.

ICD-10-CM Code(s): D02.20

ICD-10-CM Rationale: The Neoplasm Table under the main term Bronchus with subterm main. A code is selected from the Carcinoma in situ column.

6.98. ICD-9-CM Code(s): 428.0

Rationale: Acute pulmonary edema with CHF is coded to 428.0. Respiratory distress is not separately coded (*Coding Clinic* 1991, 3Q:19–21).

ICD-10-CM Code(s): I50.9

ICD-10-CM Rationale: The Alphabetic Index main term is Failure, subterm heart, congestive.

6.99. ICD-9-CM Code(s): 507.0, 482.40

Rationale: It is correct to code the aspiration pneumonia along with the superimposed staphylococcal bacterial pneumonia (*Coding Clinic* 1991, 3Q:16–17).

ICD-10-CM Code(s): J69.0, J15.20

ICD-10-CM Rationale: The Alphabetic Index main term is Pneumonia with subterms aspiration, due to, food. Another subterm under Pneumonia is staphylococcal.

6.100. a. 31622, 31625, 31636, 99144

Incorrect answer. The code for the diagnostic bronchoscopy (31622, designated as a separate procedure) should not be assigned when more extensive procedures are performed at the same session. In addition, the code for conscious sedation is included in the procedure when performed by the same physician who performs the procedure. This is indicated by the symbol ⊙ preceding the code.

b. 31628, 31632, 31636

Incorrect answer. Biopsies were taken of the walls of the bronchi, not through the walls. Code 31628 is the appropriate biopsy code. Code 31632 is also not appropriate.

c. 31625, 31636

Correct answer.

d. 31625, 31636, 99144

Incorrect answer. The endoscopic codes are appropriate, but the code for conscious sedation is included in the procedure when performed by the same physician who performs the procedure. This is indicated by the symbol ⊙ preceding the code.

6.101. ICD-9-CM and CPT Code(s): 784.42, 31526

Rationale: Code 31526 is used because an operating microscope is used during this procedure. The note below code 31526 instructs the coder that code 69990 should not be used with this code.

ICD-10-CM Code(s): R49.0

ICD-10-CM Rationale: The Alphabetic Index main term is Dysphonia.

Trauma and Poisoning

6.102. ICD-9-CM Code(s): 942.42, 945.40, 948.22, E890.3, E849.0

Rationale: The burns are third degree but are specified as deep. The burn on the leg is of an unspecified site. The percent of body surface burned is 25 percent, so the fourth digit of 2 is assigned with code 948; the percent of third-degree burn is 25 percent, so the fifth digit is 2. Because the fire was in a house, category E890 is used.

ICD-10-CM Code(s): T21.31xA, T24.301A, T31.22xA, X00.0xxA, Y92.019, Y99.8

ICD-10-CM Rationale: The Alphabetic Index main term is Burn, subterm chest wall, third degree. The burn of the right leg is found under Burn, lower, limb, right, third degree. The extent of burn is found under Burn, extent, 20–29 percent, with 20–29 percent third degree burns. A note under the burn codes directs the coder to code the source, intent, and place of the burn as appropriate. The Alphabetic Index Table of External Cause main term is Exposure, subterm fire, uncontrolled, in building or structure. The place of the injury can be found in the Table of External Causes under main term Place of occurrence, subterm residence, house, single family. The External Status code (External status) is also found in the Table of External Causes.

6.103. ICD-9-CM Code(s): 709.2, 906.7, 906.8, E929.4

Rationale: It is incorrect to assign a current burn code for a late effect. Index the term "late." The residual of a late effect is listed in the first position, followed by the late effect code. The late effect E code could also be added in this case.

ICD-10-CM Code(s): L90.5, T24.301S, T21.31xS, X00.0xxS

ICD-10-CM Rationale: The Alphabetic Index main term is Scar. The same codes for the burns and external codes are assigned as in question 6.102 with the 7th character extension being changed from A to S to indicate that this is a sequelae.

6.104. ICD-9-CM Code(s): 536.41, 682.2, 041.11, 438.82

Rationale: The infection of the gastrostomy code is listed first. The note in the tabular of the book instructs that an additional code is used to specify cellulitis and the organism, if known. Both are present here and should be coded. The dysphagia due to the old stroke is also coded.

ICD-10-CM Code(s): K94.22, L03.311, B95.6, I69.391

ICD-10-CM Rationale: The Alphabetic Index main term is Complication, subterm gastrostomy, infection. The coder is reminded to use an additional code to specify the infection such as cellulitis (L03.311). To identify the organism, reference main term Infection, infected, infective, subterm staphylococcal, as cause of disease classified elsewhere, aureus. The stroke sequelae is found at main term Sequelae, subterm stroke, dysphagia.

6.105. CPT Code(s): 14301

Rationale: CPT code 14301 describes the adjacent tissue transfer of larger dimension, regardless of location.

6.106. ICD-9-CM Code(s): 928.21, E919.3, E849.3

Rationale: This is confusing to look up in the index. If you look in the index under ankle with other parts of foot, it gives you 928.20. If you look in the index under foot, excluding toe(s) alone (with ankle), the code is 928.20. However, if you look in the index under toe(s) with foot and ankle, the code assigned is 928.21. This seems like the most specific code. In the index under crushed, by machinery, it says see accident, machine.

ICD-10-CM Code(s): S97.02xA, S97.82xA, S97.102A, W31.1xxA, Y92.69, Y99.0

ICD-10-CM Rationale: The Alphabetic Index main term is Crush, crushed, crushing, subterm ankle (S97.0-), foot (S97.8-), toe (S97.10). The codes are completed using the Tabular List. The Alphabetic Index for External Causes is used to code the place and kind of accident. The main term is Contact, subterm with, machine, metalworking. Place of occurrence, subterm industrial and construction area. The External cause status is civilian activity done for financial or other compensation.

Part III

Advanced Coding Exercises

Chapter 7. Case Studies from Inpatient Health Records

Unless otherwise stated, code set answers given in Chapter 7 are ICD-9-CM.

Disorders of the Blood and Blood-Forming Organs

7.1.   a. 428.0, 276.51, 287.30, 599.0, 250.00

Correct answer. The physician could be queried as to the use of V58.66, Long term use of aspirin.

b. 428.0, 276.51, 287.5, 599.0, 250.00

Incorrect answer. The documentation states primary thrombocytopenia, so code 287.5 is not the best choice.

c. 428.0, 511.9, 276.51, 287.30, 599.0, 250.00

Incorrect answer. Pleural effusion is not separately coded when present with CHF (*Coding Clinic* 1991, 3Q:19–20).

d. 276.51, 511.9, 428.0, 287.30, 782.7, 599.0, 250.00

Incorrect answer. The principal diagnosis should be the CHF because it was present on admission and the main focus of treatment during the inpatient stay. Pleural effusion is not separately coded when present with CHF. The petechia is not coded because it is part of the thrombocytopenia and is excluded as an additional code.

ICD-10-CM Code(s): I50.9, J91.8, E86.0, D69.49, N39.0, E11.9

ICD-10-CM Rationale: For code I50.9, the Alphabetic Index main term is Failure, subterms heart, congestive. For code J91.8, the Alphabetic Index main term is Effusion, pleura. Note: This Index entry takes you to J90 which is for pleural effusion not elsewhere classified. The entry below it, J91, contains an Excludes2 note and the correct code. For code E86.0, the Alphabetic Index main term is Dehydration. For code D69.49, the Alphabetic Index main term is Thrombocytopenia, subterm primary. For code N39.0, the Alphabetic Index main term is Infection, subterm urinary (tract). For code E11.9, the Alphabetic Index main term is Diabetes, subterm type 2.

Optional MS-DRG Exercise (for users with access to MS-DRG software or tables)

The correct MS-DRG assignment is 292, Heart Failure and Shock with CC.

a. MS-DRG assignment in this case is based on the principal diagnosis; the secondary codes do not impact the MS-DRG.

Correct answer. Urinary tract infection (599.0) impacts this MS-DRG.

b. A principal diagnosis of CHF results in a higher-paying MS-DRG than a principal diagnosis of dehydration.

Incorrect answer. This is true.

c. This patient's LOS exceeded the average length of stay for the assigned MS-DRG.

Incorrect answer. This is true.

d. All of the above are true statements.

Incorrect answer. Choice "a" is a false statement, as secondary codes do impact this MS-DRG assignment.

7.2. ICD-9-CM Principal Diagnosis: Sickle cell pain crisis, 282.62

ICD-9-CM Additional Diagnoses:

Staphylococcus aureus bacteremia, 790.7, 041.11

Priapism, 607.3

Asthma, 493.90

Gastroesophageal reflux disease, 530.81

Hemorrhoids, 455.6

ICD-9-CM Procedures:

PICC line placement, 38.93

Bone scan, 92.14

Transesophageal echocardiogram, 88.72

Injection or infusion of other therapeutic or prophylactic substance, 99.29

Rationale: Pain is included in the code for sickle cell disease with crisis. According to *Coding Clinic* (2003, 4Q:79–81), Bacteremia is defined as the presence of bacteria in the blood.

Issues to clarify: The physician should be queried about the type of crisis if the full record does not provide this detail.

ICD-10-CM Code(s): D57.00, R78.81, B95.6, N48.30, J45.909, K21.9, I84.20

ICD-10-CM Rationale: For code D57.00, the Alphabetic Index main term is Disease, subterms sickle-cell, with crisis. For code R78.81, the Alphabetic Index main term is Bacteremia. For code B95.6, the Alphabetic Index main term is Staphylococcus, subterm aureus, as cause of disease classified elsewhere. For code N48.30, the Alphabetic Index main term is Priapism. For code J45.909, the Alphabetic Index main term is Asthma. For code K21.9, the Alphabetic Index main term is Reflux, subterm gastroesophageal. For code I84.20, the Alphabetic Index main term is Hemorrhoids.

ICD-10-PCS Code(s): Codes for the PICC line, bone scan, and injection; B24BZZ4

ICD-10-PCS Rationale: There is not enough information in the summary to code the PICC line placement, bone scan, or injection. Additional documentation from the record is necessary to assign these codes. For code B24BZZ4, the Alphabetic Index main term is Ultrasonography, subterms Heart with Aorta, Transesophageal.

7.3.   ICD-9-CM Principal Diagnosis: Anemia of chronic disease, 285.29-Y

ICD-9-CM Additional Diagnoses:

   Hypertension and Chronic renal insufficiency, 403.90-Y and 585.9-Y

   Diabetes, 250.00-Y

   Long term (current use) of insulin, V58.67 (exempt)

   Coronary artery disease, 414.01-Y

   Congestive heart failure, 428.0-Y

   Hypokalemia, 276.8-N

ICD-9-CM Principal Procedure: Transfusion of packed cells, 99.04

ICD-9-CM Additional Procedures: Not applicable

Rationale: The chronic renal insufficiency is not documented as the cause of the anemia, as chronic renal insufficiency is just one of the patient's chronic conditions. A history of coronary artery bypass graft is not documented, so the disease is of the native arteries. *Coding Clinic* (2004, 1Q:24). An additional code specifying the stage of renal insufficiency needs to be added per "use additional code" instructional note under 403.90.

Procedure 99.04 is reported once in ICD-9-CM.

ICD-10-CM Code(s): Query the physician on the condition that led to anemia of chronic disease. I12.9, N18.9, E11.9, Z79.4, I25.10, I50.9, E87.6

ICD-10-CM Rationale: In order to assign the code for anemia of chronic disease, the physician must be queried on the condition that led to anemia of chronic disease. For code I12.9, the Alphabetic Index main term is Hypertension, subterm kidney. For code N18.9, the Alphabetic Index main term is Insufficiency, subterms renal, chronic. For code E11.9, the Alphabetic Index main term is Diabetes, diabetic, subterm type 2. For code Z79.4, the Alphabetic Index main term is Long-term (current) drug therapy (use of), subterm insulin. For code I25.10, the Alphabetic Index main term is Arteriosclerosis, arteriosclerotic, subterms coronary (artery). For code I50.9, the Alphabetic Index main term is Failure, subterms heart, congestive. For code E87.6, the Alphabetic Index main term is Hypokalemia.

ICD-10-PCS Code(s): 30233N1

ICD-10-PCS Rationale: The Alphabetic Index main term is Transfusion with subterms Vein, Peripheral, Blood, Red Cells.

Disorders of the Cardiovascular System

7.4.   a. 414.01, 414.05, 410.12, 411.1, V45.82, 36.11, 36.15, 39.61, 37.22, 88.53, 88.57

Correct answer.

b. 414.01, 414.05, 410.12, 411.1, V45.81, 36.12, 39.61, 37.22, 88.53, 88.57

Incorrect answer. The bypass consisted of one coronary (36.11) and one mammary (36.15). V codes indicating CABG status are redundant when the diagnosis code itself indicates that the status exists. Therefore, only code 414.05 needs to be reported. Report V45.82 for the angioplasty status.

c. 414.00, 414.05, 410.11, 411.1, 36.11, 36.15, 39.61, 37.22, 88.53, 88.57

Incorrect answer. The coronary atherosclerosis should be coded to 414.01 since there was documentation in the native marginal circumflex of 80% stenosis. The MI of the anterior wall occurred prior to transfer; therefore, code to the fifth digit of 2 (410.12).

d. 414.01, 414.05, 410.12, 411.1, 412, V45.81, 36.11, 36.15, 39.61, 37.22, 88.53, 88.57

Incorrect answer. The MI was recent, not old, so code 412 should not be coded. V codes indicating CABG status are redundant when the diagnosis code itself indicates that the status exists. Therefore, only code 414.05 needs to be reported.

Optional MS-DRG Exercise (for users with access to MS-DRG software or tables)

The principal diagnosis is 414.01, Coronary atherosclerosis of native coronary artery.

In addition to the principal diagnosis, the procedure codes are 36.11 and 37.22. This case groups to MS-DRG 234, Coronary Bypass with Cardiac Catheterization without MCC.

False: The presence or absence of the CC codes does not change the MS-DRG assignment; a major complication/comorbid condition does change the assignment.

ICD-10-CM Code(s): I25.110, I25.700, I21.09, Z95.5

ICD-10-CM Rationale: For code I25.110, the Alphabetic Index main term is Arteriosclerosis, subterms coronary (artery), native vessel, with, angina pectoris, unstable. For code I25.700, the Alphabetic Index main term is Arteriosclerosis, subterms coronary (artery), bypass graft, with, angina pectoris, unstable. For code I21.09, the Alphabetic Index main term is Infarction, subterms myocardium, ST elevation, anterior. For code Z95.5, the Alphabetic Index main term is Status, subterms angioplasty, coronary artery, with implant.

ICD-10-PCS Code(s): Procedural reports are needed to assign the codes.

ICD-10-PCS Rationale: There is not enough information in the summary to code the procedures. The remainder of the chart would need to be reviewed to accurately assign the procedure codes.

7.5. ICD-9-CM Principal Diagnosis: Acute inferior MI initial episode, 410.41-Y

ICD-9-CM Additional Diagnoses:

> Complete heart block, 426.0-Y
>
> Hematemesis, 578.0-N
>
> Acute blood loss anemia, 285.1-N
>
> Hyperlipidemia, 272.4-Y
>
> Arteriosclerotic coronary artery disease, 414.01-Y
>
> Nausea and vomiting, 787.01-N
>
> Adverse effect of anesthetics, E938.4-N
>
> History of tobacco use, V15.82
>
> Accident Occurring in Residential Institution, E849.7-N

ICD-9-CM Procedures:

> CABG × 2, 36.12
>
> PTCA, 00.66
>
> Insertion of one vascular stent, 00.45
>
> Procedure on single vessel, 00.40
>
> Insertion of non-drug-eluting stent(s), 36.06
>
> Left heart catheterization, 37.22
>
> Angiography, 88.55
>
> Ventriculography, 88.53
>
> EGD, 45.13
>
> Extracorporeal circulation, 39.61

Rationale: Acute inferior MI is documented on the 4/20 EKG. Use code 578.0 for the hematemesis because no cause was identified. Following the PTCA, the patient experienced acute blood loss anemia. The patient was found to have arteriosclerotic heart disease. Code the native artery (fifth digit of "1") because the patient has never undergone bypass surgery prior to this admission. Therefore, assume the ASHD is of the native artery. Nausea and vomiting (787.01) is the adverse effect of a drug (E938.4). Extracorporeal circulation is coded as directed by the ICD-9-CM notation. Cardioplegia would not be coded because this is included in the coronary artery bypass code.

ICD-10-CM Code(s): I21.19, I44.2, K92.0, D62, E78.5, I25.10, T41.205A, Z87.891, Y92.234

ICD-10-CM Rationale: For code I21.19, the Alphabetic Index main term is Infarction, subterms myocardium, ST elevation, inferior. For code I44.2, the Alphabetic Index main term is Block, subterms heart, complete. For code K92.0, the Alphabetic Index main term is Hematemesis. For code D62, the Alphabetic Index main term is Anemia, subterms blood loss, acute. For code E78.5, the Alphabetic Index main term is Hyperlipidemia. For code I25.10, the Alphabetic Index main term is Arteriosclerosis, arteriosclerotic, subterms coronary (artery). For code T41.205A, go to the Table of Drugs and Chemicals and locate the main term Anesthetic NEC, subterm general NEC, adverse effect column. For code Z87.891, the Alphabetic Index main term is History, subterms personal, nicotine dependence. For code Y92.234, go to the Index to External Causes and the main term is Place of occurrence, subterms hospital, operating room.

ICD-10-PCS Code(s): 021109W, 06BP4ZZ, 02703DZ, 4A023N7, B2111ZZ, B2151ZZ, 0DJ08ZZ, 5A1221Z, 5A1935Z

ICD-10-PCS Rationale: For code 021109W, the Alphabetic Index main term is Bypass, subterms Artery, Coronary, Two Sites. For code 06BP4ZZ, the Alphabetic Index main term is Excision, subterms Vein, Greater Saphenous, Right. For code 02703DZ, the Alphabetic Index main term is Dilation, subterms Artery, Coronary, One Site. For code 4A023N7, the Alphabetic Index main term is Catheterization, subterm Heart—see Measurement, Cardiac. For code B2111ZZ, the Alphabetic Index main term is Fluoroscopy, subterms Artery, Coronary, Bypass Graft, Multiple. For code B2151ZZ, the Alphabetic Index main term is Fluoroscopy, subterms Heart, Left. For code 0DJ08ZZ, the Alphabetic Index main term is EGD (Esophagogastroduodenoscopy). For code 5A1221Z, the Alphabetic Index main term is Performance, Cardiac, Continuous, Output. For code 5A1935Z, the Alphabetic Index main term is Performance, Respiratory, Continuous, Less than 24 Consecutive Hours Ventilation.

7.6. a. 00.61, 99.10, 00.63

Correct answer.

b. 00.61, 99.10, 00.64

Incorrect answer. Code 00.64 reports insertion of stents into other precerebral extracranial arteries than the carotid. Code 00.63 is specific for stenting of the carotid artery.

c. 00.61, 00.63

Incorrect answer. These codes are appropriate, but code 99.10 should also be reported as indicated in the Code Also note. Streptokinase is considered a thrombolytic agent, as are urokinase, alteplase, anistreplase, and reteplase. Note that routine injection of heparin during a procedure is not considered injection of a thrombolytic agent.

d. 00.61

Incorrect answer. The Code Also note instructs the following to be coded: injection of the thrombolytic agent (99.10) and placement of the carotid artery stent (00.63).

ICD-10-PCS Code(s): 03CJ3ZZ, 037J3DZ, code for infusion of streptokinase

ICD-10-PCS Rationale: For code 03CJ3ZZ, the Alphabetic Index main term is Atherectomy, see Extirpation, Upper Arteries. For code 037J3DZ, the Alphabetic Index main term is Dilation, subterms Artery, Common Carotid, Left. To code the infusion of Streptokinase, the body region must be determined from the medical record.

7.7.   a. 00.66, 00.40, 36.07, 36.07, 99.10

Incorrect answer. Code 36.07 is appropriate for the atherectomy, and 99.10 for the urokinase infusion, but code 36.07 should be reported only once since the descriptor for this code is "Insertion of drug-eluting coronary artery stent(s)." The code is assigned once irrespective of the number of stents placed. The code 00.46 identifies the number of stents inserted.

b. 00.66, 36.07

Incorrect answer. These codes are appropriate, but code 99.10 should also be reported for the infusion of urokinase, which is considered a thrombolytic agent. The codes for the number of vessels treated and number of stents inserted should also be assigned, 00.40 and 00.46.

c. 00.66, 00.40, 00.46, 36.07, 99.10

Correct answer.

d. 36.09, 00.40, 00.46, 36.06, 99.10

Incorrect answer. Code 00.40 and 00.46 are appropriate for the number of vessels treated and number of stents inserted and 99.10 for the urokinase infusion, but code 36.06 is used to report insertion of non-drug-eluting stents. Stents that are impregnated with sirolimus are by definition drug-eluting stents and should be reported with code 36.07. Sirolimus is an immunosuppressive drug that has been found to prevent or dramatically slow restenosis within atherectomized or angioplastied arteries. The principal procedure, atherectomy, should be coded 00.66, not 36.09.

ICD-10-PCS Code(s): 02C00ZZ, 027034Z, 3E07317

ICD-10-PCS Rationale: For code 02C00ZZ, the Alphabetic Index main term is Atherectomy, see Extirpation, Heart and Great Vessels. For code 027034Z, the Alphabetic Index main term is Dilation, subterms Artery, Coronary, One Site. For code 3E07317, the Alphabetic Index main term is Introduction, subterms Artery, Coronary.

7.8.   a. 38.44

Incorrect answer. Code 38.44 reports resection of the aneurysm of the aorta and replacement with a graft. This is an open, not a percutaneous, endovascular procedure. Code 39.71, Endovascular implantation of other graft in abdominal aorta, is the appropriate code.

b. 39.79

Incorrect answer. Code 39.79 reports an endovascular repair of vessels other than the aorta and vessels of the head and neck. Code 39.71, Endovascular implantation of other graft in abdominal aorta, is the appropriate code.

c. 39.71

Correct answer.

d. 39.7

Incorrect answer. Code 39.7 is a truncated code; a fourth digit is required. Code 39.71, Endovascular implantation of other graft in abdominal aorta, is the appropriate code.

ICD-10-PCS Code(s): 04U00JZ

ICD-10-PCS Rationale: The Alphabetic Index main term is Supplement, subterms Aorta, Abdominal.

7.9.   a. 411.1, 414.01, 250.00, 272.0, 36.12, 36.15, 39.61

Incorrect answer. The reason the patient was admitted is due to his coronary artery disease; therefore, 414.01 is sequenced as the principal diagnosis.

b. 414.01, 411.1, 250.00, 272.0, 36.12, 36.15, 39.61
Correct answer.

c. 414.00, 413.9, 995.89, 250.00, 36.12, 36.15, 39.61

Incorrect answer. The patient's coronary artery disease is identified as his native arteries. The angina is documented as being unstable. Hypothermia should not be coded as it is considered integral to the bypass surgery (*Coding Clinic* 1995, 1Q:5–6). Hypercholesterolemia meets reporting guidelines as a secondary procedure.

d. 414.01, 411.1, 272.0, 250.00, 36.13, 39.61

Incorrect answer. The patient actually had two vein graft bypass and one internal mammary artery. Therefore, the procedure code 36.13 is incorrect. The correct codes are 36.12 and 36.15.

ICD-10-CM Code(s): I25.10, I21.09, E11.9, E78.0, Z79.4

ICD-10-CM Rationale: For code I25.10, the Alphabetic Index main term is Arteriosclerosis, arteriosclerotic, subterms coronary (artery). For code I21.09, the Alphabetic Index main term is Infarct, infarction, subterms myocardium, ST elevation, anterior. For code E11.9, the Alphabetic Index main term is Diabetes, diabetic, subterm type 2. For code E78.0, the Alphabetic Index main term is Hypercholesterolemia. For code Z79.4, the Alphabetic Index main term is Long-term (current) drug therapy (use of), subterm insulin.

ICD-10-PCS Code(s): 021209W, 02100Z9, 5A1221Z, 5A1935Z, 06BQ4ZZ

ICD-10-PCS Rationale: For code 021209W, the Alphabetic Index main term is Bypass, subterms Artery, Coronary, Three Sites. For code 02100Z9, the Alphabetic Index main term is Bypass, subterms Artery, Coronary, One Site. For code 5A1221Z, the Alphabetic Index main term is Performance, subterms Cardiac, Continuous, Output. For code 5A1935Z, the Alphabetic Index main term is Performance, subterms Respiratory, Less than 24 Consecutive Hours, Ventilation. For code 06BQ4ZZ, the Alphabetic Index main term is Excision, subterms Vein, Greater Saphenous, Left.

7.10.   a. 411.1, 424.0, 429.81, 36.12, 36.15, 39.61, 35.12, 35.31
Correct answer.

b. 411.1, 424.0, 36.12, 36.15, 39.61, 35.12, 35.31

Incorrect answer. An additional code should be assigned for the papillary muscle tethering since it had to be repaired.

    c. 411.1, 424.0, 429.81, 36.13, 39.61, 35.12, 35.31

Incorrect answer. The patient had two aortocoronary vein bypass grafts and one internal mammary artery bypass graft. The correct codes are 36.12 and 36.15 and not 36.13.

    d. 411.0, 424.0, 429.81, 36.12, 36.15, 39.61, 35.12, 35.31

Incorrect answer. The documentation states "unstable postinfarct angina" which indexes to Angina—unstable—411.1.

ICD-10-CM Code(s): I20.0, I34.0, I51.89

ICD-10-CM Rationale: For code I20.0, the Alphabetic Index main term is Angina, subterm unstable. For code I34.0, the Alphabetic Index main term is Insufficiency, subterm mitral. For code I51.89, the Alphabetic Index main term is Dysfunction, subterm papillary muscle.

ICD-10-PCS Code(s): 021109W, 02100Z9, 06BQ4ZZ, 02UG0JZ. 02QD0ZZ, 5A1221Z, 5A1935Z

ICD-10-PCS Rationale: For code 021109W, the Alphabetic Index main term is Bypass, subterms Artery, Coronary, Two Sites. For code 02100Z9, the Alphabetic Index main term is Bypass, subterms Artery, Coronary, One Site. For code 06BQ4ZZ, the Alphabetic Index main term is Excision, subterms Vein, Greater Saphenous, Left. For 02UG0JZ, the Alphabetic Index main term is Supplement, subterms Valve, Mitral. For 02QD0ZZ, the Alphabetic Index main term is Valvuloplasty, subterm see Repair, Heart and Great Vessels. For code 5A1221Z, the Alphabetic Index main term is Performance, Cardiac, Continuous, Output. For code 5A1935Z, the Alphabetic Index main term is Performance, Respiratory, Continuous, Less than 24 Consecutive Hours Ventilation.

Disorders of the Digestive System

7.11.   ICD-9-CM Principal Diagnosis: Acute cholecystitis, 575.0-Y

    ICD-9-CM Additional Diagnoses:

        Acute pancreatitis, 577.0-Y

        Bile duct obstruction, 576.2-Y

    ICD-9-CM Rationale: The cholecystitis is documented as acute. Though the physician suspected a stone in the bile duct, none was found and the diagnosis after study was "evidence of bile duct obstruction." The POA indicator Y (yes) is assigned to the diagnosis codes as all conditions were present on admission.

    ICD-9-CM Principal Procedure: Cholecystectomy, 51.22

    ICD-9-CM Additional Procedures:

        Common duct exploration for relief of obstruction, 51.42

        Feeding jejunostomy, 46.39

        Intraoperative cholangiogram, 87.53

    Rationale: The cholecystectomy was performed open, not laparoscopically.

ICD-10-CM Code(s): K80.01, K85.1

ICD-10-CM Rationale: For code K80.01, the Alphabetic Index main term is Calculus, subterms gallbladder, with, cholecystitis, acute, with, obstruction. For code K85.1, the Alphabetic Index main term is Pancreatitis, acute, gallstone.

ICD-10-PCS Code(s): 0FT40ZZ, 0FJB0ZZ, 0DHA0UZ, BF101ZZ

ICD-10-PCS Rationale: For code 0FT40ZZ, the Alphabetic Index main term is Cholecystectomy—see Resection, Gallbladder. For code 0FJB0ZZ, the Alphabetic Index main term is Inspection, subterms Duct, Hepatobiliary. For code 0DHA0UZ, the Alphabetic Index main term is Insertion of device in, subterm Jejunum. For code BF101ZZ, the Alphabetic Index main term is Fluoroscopy, subterm Bile Duct. Note: Temporary postoperative wound drains are considered integral to the performance of a procedure and are not coded as devices. Therefore, the placement of the Jackson-Pratt drain is not coded.

7.12. ICD-9-CM Principal Diagnosis: Acute gastric ulcer with hemorrhage, 531.00-Y

ICD-9-CM Additional Diagnoses:

Chronic pancreatitis, 577.1-Y

Alcoholic cirrhosis of liver, 571.2-Y

Alcoholism, 303.90-Y

Chronic hepatitis C without mention of hepatic coma, 070.54 -Y

ICD-9-CM Rationale: When cirrhosis is due to both alcohol and chronic hepatitis C, it is not necessary to report code 571.5 since the cirrhosis is reported with code 571.2 and nonalcoholic liver disease is included in code 070.54 (*Coding Clinic* 2011, 1Q:23). The POA indicator Y (yes) is assigned to the diagnosis codes as all conditions were present on admission.

ICD-9-CM Principal Procedure: Partial gastrectomy with anastomosis to jejunum, 43.7

ICD-9-CM Additional Procedures:

Feeding jejunostomy, 46.39

ICD-10-CM Code(s): K25.0, K86.1, K70.30, F10.20, B18.2

ICD-10-CM Rationale: For code K25.0, the Alphabetic Index main term is Ulcer, subterms stomach, acute, with, hemorrhage. For code K86.1, the Alphabetic Index main term is Pancreatitis, subterm chronic. For code K70.30, the Alphabetic Index main term is Cirrhosis, subterm alcoholic. For code F10.20, the Alphabetic Index main term is Alcoholism. For code B18.2, the Alphabetic Index main term is Hepatitis, subterms C, chronic.

ICD-10-PCS Code(s): 0DB60ZZ, 0D160ZA, 0DHA0UZ

ICD-10-PCS Rationale: For code 0DB60ZZ, the Alphabetic Index main term is Excision, subterm Stomach. For code 0D160ZA, the Alphabetic Index main term is Bypass, subterm Stomach. For code 0DHA0UZ, the Alphabetic Index main term is Insertion of device in, subterm Jejunum.

Optional MS-DRG Exercise (for users with access to MS-DRG software or tables)

MS-DRG 327 is the correct MS-DRG assignment.

The code 577.1 is a CC, which affects the MS-DRG assignment.

7.13. ICD-9-CM Principal Diagnosis: Morbid obesity, 278.01-Y

ICD-9-CM Additional Diagnoses:

Gastroesphogeal reflux, 530.81-Y

Obstructive sleep apnea, 327.23-Y

ICD-9-CM Principal Procedure: Revision gastroplasty converted to Roux-en-Y, 44.39

ICD-9-CM Additional Procedures:

Removal of ring, 44.99

Liver biopsy, 50.11

Gastroscopy, 44.13

The eroded ring is not a complication because the reason the ring eroded was due to her increased weight. See *Coding Clinic* (2003, 3Q:3–8) for reference. Code 278.01 is reported for the morbid obesity. Code 327.23 is reported for Obstructive sleep apnea. Code 44.39, Other gastroenterostomy, is reported when a gastroplasty is converted to Roux-en-Y procedure per *Coding Clinic* (2003, 3Q:3–8). The endoscopy procedure and the procedure to remove the ring should also be coded, 44.99. A liver biopsy was also performed in addition to removal of the ring and endoscopy.

ICD-10-CM Code(s): E66.01, K21.9, G47.33

ICD-10-CM Rationale: For code E66.01, the Alphabetic Index main term is Obesity, subterm morbid. For code K21.9, the Alphabetic Index main term is Reflux, subterm gastroesophageal. For code G47.33, the Alphabetic Index main term is Apnea, subterms sleep, obstructive.

ICD-10-PCS Code(s): 0D160ZA, 0DP60CZ, 0FB00ZX, 0DJ68ZZ

ICD-10-PCS Rationale: For code 0D160ZA, the Alphabetic Index main term is Bypass, subterm Stomach. For code 0DP60CZ, the Alphabetic Index main term is Removal of device from, subterm Stomach. For code 0FB20ZX, the Alphabetic Index main term is Excision, subterm Liver, Left Lobe. For code 0DJ68ZZ, the Alphabetic Index main term is Gastroscopy.

Optional MS-DRG Exercise (for users with access to MS-DRG software or tables)

MS-DRG 621, OR Procedures for Obesity without CC/MCC

a. Secondary diagnosis of a complication/comorbid condition or a major complication/comorbid condition

Correct answer. Addition of a CC/MCC would change the current MS-DRG.

b. Additional procedure codes

Incorrect answer. The principal procedure in addition to principal diagnosis is generating the MS-DRG.

c. If one of the current diagnoses was not present on admission

Incorrect answer. The secondary diagnoses are not designated as a CC/MCC, so if they were identified as hospital-acquired conditions in addition to being *not* present on admission, the MS-DRG would remain the same.

d. All of the above

Incorrect answer. Only "a" would change the MS-DRG assignment of this admission.

Endocrine, Nutritional, and Metabolic Diseases and Immunity Disorders

7.14.   a. 239.7, 255.0, 401.9, 785.1, 07.21

Incorrect answer. The alphabetic index directs the coder accordingly: Tumor, cortical (benign), 227.0, malignant cortical, 194.0, and rest—see Neoplasm by site benign. Code 239.7 is coded to an adrenal neoplasm of uncertain behavior. There is no documentation to support this code selection.

b. 194.0, 401.9, 785.1, 07.22

Incorrect answer. The alphabetic index directs the coder accordingly: Tumor, cortical (benign), 227.0, malignant cortical, 194.0, and rest—see Neoplasm by site benign. The type of tumor has not been identified and thus 194.0, malignant tumor of the adrenal, is incorrectly reported. Cushing Syndrome meets secondary reporting as it is not inherent to the tumor. The tumor is unilateral, but there is no indication that a unilateral adrenalectomy was performed. Code 07.21 is correct.

c. 227.0, 255.0, 401.9, 785.1, 07.21

Correct answer.

d. 227.0, 255.0, 07.29

Incorrect answer. Hypertension 401.9 and palpitations 785.1 meet reporting guidelines as secondary diagnoses as patient discharged on Toprol used to treat both hypertension and palpitations. Code 07.21 is correct for excision of lesion of adrenal gland and thus other partial adrenalectomy, 07.29, is incorrect reporting.

ICD-10-CM Code(s): D35.01, E24.8, I10, R00.2

ICD-10-CM Rationale: For code D35.01, go to the Neoplasm Table and locate the main term Neoplasm, subterms adrenal, cortex, benign. For code E24.8, the Alphabetic Index main term is Cushing's syndrome or disease, subterm specified NEC. For code I10, the Alphabetic Index main term is Hypertension. For code R00.2, the Alphabetic Index main term is Palpitations. Note: The physician should be queried regarding whether or not the Cushing's is related to the ACTH. The patient is also on various medications. The physician could be queried as to whether the underlying conditions are pertinent to this encounter.

ICD-10-PCS Code(s): 0GB30ZZ

ICD-10-PCS Rationale: The Alphabetic Index main term is Excision, subterms Gland, Adrenal, Right.

Optional MS-DRG Exercise (for users with access to MS-DRG software or tables)

a. 644, Endocrine Disorders with CC

Incorrect answer. The procedure code 07.21 was performed.

b. 615, Adrenal and Pituitary Procedures without CC/MCC

Incorrect answer. This admission has a CC (255.0).

c. 614, Adrenal and Pituitary Procedures with CC/MCC

Correct answer.

d. 628, Other Endocrine, Nutritional and Metabolic OR Procedures with MCC

Incorrect answer. The procedure code is 07.21, which groups in this instance to 614.

7.15. ICD-9-CM Principal Diagnosis: Diabetic hypoglycemia, 250.82-Y

ICD-9-CM Additional Diagnoses:

Diabetic neuropathy, 250.62-Y, 357.2-Y

Diabetic nephropathy, 250.42-Y, 583.81-Y

Long term (current use) of insulin, V58.67

Lung cancer, 162.9-Y

Hepatomegaly, 789.1-Y

ICD-9-CM Rationale: According to the *ICD-9-CM Official Guidelines for Coding and Reporting*, when a patient is admitted for the purpose of chemotherapy and develops complications, the principal diagnosis is V58.11, Encounter for chemotherapy. In this case, the patient initially presented to the facility as an outpatient for chemotherapy, but then was admitted as an inpatient to control his diabetes. The same fifth digit for diabetes mellitus should be used for all of the applicable diabetic manifestations coded in the hospital admission. According to *Coding Clinic* (2002, 2Q:13), a physician statement of "poorly controlled" diabetes should be clarified to determine if the diabetes is, in fact, uncontrolled. Query the physician to determine if "not controlled," "Admitted for control of his diabetes," and "due to poor diabetes control" means uncontrolled before fifth-digit assignment is made. If physician responds to the query as "uncontrolled," then the fifth digit of 2 (type II or unspecified, uncontrolled) is assigned to all three diabetes codes. Otherwise, all three diabetes codes are assigned a fifth digit of 1 (type II diabetes not stated as uncontrolled). Manifestation codes for the diabetic neuropathy and diabetic nephropathy are assigned as secondary diagnoses. According to *Coding Clinic* (2005, 1Q:43–45), V58.67 is reported for type II patients who routinely use insulin.

The documentation states, "He has been on 70/30 insulin, 25 units in the morning and 15 units in the evening." A physician query may be appropriate to determine if the hypoglycemia is due to chemotherapy treatment based on the documentation, "One difficulty here is the cyclic nature of his chemo treatment regimen, likely to produce major shifts in his glucose, which is already difficult to control. Patient will need to monitor his glucose levels closely." See instructional note under 250.8x, "Use Additional E code to identify cause if drug induced." If physician response to the query is that the chemotherapy is the cause of the hypoglycemia, then add E933.1. If not, then do not assign the E code. The patient has previously had surgery for the lung cancer; however, the cancer is still under treatment, so the V code for "history of" is not appropriate and the cancer code of 162.9 is reported. Hyperlipidemia is not reported, as it was not evaluated or treated in the hospital and did not meet reporting guidelines for additional diagnoses. See *ICD-9-CM Official Guidelines for Coding and Reporting* and *Coding Clinic* (2006, 4Q:234–235). All diagnosis codes are present on admission and require a POA indicator of Y (yes), except V58.67. No POA indicator is assigned as category V58 is listed on the POA Exempt list.

ICD-9-CM Procedures: No reportable procedure; medical treatment only.

Rationale: There is no documentation to indicate that chemotherapy (99.25) was administered during this inpatient hospitalization.

Issues to clarify: The coding professional is advised to review the health record on this case to verify that physician documentation is consistent and supports the assignment of the fifth digit for uncontrolled diabetes. If there is any uncertainty, the physician should be queried for clarification.

ICD-10-CM Code(s): E11.649, E11.40, E11.21, Z79.4, C34.90, R16.0

ICD-10-CM Rationale: For code E11.649, the Alphabetic Index main term is Diabetes, subterms type 2, with, hypoglycemia. For code E11.40, the Alphabetic Index main term is Diabetes, subterms type 2, with, neuropathy. For code E11.21, the Alphabetic Index main term is Diabetes, subterms type 2, with, nephropathy. For code Z79.4, the Alphabetic Index main term is Long-term (current) drug therapy (use of), subterm insulin. For code C34.90, go to the Neoplasm Table and locate the main term Neoplasm, subterms lung, malignant primary. For code R16.0, the Alphabetic Index main term is Hypertrophy, subterm liver.

7.16. ICD-9-CM Principal Diagnosis: Diabetes with ketoacidosis, type I, 250.13-Y

ICD-9-CM Additional Diagnoses:

Dehydration, 276.51-Y

Congestive heart failure, 428.0-Y

Aortic valve disorder, 424.1-Y

Urinary tract infection, 599.0-Y

E. coli infection, 041.49-Y

Hyperkalemia, 276.7-Y

Peripheral vascular disease, 443.9-Y

Hypertension, 401.9-Y

Hyperlipidemia, 272.4-Y

Renal ureteral disease, 593.9-Y

Old myocardial infarction, 412-Y

Tobacco use, 305.1-Y

Coronary artery disease, 414.01-Y

Issues to clarify: According to *Coding Clinic* (2006, 2Q), "Diabetic ketoacidosis is by definition uncontrolled and code 250.13 is the default."

ICD-10-CM Code(s): E10.10, E86.0, I50.9, I35.0, N39.0, B96.2, E87.5, I73.9, I10, E78.5, N28.9, I25.2, F17.210, I25.10

ICD-10-CM Rationale: For code E10.10, the Alphabetic Index main term is Diabetes, subterms type 1, with ketoacidosis. For code E86.0, the Alphabetic Index main term is Dehydration. For code I50.9, the Alphabetic Index main term is Failure, subterms heart, congestive. For code I35.0, the Alphabetic Index main term is Stenosis, subterm aortic. For code N39.0, the Alphabetic Index main term is Infection, subterm urinary (tract). For code B96.2, the Alphabetic Index main term is *Escherichia (E.) coli*, as cause of disease classified elsewhere. For code E87.5, the Alphabetic Index main term is Hyperkalemia. For code I73.9, the Alphabetic Index main term is Disease, subterms peripheral, vascular NOS. For code I10, the Alphabetic Index main term is Hypertension. For code E78.5, the Alphabetic Index main term is Hyperlipidemia. For code N28.9, the Alphabetic Index main term is Disease, subterm ureter. For code I25.2, the Alphabetic Index main term is Infarction, subterms myocardium, healed or old. For code F17.210, the Alphabetic Index main term is Smoker—see Dependence, drug, nicotine; Dependence, drug, nicotine, cigarettes. For code I25.10, the Alphabetic Index main term is Arteriosclerosis, arteriosclerotic, subterms coronary (artery).

Disorders of the Genitourinary System

7.17. ICD-9-CM Principal Diagnosis: Bleeding, postmenopausal, 627.1-Y

ICD-9-CM Additional Diagnoses:

Anemia due to blood loss, 280.0-Y

Long-term current use of anticoagulants, V58.61 (exempt)

Status heart valve, V43.3 (exempt)

ICD-9-CM Procedures:

Endometrial ablation; Dilation and curettage, 68.23

Transfusion packed cells, 99.04

Issues to clarify: Query the physician with regard to the anemia in order to select the best code for the patient's condition. Per *Coding Clinic* (1993, 4Q:3), if the physician clearly documents the anemia is due to acute blood loss, code 285.1 should be assigned. Anemia due to chronic blood loss is coded to 280.0, Secondary to blood loss (chronic). The physician should always be queried if there is a lack of sufficient documentation.

ICD-9-CM Rationale: History of present illness states "bleeding after being menopausal for approximately one year." The endometrial biopsy was performed prior to admission. The code for the endometrial ablation includes D&C.

ICD-10-CM Code(s): N95.0, D50.0, Z79.01, Z95.2

ICD-10-CM Rationale: For code N95.0, the Alphabetic Index main term is Bleeding, subterm postmenopausal. For code D50.0, the Alphabetic Index main term is Anemia, subterm blood loss. For code Z79.01, the Alphabetic Index main term is Long-term drug therapy, subterm anticoagulants. For code Z95.2, the Alphabetic Index main term is Presence, subterm heart valve implant.

ICD-10-PCS Code(s): 0UDB7ZZ, 0U5B7ZZ, 30233N1

ICD-10-PCS Rationale: For code 0UDB7ZZ, the Alphabetic Index main term is Extraction, subterm Endometrium. For code 0U5B7ZZ, the Alphabetic Index main term is Destruction, subterm Endometrium. For code 30233N1, the Alphabetic Index main term is Transfusion with subterms Vein, Peripheral, Blood, Red Cells.

Optional MS-DRG Exercise (for users with access to MS-DRG software or tables)

MS-DRG assignment with the acute blood loss anemia code: MS-DRG 742—UTERINE & ADNEXA PROC FOR NON-MALIGNANCY W CC/MCC

MS-DRG assignment with anemia due to blood loss code: MS-DRG 743—UTERINE & ADNEXA PROC FOR NON-MALIGNANCY W/O CC/MCC

MS-DRG appropriate for this case: MS-DRG 743

7.18. Note: The *Official Coding Guidelines* state: "If the diagnosis documented at the time of discharge is qualified as 'probable,' 'suspected,' 'likely,' 'questionable,' 'possible,' 'still to be ruled out,' or other similar terms indicating uncertainty, code the condition as if it existed or was established."

ICD-9-CM Principal Diagnosis: Probable urosepsis with streptococcal bacteremia, 599.0-Y, 041.03-Y

ICD-9-CM Rationale: According to *Coding Clinic* (2003, 4Q:79–81), Bacteremia is defined as the presence of bacteria in the blood.

Additional diagnoses:

Left lower extremity cellulitis, 682.6-Y

Status post acute renal failure likely secondary to acute tubular necrosis, 584.5-Y

Insulin requiring diabetes mellitus, 250.00-Y, V58.67 (exempt)

Probable chronic obstructive pulmonary disease, 496-Y

Hypothyroidism, 244.9-Y

Hypertension, 401.9-Y

Probable iron deficiency anemia, 280.9-Y

ICD-9-CM Procedures: Doppler ultrasound of the left lower extremity, which showed no evidence of DVT, 88.77

Issues to clarify: The physician should be queried to determine if a code should be assigned for the pulmonary edema and, if so, whether it is acute (of cardiac origin or not) or chronic (*Coding Clinic* 1988, 4Q:3–5).

ICD-10-CM Code(s): Query the physician for clarification on probable urosepsis with streptococcal bacteremia, L03.116, N17.0, E11.9, Z79.4, J44.9, E03.9, I10, D50.9

ICD-10-CM Rationale: Per ICD-10-CM Coding and Reporting Guidelines, the term urosepsis is a nonspecific term. It is not to be considered synonymous with sepsis. It has no default code in the Alphabetic Index. Should a provider use this term, he/she must be queried for clarification. For code L03.116, the Alphabetic Index main term is Cellulitis, subterm lower limb. For code N17.0, the Alphabetic Index main term is Failure, subterms renal, acute, with, tubular necrosis. For code E11.9, the Alphabetic Index main term is Diabetes, diabetic, subterm type 2. For code Z79.4, the Alphabetic Index main term is Long-term (current) drug therapy (use of), subterm insulin. For code J44.9, the Alphabetic Index main term is Disease, subterms lung, obstructive (chronic). For code E03.9, the Alphabetic Index main term is Hypothyroidism. For code I10, the Alphabetic Index main term is Hypertension. For code D50.9, the Alphabetic Index main term is Anemia, subterms deficiency, iron.

ICD-10-PCS Code(s): B54CZZ3

ICD-10-PCS Rationale: The Alphabetic Index main term is Ultrasonography, subterms Vein, Lower Extremity, Left, Intravascular.

7.19.   a. 996.81, 586, 55.53, 55.69, 39.95 × 2

Correct answer.

b. 586, 996.81, 55.69, 39.95 × 2

Incorrect answer. The complication of the transplanted organ is reported as the principal diagnosis in accordance with the *ICD-9-CM Official Guidelines for Coding and Reporting* and *Coding Clinic* (2006, 4Q:231–232), which states, "When the admission is for treatment of a complication resulting from surgery or other medical care, the complication code is sequenced as the principal diagnosis." Removal of the previously transplanted or rejected kidney is reported.

c. 586, V42.0, 55.53, 55.69, 39.95

Incorrect answer. Code V42.0 is used only to report transplant organ status when there are no complications. In this case, the principal diagnosis is the complication of the transplanted organ (996.81). Dialysis was done before and after surgery; therefore, it is reported twice.

d. 584.9, V42.0, 55.69, 39.95

Incorrect answer. Coding is based on physician documentation and there is no documentation of "acute" renal failure (584.9); therefore, renal failure unspecified (586) is coded to report the renal failure. Code V42.0 is used to report transplant organ status when there are no complications. In this case, the first-listed code should be complication of the transplanted organ (996.81). Removal of the previously transplanted or rejected kidney is reported. Dialysis was done before and after surgery; therefore, it is reported twice.

ICD-10-CM Code(s): T86.12, N19

ICD-10-CM Rationale: For code T86.12, the Alphabetic Index main term is Complication, subterms transplant, kidney, failure. For code N19, the Alphabetic Index main term is Failure, subterm renal.

ICD-10-PCS Code(s): 0TY10Z0, 5A1D00Z

ICD-10-PCS Rationale: For code 0TY10Z0, the Alphabetic Index main term is Transplantation, subterms Kidney, Left. For code 5A1D00Z, the Alphabetic Index main term is Hemodialysis.

7.20 a. 584.9, 428.0, 496, 345.90, 459.81, 721.90, 715.09, 278.01, 275.49, 712.37, 401.9

Correct answer.

b. 403.90, 584.9, 428.0, 496, 345.90, 459.81, 721.90, 715.09, 278.01, 275.49, 712.37

Incorrect answer. Category 403 may only be used in instances of chronic kidney disease. This patient has acute renal failure and hypertension, which are not classified to category 403. Hypertension must be coded separately.

c. 586, 428.0, 496, 345.90, 459.81, 721.90, 715.09, 278.01, 275.49, 712.37

Incorrect answer. The renal failure is specified as acute. The patient has a history of hypertension and is currently on medication for hypertension, so this should be coded.

d. 404.90, 584.9, 428.0, 496, 345.90, 459.81, 721.90, 715.09, 278.01, 275.49, 712.37

Incorrect answer. There is not an assumed causal relationship between hypertension and congestive heart failure, nor is there a relationship between acute renal failure and hypertension.

Issue to clarify: Is the renal failure also chronic as noted in chief complaint since it's not documented anywhere else?

ICD-10-CM Code(s): N17.9, I50.9, J44.9, G40.909, I87.2, M47.819, M15.0, E66.01, M11.271, I10

ICD-10-CM Rationale: For code N17.9, the Alphabetic Index main term is Failure, subterms renal, acute. For code I50.9, the Alphabetic Index main term is Failure, subterms heart, congestive. For code J44.9, the Alphabetic Index main term is Disease, subterms lung, obstructive (chronic). For code G40.909, the Alphabetic Index main term is Seizure, subterm disorder. For code I87.2, the Alphabetic Index main term is Insufficiency, subterm venous. For code M47.819, the Alphabetic Index main term is Osteoarthritis, subterm spine—see Spondylosis; Spondylosis, subterm without myelopathy or radiculopathy. For code M15.0, the Alphabetic Index main term is Osteoarthritis, subterm primary. For code E66.01, the Alphabetic Index main term is Obesity, subterm morbid. For code M11.271, the Alphabetic Index main term is Chondrocalcinosis, subterm ankle. For code I10, the Alphabetic Index main term is Hypertension.

Optional MS-DRG Exercise (for users with access to MS-DRG software or tables)

False: The MS-DRG for this admission is 684, Renal Failure without CC/MCC.

Infectious Diseases

7.21.   ICD-9-CM Principal Diagnosis: Septicemia due to E. coli, 038.42-Y

ICD-9-CM Additional Diagnoses:

UTI, 599.0-Y

Group D strep, 041.04-Y

Renal insufficiency, 593.9-Y

Chronic obstructive lung disease, 496-Y

Previous CVA with residual of hemiplegia, 438.20

Previous CVA with aphasia, 438.11

Issues to clarify: According to *Coding Clinic* (2003, 4Q:79–81) and *Coding Clinic* (2006, 4Q:154–160), septicemia is often used interchangeably by physicians. However, the terms septicemia and sepsis are no longer synonymous. A query is appropriate for this record. The physician should also be queried to confirm if the E. coli as well as Group D strep were causative agents for the UTI. During the course of stay in the hospital, the patient underwent "fluid rehydration." The coding professional may want to initiate a separate query to the physician to determine if dehydration meets secondary diagnosis reporting. The EKG showed sinus tachycardia; unless the physician indicates this is a significant finding, it is not coded. The patient is on tube feedings; therefore, review the remainder of the health record to determine if the patient has a gastrostomy (V44.1).

ICD-10-CM Code(s): Query the physician, N39.0, B95.2, N28.9, J44.9, I69.359, I69.320

ICD-10-CM Rationale: Sepsis and septicemia are often used interchangeably by physicians. However, the terms septicemia and sepsis are not synonymous. A query is appropriate for this record. For code N39.0, the Alphabetic Index main term is Infection, subterm urinary (tract). For code B96.2, the Alphabetic Index main term is *Escherichia (E.) coli*, as cause of disease classified elsewhere. For code N28.9, the Alphabetic Index main term is Insufficiency, subterm renal. For code J44.9, the Alphabetic Index main term is Disease, subterms lung, obstructive (chronic). For code I69.359, the Alphabetic Index main term is Hemiplegia, subterms following, cerebrovascular disease, cerebral infarction. For code I69.320, the Alphabetic Index main term is Aphasia, subterms following, cerebrovascular disease, cerebral infarction.

Optional MS-DRG Exercise (for users with access to MS-DRG software or tables)

The MS-DRG assignment is 872, Septicemia without Mechanical Ventilation 96+Hours without MCC.

7.22.   a. 042, 136.3, 276.2, 581.89, 585.9, 280.0, 305.61, 305.51, 455.5, 305.1, 33.24, 99.04
Correct answer.

b. 042, 136.3, 276.2, 581.89, 585.9, 280.0, 455.5, 33.24, 99.04
Incorrect answer. The heroin, cocaine, and tobacco abuse should be assigned codes to describe these additional conditions.

c. 042, 136.3, 581.89, 585.9, 280.0, 305.61, 305.51, 305.1, 33.24, 99.04
Incorrect answer. The metabolic acidosis and bleeding external hemorrhoids should be assigned codes to describe these additional conditions.

d. 136.3, 042, 581.89, 585.9, 280.0, 305.61, 305.51, 305.1, 33.24, 99.04

Incorrect answer. The principal diagnosis is AIDS, 042. In accordance with *ICD-9-CM Official Guidelines for Coding and Reporting* and *Coding Clinic* (2006, 4Q:152), report code 042 as the principal diagnosis when a patient is admitted for an HIV-related condition. The HIV-related conditions are reported as secondary diagnoses. The metabolic acidosis and bleeding external hemorrhoids should be assigned codes to describe these additional conditions.

ICD-10-CM Code(s): B20, B59, N12, N18.9, D50.0, F14.10, F11.10, I84.121, F17.200

ICD-10-CM Rationale: For code B20, the Alphabetic Index main term is Human, subterm immunodeficiency virus. For code B59, the Alphabetic Index main term is Pneumonia, subterm Pneumocystits (carinii). For code N12, the Alphabetic Index main term is Nephritis, subterm interstitial—see Nephritis, tubulo-interstitial. For code N18.9, the Alphabetic Index main term is Failure, subterms renal, chronic. For code D50.0, the Alphabetic Index main term is Anemia, subterms normocytic, due to blood loss. For code F14.10, the Alphabetic Index main term is Abuse, subterms drug, cocaine. For code F11.10, the Alphabetic Index main term is Abuse, subterms drug, opioid. For code I84.121, the Alphabetic Index main term is Hemorrhoids, subterm external. Note: The Index refers to code I84.22 but this code is for hemorrhoids without complications. Documentation states the external hemorrhoid bleeding. For code F17.200, the Alphabetic Index main term is Dependence, subterms drug, nicotine.

ICD-10-PCS Code(s): 0BB68ZX, 0BBB8ZX, 30233N1

ICD-10-PCS Rationale: For code 0BB68ZX, the Alphabetic Index main term is Excision, subterms Bronchus, Lower Lobe, Right. For code 0BBB8ZX, the Alphabetic Index main term is Excision, subterms Bronchus, Lower Lobe, Left. For code 30233N1, the Alphabetic Index main term is Transfusion with subterms Vein, Peripheral, Blood, Red Cells.

7.23. a. 523.10, 054.9, 745.4, 446.1, 034.0

Incorrect answer. There is a combination code for the herpetic gingivostomatitis.

b. 054.2, 745.4, 034.0, 446.1, 785.6, 372.30, 782.1

Incorrect answer. Kawasaki's disease includes the lymphadenopathy, conjunctivitis, and rash, so these would not be coded separately.

c. 054.2, 745.4, 446.1, 034.0

Correct answer.

d. 054.2, 446.1, 034.0

Incorrect answer. The ventriculoseptal defect (VSD) should also be coded.

ICD-10-CM Code(s): B00.2, Q21.0, M30.3, J02.0

ICD-10-CM Rationale: For code B00.2, the Alphabetic Index main term is Gingivostomatitis, subterm herpesviral. For code Q21.0, the Alphabetic Index main term is Defect, subterm ventricular septal. For code M30.3, the Alphabetic Index main term is Kawasaki's syndrome. For code J02.0, the Alphabetic Index main term is Pharyngitis, subterm streptococcal.

7.24. a. 038.9, 995.91, 599.0, 434.11, 394.1, 397.0, 398.91, 427.31, 287.5, 285.9

Incorrect answer. Because organ dysfunction (renal failure) is present with the sepsis, 995.92 is reported as Severe Sepsis.

b. 995.91, 599.0, 586, 434.11, 424.0, 397.0, 428.0, 427.31, 287.5, 285.9

Incorrect answer. Code 038.9 is reported as the principal diagnosis per the Excludes note under 995.91 that instructs the coder to Code First underlying infection (038.9). Because organ dysfunction (renal failure) is present with the sepsis, 995.92 is reported as Severe Sepsis. The congestive heart failure is presumed to be rheumatic in nature per *Coding Clinic* (1995, 1Q:6) when mitral valve and aortic valve insufficiency is present with congestive heart failure. ICD-9-CM classifies the congestive heart failure as rheumatic 398.91.

c. 038.9, 995.92, 599.0, 586, 434.11, 396.3, 397.0, 398.91, 427.31, 287.5, 285.9

Correct answer.

d. 434.11, 038.9, 995.92, 586, 428.0, 424.0, 397.0, 427.31, 287.5, 285.9

Incorrect answer. Sepsis is the reason the patient was admitted to the facility. The code 599.0 for urinary tract infection meets additional diagnosis reporting. Per *Coding Clinic* (1995, 1Q:6), the congestive heart failure is presumed to be rheumatic in nature when mitral valve and aortic value insufficiency is present with congestive heart failure. ICD-9-CM classifies the congestive heart failure as rheumatic 398.91.

ICD-10-CM Code(s): A41.9, R65.20, N39.0, N19, I63.40, I08.3, I50.9, I48.0, D69.6, D64.9

ICD-10-CM Rationale: For code A41.9, the Alphabetic Index main term is Sepsis. For code R65.20, the Alphabetic Index main term is Sepsis, subterms with, acute organ dysfunction. For code N39.0, the Alphabetic Index main term is Infection, subterm urinary (tract). For code N19, the Alphabetic Index main term is Failure, subterm renal. For code I63.40, the Alphabetic Index main term is Embolism, subterms artery, cerebral—see Occlusion, artery, cerebral; Occlusion, artery, cerebral, with infarction, due to, embolism. For code I08.3, the Alphabetic Index main term is Insufficiency, mitral, with aortic valve disease, with tricuspid disease. For code I50.9, the Alphabetic Index main term is Failure, subterms heart, congestive. For code I48.0, the Alphabetic Index main term is Fibrillation, subterm atrial or auricular. For code D69.6, the Alphabetic Index main term is Thrombocytopenia. For code D64.9, the Alphabetic Index main term is Anemia.

Optional MS-DRG Exercise (for users with access to MS-DRG software or tables)

a. 064, Intracranial Hemorrhage or Cerebral Infarction with MCC
Incorrect answer as the patient's cerebral infarct developed after admission.

b. 871, Septicemia without mechanical ventilation 96+hours with MCC
Correct answer.

c. 872, Septicemia without mechanical ventilation 96+hours without MCC
Incorrect answer as an MCC is present (434.11).

d. 868, Other Infectious and Parasitic Disease Diagnoses with CC
Incorrect answer as the correct diagnosis codes group to MS-DRG 871.

7.25. ICD-9-CM Principal Diagnoses:

038.42-Y, *Escherichia coli* sepsis (either this or 038.11 may be the principal diagnosis)

038.11-Y, Staphylococcus aureus sepsis (either this or 038.42 may be the principal diagnosis)

ICD-9-CM Secondary Diagnoses:

995.91, Sepsis

599.0-Y, Urinary tract infection

294.20-Y, Dementia

244.9-Y, Hypothyroidism

401.9-Y, Hypertension

263.9-Y, Protein calorie malnutrition

787.20-Y, Dysphagia

ICD-10-CM Code(s): A41.51, A41.0, N39.0, B96.2, B95.6, F03, E03.9, I10, E46, R13.10

ICD-10-CM Rationale: For code A41.51, the Alphabetic Index main term is Sepsis, subterm *Escherichia coli*. For code A41.0, the Alphabetic Index main term is Sepsis, subterms Staphylococcus, aureus. For code N39.0, the Alphabetic Index main term is Infection, subterm urinary (tract). For code B96.2, the Alphabetic Index main term is *Escherichia (E.) coli*, subterm as cause of disease classified elsewhere. For code B95.6, the Alphabetic Index main term is Staphylococcus, subterm as cause of disease classified elsewhere. For code F03, the Alphabetic Index main term is Dementia. For code E03.9, the Alphabetic Index main term is Hypothyroidism. For code I10, the Alphabetic Index main term is Hypertension. For code E46, the Alphabetic Index main term is Malnutrition, subterm protein. For code R13.10, the Alphabetic Index main term is Dysphagia.

Behavioral Health Conditions

7.26.   a. 296.24, V62.84, 94.27, 94.22, 94.08

Correct answer.

b. 296.23, V62.84, 94.27, 94.22, 94.08

Incorrect answer. The admitting diagnosis specified the major depressive disorder as with psychotic features; therefore, the fifth digit of 3 (without psychotic features) is incorrect.

c. 296.24, V62.84, 427.9, 94.26, 94.22, 94.08

Incorrect answer. The cardiac arrhythmia may be an incidental symptom or a complication that should be reported. The physician may be queried for clinical significance and impact to the patient's care. ECT is coded 94.27.

d. 296.23, V62.84, 997.1, 427.9, 94.27, 94.22, 94.08

Incorrect answer. The admitting diagnosis specified the major depressive disorder as with psychotic features; therefore, the fifth digit of 3 (without psychotic features) is incorrect. The cardiac arrhythmia may be an incidental symptom or a complication that should be reported. The physician may be queried for clinical significance and impact to the patient's care.

ICD-10-CM Code(s): F32.3, R45.851

ICD-10-CM Rationale: For code F32.3, the Alphabetic Index main term is Disorder, subterms depressive, major, with psychotic symptoms. For code R45.851, the Alphabetic Index main term is Ideation, subterm suicidal.

ICD-10-PCS Code(s): GZB0ZZZ, GZ3ZZZZ, GZ11ZZZ, GZ13ZZZ

ICD-10-PCS Rationale: For code GZB0ZZZ, the Alphabetic Index main term is Electroconvulsive Therapy, subterm electroconvulsive therapy, unilateral-single seizure. For code GZ3ZZZZ, the Alphabetic Index main term is Medication Management. For code GZ11ZZZ, the Alphabetic Index main term is Psychological Tests, subterm personality and behavioral. For code GZ13ZZZ, the Alphabetic Index main term is Psychological Tests, subterm neuropsychological.

7.27. a. 295.34, 425.4, 401.9, 496, 250.01, 94.25

Incorrect answer. Alphabetical index: Cardiomyopathy, due to, hypertension—see Hypertension with heart involvement. A combination code exists for cardiomyopathy due to hypertension; code 402.90 is reported rather than 425.4 and 401.9. The diabetes is specified as type II; therefore, the fifth digit of 1 (type I) is incorrect.

b. 295.32, 402.90, 496, 250.01, 94.25

Incorrect answer. The correct fifth digit for schizophrenia is 4, as the physician documented chronic with acute exacerbation. The diabetes is specified as type II; therefore, the fifth digit of 1 (type I) is incorrect.

c. 295.34, 402.90, 496, 250.00, 94.25

Correct answer.

d. 295.84, 402.90, 496, 250.00, 94.25

Incorrect answer. The schizophrenia was specified as paranoid type, which is coded to subcategory 295.3.

ICD-10-CM Code(s): F20.0, I11.9, J44.9, E11.9

ICD-10-CM Rationale: For code F20.0, the Alphabetic Index main term is Schizophrenia, subterm paranoid (type). For code I11.9, the Alphabetic Index main term is Cardiomyopathy, subterm hypertensive—see Hypertension, heart. For code J44.9, the Alphabetic Index main term is Disease, subterms lung, obstructive (chronic). For code E11.9, the Alphabetic Index main term is Diabetes, diabetic, subterm type 2.

ICD-10-PCS Code(s): GZ3ZZZZ

ICD-10-PCS Rationale: The Alphabetic Index main term is Medication Management.

7.28. a. 969.72, 785.0, 304.40, E950.3, 980.0, 303.00, E950.9, 314.01, 312.00

Correct answer. In real practice, the coding professional would review the consultation report and other relevant documentation in the health record for confirmation of the ADHD, aggressive behavior, or other applicable psychiatric diagnoses. The coding professional may also want to query the physician to determine if the diagnosis of dehydration is applicable.

b. 785.0, E939.7, 305.90, 314.01, 312.00

Incorrect answer. The coding guidelines for a poisoning, rather than adverse effect, should be followed. The amphetamine poisoning and drug dependence should be coded. Any time alcohol is involved with another drug, it is coded as a poisoning. The alcohol code is incorrect; when there is documentation of drug dependence, drug abuse codes are not used.

c. 969.72, 785.0, 304.00, E980.3, 303.00, 314.01, 312.00

Incorrect answer. The E code for suicide attempt should be assigned. Any time alcohol is involved with another drug, it is coded as a poisoning. The drug the patient was dependent on was amphetamines.

d. 785.0, 303.00, 304.40, 969.72, E950.3, 980.0, E950.9, 314.01, 312.00

Incorrect answer. The poisoning codes are incorrectly sequenced as secondary diagnoses.

ICD-10-CM Code(s): T43.622A, T51.0x2A, R00.0, F15.229, F10.229, F90.9, F91.1

ICD-10-CM Rationale: For code T43.622A, the Alphabetic Index main term in the Table of Drugs and Chemicals is Amphetamine, subterm poisoning, intentional self harm. For code T51.0x2A, the Alphabetic Index main term in the Table of Drugs and Chemicals is Alcohol, subterms beverage, poisoning, intentional self harm. For code R00.0, the Alphabetic Index main term is Tachycardia. For code F15.229, the Alphabetic Index main term is Dependence, subterm amphetamine—see Dependence, drug, stimulant NEC, with, intoxication. For code F10.229, the Alphabetic Index main term is Dependence, subterm alcohol, with, intoxication. For code F90.9, the Alphabetic Index main term is Disorder, subterm attention-deficit hyperactivity. For code F91.1, the Alphabetic Index main term is Disorder, subterm solitary aggressive type.

Disorders of the Musculoskeletal System and Connective Tissue

7.29. ICD-9-CM Principal Diagnosis: Bucket-handle tear, medial meniscus, 836.0-Y

ICD-9-CM Additional Diagnoses:

    Tackle in sport, E886.0

    Accident, occurring, football field, E849.4

    Activity, football, tackle, E007.0

    External cause status, sport not for income, E000.8

ICD-9-CM Procedures: Meniscectomy, 80.6

ICD-10-CM Code(s): S83.212D, W03.xxxD, Y92.321, Y93.61, Y99.8

ICD-10-CM Rationale: For code S83.212D, the Alphabetic Index main term is Tear, subterms meniscus, medial, bucket-handle. For code W03.xxxD, the Alphabetic Index to External Cause main term is Tackle in sport. For code Y92.321, the Alphabetic Index to External Cause main term is Place of occurrence, subterm football field. For code Y93.61, the Alphabetic Index to External Cause main term is Activity, subterms football, tackle. For code Y99.8, the Alphabetic Index to External Cause main term is External cause status, subterm recreation or sport not for income or while a student.

ICD-10-PCS Code(s): OSBD4ZZ

ICD-10-PCS Rationale: For code OSBD4ZZ, the Alphabetic Index main term is Excision, subterms Joint, Knee, Left.

7.30.   a. 715.16, 81.54

Correct answer.

b. 715.36, 81.47

Incorrect answer. The osteoarthritis was localized to the right knee. Total knee arthroplasty was performed.

c. 715.16, 81.55

Incorrect answer. The knee replacement was not a revision.

d. 715.36, 81.54

Incorrect answer. The osteoarthritis was localized to the right knee.

ICD-10-CM Code(s): M17.11

ICD-10-CM Rationale: The Alphabetic Index main term is Osteoarthritis, subterms primary, knee.

ICD-10-PCS Code(s): 0SRC0JZ

ICD-10-PCS Rationale: The Alphabetic Index main term is Replacement, subterms Joint, Knee, Right.

7.31.   a. 812.52, 401.9, 250.01, 79.32

Incorrect answer. The diagnosis code is for an open fracture, which is not described here. The hypertension should be specified as malignant. The procedure code is not specific to the humeral condyle.

b. 812.42, 401.0, 250.01, 79.31

Correct answer.

c. 812.42, 401.0, 250.01, 78.52

Incorrect answer. The procedure code is for internal fixation without fracture reduction. In this case, a fracture was manually reduced.

d. 812.52, 401.9, 250.00, 79.32

Incorrect answer. The diagnosis code is for an open fracture, which is not described here. The hypertension should be specified as malignant. The diabetes should be specified as type I. The procedure code is not specific to the humeral condyle.

ICD-10-CM Code(s): S42.451A, I10, E10.9

ICD-10-CM Rationale: For code S42.451A, the Alphabetic Index main term is Fracture, subterm humerus, lower end, condyle, lateral. For code I10, the Alphabetic Index main term is Hypertension (malignant). For code E10.9, the Alphabetic Index main term is Diabetes, subterm type 1.

ICD-10-PCS Code(s): 0PSF04Z

ICD-10-PCS Rationale: The Alphabetic Index main term is Reposition, subterms Humeral Shaft, Right.

7.32. ICD-9-CM Principal Diagnosis: 722.10-Y

ICD-9-CM Additional Diagnoses: 338.18-N, 349.31-N, 722.52-Y, E870.0-N

ICD-9-CM Procedures: 80.51, 84.82, 03.59

ICD-9-CM Rationale: Displacement of L5–S1 intervertebral disc meeting reporting guidelines for principal diagnosis. The acute pain documented as occurring after surgery and the laceration during surgery meet reporting guidelines for secondary diagnoses along with the degenerative lumbar disc disease. For diagnoses 338.18, 349.31, and E870.0, a POA indicator of N (no) is assigned, as the pain occurred postoperatively, and accidental laceration occurred during the procedure and was not present at the time of admission. Diagnoses 722.10 and 722.52 were present at the time of admission and are assigned a POA indicator of Y (yes).

ICD-10-CM Code(s): M51.17, G89.18, G97.41, Y65.8

ICD-10-CM Rationale: For code M51.17, the Alphabetic Index main term is Displacement, subterms intervertebral disc, lumbosacral region, with, neuritis, radiculitis, radiculopathy or sciatica. For code G89.18, the Alphabetic Index main term is Pain, subterm postoperative NOS. For code G97.41, the Alphabetic Index main term is Tear, subterm dural. For code Y65.8, the External Cause Index main term is Misadventure to patient during surgical or medical care, subterm cut.

ICD-10-PCS Code(s): 0SB40ZZ, 0QH004Z, 00QT0ZZ

ICD-10-PCS Rationale: For code 0SB40ZZ, the Alphabetic Index main term is Excision, subterms Disc, Lumbosacral. For code 00QT0ZZ, the Alphabetic Index main term is Repair, subterm Spinal Meninges.

Neoplasms

7.33. ICD-9-CM Principal Diagnosis: Admission for chemotherapy, V58.11

ICD-9-CM Additional Diagnoses:

Peritoneal carcinomatosis, 197.6-Y

Malignant ascites, 789.51-Y

History of colon carcinoma (organ removed), V10.05

Status colostomy, V44.3

Family history of colon cancer, V16.0

History of radiation therapy, V15.3

History of tobacco use, V15.82

ICD-9-CM Procedures:

Other venous catheterization, 38.93

Chemotherapy, 99.25

ICD-9-CM Rationale: The patient is admitted for chemotherapy, as documented in the discharge summary and reflected in the physician orders, so V58.11 is the principal diagnosis. The organ of origin (colon) has been removed. Therefore, code the history of malignant neoplasm of the colon. Whenever there is a secondary neoplasm code, the primary site must be designated either with a code for the primary site or a V code. The breast cyst is not mentioned except in the History and Physical. Before coding, the physician would need to be queried.

ICD-10-CM Code(s): Z51.11, C78.6, R18.0, Z85.038, Z93.3, Z93.3, Z92.3, Z87.891

ICD-10-CM Rationale: For code Z51.11, the Alphabetic Index main term is Chemotherapy, subterm cancer. For code C78.6, go to the Neoplasm Table and locate the main term Neoplasm, subterm peritoneum, malignant secondary. For code R18.0, the Alphabetic Index main term is Ascites, subterm malignant. For code Z85.038, the Alphabetic Index main term is History, subterms personal, malignant neoplasm, colon NEC. For code Z93.3, the Alphabetic Index main term is Status, subterm colostomy. For code Z87.891, the Alphabetic Index main term is History, subterms personal, nicotine dependence.

ICD-10-PCS Code(s): 02HV33Z, 3E04305

ICD-10-PCS Rationale: For code 02HV33Z, the Alphabetic Index main term is Insertion of device in, subterm Vena Cava, Superior. For code 3E04305, the Alphabetic Index main term is Introduction, subterms Vein, Central.

7.34.   ICD-9-CM Principal Diagnosis: Recurrent lung carcinoma, 162.5-Y

ICD-9-CM Additional Diagnoses:

Intra-operative myocardial infarction (MI), 997.1-N

Non-transmural MI, 410.71-N

Hypertension, 401.9-Y

Iatrogenic hypotension, 458.29-N

COPD, 496-Y

DJD of lumbar spine, 721.3-Y

Hemiparesis of dominant side, late effect of stroke, 438.21

History of tobacco use, V15.82

Surgical absence lung, V45.76

ICD-9-CM Procedure:

Pneumonectomy, 32.59

ICD-9-CM Rationale: The coder needs to differentiate if the myocardial infarction caused the hypotension or if the hypotension caused the myocardial infarction. In this case, the intraoperative hypotension occurred, which resulted in an MI. Codes 496, 721.3, 438.21, V15.82, and V45.76 should be coded because they are documented in the medical record and are relevant to the admission.

ICD-10-CM Code(s): C34.12, I97.791, I21.4, I10, I95.89, J44.9, M43.06, I69.951, Z87.891, Z90.2

ICD-10-CM Rationale: For code C34.12, go to the Neoplasm Table and locate the main term Neoplasm, subterms lung, upper lobe, malignant primary. For code I97.791, the Alphabetic Index main term is Infarct, subterms myocardium, intraoperative, during other surgery. For code I21.4, the Alphabetic Index main term is Infarct, subterm non-ST elevation. For code I10, the Alphabetic Index main term is Hypertension. For code I95.89, the Alphabetic Index main term is Hypotension, subterm iatrogenic. For code J44.9, the Alphabetic Index main term is Disease, subterms lung, obstructive (chronic). For code M43.06, the Alphabetic Index main term is Disease, subterms joint, degenerative, spine—see Spondylosis; Spondylosis, subterm lumbar region. For code I69.951, the Alphabetic Index main term is Hemiplegia, subterms following, cerebrovascular disease, cerebral infarction. For code Z87.891, the Alphabetic Index main term is History, subterms personal, nicotine dependence. For code Z90.2, the Alphabetic Index main term is Absence, subterms lung, acquired.

ICD-10-PCS Code(s): 0BTL0ZZ

ICD-10-PCS Rationale: The Alphabetic Index main term is Resection, subterms Lung, Left.

7.35. ICD-9-CM Principal Diagnosis: Fibroadenoma, 217-Y

ICD-9-CM Additional Diagnoses:

    Bone metastasis, 198.5-Y

    Pulmonary metastasis, 197.0-Y

    History breast cancer, V10.3

    Absent breast, V45.71

ICD-9-CM Procedures:

    Mastectomy, 85.41

    Insertion of tissue expander, 85.95

ICD-9-CM Rationale: The patient is currently still under treatment for both the bone and lung metastases and therefore both should be coded as active conditions. The patient also has a history of right breast carcinoma, and an acquired absence of the right breast due to a previous mastectomy. When a primary malignancy has been previously excised or eradicated from its site and there is no further treatment directed to that site and there is no evidence of any existing primary malignancy, a code from category V10, Personal history of malignant neoplasm, should be used (*ICD-9-CM Official Guidelines for Coding and Reporting*).

ICD-10-CM Code(s): D24.2, C79.51, C78.00, Z85.3, Z90.11

ICD-10-CM Rationale: For code D24.2, the Alphabetic Index main term is Fibroadenoma, subterm specified site—see Neoplasm, by site, benign. For code C79.51, go to the Neoplasm Table and access the main term Neoplasm, subterms bone, malignant secondary. For code C78.00, go to the Neoplasm Table and access the main term Neoplasm, subterms pulmonary, malignant secondary. For code Z85.3, the Alphabetic Index main term is History, subterms personal, malignant neoplasm, breast. For code Z90.11, the Alphabetic Index main term is Absence, breast.

ICD-10-PCS Code(s): 0HTU0ZZ, 0HHV0NZ

ICD-10-PCS Rationale: For code 0HTU0ZZ, the Alphabetic Index main term is Resection, subterms Breast, Left. For code 0HHV0NZ, the Alphabetic Index main term is Insertion of device in, subterms Breast, Bilateral.

7.36. ICD-9-CM Principal Diagnosis: Pathological fracture L2, 733.13-Y

ICD-9-CM Additional Diagnoses:

Metastasis to the bone, 198.5-Y

Metastasis to the lung, 197.0-Y

Metastasis left celiac ganglion node plexus, 198.89-Y

History of primary colon cancer, V10.05

Cord compression from underlying neoplastic disease, 336.3-Y

UTI, 599.0-Y

Pseudomonas aeruginosa, 041.7-Y

Hypertension, 401.9-Y

Colostomy from previous colon cancer surgery, V44.3

ICD-9-CM Procedures:

Anterior allograft bone fusion at L2, 81.06

L2 laminectomy with decompression, 03.09

Physical therapy, 93.39

ICD-9-CM Rationale: All diagnoses are assigned POA indicator Y (yes) except V10.05 and V44.3, as these codes are on the POA Exempt List; therefore, no indicator is attached.

ICD-10-CM Code(s): M84.58xA, C79.51, C78.01, C81.02, C79.89, Z85.038, N39.0, B96.5, I10, Z93.3

ICD-10-CM Rationale: For code M84.58xA, the Alphabetic Index main term is Fracture, pathological, subterm due to, neoplastic disease, vertebra. For code C79.51, go to the Neoplasm Table and locate the main term Neoplasm, subterms bone, malignant secondary. For codes C78.01 and C81.02, go to the Neoplasm Table and locate the main term Neoplasm, subterms lung, malignant secondary. For code C79.89, go to the Neoplasm Table and locate the main term Neoplasm, subterms specified site NEC, malignant secondary. For code Z85.038, the Alphabetic Index main term is History, subterms personal, malignant neoplasm, colon NEC. For code N39.0, the Alphabetic Index main term is Infection, subterm urinary (tract). For code B96.5, the Alphabetic Index main term is Pseudomonas, subterm aeruginosa, as cause of disease classified elsewhere. For code I10, the Alphabetic Index main term is Hypertension. For code Z93.3, the Alphabetic Index main term is Status, subterm colostomy.

ICD-10-PCS Code(s): 0SG00K0, 0SB00ZZ, code for the physical therapy

ICD-10-PCS Rationale: For code 0SG00K0, the Alphabetic Index main term is Fusion, subterm Lumbar Vertebral. For code 0SB00ZZ, the Alphabetic Index main term is Excision, subterms Joint, Lumbar Vertebral. The physical therapy (F07) cannot be coded without further detail from the medical record.

7.37.   a. 198.3, 189.0, 780.39, 414.01
   Correct answer.

   b. 780.39, 198.3, 189.0, 414.01
   Incorrect answer. The seizures are a result of the metastatic brain cancer; therefore, the metastatic brain cancer should be the principal diagnosis.

   c. 189.0, 198.3, 780.39, 414.01
   Incorrect answer. This admission is directed at the metastatic brain cancer rather than the kidney carcinoma; therefore, the metastatic brain cancer should be the principal diagnosis.

   d. 198.3, 189.0, 414.01
   Incorrect answer. The patient is experiencing seizures due to the metastatic brain cancer; therefore, the seizure disorder should be coded as a secondary diagnosis.

   ICD-10-CM Code(s): C79.31, C64.1, R56.9, I25.10

   ICD-10-CM Rationale: For code C79.31, go to the Neoplasm Table and locate the main term Neoplasm, subterms brain NEC, malignant secondary. For code C64.1, the Alphabetic Index main term is Hypernephroma. For code R56.9, the Alphabetic Index main term is Seizure. For code I25.10, the Alphabetic Index main term is Arteriosclerosis, arteriosclerotic, subterms coronary (artery).

Optional MS-DRG Exercise (for users with access to MS-DRG software or tables)

   055, Nervous System Neoplasms without MCC
   MDC 1, Diseases and Disorders of the Nervous System (medical)

Disorders of the Nervous System and Sense Organs

7.38.   ICD-9-CM Principal Diagnosis: Transient vertigo versus posterior circulation transient ischemic attack, 780.4, 435.9

   ICD-9-CM Rationale: Official Coding Guidelines for two or more comparative or contrasting conditions state, "In those rare instances when two or more contrasting or comparative diagnoses are documented as 'either/or' (or similar terminology), they are coded as if the diagnoses were confirmed and the diagnoses are sequenced according to the circumstances of the admission. If no further determination can be made as to which diagnosis should be principal, either diagnosis may be sequenced first."

ICD-9-CM Additional Diagnoses:

Noninsulin dependent diabetes, 250.00

Coronary artery disease status post coronary bypass grafting, 414.00

Hyperlipidemia, 272.4

Smoker, 305.1

Past MI, 412

Hypertension, 401.9

Old lacunar infarct, V12.54

ICD-9-CM Rationale: According to *Coding Clinic* (1997, 3Q:15), assign 414.00 when a patient has coronary artery disease and has had a previous CABG. Code 414.05 would be used if the physician confirmed that CAD had developed over the previous bypass graft. As stated in *Coding Clinic* (1994, 4Q:49), CAD of bypass graft should not be assigned based solely on the fact that the patient has atherosclerosis and has a history of bypass surgery.

Issues to clarify: ER note lists mild neuropathy secondary to his diabetes mellitus. The physician should be queried if the full record does not provide further substantiation of this diagnosis.

ICD-10-CM Code(s): R42, G45.9, E11.9, I25.10, E78.5, F17.210, I25.2, I10, Z86.73

ICD-10-CM Rationale: For code R42, the Alphabetic Index main term is Vertigo. For code G45.9, the Alphabetic Index main term Attack, subterm transient ischemic. For code E11.9, the Alphabetic Index main term is Diabetes, diabetic, subterm type 2. For code I25.10, the Alphabetic Index main term is Arteriosclerosis, arteriosclerotic, subterms coronary (artery). For code E78.5, the Alphabetic Index main term is Hyperlipidemia. For code F17.210, the Alphabetic Index main term is Smoker—see Dependence, drug, nicotine; Dependence, drug, nicotine, cigarettes. For code I25.2, the Alphabetic Index main term is Infarction, subterms myocardium, healed or old. For code I10, the Alphabetic Index main term is Hypertension. For code Z86.73, the Alphabetic Index main term is History, subterms personal, cerebral infarction without residual deficit.

7.39.   a. 722.52, 721.3, 724.02, 724.4, 414.00, 401.9, V45.81, V45.82, 03.92, 99.23, 88.93

Incorrect answer. The codes from category 724 should not be reported. Per *Coding Clinic* (1989, 2Q:14), pain or neuritis due to spondylosis or intervertebral disc disorder is included in the 721–722 categories. Spinal stenosis due to degeneration (arthritic) of the intervertebral disc is classified to the 722 category. Review excludes notes.

b. 724.4, 414.00, 401.9, V45.81, V45.82, 03.92, 99.23, 88.93

Incorrect answer. Degenerative disc disease is the principal diagnosis and is coded 722.52. The lumbar arthropathy should also be reported, 721.3. Lumbar radiculopathy (724.4) is included in the codes in category 722–721. See *Coding Clinic* reference and rationale above.

c. 722.52, 721.3, 414.00, 401.9, V45.81, V45.82, 03.92, 99.23, 88.93

Correct answer.

d. 722.52, 721.3, 414.00, 401.9, V45.81, V45.82, 03.91, 88.93

Incorrect answer. The procedure codes for lumbar epidural steroid injection are 03.92 and 99.23.

Optional MS-DRG Exercise (for users with access to MS-DRG software or tables)

a. True

b. False. The correct MS-DRG assignment is 552, Medical Back Problems without MCC.

c. False. MS-DRG assignment is the same with or without this procedure code.

d. False. MS-DRG 552, Medical Back Problems without MCC, is in MDC 8, diseases and disorders of the musculoskeletal system and connective tissue.

ICD-10-CM Code(s): M51.16, M46.96, I25.10, I10, Z95.1, Z95.5

ICD-10-CM Rationale: For code M51.16, the Alphabetic Index main term is Degeneration, subterm intervertebral disc, lumbar, with, neuritis, radiculitis, radiculopaty, or sciatica. For code M46.96, the Alphabetic Index main term is Arthropathy (see also Arthritis); Arthritis, subterm spine (see also Spondylopathy, inflammatory); Spondylopathy, subterms inflammatory, lumbar region. For code I25.10, the Alphabetic Index main term is Arteriosclerosis, arteriosclerotic, subterms coronary (artery). For code I10, the Alphabetic Index main term is Hypertension. For code Z95.1, the Alphabetic Index main term is Status, subterm aortocoronary bypass. For code Z95.5, the Alphabetic Index main term is Status, subterms angioplasty, coronary artery, with implant. Code M99.53, Intervertebral disc stenosis or neural canal of lumbar region, is not coded. A note under category M99 states: This category should not be used if the condition can be classified elsewhere.

ICD-10-PCS Code(s): 3E0S33Z, BR39ZZZ

ICD-10-PCS Rationale: For code 3E0S33Z, the Alphabetic Index main term is Introduction, subterm epidural space, anti-inflammatory. For code BR39ZZZ, the Alphabetic Index main term is Magnetic Resonance Imaging, subterms spine, lumbar.

Newborn/Congenital Disorders

7.40.   a. 771.2, 041.09

Incorrect answer. This is not a specific umbilical cord infection code. Staphylococcus aureus should also be coded.

b. 686.9, 041.11, 041.09

Incorrect answer. This code, 686.9, is for omphalitis, but not of a newborn.

c. 771.4

Incorrect answer. The organisms identified in the culture would be separately coded.

d. 771.4, 041.11, 041.09

Correct answer.

ICD-10-CM Code(s): P38.9, B95.6, B95.4

ICD-10-CM Rationale: For code P38.9, the Alphabetic Index main term is Omphalitis. For code B95.6, the Alphabetic Index main term is Staphylococcus, subterm aureus, as cause of disease classified elsewhere. For code B95.4, the Alphabetic Index main term is Streptococcus, subterm specified NEC, as cause of disease classified elsewhere.

7.41. a. 770.6, V30.10, V50.2, 96.04

Incorrect answer. The birth code should be the principal diagnosis code, and the fifth digit of 0 only applies to V30.0. The correct code is V30.1. There is no documentation to indicate the baby was intubated. Manual resuscitation (93.93) and oxygen therapy (93.96) should be coded. The circumcision should also be coded.

b. V30.1, 770.6, V50.2, 64.0, 93.93, 93.96

Correct answer.

c. V30.1, 769, V50.2, 64.0, 96.04

Incorrect answer. Because the chest x-ray stated wet lungs and the patient was only in NICU for about one day, the code 770.6 for wet lung syndrome is more appropriate than the 769 code for respiratory distress syndrome. There is no documentation to indicate the baby was intubated. Manual resuscitation (93.93) and oxygen therapy (93.96) should be coded.

d. V30.10, 768.6, V50.2, 64.0, 96.05, 93.96

Incorrect answer. The correct birth code is V30.1, as the fifth digit only applies to V30.0. Code 768.6 is incorrect, as there is no mention of asphyxia at the time of birth. The documentation does not support intubation, only resuscitation (93.93).

ICD-10-CM Code(s): Z38.1, P22.1

ICD-10-CM Rationale: For code Z38.1, the Alphabetic Index main term is Newborn, subterm born outside hospital. For code P22.1, the Alphabetic Index main term is Syndrome, subterms wet, lung, newborn. For code Z41.2, the Alphabetic Index main term is Circumcision.

ICD-10-PCS Code(s): 0VTT0ZZ, 5A19054, 3E0F7GC

ICD-10-PCS Rationale: For code 0VTT0ZZ, the Alphabetic Index main term is Resection, subterm Prepuce. For code 5A19054, the Alphabetic Index main term is Resuscitation, subterm Pulmonary. For code 3E0F7GC, the Alphabetic Index main term is Introduction, subterm Respiratory Tract.

Optional MS-DRG Exercise (for users with access to MS-DRG software or tables)

   a. Complication or comorbid condition

   Incorrect answer as this MS-DRG is not subdivided based upon a CC.

   b. Major complication or comorbid condition

   Incorrect answer as this MS-DRG is not subdivided based upon an MCC.

   c. Procedure code

   Incorrect answer as this MS-DRG is not subdivided based upon a procedure.

   d. Other significant problems

   Correct answer; other significant problems also drive this MS-DRG assignment.

7.42.   a. 747.0, 765.10, 765.27, 38.85

   Incorrect answer. Codes in category 765 are assigned for conditions arising in the perinatal period. The includes note at category 765 also indicates that the listed conditions are reported in a fetus or newborn. The codes are not applicable on this three-year-old's admission.

   b. 745.9, 35.39

   Incorrect answer. Patent ductus arteriosus is a specific congenital anomaly that is reported with code 747.0. Procedure code 38.85 is a more specific code to reflect the procedure described.

   c. 747.0, 38.85

   Correct answer.

   d. 745.0, 38.85

   Incorrect answer. The patient's condition is specified as patent ductus arteriosus (747.0).

   ICD-10-CM Code(s): Q25.0

   ICD-10-CM Rationale: The Alphabetic Index main term is Patent, subterm ductus arteriosus or Botallo's.

   ICD-10-PCS Code(s): 02LR0ZT

   ICD-10-PCS Rationale: The Alphabetic Index main term is Occlusion, subterms Artery, Pulmonary, Left.

7.43.   a. 996.75, 741.03, 02.42

   Correct answer.

   b. 996.2, 741.03, 02.41, 02.42

   Incorrect answer. This is not a mechanical complication; the shunt is occluded. Code 996.75 is more appropriate. The irrigation was unsuccessful; therefore, it is not coded.

c. 741.03, V45.2, 02.42, 02.43

Incorrect answer. The plugged shunt is the reason for admission and should be coded and sequenced first (996.75). V45.2 reflects status only and is not used, as there is a complication present. Removal of the old shunt is assumed in the replacement code and does not need to be coded separately, so the 02.43 code is not needed.

d. 996.75, 742.3, 741.00, 02.42

Incorrect answer. The spina bifida can be classified at the lumbar region because the physician states that the defect is at the bottom of the spine. The hydrocephalus is included in code 741.0x and would not be separately reported.

ICD-10-CM Code(s): T85.81xA, Q05.2

ICD-10-CM Rationale: For code T85.81xA, the Alphabetic Index main term is Complication, subterm ventricular shunt, embolism. For code Q05.2, the Alphabetic Index main term is Spina bifida, subterm lumbar, with hydrocephalus.

ICD-10-PCS Code(s): 00H602Z, 00P602Z

ICD-10-PCS Rationale: For code 00H602Z, the Alphabetic Index main term is Insertion of device in, subterm cerebral ventricle. For code 00P602Z, the Alphabetic Index main term is Removal of device from, subterm cerebral ventricle.

Pediatric Conditions

7.44.   a. 752.61, 550.91, 752.69, 58.49, 53.02, 64.0, 57.94

Incorrect answer. The hernia is not specified as recurrent, so a fifth digit of 0 should be used (550.90). Redundant preputial tissue is coded 605. Hypospadias repair is coded 58.45. Excision of the nevus is also reported (222.1, 64.2).

b. 752.61, 605, 550.90, 239.5, 58.47, 53.01, 64.2, 57.94

Incorrect answer. A nevus is coded as a benign neoplasm of the skin (222.1). In real practice, the coding professional would, of course, confirm this by checking the pathology report. Hypospadias repair is coded 58.45. This is an indirect hernia (determined because descriptions of the hernia sac, external oblique, and inguinal ring are mentioned; a direct hernia would be between the inferior epigastric artery and the edge of the rectus muscle). Code 53.02 is reported. The circumcision is also reported, 64.0.

c. 752.61, 550.91, 752.69, 58.49, 53.00, 57.94

Incorrect answer. The hernia is not specified as recurrent, so a fifth digit of 0 should be used (550.90). Redundant preputial tissue is coded 605. Excision of the nevus is also reported (222.1, 64.2). Hypospadias repair is coded 58.45. This is an indirect hernia (determined because descriptions of the hernia sac, external oblique, and inguinal ring are mentioned; a direct hernia would be between the inferior epigastric artery and the edge of the rectus muscle). Code 53.02 is reported. The circumcision is also reported, 64.0.

d. 752.61, 605, 550.90, 222.1, 58.45, 53.02, 64.0, 64.2, 57.94

Correct answer.

ICD-10-CM Code(s): Q54.1, N47.8, K40.90, D29.0

ICD-10-CM Rationale: For code Q54.1, the Alphabetic Index main term is Hypospadias, subterm penile. For code N47.8, the Alphabetic Index main term is Redundant, subterm prepuce. For code K40.90, the Alphabetic Index main term is Hernia, subterm inguinal, unilateral. For code D29.0, the Alphabetic Index main term is Nevus, subterm male genital organ.

ICD-10-PCS Code(s): 0TSD0ZZ, 0YQ50ZZ, 0VTT0ZZ, 0VBS0ZX, 0T9B70Z

ICD-10-PCS Rationale: For code 0TSD0ZZ, the Alphabetic Index main term is Reposition, subterm Urethra. For code 0YQ50ZZ, the Alphabetic Index main term is Repair, subterms Inguinal Region, Right. For code 0VTT0ZZ, the Alphabetic Index main term is Resection, subterm Prepuce. For code 0VBS0ZX, the Alphabetic Index main term is Excision, subterm Penis. For code 0T9B70Z, the Alphabetic Index main term is Urethral catheterization, indwelling.

7.45. a. 170.4, 758.0, 77.41

Incorrect answer. A vascular access device is implanted, 86.07.

b. 170.4, 170.3, 170.2, 77.81

Incorrect answer. The bone scan showed some questionable areas, but the physician does not document a diagnosis of sarcoma of the ribs and vertebra. The physician would have to be queried before these additional diagnosis codes could be added. The biopsy is not specified as excisional; code 77.41 is correct. Down syndrome is also reported, 758.0. A vascular access device is implanted, 86.07.

c. 170.4, 758.0, 77.61, 86.07

Incorrect answer. The biopsy is not specified as excisional, so code 77.41 is correct.

d. 170.4, 758.0, 77.41, 86.07

Correct answer.

ICD-10-CM Code(s): C40.02, Q90.9

ICD-10-CM Rationale: For code C40.02, the Alphabetic Index main term is Sarcoma, subterm Ewing's—see Neoplasm, bone malignant; Neoplasm, bone, scapula, malignant primary. For code Q90.9, the Alphabetic Index main term is Down syndrome.

ICD-10-PCS Code(s): 0PB60ZX, 0JH80XZ

ICD-10-PCS Rationale: For code 0PB60ZX, the Alphabetic Index main term is Excision, subterms Scapula, Left. For code 0JH80XZ, the Alphabetic Index main term is Insertion of device in, subterms Subcutaneous Tissue and Fascia, Abdomen.

Optional MS-DRG Exercise (for users with access to MS-DRG software or tables)

a. 517, Other musculoskeletal system and connective tissue OR procedure without CC/MCC

Incorrect answer as the procedure code is 77.41.

b. 497, Local excision and removal internal fixation devices except hip and femur without CC/MCC

Incorrect answer as the procedure code is 77.41.

c. 479, Biopsies of musculoskeletal system and connective tissue without CC/MCC

Correct answer.

d. 477, Biopsies of musculoskeletal system and connective tissue with MCC

Incorrect answer as neither a CC nor an MCC are present on this admission.

Conditions of Pregnancy, Childbirth, and the Puerperium

7.46. ICD-9-CM Principal Diagnosis: Occiput posterior position, 660.31, 652.81

ICD-9-CM Additional Diagnoses:

Arrest of descent, 661.11

Premature rupture of membranes, 658.11

Failed attempt at vaginal birth after C-section, 659.11

Onset of labor after 37 weeks, with delivery by C-section, 649.81

Previous cesarean section, 654.21

Positive group B strep, 648.91, V02.51

Delivery of a live infant, V27.0

ICD-9-CM Rationale: According to *Coding Clinic* (2006, 3Q:14), assign code 648.9X, Other current conditions in the mother, classifiable elsewhere, but complicating pregnancy, childbirth, or the puerperium, and code V02.51, Carrier or suspected carrier of infectious diseases, Group B streptococcus, to identify group B strep carriers in pregnancy.

ICD-9-CM Procedures:

Low transverse cesarean delivery, 74.1

Pitocin for induction of labor, 73.4

ICD-10-CM Code(s): O64.0xx0, O42.02, O66.41, O34.21, O99.824, Z37.0

ICD-10-CM Rationale: For code O64.0xx0, the Alphabetic Index main term is Delivery, subterms complicated, by, obstruction, due to, persistent, occipitoposterior. For code O42.02, the Alphabetic Index main term is Pregnancy, subterms complicated by, premature rupture of membranes, with onset of labor, within 24 hours, after 37 weeks gestation. For code O66.41, the Alphabetic Index main term is Delivery, subterms complicated, by, failed, attempted vaginal birth after previous cesarean delivery. For code O34.21, the Alphabetic Index main term is Delivery, subterms cesarean, previous, cesarean delivery. For code O99.824, the Alphabetic Index main term is Delivery, subterms cesarean, streptococcus B carrier state. For code Z37.0, the Alphabetic Index main term is Outcome of delivery, subterms single NEC, liveborn.

ICD-10-PCS Code(s): 10D00Z1, 3E033VJ

ICD-10-PCS Rationale: For code 10D00Z1, the Alphabetic Index main term is Cesarean section. For code 3E033VJ, the Alphabetic Index main term is Introduction, subterms Vein, Peripheral.

7.47. ICD-9-CM Principal Diagnosis: Delivery complicated by nuchal cord without compression, 663.31-Y

ICD-9-CM Additional Diagnoses:

    Outcome of newborn, V27.0

    Mitral valve prolapsed in pregnancy, 648.61-Y

    Mitral valve prolapsed, 424.0-Y

ICD-9-CM Procedure: Episiotomy with episiorrhaphy repair, 73.6

Rationale: As per the delivery note, this is a delivery with a nuchal cord wrapped around the baby's neck. Codes 648.61 and 424.0 must be coded because they affected the monitoring of the patient and were documented in the medical record.

ICD-10-CM Code(s): O69.81x0, Z37.0, O99.413, I34.1

ICD-10-CM Rationale: For code O69.81x0, the Alphabetic Index main term is Delivery, subterms complicated, by, cord, around neck, without compression. For code Z37.0, the Alphabetic Index main term is Outcome of delivery, subterms single NEC, liveborn. For code O99.413, the Alphabetic Index main term is Pregnancy, subterms complicated by, cardiovascular diseases. For code I34.1, the Alphabetic Index main term is Prolapse, subterm mitral (valve).

ICD-10-PCS Code(s): 0W8NXZZ

ICD-10-PCS Rationale: The Alphabetic Index main term is Division, subterm Perineum, Female.

7.48. ICD-9-CM Principal Diagnosis: Premature delivery, 644.21-Y

ICD-9-CM Additional Diagnoses:

    Twin delivery, 651.01-Y

    Chorioamnionitis, 658.41-Y

    Cord around neck, 663.11-Y

    Outcome of delivery, V27.2

    Multiple gestation placenta status, V91.00

ICD-9-CM Procedure:

    Low cervical cesarean section, 74.1

Rationale: Code 644.21, preterm delivery at 33 weeks, is sequenced as the principal diagnosis. When a delivery occurs, the principal diagnosis should correspond to the main circumstances or complication of the delivery. In cases of cesarean delivery, the selection of the principal diagnosis should correspond to the reason the cesarean delivery was performed unless the reason for admission/encounter was unrelated to the condition resulting in the cesarean delivery (*ICD-9-CM Official Guidelines for Coding and Reporting*). In this case the reason for the admission was the preterm labor that could not be stopped. The medical record should be reviewed for the number of placenta and number of amniotic sacs in order to assign a more specified code than V91.00.

ICD-10-CM Code(s): O60.14x0, O30.003, O41.1230, O69.1xx1, Z37.2

ICD-10-CM Rationale: For code O60.14x0, the Alphabetic Index main term is Pregnancy, subterms complicated by, preterm labor, third trimester, with third trimester preterm delivery. For code O30.003, the Alphabetic Index main term is Pregnancy, subterm twin. For code O41.1230, the Alphabetic Index main term is Chorioamnionitis. For code O69.1xx1, the Alphabetic Index main term is Compression, subterms umbilical cord, complicating delivery, cord around neck. For code Z37.2, the Alphabetic Index main term is Outcome of delivery, subterms twin, both liveborn.

ICD-10-PCS Code(s): 10D00Z1

ICD-10-PCS Rationale: The Alphabetic Index main term is Cesarean section. Although most hospitals do not code the magnesium sulfate tocolysis it would not be incorrect to also assign a code for this procedure. If coded, the code would be assigned from the Administration section, root operation Introduction.

7.49.　ICD-9-CM Principal Diagnosis: Long labor, prolonged second stage, delivered, 662.21-N

ICD-9-CM Additional Diagnoses:

　　Problem amniotic membrane delayed delivery after AROM, 658.31-N

　　Septic thrombophlebitis, PP, delivered w/ PP comp, 670.32-N

　　Endomyometritis, delivered w/ PP comp, 670.12-N

　　Anemia, delivered w/ postpartum complication, 648.22-N, 285.9-N

　　Obstetrical surgery, delivered w/ PP complication, 669.42-N

　　Onset of labor after 37 weeks, with delivery by C-section, 649.81

　　Ileus, 560.1-N

　　Comp of L&D, delivered w/ postpartum complication, 669.82-N

　　Hypokalemia, 276.8-N

　　Comp obstetrical surgical wounds, del w/ PP comp, 674.32-N

　　Outcome of delivery, single liveborn, V27.0 (exempt list)

ICD-9-CM Procedures: 74.0, 73.09

ICD-10-CM Code(s): O63.1, O75.5, O86.81, O86.12, O90.81, O75.4, K56.7, O75.81, E87.6, O90.2, Z37.0

ICD-10-CM Rationale: For code O63.1, the Alphabetic Index main term is Delivery, subterms complicated, by, prolonged labor, second stage. For code O75.5, the Alphabetic Index main term is Delivery, subterms delayed, following rupture of membranes, artificial. For code O86.81, the Alphabetic Index main term is Thrombophlebitis, subterm puerperal, postpartum, childbirth, septic. For code O86.12, the Alphabetic Index main term is Endometritis, subterm puerperal, postpartum, childbirth. For code O90.81, the Alphabetic Index main term is Pregnancy, subterms complicated, by, anemia, postpartum. For code O75.4, the Alphabetic Index main term is Complication, subterm obstetric, procedure, specified NEC. For code K56.7, the Alphabetic Index main term is Ileus. For code O75.81, the Alphabetic Index main term is Exhaustion, subterm maternal, complicating delivery. For code E87.6, the Alphabetic Index main term is Hypokalemia. For code O90.2, the Alphabetic Index main term is Seroma—see also Hematoma; Hematoma, cesarean delivery wound. For code Z37.0, the Alphabetic Index main term is Outcome of delivery, subterms single NEC, liveborn.

ICD-10-PCS Code(s): 10D00Z0, 10907ZC

ICD-10-PCS Rationale: For code 10D00Z0, the Alphabetic Index main term is Cesarean section. For code 10907ZC, the Alphabetic Index main term is Drainage, subterms Product of Conception, Amniotic Fluid, Therapeutic.

Disorders of the Respiratory System

7.50. ICD-9-CM Principal Diagnosis: Calf skin ulcer, 707.12-Y

ICD-9-CM Additional Diagnoses:

> Bone necrosis, 730.16
>
> *E. coli* sepsis, 038.42
>
> Severe sepsis, 995.92
>
> Acute respiratory failure, 518.81
>
> Disseminated intravascular coagulation, 286.6

ICD-9-CM Procedure:

> Right below-the-knee amputation, 84.15

ICD-9-CM Rationale: The coding of severe sepsis requires a minimum of two codes: first a code for the underlying systemic infection, followed by a code for severe sepsis. Additional code(s) for the associated organ dysfunction are also required (*ICD-9-CM Official Guidelines for Coding and Reporting*). Following the guidelines, 995.92 (severe sepsis), 518.81 (acute respiratory failure), and 286.6 (DIC) are also coded.

ICD-10-CM Code(s): L97.214, A41.51, R65.20, J96.00, D65

ICD-10-CM Rationale: For code L97.214, the Alphabetic Index main term is Ulcer, subterms lower limb, calf, right, with bone necrosis. For code A41.51, the Alphabetic Index main term is Sepsis, subterm *Escherichia coli (E. coli)*. For code R65.20, the Alphabetic Index main term is Sepsis, subterm severe. For code J96.00, the Alphabetic Index main term is Failure, subterm respiration, respiratory, acute. For code D65, the Alphabetic Index main term is Defibrination (syndrome).

ICD-10-PCS Code(s): 0Y6H0Z1

ICD-10-PCS Rationale: The Alphabetic Index main term is Detachment, Leg, Lower, Right.

Optional MS-DRG Exercise (for users with access to MS-DRG software or tables)

579, Other skin, subcutaneous tissue & breast procedures with MCC

7.51.   ICD-9-CM Principal Diagnosis:

Pneumonia, due to gram-negative bacteria, 482.83-Y

ICD-9-CM Additional Diagnoses:

Acute respiratory failure, 518.81-N

Cardiac arrest, 427.5-N

Cryptococcal meningitis, 117.5-N [321.0-N]

Severely malnourished, 261-Y

ICD-9-CM Rationale: It is important that the coding professional confirm that the cryptococcal organism caused the meningitis only and not systemic or a causative agent of the pneumonia. The pneumonia is coded differently if caused by the cryptococcus. Streptococcus A as well as Proteus mirabilis are mentioned on the culture from the bronchoalveolar lavage. The coding professional may want to query the physician to determine if this was also a causative agent of the pneumonia before assigning code 482.31. Results of the open lung biopsy showed advanced fibrosis. The coder should query the physician to determine if pulmonary fibrosis (515) should also be coded. The patient was rehydrated and treated for a low albumin, so the coder would also need physician input to assign codes for dehydration (276.51) and low albumin (273.8).

ICD-9-CM Procedures:

Open lung biopsy, 33.28

Continuous mechanical ventilation, 96.70

Intubation, 96.04

Bronchoalveolar lavage, 33.24

Spinal tap, 03.31

ICD-9-CM Rationale: The discharge summary does not indicate how long the patient was on continuous mechanical ventilation. The coding professional would check the ventilation flow sheet, or another source document within the health record, to determine how long the patient was on continuous ventilatory support in order to assign a more specific code.

ICD-10-CM Code(s): J15.6, J96.00, I46.9, B45.1, E43

ICD-10-CM Rationale: For code J15.6, the Alphabetic Index main term is Pneumonia, subterm gram-negative bacteria NEC. For code J96.00, the Alphabetic Index main term is Failure, subterms respiratory, acute. For code I46.9, the Alphabetic Index main term is Arrest, subterm cardiac. For code B45.1, the Alphabetic Index main term is Meningitis, subterm cryptococcal. For code E43, the Alphabetic Index main term is Malnutrition, subterm severe.

ICD-10-PCS Code(s): 0BBK0ZX, 0BH17EZ, Mechanical Ventilation code based on hours on ventilation, 009Y3ZX, 0B9L80Z

ICD-10-PCS Rationale: For code 0BBK0ZX, the Alphabetic Index main term is Excision, subterms Lung, Right. For code 0BH17EZ, the Alphabetic Index main term is Insertion of device in, subterm trachea. For code 009Y3ZX, the Alphabetic Index main term is Drainage, subterms spinal cord, lumbar. For code 0B9L80Z, the Alphabetic Index main term is Drainage, subterms lung, left.

Optional MS-DRG Exercise (for users with access to MS-DRG software or tables)

    a. 163, Major Chest Procedure with MCC

Correct answer.

    b. 853, Infectious and Parasitic Diseases with OR Procedure with MCC

Incorrect answer. Without further information from the physician, this case is assigned to MS-DRG 163. If the physician indicated that the pneumonia was due to a cryptococcal organism, then the principal diagnosis code would change, perhaps to 117.5, and the MS-DRG would likely be 853. From the information provided here, the cryptococcal organism appears to have caused the meningitis only.

    c. 178, Respiratory Infections and Inflammations with CC

Incorrect answer. The MS-DRG is 163, based on the open lung biopsy.

    d. MS-DRG 003, ECMO or Tracheostomy with Mechanical Ventilation 96+ Hours or Principal Diagnosis Except Face, Mouth and Neck with Major OR

Incorrect answer. MS-DRG assignment is based on the open lung biopsy and is unaffected by the length of time the patient was on continuous mechanical ventilation.

7.52. ICD-9-CM Principal Diagnosis: Gram-negative pneumonia, 482.83-Y

ICD-9-CM Additional Diagnoses:

    Non-insulin-dependent diabetes (insulin requiring), uncontrolled, 250.52-Y

    Retinopathy, 362.01-Y

    Hypertension, 401.9-Y

    Resistant gram-negative bacteria, V09.2-Y

    Degenerative joint disease of knees, 715.36-Y

    Aortic stenosis, 424.1-Y

    Long-term use of insulin, V58.67

ICD-9-CM Rationale: The patient has gram-negative pneumonia documented in the History and Physical and 2/2 Progress Note. The organism causing the pneumonia needs to be specified in the medical record in areas other than just the sputum culture to code. *Coding Clinic* (1988, 3Q:11). Use non-insulin-dependent diabetes mellitus (insulin requiring), uncontrolled because the History and Physical states "Diabetes mellitus—uncontrolled." Progress notes also support: 1/31 progress note addresses treatment plan for diabetes out of control. Orders of 1/31 and 2/1 reflect treatment. *Coding Clinic* (2002, 2Q:13). Code V09.2 is reported because the resistant organism is documented in the discharge summary.

ICD-10-CM Code(s): J15.6, E11.319, E11.65, I10, Z16, M17.0, I35.0, Z79.4

ICD-10-CM Rationale: For code J15.6, the Alphabetic Index main term is Pneumonia, subterm gram-negative bacteria NEC. For code E11.319, the Alphabetic Index main term is Diabetes, subterms type 2, with, retinopathy. For code E11.65, the Alphabetic Index main term is Diabetes, subterms inadequately controlled—code to Diabetes, by type, with hyperglycemia; Diabetes, type 2, with, hyperglycemia. For code I10, the Alphabetic Index main term is Hypertension. For code Z16, the Alphabetic Index main term is Drug, subterm resistant organism infection. For code M17.0, the Alphabetic Index main term is Degeneration, subterm joint—see Osteoarthritis; Osteoarthritis, knee, bilateral. For code I35.0, the Alphabetic Index main term is Stenosis, subterm aortic. For code Z79.4, the Alphabetic Index main term is Long-term (current) drug therapy (use of), subterm insulin.

7.53. ICD-9-CM Principal Diagnosis: Acute respiratory failure, 518.81-Y

ICD-9-CM Additional Diagnoses:

MRSA Pneumonia, 482.42-Y

Congestive heart failure, 428.0-Y

Cerebral vascular accident with infarction, 433.11-N

Acute renal failure, 584.9-N

Hemiplegia secondary to stroke, 342.90-N

ICD-9-CM Procedures:

Mechanical ventilation, 96.72

TPN, 99.15

Packed red blood cell transfusion, 99.04

ICD-9-CM Rationale: Per *ICD-9-CM Official Guidelines for Coding and Reporting* and *Coding Clinic* (2007, 4Q:178–179), the acute respiratory failure may be assigned as the principal diagnosis if it is responsible for occasioning the admission to the hospital, which it was in this particular case. The chart should be reviewed to determine the cause of the lung mass for a more specific code or if it is incidental to the patient's CHF or pneumonia. More information is needed to code the placement of the central venous line. The coding of transfusions is facility-specific and may not be coded at all hospitals. Do not assign a code from category V09, since code 482.42 includes information about the organism being resistant to Methicillin (*ICD-9-CM Official Coding Guidelines*). Per *Coding Clinic* (1998, 4Q:87), code 342.90, Hemiplegia, unspecified may be assigned as an additional diagnosis to identify the current neurologic deficits that resulted from the cerebral infarction. When codes from the 430–437 series are used, additional codes are needed to identify any sequelae present, such as category 342 for any associated hemiplegia.

ICD-10-CM Code(s): J96.00, J15.21, Z16, I50.9, I63.232, G81.91, N17.9

ICD-10-CM Rationale: For code J96.00, the Alphabetic Index main term is Failure, subterms respiratory, acute. For code J15.21, the Alphabetic Index main term is Pneumonia, subterms in, staphylococcus, aureus. For code Z16, the Alphabetic Index main term is Drug, subterm resistant organism infection. For code I50.9, the Alphabetic Index main term is Failure, subterms heart, congestive. For code I63.232, the Alphabetic Index main term is Infarction, subterms cerebral, due to, stenosis NEC, precerebral artery. For code G81.91, the Alphabetic Index main term is Hemiplegia. (Note: *ICD-10-CM Official Guidelines for Coding and Reporting* state the default is dominant for the right side when the side is documented but not specified as dominant or nondominant.) For code N17.9, the Alphabetic Index main term is Failure, subterms renal, acute.

ICD-10-PCS Code(s): 0BH17EZ, 5A1955Z, 3E0336Z, 30233N1

ICD-10-PCS Rationale: For code 0BH17EZ, the Alphabetic Index main term is Insertion of device in, subterm trachea. For code 5A1955Z, the Alphabetic Index main term is Performance, Respiratory, Continuous, Greater than 96 Consecutive Hours Ventilation. For code 3E0336Z, the Alphabetic Index main term is Introduction, subterms Vein, Peripheral, Nutritional Substance. For code 30233N1, the Alphabetic Index main term is Transfusion with subterms Vein, Peripheral, Blood, Red Cells.

Optional MS-DRG Exercise (for users with access to MS-DRG software or tables)

a. 189, Pulmonary Edema and Respiratory Failure

Incorrect answer. The principal diagnosis is Respiratory Failure and with the ventilator, the correct MS-DRG is 207, Respiratory System Diagnosis with Ventilator Support 96+ Hours.

b. 291, Heart Failure and Shock with MCC

Incorrect answer. The principal diagnosis is Respiratory Failure and with the ventilator, the correct MS-DRG is 207, Respiratory System Diagnosis with Ventilator Support 96+ Hours.

c. 207, Respiratory System Diagnosis with Ventilator Support 96+ Hours

Correct answer.

d. 064, Intracranial Hemorrhage or Cerebral Infarction with MCC

Incorrect answer. The principal diagnosis is Respiratory Failure and with the ventilator, the correct MS-DRG is 207, Respiratory System Diagnosis with Ventilator Support 96+ Hours.

7.54.   a. 466.0, 515, 428.0

Correct answer.

b. 491.22, 428.0

Incorrect answer. Pulmonary fibrosis is not considered to be COPD; therefore, the codes are reported separately.

c. 491.22, 466.0, 515, 428.0

Incorrect answer. Pulmonary fibrosis is not considered to be COPD; therefore, the codes are reported separately.

d. 428.0, 466.0, 515

Incorrect answer. Bronchitis is the reason for admission after study. The pneumonia was ruled out.

ICD-10-CM Code(s): J20.9, J84.1, I50.9

ICD-10-CM Rationale: For code J20.9, the Alphabetic Index main term is Bronchitis, subterm acute. For code J84.1, the Alphabetic Index main term is Fibrosis, subterm lung. For code I50.9, the Alphabetic Index main term is Failure, subterms heart, congestive.

7.55. ICD-9-CM Principal Diagnosis: 486-Y, pneumonia

ICD-9-CM Rationale: Query physician for presence of respiratory failure at the time of admission based on the following documentation: Discharge diagnosis: respiratory failure. Admitted to the hospital for treatment of pneumonia and hypoxemia. Her pO_2 in the ER was 50 on room air. Quadriplegia affects her ability to breath and contributes to respiratory infections. ABG pH 7.482, pCO_2 33, pO_2 low at 50, HCO_3 324 and total CO_2 was 55. Her O_2 sat was only 88% on room air. Do not code the respiratory failure without further clarification from the physician, as it clinically does not appear that the patient was in failure.

ICD-9-CM Secondary Diagnoses:

276.51-Y, Dehydration

344.00-Y, Quadriplegia (fifth digit of 0 unspecified as documentation does not state complete or incomplete)

596.4-Y, Atonic bladder

305.1-Y, Tobacco use

276.8-Y, Hypokalemia

799.02-Y, Hypoxemia

ICD-9-CM Rationale: According to *Coding Clinic* (2006, 2Q:24–25), it is appropriate to code hypoxemia along with pneumonia as it is not inherent to pneumonia and it indicates a deficient oxygenation of the blood. However, if the physician is queried for the presence of acute respiratory failure and the physician confirms this diagnosis, hypoxemia is not coded since it is inherent to respiratory failure.

ICD-10-CM Code(s): J18.9, E86.0, G82.50, N31.2, F17.210, E87.6, R09.02

ICD-10-CM Rationale: For code J18.9, the Alphabetic Index main term is Pneumonia. For code E86.0, the Alphabetic Index main term is Dehydration. For code G82.50, the Alphabetic Index main term is Quadraplegia. For code N31.2, the Alphabetic Index main term is Atonia, subterm bladder. For code F17.210, the Alphabetic Index main term is Smoker—see Dependence, drug, nicotine; Dependence, drug, nicotine, cigarettes. For code E87.6, the Alphabetic Index main term is Hypokalemia. For code R09.02, the Alphabetic Index main term is Hypoxemia. (Note: Do not code the respiratory failure without further clarification from the physician.)

7.56. a. 493.91, 305.1, V07.4

Incorrect answer. The asthma and COPD is a combination code, 493.22.

b. 466.0, 493.22, 305.1, V07.4

Incorrect answer. The acute bronchitis is included in the asthma and COPD combination code.

c. 493.22, 491.22, 305.1, V07.4

Correct answer.

d. 493.21

Incorrect answer. The patient was not admitted as an inpatient with status asthmaticus. Status asthmaticus (fifth digit of 1) was documented in the ER and the patient was initially admitted to observation. When the patient's condition did not resolve as an observation, the H&P documents acute exacerbation of asthma/chronic obstructive pulmonary disease/acute bronchitis (fifth digit of 2). See *Coding Clinic* (2006, 3Q:20). Codes for tobacco use and hormone replacement therapy meet additional diagnoses reporting guidelines.

ICD-10-CM Code(s): J44.1, J44.0, J45.901, F17.210, Z79.890

ICD-10-CM Rationale: For code J44.1, the Alphabetic Index main term is Asthma, subterms with, chronic obstructive pulmonary disease, with, acute exacerbation. For code J44.0, the Alphabetic Index main term is Bronchitis, subterms acute or subacute, with chronic obstructive pulmonary disease. For code J45.901, the Alphabetic Index main term is Asthma, subterms with, exacerbation. For code F17.210, the Alphabetic Index main term is Smoker— see Dependence, drug, nicotine; Dependence, drug, nicotine, cigarettes. For code Z79.890, the Alphabetic Index main term is Therapy, subterms drug, long-term, hormone replacement.

7.57. ICD-9-CM Code(s): 486-Y, 491.21-Y, V15.82, 33.24

This patient was admitted primarily for postobstructive pneumonia according to the source document. The patient was admitted with an additional diagnosis of a lung mass; however, this was ruled out by bronchoscopy. The COPD is exacerbated as documented in the discharge summary. The two conditions are reported separately even though the physician documents postobstructive pneumonia as a diagnosis. See *Coding Clinic* (1998, 1Q:8 and 1997, 3Q:9). Pneumonia and COPD were present on admission and therefore a Y (yes) indicator is attached to each code. Code V15.82 is POA exempt.

ICD-10-CM Code(s): J18.9, J44.1, Z87.891

ICD-10-CM Rationale: For code J18.9, the Alphabetic Index main term is Pneumonia. For code J44.9, the Alphabetic Index main term is Disease, subterms lung, obstructive (chronic). For code Z87.891, the Alphabetic Index main term is History, subterms personal, nicotine dependence.

ICD-10-PCS Code(s): 0BB68ZX

ICD-10-PCS Rationale: The Alphabetic Index main term is Excision, subterms Bronchus, Lower Lobe, Right.

Optional MS-DRG Exercise (for users with access to MS-DRG software or tables)

194, Simple Pneumonia and Pleurisy with CC

Trauma and Poisoning

7.58.   a. 709.2, 909.1, E929.2

Incorrect answer. This is a late effect of a poisoning; however, there is a more specific code for scar of the trachea (478.9), and the late effect of a burn should also be assigned (906.8).

b. 478.9, 909.1, 906.8, E929.2

Correct answer.

c. 709.2, 909.5, 906.8, E864.2

Incorrect answer. This code sequence reflects an adverse effect, and this scenario represents a late effect of a poisoning. Also, there is a more specific code for scar of the trachea. (See scar, trachea, in the Alphabetic Index.)

d. 478.9, 909.5, E864.2

Incorrect answer. This code sequence reflects an adverse effect, and this scenario represents a late effect of a poisoning. You'll notice in trying to assign the E code for an adverse effect of drain cleaner that there is no code in the therapeutic use column of the table of drugs and chemicals. If there is no therapeutic use of a drug/chemical, there cannot be an adverse effect.

ICD-10-CM Code(s): J39.8, T54.3x1S, T28.5xxS, T27.4xxS, T28.6xxS

ICD-10-CM Rationale: For code J39.8, the Alphabetic Index main term is Scar, subterm trachea. For code T54.3x1S, the Alphabetic Index main term is Drugs and Chemical Table, Drano. For code T28.5xxS, the Alphabetic Index main term is Corrosion, subterm mouth and Corrosion, subterm throat. For code T27.4xxS, the Alphabetic Index main term is Corrosion, subterm trachea. For code T28.6xxS, the Alphabetic Index main term is Corrosion, subterm esophagus.

Optional MS-DRG Exercise (for users with access to MS-DRG software or tables)

153, Otitis Media and Upper Respiratory Infection without MCC

7.59.   ICD-9-CM Principal Diagnosis: Skull fracture, 801.05-Y

ICD-9-CM Additional Diagnoses:

Zygomatic arch fracture, 802.4-Y

Cerebral edema, 348.5-Y

Motorcycle accident, E822.0

Mountain accident, E849.8

ICD-9-CM Procedures:

Endotracheal intubation, 96.04

Mechanical ventilation, 96.72

Monitoring intracranial pressure, 01.10

Brain wave measurement, 89.14

ICD-9-CM Rationale: The hypotension, hypoxemia, and apnea are all symptoms of the severe intracranial injury and are not coded separately. An activity code was not coded as there is no applicable activity code for driving a motorcycle. Additionally, a status code was not coded due to the fact that this information was not documented.

ICD-10-CM Code(s): S02.19xA, S02.402A, S06.1x7A, R40.2312, R40.2112, R40.2212, V20.0xxA, Y92.828

ICD-10-CM Rationale: For code S02.19xA, the Alphabetic Index main term is Fracture, subterms traumatic, skull, temporal bone. For code S02.402A, the Alphabetic Index main term is Fracture, subterms traumatic, zygoma. For code S06.1x7A, the Alphabetic Index main term is Injury, subterms intracranial, cerebral edema, traumatic. For code R40.2312, the Alphabetic Index main term is Coma, subterms with, motor response (none). For code R40.2112, the Alphabetic Index main term is Coma, subterms with opening of eyes (never). For code R40.2212, the Alphabetic Index main term is Coma, subterms with, verbal response (none). For code V20.0xxA, the Alphabetic Index to External Causes main term is Accident, subterms transport, motorcyclist. For code Y92.828, the Alphabetic Index to External Causes main term is Place of occurrence, subterm mountain.

ICD-10-PCS Code(s): 0BH17EZ, 5A1955Z, 4A103BD, 4A00X4Z

ICD-10-PCS Rationale: For code 0BH17EZ, the Alphabetic Index main term is Insertion of device in, subterm Trachea. For code 5A1955Z, the Alphabetic Index main term is Performance, subterms Respiratory, Greater than 96 Consecutive Hours, Ventilation. For code 4A103BD, the Alphabetic Index main term is Monitoring, subterms Central Nervous, Pressure, Intracranial. For code 4A00X4Z, the Alphabetic Index main term is Measurement, subterms Central Nervous, Electrical Activity.

7.60.   ICD-9-CM Principal Diagnosis: Laceration of liver, 2 cm deep, 864.03-Y

ICD-9-CM Additional Diagnoses:

Dehiscence of operative wound, 998.32-N

Infection of operative wound, 998.59-N

Passenger in MVA, E812.1 (exempt list)

Place of occurrence highway or street, E849.5 (exempt list)

ICD-9-CM Procedures:

Liver lobectomy, 50.3

Reopening and drainage of operative wound, 54.12

Issues to clarify: It is unknown from this brief case summary whether the dehiscence was internal or external. In real practice, the coding professional would review the operative report and other documentation to discern this and assign the most specific code. The coder would also look for documentation that might indicate the causative organism of the infection in the operative wound.

ICD-9-CM Rationale: The coder would not assign a code for an organism based on culture results alone; the physician must document the causative agent.

ICD-10-CM Code(s): S36.115A, T81.31xA, T81.4xxA, V49.50xA, Y92.411

ICD-10-CM Rationale: For code S36.115A, the Alphabetic Index main term is Laceration, subterms liver, moderate. For code T81.31xA, the Alphabetic Index main term Dehiscence, subterm operation wound NEC. For code T81.4xxA, the Alphabetic Index main term Infection, subterm postoperative wound. For code V49.50xA, the Alphabetic Index to External Causes main term Accident, subterms transport, car occupant, passenger, collision, motor vehicle. For code Y92.411, the Alphabetic Index to External Causes main term is Place of occurrence, subterm freeway.

ICD-10-PCS Code(s): 0FT10ZZ, 0W9F0ZZ

ICD-10-PCS Rationale: For code 0FT10ZZ, the Alphabetic Index main term is Resection, subterms liver, right lobe. For code 0W9F0ZZ, the Alphabetic Index main term Drainage, subterm abdominal wall.

7.61. a. 865.11

Incorrect answer. In this case, there is no documentation of open wound into cavity. Also, because there is a laceration, 865.02 would be assigned. It would also be appropriate to code the concussion, the E code for the cause of the accident, and the E code for the place of occurrence.

b. 865.02, 850.9, E816.1, E849.5

Incorrect answer. The concussion was documented with a loss of consciousness of 10 minutes.

c. 865.02, 850.11, E816.1, E849.5

Correct answer.

d. 865.01, 865.02, 850.11, E816.1, E849.5

Incorrect answer. In this case, when the spleen has a hematoma and a laceration, only one code is used because code 865.01 states hematoma without rupture of capsule.

ICD-10-CM Code(s): S36.039A, S06.0x1A, V47.62xA, Y92.411

ICD-10-CM Rationale: For code S36.039A, the Alphabetic Index main term is Laceration, subterm spleen. For code S06.0x1A, the Alphabetic Index main term is Concussion. For code V47.62xA, the Alphabetic Index to External Causes main term Accident, subterms transport, car occupant, passenger, collision, stationary object. For code Y92.411, the Alphabetic Index to External Causes main term is Place of occurrence, subterm freeway.

Chapter 8. Case Studies from Ambulatory Health Records

Unless otherwise stated, code set answers given in Chapter 8 are ICD-9-CM and/or CPT.

Disorders of the Blood and Blood-Forming Organs

8.1. a. 282.61, 789.09, 427.31, 250.00, 99285

Incorrect answer. The sickle-cell anemia is in crisis, so 282.61 is not correct. It would not be necessary to code the inguinal pain because pain, fever, and so on are part of a sickle-cell crisis. The level is four for the E/M code per the documentation, so code 99285 is not correct. It is correct to add the x-ray codes.

b. 282.62, 733.42, 99284, 73550, 73510

Incorrect answer. The avascular necrosis was not confirmed, but only documented as "rule out." This would not be coded in the outpatient setting. The atrial fib and diabetes should be coded. A modifier of -25 should be appended to the 99284 code.

c. 282.62, 427.31, 250.00, 73550, 73510

Incorrect answer. The emergency department service should be reported with 99284-25.

d. 282.62, 427.31, 250.00, 99284-25, 73550, 73510

Correct answer.

Rationale: The CMS Web site (http://www.cms.gov/manuals) states that modifier -25 should be appended to an evaluation and management code when reported with a significant procedure (status indicator S or T) on the same day of service. Different fiscal intermediaries may have varying requirements for use of modifier -25.

ICD-10-CM Code(s): D57.00, E11.9, I48.0

ICD-10-CM Rationale: The Alphabetic Index main term is Crisis, subterm sickle-cell. The diabetes is found under main term Diabetes, subterm type 2. Main term Fibrillation, subterm atrial gives code I48.0.

8.2. a. 280.0, 792.1, 414.01, 250.00, V45.81, V17.49, 36430, P9051 (× 3 units)

Correct answer.

Rationale: The physician may be queried for the underlying cause of the chronic blood loss.

b. 285.9, 780.79, 36430, P9051 (3 units)

Incorrect answer. The anemia is specified as severe chronic blood loss anemia, so code 285.9 is not the correct answer. Indexing Anemia, blood loss, chronic results in code 280.0. It is not correct to code the weakness because it is a symptom of the more definitive diagnosis of anemia. The additional diagnoses of diabetes, ASHD, status bypass, and family history of cardiovascular disease may be coded because they were treated and/or are applicable to the case.

c. 280.0, 578.1, 414.01, 250.00, V45.81, V17.49, 36430

Incorrect answer. It is not correct to assume that the patient has GI bleeding, and the physician should be asked to add occult blood as a final diagnosis, if appropriate, which is coded to 792.1. The HCPCS Level II code with the number of units should also be added to account for the purchase of the packed cells from the blood bank. This code may generate an additional reimbursement under the APC system.

d. 285.9, 792.1, 414.01, 250.00, V45.81, V17.49, P9051 (3 units)

Incorrect answer. The anemia is specified as severe chronic blood loss anemia, so code 285.9 is not the correct answer. The transfusion administration code must be assigned with a CPT code in order for the APC to be generated. The physician should be asked to add occult blood as a final diagnosis, if appropriate.

ICD-10-CM Code(s): D50.0, E11.9, R19.5, I25.10, Z95.1, Z82.49

ICD-10-CM Rationale: The Alphabetic Index main term is Anemia with subterm blood loss. Main term is Diabetes with subterm type 2. Main term is Occult with subterm blood in feces (stools). Main term is Arteriosclerosis with subterm coronary (artery). Main term is Status (post) with subterm aortocoronary bypass. Main term is History with subterms family (of), disease or disorder (of), cardiovascular.

8.3.   a. 599.0, 276.51, 428.0, 287.5, 250.00

Incorrect answer. The thrombocytopenia was specified as primary, so code 287.5 is not the best choice.

b. 599.0, 276.51, 428.0, 511.9, 287.5, 250.00

Incorrect answer. Pleural effusion is not separately coded when present with CHF. *Coding Clinic* (1991, 3Q:19–20). The thrombocytopenia was specified as primary, so code 287.5 is not the best choice.

c. 599.0, 276.51, 428.0, 287.30, 250.00

Correct answer.

d. 599.0, 276.51, 428.0, 511.9, 287.30, 782.7, 250.00

Incorrect answer. Pleural effusion is not separately coded when present with CHF. The petechia is not coded. It is part of the thrombocytopenia and is excluded as an additional code.

ICD-10-CM Code(s): N39.0, E86.0, I50.9, D69.49, E11.9

ICD-10-CM Rationale: The Alphabetic Index main term is Infection, subterm urinary (tract). The dehydration is found under main term Dehydration. The CHF is found under main term Failure, subterm heart, congestive. Main term Thrombocytopenia, subterm primary gives code D69.49. The diabetes mellitus is coded by finding main term Diabetes, subterm type 2.

8.4.   a. 285.22, 285.3, 197.7, V10.3, E933.1

Correct answer.

b. 285.9, 197.7, V10.3, E933.1

Incorrect answer. The anemia is documented as in neoplastic disease, so code 285.9 is not the most specific choice. The anemia in neoplastic disease code (285.22) would be a better choice. The anemia is also documented as due to chemotherapy. Code 285.3 is required to report this condition. The *ICD-9-CM Official Guidelines for Coding and Reporting of Outpatient Services,* Section 1.C.2.c.1, states that code 285.22, Anemia in neoplastic disease, and code 285.3, Antineoplastic chemotherapy induced anemia, may both be assigned if anemia in neoplastic disease and anemia due to antineoplastic chemotherapy are both documented.

c. 197.7, 285.22, V10.3, E933.1

Incorrect answer. The patient is admitted for blood transfusion, so the anemia would be listed as the first diagnosis. The anemia is also documented as due to chemotherapy. Code 285.3 is required to report this condition. The *ICD-9-CM Official Guidelines for Coding and Reporting of Outpatient Services,* Section 1.C.2.c.1, states that code 285.22, Anemia in neoplastic disease, and code 285.3, Antineoplastic chemotherapy induced anemia, may both be assigned if anemia in neoplastic disease and anemia due to antineoplastic chemotherapy are both documented.

d. 285.9, 197.7, V10.3

Incorrect answer. The anemia is documented as in neoplastic disease, so code 285.9 is not the most specific choice. The anemia in neoplastic disease code (285.22) would be a better choice. The anemia is also documented as due to chemotherapy. Code 285.3 is required to report this condition. The *ICD-9-CM Official Guidelines for Coding and Reporting of Outpatient Services,* Section 1.C.2.c.1, states that code 285.22, Anemia in neoplastic disease, and code 285.3, Antineoplastic chemotherapy induced anemia, may both be assigned if anemia in neoplastic disease and anemia due to antineoplastic chemotherapy are both documented. It would also be appropriate to add the E code to show that the chemotherapy also helped cause the anemia.

ICD-10-CM Code(s): C78.7, D64.81, D63.0, Z85.3, T45.1x5A

ICD-10-CM Rationale: The code for the current liver metastasis is assigned as the principal diagnosis according to ICD-10-CM Coding Guideline I.C.2.C.1. Access the Neoplasm Table and go to the subterm liver and select a code from the Malignant Secondary column since the liver is a metastatic site. The Alphabetic Index main term is Anemia with subterms in (due to), neoplastic disease and due to antineoplastic chemotherapy to get codes D64.81 and D63.0. The Alphabetic Index main term is History with subterms personal (of) malignant neoplasm, breast. The main term in the Drug and Chemical Table is antineoplastic NEC, then select a code from the Adverse Effect column with a seventh character extension of A for initial encounter.

Disorders of the Cardiovascular System

8.5.   a. 786.50, 796.3, 93015

Incorrect answer. The patient's presenting symptom was arm pain, not chest pain, so code 729.5 is the primary diagnosis. The correct code is 458.9, not 796.3, according to the index. Low, blood pressure takes you to code 458.9. The hospital is providing only the technical component of the test, so code 93015 is inappropriate. Code 93017 is correct.

   b. 729.5, 796.3, 93015

Incorrect answer. The correct code is 458.9, not 796.3, according to the index. Low, blood pressure takes you to code 458.9. The hospital is providing only the technical component of the test, so code 93015 is inappropriate. Code 93017 is correct.

   c. 414.8, 458.29, 93017

Incorrect answer. The procedure code is correct, but the diagnosis codes are not. The patient's presenting symptom was arm pain, not chest pain, indicating ischemic heart disease, so code 729.5 is the primary diagnosis. Although it appears that the hypotension may have been iatrogenic (induced by the stress test), physician query would be required. Code 458.9 is more appropriate for this documentation.

   d. 729.5, 458.9, 93017

Correct answer.

ICD-10-CM Code(s): M79.602, I95.9

ICD-10-CM Rationale: The Alphabetic Index main term is Pain, subterm limb, upper. The code is completed using the Tabular List. The Alphabetic Index main term is Hypotension.

8.6.   a. 404.92, 36830

Incorrect answer. The documentation supports heart failure, so the correct combination fifth-digit code is 3 (404.93). Additional codes are reported to specify the type of heart failure, in this case, congestive (428.0), and stage of chronic kidney disease (585.6).

   b. 404.93, 585.6, 428.0, 36830
Correct answer.

   c. 585.6, 428.0, 401.9, 36821

Incorrect answer. There is a combination code for the hypertensive heart and chronic kidney disease with heart failure. Code 36821 is incorrect because a Gore-Tex graft was required. Because direct connection was not possible, code 36830 is the correct CPT code.

   d. 404.93, 36821

Incorrect answer. Additional codes are reported to specify the type of heart failure, in this case, congestive (428.0), and stage of chronic kidney disease (585.6). A Gore-Tex graft was required and direct connection was not possible; code 36830 is the correct CPT code.

ICD-10-CM Code(s): I13.2, I50.9, N18.6

ICD-10-CM Rationale: The Alphabetic Index main term is Hypertension with subterms cardiorenal, with heart failure, with stage 5 or end stage renal disease. There are two notes to "Use additional code to identify type of heart failure (I50-)" and "Use additional code to identify the stage of chronic kidney disease (N18.5; N18.6)."

8.7.   a. 414.00, 413.9, V45.81, 93461

Correct answer.

b. 414.01, 414.02, 93453, 93460

Incorrect answer. It is not known if arteriosclerosis was found in the native arteries or the grafts. Because grafts are examined, it can be assumed that the patient is post CABG, so that should be coded also, but 414.00 is as specific as we can get without further physician clarification. The angina should be coded. Code 93460 should not be used because the CPT code book directs the coder to not report this code along with 93453.

c. 414.00, 413.9, V45.81, 93453, 93462

Incorrect answer. The diagnosis codes are correct, but the imaging CPT codes have been omitted. The catheterization was not done by transseptal puncture; therefore 93462 is incorrect.

d. 414.01, 414.02, 413.9, V45.81, 93461

Incorrect answer. It is not known if arteriosclerosis was found in the native arteries or the grafts. Because grafts are examined, it can be assumed that the patient is post CABG, so that should be coded also, but 414.00 is as specific as we can get without further physician clarification.

ICD-10-CM Code(s): I25.119, Z95.1

ICD-10-CM Rationale: The Alphabetic Index main term is Arteriosclerosis, subterm coronary, native vessel, with angina pectoris. The patient has a history of CABG. The main term is Presence, subterm aortocoronary (bypass) graft.

8.8.   a. 279.3, 558.9, 748.3, V13.69, V15.1, V44.1

Correct answer.

b. 558.9, 790.7, V15.1, V44.1

Incorrect answer. Differential diagnoses of bacteremia or septicemia are not coded until confirmed. Personal history of congenital malformation, V13.69, should be coded once the congenital malformation is repaired. In addition, V15.1 should be coded to specify that the surgery was of the heart and great vessels. Both larygnomalacia, 748.3, and unspecified immunodeficiency, 279.3, should be reported.

c. 787.01, 558.9, V44.1

Incorrect answer. Nausea and vomiting are integral to acute gastroenteritis and are therefore not coded. Personal history of congenital malformation, V13.69, should be coded once the congenital malformation is repaired. In addition, V15.1 should be coded to specify that the surgery was of the heart and great vessels. Both larygnomalacia, 748.3, and unspecified immunodeficiency, 279.3, should be reported.

d. 787.03, 780.60, 558.9, 745.2, V15.1, V44.1

Incorrect answer. Vomiting and fever are integral to acute gastroenteritis and are therefore not coded. Personal history of congenital malformation, V13.69, should be coded once the congenital malformation is repaired. Tetralogy of Fallot is no longer coded once the malformation is repaired. Both larygnomalacia, 748.3, and unspecified immunodeficiency, 279.3, should be reported.

Rationale: Some children's hospitals do continue to report the congenital malformations once they are repaired, for research purposes.

ICD-10-CM Code(s): D84.9, K52.9, Q31.5, Z84.74, Z98.89, Z93.1

ICD-10-CM Rationale: The Alphabetic Index main term is Immunodeficiency. The main term is Gastroenteritis (acute). Another main term is Laryngomalacia (acute). The main term is History with subterms personal (of), congenital malformation (corrected), heart, and History, personal (of), surgery NEC. Another main term is Status (post) with subterm gastrostomy.

8.9. a. 32110-CA

Incorrect answer. Open heart massage should be reported as 32160-CA.

b. 32110, 32160

Incorrect answer. The CPT codes are correct, but to obtain payment from Medicare for procedures listed on the inpatient list when the patient dies prior to being admitted, modifier -CA must be applied to each code. See *Coding Clinic for HCPCS* (2003, 1Q:10) and *Coding Clinic for HCPCS* (2004, 4Q:11) for a complete discussion of the -CA modifier.

c. 32160-CA

Incorrect answer. The thoractomy for control of traumatic hemorrhage should be coded with 32110-CA.

d. 32110-CA, 32160-CA

Correct answer.

8.10. ICD-9-CM and CPT Code(s): 427.41, 427.5, 412, 414.01, 99291, 92960, 92950-59

Symptoms of palpitations, lightheadedness, syncope, and hypotension are all symptoms of ventricular arrythmia and ventricular fibrillation and are therefore not coded. Cardiac arrest is coded based on *Coding Clinic* guidance (1988, 2Q:8). CPR, 92950, is coded separately from the provision of critical care services.

ICD-10-CM Code(s): I47.2, I46.2, I25.2, I25.10, I49.01

ICD-10-CM Rationale: The Alphabetic Index main term is Tachycardia. The main term is Arrest, arrested with subterm cardiac. Another main term is Old (previous) myocardial infarction. Another main term is Arteriosclerosis, arteriosclerotic with subterm coronary (artery). Another main term is Fibrillation with subterm ventricular.

8.11. a. 437.3, 36100, 37204, 75894

Incorrect answer. The diagnosis code is for the intracranial internal carotid. The correct code is 442.81. Code 37204 is for a nonhead and neck vessel, so code 61626 is required.

b. 442.81, 36620

Incorrect answer. The correct CPT codes are 61626 and 36100 for the injection of the contrast media, with code 75894 added from the chargemaster for the x-ray component.

c. 442.81, 36100, 37204, 75894

Incorrect answer. Code 37204 is for nonhead and neck vessels. Code 61626 is used in this case.

d. 442.81, 61626, 36100, 75894

Correct answer.

ICD-10-CM Code(s): I72.0

ICD-10-CM Rationale: The Alphabetic Index main term is Aneurysm, subterm carotid (artery) (common) (external), internal, extracranial portion.

8.12. ICD-9-CM First-Listed Diagnosis: 414.01

ICD-9-CM Additional Diagnoses: 997.1, 414.12, V45.82, E870.6, E849.7

CPT Code(s): 92980-RC, 93458

Rationale: Since a diagnostic cardiac catheterization with injections and imaging was performed prior to the stent placement, it is necessary to code the diagnostic procedures in addition to the stent. Diagnosis code 414.12, dissection, is not a normal result of a PTCA procedure and the physician inserted a stent to cover/protect the dissection; therefore, this condition is reported as a secondary diagnosis that impacted care. Infusion codes integral to surgery/anesthesia would not be reported separately; however, if an infusion provided to a patient is not routinely part of the procedure, then an appropriate infusion code with modifier -59 may be added to show that it was a separate procedure. The HCPCS Level II C-code for the stent device is also reported and is not included in this example.

ICD-10-CM First-Listed Diagnosis: I25.119

ICD-10-CM Rationale: The Alphabetic Index main term is Arteriosclerosis, arteriosclerotic with subterms coronary (artery), native vessel, with ischemic chest pain.

ICD-10-CM Additional Diagnoses: I97.88, I25.42, Z98.61, Y65.8

ICD-10-CM Rationale: The Alphabetic Index main term is Complication with subterms intraoperative, specified NEC, circulatory system. The main term is Dissection with subterms artery, coronary. Another main term is Status (post) with subterms angioplasty, coronary artery. The main term in the Index to External Cause is Misadventure (to) patients during surgical or medical care, specified type NEC.

8.13. a. 427.5, 782.5, 92950, 92960, 99291, J0171

Incorrect answer. Cyanosis would not be coded separately. This is integral to the cardiac arrest.

b. 427.5, 92950, 92960, 99291, J0171

Correct answer.

c. 427.5, 782.5, 92950, 92960, 99291

Incorrect answer. The cyanosis is not coded separately. Also, the J codes for the epi should be coded.

d. 427.5, 99291, J0171

Incorrect answer. The CPR and the defibrillation should both be coded. They are not included in the critical care code 99291.

ICD-10-CM Code(s): I46.9

ICD-10-CM Rationale: The Alphabetic Index main term is Arrest, subterm cardiac.

Disorders of the Digestive System

8.14. a. 578.0, 553.3, V49.86, 43281

Incorrect answer. The cause of the hematemesis was determined by previous endoscopy to be the paraesophageal hernia. Therefore, the hematemesis is not coded. The hernia repair took place with the implantation of mesh, described in CPT code 43282.

b. 553.3, 49652

Incorrect answer. CPT code 49652 describes laparoscopic repair of a variety of hernias but not a paraesophageal hernia. Code 43282 correctly describes the repair of this hernia with the implantation of mesh. In addition, the code for DNR status, V49.86, should be added to the case.

c. 553.3, V49.86, 43282

Correct answer.

d. 578.0, 553.3, 43659

Incorrect answer. The cause of the hematemesis was determined by previous endoscopy to be the paraesophageal hernia. Therefore, the hematemesis is not coded. CPT code 43282, new in 2010, describes the repair of the paraesophageal hernia with implantation of mesh. In the past, coding of this procedure did require the use of an unlisted code. In addition, the code for DNR status, V49.86, should be added to the case.

ICD-10-CM Code(s): Q40.1, Z66

ICD-10-CM Rationale: The Alphabetic Index main term is Hernia with subterm paraesophageal. ICD-10-CM classifies this type of hernia as congenital. Another main term is DNR (Do Not Resuscitate).

8.15. a. 550.90, 562.10, V10.05, 49505-RT, G0105

Incorrect answer. Although the header did not include screening colonoscopy, this information was available in the body of the report. Diverticulosis was not confirmed, so it is not appropriate to report. Because the resection at the rectosigmoid junction was mentioned, code V10.06 was used for the history of CA. Although the HCPCS Level II code is correct for Medicare reporting, there is no information indicating that this is a Medicare patient, so CPT code 45378 is the correct choice.

b. 550.90, V76.51, V10.06, 49505-RT, 45378

Correct answer. If the patient were specified as Medicare, an HCPCS Level II procedure code (G0105) would be used, rather than the CPT code, for the colonoscopy. Because the resection at the rectosigmoid junction was mentioned, code V10.06 was used for the history of CA.

c. 550.91, V76.51, V10.05, 49505-RT, 49568-RT

Incorrect answer. The fifth digit used for the hernia code should be 0 because there is no documentation in this report of previous surgical repair. The V10.05 is for a history of colon cancer. Because the anastomosis examined is at the rectosigmoid junction, code V10.06 is more accurate. Code 49568 is never reported with inguinal hernia repair, so it should not appear. Lastly, the colonoscopy procedure code does not appear in the list, and it should be reported even though the physician did not list it in the procedure heading.

d. 550.90, V10.06, 49520-RT, 45330

Incorrect answer. Because the colonoscopy was performed for screening to rule out recurrent malignancy, code V76.51 should be added. The CPT code for the hernia repair is for a recurrent hernia that was not documented in this record, so code 49505 is used. The CPT code 45330 is for a sigmoidoscopy, and the documentation clearly described an exam to the ileocecal valve, which is a colonoscopy (45378).

ICD-10-CM Code(s): K40.90, Z12.11, Z85.048

ICD-10-CM Rationale: The Alphabetic Index main term is Hernia, subterm inguinal. The Alphabetic Index main term is Screening, subterm neoplasm, intestinal tract, colon. The Alphabetic Index main term is History, subterm rectum.

8.16.   a. 574.50, 43262, 43273

Incorrect answer. The documentation states that the Choledocholithiasis is associated with obstruction, and therefore 574.51 is the correct code. CPT code 43264 is required to describe the stone extraction. Assignment of CPT code 74330 may be necessary if radiology procedures are not assigned via the chargemaster.

b. 574.50, 43262, 43264

Incorrect answer. The documentation states that the Choledocholithiasis is associated with obstruction, and therefore 574.51 is the correct code. CPT code 43273 is also required to describe the endoscopic visualization of the common bile duct. Assignment of CPT code 74330 may be necessary if radiology procedures are not assigned via the chargemaster.

c. 574.51, 43262, 43264, 43273

Correct answer. Assignment of CPT code 74330 may be necessary if radiology procedures are not assigned via the chargemaster.

d. 574.51, 43262

Incorrect answer. CPT code 43264 is required to describe the stone extraction. CPT code 43273 is also required to describe the endoscopic visualization of the common bile duct. Assignment of CPT code 74330 may be necessary if radiology procedures are not assigned via the chargemaster.

ICD-10-CM Code(s): K80.51

ICD-10-CM Rationale: The Alphabetic Index main term is Calculus with subterms bile duct, with, obstruction.

8.17.   a. 211.3, 211.4, 562.10, 45385, 45384-59, 45380-59

Correct answer.

b. 211.3, 569.0, 45384

Incorrect answer. The code for adenomatous rectal polyp (211.4) is added because the polyp at 20 cm is from the rectum. Each procedure performed by a separate technique is reported in CPT. Code 45384 is reported for the polyp removal via cautery at 60 cm. Code 45385 is reported for the polyp removal via snare at 20 cm. Code 45380 is reported for the biopsy at 80 cm. Modifier -59 is applied to the subsequent CPT codes to show distinct and separate sites were involved.

c. 211.3, 569.0, 45385, 45384-59, 45380-59

Incorrect answer. Adenomatous rectal polyp should be coded. The diverticulosis code, 562.10, was omitted from this list.

d. 792.1, 211.3, 569.0, 562.10, 45385, 45384

Incorrect answer. Code 792.1 is not reported when the etiology (polyps) is known. Code 211.4 should be assigned for the adenomatous polyp from the 20-cm location. Also, modifier -59 should be added to all subsequent CPT codes to show that they are distinct from each other due to separate sites and techniques involved. CPT code 45380-59 is needed to report the biopsy of the lesion mentioned. When a biopsy and a polypectomy are not of the same location, they may be separately reported.

ICD-10-CM Code(s): D12.4, D12.3, K57.30

ICD-10-CM Rationale: The Alphabetic Index main term is Polyp, subterm colon, descending (D12.4). (This is the polyp at 60 cm.) The 80 cm is at the transverse or D12.3. The diverticulosis is found at main term Diverticulosis, subterm large intestine.

8.18.   a. 550.93, 49650, 49651, J0290 × 2
Correct answer.

b. 550.92, 49650, 49651, 49568

Incorrect answer. According to *Coding Clinic*, November/December 1985, a bilaterial hernia with one side recurrent is coded as 550.93: Code 49568, insertion of mesh, is not recorded with codes representing inguinal herniorrhaphy. The J code for the Ampicillin should be reported.

c. 550.93, 49650, 49651

Incorrect answer. The J code for the Ampicillin should be reported.

d. 550.91, 550.90, 49650-50, J0290 × 2

Incorrect answer. According to *Coding Clinic*, November/December 1985, a bilaterial hernia with one side recurrent is coded as 550.93. There were two different procedures done so a bilateral modifier should not be attached to 49650. This would not capture the repair of the recurrent hernia.

ICD-10-CM Code(s): K40.91, K40.90

ICD-10-CM Rationale: The Alphabetic Index main term is Hernia with subterms inguinal, unilateral (left), recurrent. Another main term is Hernia with subterms inguinal, unilateral (right), not specified as recurrent.

8.19.   a. 237.4, 573.8, 275.42, 276.51, 787.91, 276.8, 275.2, 626.0
Correct answer.

b. 211.6, 227.3, 197.7, 275.42, 276.51, 787.91, 276.8, 275.2, 626.0

Incorrect answer. Codes 211.6 and 227.3 are incorrect because the Alphabetic Index instructs the coding professional to code adenoma, multiple, endocrine two or more specified sites, to 237.4. In addition, the lesions in the liver are not yet confirmed as metastatic neoplasms, so code 573.3 is used rather than 197.7 in the outpatient setting.

c. 235.5, 237.0, 197.7, 275.42, 276.51, 787.91, 276.8, 275.2, 626.0

Incorrect answer. Codes 235.5 and 237.0 are incorrect because the Alphabetic Index instructs the coding professional to code adenoma, multiple, endocrine two or more specified sites, to 237.4. In addition, the lesions in the liver are not yet confirmed as metastatic neoplasms, so code 573.3 is used rather than 197.7 in the outpatient setting.

d. 237.4, 573.8, 259.2, 275.42, 276.51, 787.91, 276.8, 275.2, 626.0

Incorrect answer. The carcinoid syndrome is documented as "probable" at this point and has not been confirmed. Outpatient coding guidelines direct not to code probable diagnoses as if confirmed. Code 259.2 is not reported until the MEN-1 has been confirmed.

ICD-10-CM Code(s): D44.3, D37.8, K76.8, E83.52, E86.0, K52.9, E87.6, E83.42, N91.2

ICD-10-CM Rationale: The Alphabetic Index main term is Adenoma, subterm endocrine, single specified—see neoplasm, uncertain behavior by site. The code for the pancreas is found under Pancreas, tail, uncertain. Liver lesions, not mets, are coded since the mets is not confirmed. Main term Lesion, liver directs the coder to K76.9 but a review of the Tabular List reveals that the correct code is K76.8. The Alphabetic Index main term for hypercalcemia is Hypercalcemia. The patient's dehydration is found at Dehydration. The Alphabetic Index main term is Diarrhea, subterm chronic. The Alphabetic Index main term is Hypokalemia. The Alphabetic Index main term is Hypomagnesemia. The Alphabetic Index main term is Amenorrhea.

8.20. a. 162.9, 250.62, 357.2, 250.42, 583.81, V58.67, 272.4, 789.1

Incorrect answer. The patient was admitted for chemotherapy. Code V58.11 should be reported as the principal diagnosis. See *Coding Clinic* (2003, 4Q).

b. V58.11, 250.62, 250.42, V58.67, 272.4, 789.1

Incorrect answer. The reason for the chemotherapy, lung cancer, should also be coded. Diabetic neuropathy and nephropathy both require two codes to report both the diabetes with the specific complications and the manifestations of the diabetic complications.

c. V58.11, 162.9, 250.62, 357.2, 250.42, 583.81, V58.67, 272.4, 789.1

Correct answer.

d. 162.9, 250.02, V58.67, 272.4, 789.1

Incorrect answer. The patient was admitted for chemotherapy. Code V58.11 should be reported as the principal diagnosis. See *Coding Clinic* (2003, 4Q). Diabetic neuropathy and nephropathy are documented, were addressed during the stay, and should be coded as 250.62 with 357.2, and 250.42 with 583.81, respectively.

ICD-10-CM Code(s): Z51.11, C34.90, E11.40, E11.21, Z79.4, E78.5, R16.0

ICD-10-CM Rationale: The Alphabetic Index main term is Encounter (for) with subterm chemotherapy for neoplasm. In the Neoplasm Table, the subterm is lung and a code is chosen from the Malignant Primary column. The Alphabetic

Index main term is Diabetes with subterms type 2, with neuropathy and also nephropathy. In the Alphabetic Index, the main term is Long-term drug therapy with subterm insulin. The main term is Hyperlipemia, hyperlipidemia. The main term is Hepatomegaly—there is a note to "See hypertrophy, liver." Under main term Hypertrophy, the subterm is liver.

Disorders of the Genitourinary System

8.21.   a. 585.6, 401.1, 36830, 90935

Incorrect answer. There is a combination diagnosis code for chronic kidney disease associated with hypertension in code 403.11. ICD-9-CM presumes a cause-and-effect relationship. See *Coding Clinic* (2002, 4Q). An additional procedure code is required for the replacement of the centrally inserted central venous access device (CPT code 36581). Modifier -59 may be needed on code 36581 to show that the procedure was distinct and not a component of the other procedure.

b. 403.90, 36825, 90935

Incorrect answer. Because we know that the hypertension is benign, we can use code 403.11 for this condition. A fifth digit of 1 is required to report the type of chronic kidney disease. An additional diagnosis code is reported to identify the stage of chronic kidney disease requiring dialysis (585.6). An additional procedure code is required for the replacement of the centrally inserted central venous access device (CPT code 36581).

c. 403.11, 585.5, 36830, 36581-59

Incorrect answer. When dialysis is provided during the same encounter, it is reported separately (90935). Stage V chronic kidney disease requiring chronic dialysis is reported with code 585.6.

d. 403.11, 585.6, 36830, 36581-59, 90935

Correct answer. The replacement of the Quinton catheter is reported with code 36581 because it is a venous catheter. The new replacement code includes the removal and the insertion of the new catheter.

ICD-10-CM Code(s): I12.0, N18.6

ICD-10-CM Rationale: The Alphabetic Index main term is Hypertension, subterm kidney, with, stage 5 CKD or ESRD. The coder is reminded to use an additional code for the CKD (N18.5, N18.6). The correct code is N18.6.

8.22.   a. V55.6, V45.74, V10.51, 50684, 74425

Correct answer.

b. V55.2, V10.51, 74425

Incorrect answer. An ileal conduit is an artificial opening for the urinary tract, not the digestive tract, although the urine is diverted into an isolated segment of the ileum following cystectomy (bladder removal). Code 50684 is required for injection of the contrast material. Diagnosis code V45.74 can be added to reflect the acquired absence of the bladder.

c. 596.8, 188.9, 74425

Incorrect answer. The reason for the test was to check on the patency of the ileal conduit. ICD-9-CM provides V codes for attention to artificial openings. Because an ileal conduit is an artificial opening for the urinary tract, code V55.6 is reported along with code V45.74 to reflect the acquired absence of the bladder. Code 188.9 presumes that the patient still has the disease. When the malignancy has been eradicated, a V code for "personal history of malignancy" should be assigned: in this case, V10.51. Code 50684 is required for injection of the contrast material, in addition to the radiology code, which can be assigned by the hospital chargemaster.

d. Contact the ordering physician to obtain a diagnosis before coding this encounter.

Incorrect answer. If the indication for the test was to check for patency of the conduit, then the code for attention to artificial opening can be assigned. If there were any other results documented following the test, then they could be coded as well. See *Coding Clinic* (2000, 1Q) for more information about reporting reason for visit vs. results available from the radiologist. Diagnosis codes V55.6, V45.74, and V10.51 would be appropriate in this case, based upon the information available.

ICD-10-CM Code(s): Z43.6, Z90.6, Z85.51

ICD-10-CM Rationale: The Alphabetic Index main term is Attention (to) with subterms artificial, opening (of), ureterostomy. The Alphabetic Index main term is Absence (of) with subterm bladder (acquired). The main term is History with subterms personal (of), malignant neoplasm, bladder.

8.23. a. 626.2, 618.4, 618.6, 616.0, 58558

Correct answer.

b. 626.2, 58558

Incorrect answer. Additional conditions were identified in the body of the operative report that merit coding. Codes 618.4 and 618.6 should be added for the cystocele/rectocele and cervical erosion because the surgeon documented these conditions and they were not simply incidental findings noted on pathological examination. The documentation indicates "uterine prolapse."

c. 626.2, 618.4, 618.6, 616.0, 58100, 58120

Incorrect answer. A combination code is available in CPT for an endometrial biopsy, D&C, and hysteroscopy examination in code 58558. To report separate codes for the components of the procedure would constitute unbundling.

d. 618.4, 618.6, 616.0, 58558

Incorrect answer. The focus of the procedure was to investigate and/or treat the menorrhagia. The other conditions were not the cause of the bleeding but are documented findings that merit coding as secondary diagnoses.

ICD-10-CM Code(s): N92.0, N81.4, N81.6, N72

ICD-10-CM Rationale: The Alphabetic Index main term is Menorrhagia. The uterine prolapse is found at main term Prolapse, subterm uterus. The cystocele is included in the uterine prolapse code. The rectocele is also included but the excludes 2 note indicates that the code for rectocele should be included as well. The Alphabetic Index main term is Erosions, subterm cervix, with cervicitis.

8.24. a. 188.9, 599.72, 52000, 52235

Incorrect answer. Code 52000 is a separate procedure code and should not be reported with code 52335.

b. 233.7, 599.71, 52214

Incorrect answer. A papillary transitional cell carcinoma is a malignant carcinoma. Code 52214 does not report the removal of the medium size bladder tumor.

c. 188.9, 599.71, 52235

Correct answer.

d. 188.9, 52214, 52235

Incorrect answer. The hematuria is not integral to the bladder tumor and should be coded separately.

ICD-10-CM Code(s): C67.9, R31.0

ICD-10-CM Rationale: In the Neoplasm Table, the subterm is bladder—use a code from the Malignant Primary column. The Alphabetic Index main term is Hematuria with subterm gross.

8.25. a. 233.1, 57420

Incorrect answer. CIN I is not considered a malignant condition as code 233.1 implies. A colposcopy was not performed.

b. 622.10, 57023, 57513

Incorrect answer. Code 622.10 does not demonstrate that the condition is a grade I CIN. The patient had a vaginal cyst not a vaginal hematoma as code 57023 represents.

c. 622.11, 57420, 57513

Incorrect answer. Code 57513 is the correct code for the laser ablation of the cervix. A colposcopy was not done.

d. 622.11, 623.8, 57513, 57010

Correct answer.

ICD-10-CM Code(s): N87.0, N89.8

ICD-10-CM Rationale: The Alphabetic Index main term is Dysplasia, subterm cervix, mild. The Alphabetic Index main term is Cyst, subterm vagina.

Infectious Diseases/Disorders of the Skin and Subcutaneous Tissue

8.26.　a. 173.3, V10.42, 30118, 30400

Incorrect answer. The cancer is on the inside of the nose at the very tip and requires an extensive resection to treat, with a composite skin graft for reconstruction. Code 173.3 is the code to report malignancy of the skin of the nose. Code 160.0, Malignant neoplasm of nasal cavities, is the more appropriate code. Code 30118 describes excision of a lesion but is generally limited to laser or cryosurgery, without any wound repair required. Code 30150 is more descriptive of the procedure required in this case because a full-thickness resection was done and grafting was required. The reconstruction code 30400 is for plastic repair of this area not involving a skin graft.

b. 160.0, V10.42, 305.1, 30150, 15760

Correct answer.

c. 160.0, 15760, 30150

Incorrect answer. Although the history of carcinoma and the tobacco abuse do not directly affect this episode of care, they may be important data elements for research or patient care tracking. Code V10.42 is assigned for the history of uterine cancer, and tobacco abuse is reported with code 305.1. The CPT code for the resection is correct, but an additional code is required to reflect the skin graft needed for closure of the defect (15760).

d. 173.3, V10.42, 305.1, 14060

Incorrect answer. The cancer is on the inside of the nose at the very tip and requires an extensive resection to treat, with a composite skin graft for reconstruction. Code 173.3 is the code to report malignancy of the skin of the nose. Code 160.0, Malignant neoplasm of nasal cavities, is the more appropriate code. The procedure codes listed here are for adjacent tissue transfer rather than full-thickness composite grafting. Skin grafting to the nose is coded in the respiratory system rather than in the integumentary system in CPT.

ICD-10-CM Code(s): C30.0, Z85.42, F17.210

ICD-10-CM Rationale: In the Neoplasm Table, the subterms are nose, internal. Select a code from the Malignant Primary column. In the Alphabetic Index, the main term is History with subterms personal (of), malignant neoplasm (of), uterus. In the Alphabetic Index, the main term is Dependence with subterms drug, nicotine, cigarettes.

8.27.　a. 998.59, E878.8, 15100

Incorrect answer. No mention is made of a wound infection, but rather, that the wound was failing to heal (998.83). The CPT code for the preparation of the recipient site is reported as code 15002 and is reported in addition to the grafting code.

b. 998.59, 15002, 15100

Incorrect answer. No mention is made of wound infection, but rather, failure to heal (998.83). The primary procedure 15100 should be listed before the preparation in sequence to reflect the most resource-intensive procedure. An E code to report the surgical procedure as a cause of abnormal reaction in a patient may be added when consistent with regulatory or hospital policy.

c. 998.83, E878.8, 15100, 15002

Correct answer.

d. 998.83, 278.01, 15200

Incorrect answer. A code for morbid obesity (278.01) is not warranted because the patient may no longer be overweight. The codes reported for the procedure are for full-thickness grafts, and this is a split-thickness graft procedure. Use of full-thickness grafts is generally reserved for the face and other cosmetically sensitive areas. Codes 15100 and 15002 are appropriate. An E code to report the surgical procedure as a cause of abnormal reaction in a patient may be added when consistent with regulatory or hospital policy.

ICD-10-CM Code(s): K91.89, Y93.8

ICD-10-CM Rationale: The Alphabetic Index main term is Complication, subterm gastrointestinal, post-operative, specified NEC. Use the Index to External Cause to find main term Complication, subterm surgical operation, specified.

8.28.   a. 172.6, 216.7, 14001, 15002

Incorrect answer. A pigmented nevus is reported as a neoplasm of uncertain behavior with code 238.2. Code 15002 is used for site preparation for free skin grafts, not advancement flaps. CPT code 11423 is reported for the removal of the heel lesion with an additional code for the layer closure (12041).

b. 216.7, 216.6, 14000

Incorrect answer. The melanoma is the reason for excision of further tissue, so it should be reported (172.6) even though the pathology report does not mention the malignancy. A pigmented nevus is reported as a neoplasm of uncertain behavior with code 238.2. Because the surgeon documented that the graft was over 10.2 sq cm, the code to report is 14001. Code 11423 must be reported for the heel lesion excision performed separately from the shoulder graft, and code 12041 should be reported for the layer closure of this excision site.

c. 216.6, 238.2, 14001, 11606, 11423

Incorrect answer. The melanoma is the reason for excision of further tissue, so it should be reported (172.6) even though the pathology report does not mention the malignancy. It is documented that this diagnosis had been confirmed by biopsy. It is incorrect to report lesion removal when the resultant defect is repaired with an advancement flap closure because any excision is included in the codes in this section. See instructional note preceding code 14000. An additional code is required for the layered closure of the excision site of the heel lesion. Although the surgeon did not document the length of this repair, the pathology report shows us that it was less than 2.5 cm, so code 12041 is reported.

d. 172.6, 238.2, 14001, 11423-59, 12041

Correct answer.

Rationale: A modifier is necessary for code 11423, as the excision of lesions is usually included in 14001. Modifier -59 is reported to indicate a different site or lesion. The documentation in the description of the procedure does not support the advancement flap of the heel lesion although the name of the operation stated advancement flap reconstruction. Coding is based on the detailed description of the operation as documented in the body of the operative report.

ICD-10-CM Code(s): C43.61, D22.72

ICD-10-CM Rationale: The Alphabetic Index main term is Melanoma (malignant) with subterm skin, shoulder. The main term is Nevus with subterms skin, heel.

8.29.   a. 216.8, 15240, 15004, 12051

Incorrect answer. The lesion is located on the auricle of the ear, not the skin of the neck/scalp behind it. The skin graft was taken from this area. Although a layer closure was used to repair the defect from the donor site, no skin graft or local flap was used, so no additional code is warranted for this repair. Note that the size of the lesion and the graft are documented in millimeters, which are 1/10 the size of the centimeters used in the CPT system.

b. 216.2, 15260, 11442

Correct answer.

c. 173.2, 15260, 11442

Incorrect answer. The pathology report confirms that the lesion was benign, even though margins were taken and the resultant defect required a skin graft. The lesion code is 216.2.

d. 216.2, 14060

Incorrect answer. This was a full-thickness graft rather than an advancement graft. The appropriate codes are 15260 and 11442.

ICD-10-CM Code(s): D22.22

ICD-10-CM Rationale: The Alphabetic Index main term is Nevus, skin, ear (external).

8.30. a. 054.10, 782.4, 790.6, 042, 99284

Incorrect answer. Documentation of lesions of both the penis and the scrotum is present, so codes 054.13 and 054.19 should be reported. Febrile jaundice is assigned code 070.1, so this is appropriate to report because the physician has used "suspected" with the hepatitis. Testing positive for HIV is not assigned to category 042 without confirmation of symptoms and infection. 795.71 is the appropriate code at this stage. Additional codes should be assigned for the drug addiction (opiates, continuous) and the lifestyle risks because they are clearly delineated by the attending physician and affect the management of the patient.

b. 054.19, 573.3, 795.71, 305.51, V69.8, 99214

Incorrect answer. Two codes from the 054 category should be used to show that both the penis and the scrotum were involved with the herpes outbreak. Code 573.3 is for noninfective hepatitis, but the documentation states that the patient had experienced febrile jaundice with "suspected" hepatitis. Code 070.1 should be used to report the febrile jaundice. Code 790.6 should also be added because the type of hepatitis is not confirmed.

Code V69.2 is more specific than code V69.8. Because the drug dependence is already coded, the V code indicates the high-risk sexual behavior. Type A provider-based emergency room visits are reported with codes from the range 99281–99285, so code 99214 is not appropriate. This code would be used for a facility clinic visit.

c. 054.13, 054.19, 070.1, 790.6, 795.71, 305.51, V69.2, 99284

Correct answer. The use of two codes from the 054 category shows that both the penis and the scrotum were involved with the herpes outbreak. Hepatitis is not coded because it is not confirmed; instead, the symptoms are coded (febrile jaundice and abnormal liver function tests).

d. 042, 305.51, 070.1, 99291

Incorrect answer. No diagnosis of HIV has been made, based upon the documentation present. If additional information were available, or symptoms of HIV could be confirmed, then the 042 code could be used. When a patient is HIV seropositive, the correct code to report is 795.71.

The patient does have HSV-2, or genital herpes, which is reported with 054.13 and 054.19. These are reported in the first position because they were the reason that the patient sought care. The code for febrile jaundice is correct, but the additional code 790.6 should also be reported because the type of hepatitis is not confirmed. A V69.2 code may be added for the high-risk sexual behavior, and code 305.51 is justified because the heroin addiction affected the management and treatment plans of the patient. Code 99291 should not be reported without additional documentation because critical care requirements were apparently not met. An emergency department visit code, 99284, is the appropriate code to report.

ICD-10-CM Code(s): A60.61, A60.02, R94.5, R75, F11.10, Z72.51

ICD-10-CM Rationale: The Alphabetic Index main term is Herpes, herpes virus, herpetic with subterms penis and scrotum. The Alphabetic Index main term is Hepatitis with subterm herpes viral. The Alphabetic Index main term is Abnormal, abnormality, abnormalities with subterms function studies, liver. Another main term is HIV with subterm nonconclusive. The Alphabetic Index main term is Abuse with subterms drug, opioid. Another main term is Problem with subterms life-style, high-risk sexual behavior.

Behavioral Health Conditions

8.31.   a. 296.24, 90870

Correct answer.

b. 296.24, 90870, 95812, 93040

Incorrect answer. The EEG and EKG are integral to the electroconvulsive therapy and should not be reported separately. Note that the description for code 90870 reads "includes necessary monitoring."

c. 296.24, 298.9, 90870, 99211-25

Incorrect answer. Code 298.9 for psychotic disorder, NOS is not necessary on this case. The psychotic features of the patient's major depressive disorder are included in code 296.24. Without further documentation of a distinct evaluation and management service, separately identifiable from the procedure, code 99211 should not be reported, even with a modifier.

d. 296.24, 90870, 95812, 93040, 99234-25

Incorrect answer. Code 90870 is correct. The EEG and EKG are integral to the electroconvulsive therapy and should not be reported separately. Without further documentation of a distinct evaluation and management service, separately identifiable from the procedure, code 99211 should not be reported, even with a modifier.

ICD-10-CM Code(s): F32.3

ICD-10-CM Rationale: The Alphabetic Index main term is Disorder, subterm major, with psychotic features.

8.32.   a. 295.34, 428.0, 99201

Incorrect answer. The evaluation and management service selected should be 99284 because this was an ED visit. In addition, a code might be required for the observation services. Individual payers have different requirements for reporting of observation services, and payer guidelines should be followed. Medicare has issued several program memoranda describing reporting of observation services for Medicare patients. These can be accessed on the CMS website at http://www.cms.gov.

b. 295.32, 99283

Incorrect answer. The appropriate fifth digit for the schizophrenia is 4 because the attending physician documented chronic with acute exacerbation. The emergency department evaluation and management service code is one level too low; 99284 would be reported with an acuity level of 4 documented. In addition, a code might be required for the observation services. Individual payers have different requirements for reporting of observation services and payer guidelines should be followed.

c. 295.34, 428.0, 99284

Correct answer. A code for the observation services might also be appropriate, depending upon the payer. More information regarding observation is located in the *2005 OPPS Final Rule,* which can be accessed at http://www.cms.gov.

d. 295.84, 99234

Incorrect answer. The schizophrenia is documented as paranoid type, which is coded to subcategory 295.3. The diagnosis of CHF should be added because a digoxin level was mentioned to evaluate the patient's management. The appropriate emergency department evaluation and management code to assign is 99284. In addition, a code might be required for the observation services. Individual payers have different requirements for reporting of observation services, and payer guidelines should be followed. Medicare has issued several program memoranda describing reporting of observation services for Medicare patients. These can be accessed at http://www.cms.gov.

ICD-10-CM Code(s): F20.00, I50.9

ICD-10-CM Rationale: The Alphabetic Index main term is Schizophrenia with subterm paranoid (type). Another main term is Failure with subterms heart, congestive.

8.33. a. 296.20, 309.81, 303.92, 301.83, 300.9, 90819

Incorrect answer. The code for psychotherapy with medical evaluation and management services is not appropriate because there is no documentation of E/M services in addition to the psychotherapy in this note. Code 296.30 is appropriate because the diagnostic statement specifies the major depressive disorder as recurrent. Also, code 303.90 is reported rather than 303.92 because the alcohol dependence is not specified as episodic.

b. 296.30, 309.81, 303.90, 301.83, 300.9, 90845

Incorrect answer. The service provided was specified to be individual dialectical behavior therapy, which is a type of psychotherapy, not psychoanalysis.

c. 296.30, 309.81, 303.90, 301.83, 90818

Incorrect answer. The attending physician noted 45 minutes spent with the patient one-on-one (1:1). Also, the suicidal risk, which affected the patient's management, is reported with code 300.9.

d. 296.30, 309.81, 303.90, 301.83, 300.9, 90818

Correct answer.

ICD-10-CM Code(s): F33.9, F43.10, F10.20, F60.3, R45.851

ICD-10-CM Rationale: The Alphabetic Index main term is Disorder, subterm depressive, major, recurrent. The main term is Disorder, subterm post-traumatic stress. Main term Alcohol, alcoholic, alcohol-induced, subterm addiction. Main term Disorder, subterm personality, borderline. Main term Ideation, subterm suicidal.

8.34. a. 295.33, 272.0, 90862

Correct answer.

b. 295.30, 272.0, 90862

Incorrect answer. The physician specified subchronic schizophrenia in the body of the note, and the diagnostic statement specified acute exacerbation. The fifth digit of 3 is appropriate. Code 295.33 is correct.

c. 295.30, 272.0, 90862, 99231

Incorrect answer. Neither 90862 nor M0064 is reported along with the evaluation and management service codes. In this case, code 90862 is the most appropriate code, particularly because the physician specifies that the purpose of the visit was a 20-minute medication review. Also, the physician specified subchronic schizophrenia in the body of the note, and the diagnostic statement specified acute exacerbation. The fifth digit of 3 is appropriate. Code 295.33 is correct.

d. 295.33, 272.0, M0064, 99231

Incorrect answer. Neither 90862 nor M0064 is reported along with the evaluation and management service codes. In this case, code 90862 is the most appropriate code, particularly because the physician specifies that the purpose of the visit was a 20-minute medication review.

ICD-10-CM Code(s): F20.0, E78.0

ICD-10-CM Rationale: The Alphabetic Index main term is Schizophrenia with subterm paranoid (type). Another main term is Hypercholesterolemia.

8.35. a. 301.83, 296.30, 304.31, 99214

Incorrect answer. Time is not a determining factor in assigning an evaluation and management level unless counseling and coordination of care constitute more than 50 percent of the encounter. Code 99212 is assigned according to the documented extent of the three key elements (history, physical examination, and medical decision making). Also, the cannabis dependence is not specified as continuous. Even though the physician notes recent use of marijuana, the coding professional cannot assume continuous vs. episodic. The fifth digit for unspecified is used; code 304.30 is appropriate.

b. 301.83, 296.30, 304.30, 99212

Correct answer.

c. 301.83, 296.30, 304.30, 90805

Incorrect answer. Psychotherapy services were not provided. The focus of this visit was not to attempt to change maladaptive behavior patterns, and there is no mention of specific treatment goals or progress toward goals. This is a hospital outpatient visit summarizing the patient's progress to date. Based upon the documented extent of history, physical examination, and medical decision making, the evaluation and management code 99212 is reported with the diagnoses listed.

d. 301.83, 296.30, 304.31, 90805

Incorrect answer. The patient is an outpatient (CMHC), but the psychotherapy code is not appropriate because psychotherapy services were not provided. The focus of this visit was not to attempt to change maladaptive behavior patterns, and there is no mention of specific treatment goals or progress toward goals. This is a hospital outpatient visit summarizing the patient's progress to date. The evaluation and management code 99212 is reported. Also, the cannabis dependence is not specified as continuous. Even though the physician notes recent use of marijuana, the coding professional cannot assume continuous vs. episodic. The fifth digit for unspecified is used; code 304.30 is appropriate.

ICD-10-CM Code(s): F60.3, F33.9, F12.20

ICD-10-CM Rationale: The Alphabetic Index main term is Disorder, subterm personality, borderline. The Alphabetic Index main term is Disorder, subterm depressive, major, recurrent. The Alphabetic Index main term is Dependence, subterm drug, cannabis.

Disorders of the Musculoskeletal System and Connective Tissue

8.36.   a. 844.9, 27385-RT

Incorrect answer. The location of the rupture (sprain) is specified as the quadriceps tendon and therefore 844.8 is the most appropriate diagnosis code. CPT 27385 describes the repair of the quadriceps muscle rather than the tendon. The quadriceps tendon is an extensor tendon and therefore, CPT code 27664 is the correct code.

b. 844.9, 27430-RT

Incorrect answer. The location of the rupture (sprain) is specified as the quadriceps tendon and therefore 844.8 is the most appropriate diagnosis code. CPT 27430 describes the quadricepsplasty procedure rather than the repair. CPT code 27664 describes the repair as it is documented in the operative report.

c. 844.8, 27658-RT, 27685-RT

Incorrect answer. CPT code 27658 describes the repair of a flexor tendon and code 27685 describes the lengthening of the tendon. The lengthening procedure is not documented in the operative report and the quadriceps tendon is an extensor tendon. Therefore, CPT code 27664 is the correct code.

d. 844.8, 27664-RT

Correct answer.

ICD-10-CM Code(s): S76.111A

ICD-10-CM Rationale: The Alphabetic Index main term is Injury with subterms muscle, quadriceps (thigh), strain. A seventh character extension of A is added to indicate that this is the initial encounter for this injury.

8.37.   a. 717.2, 717.6, 715.96, 29881-RT

Correct answer. The presence of degenerative disease implies that this is not a current injury; however, the coding professional would review the history and other portions of the health record to verify that the torn meniscus is not the result of a current injury. If the tear is due to a current injury, code 836.0 is reported rather than code 717.2. If there is any inconsistency or uncertainty, the physician should be queried for clarification. The physician may also be queried to clarify if the arthritis is localized to the knee joint. If documentation supports this, code 715.36 is more specific than code 715.96. See *Coding Clinic* (1995, 2Q) for an article on the coding of arthritis.

b. 717.43, 718.16, 29881-RT, 29874-RT

Incorrect answer. Code 717.43 describes derangement of the posterior horn of the lateral meniscus, and the medial meniscus was the structure involved. Codes in subcategory 718.1X are used to report a loose body of joints other than the knee. A fifth digit of 6 is not applicable to this subcategory. See the excludes note, which refers the coder to code 717.6 for knee. CPT code 29874 is included in 29881 except when different compartments of the knee are involved per National Correct Coding Initiative edits.

c. 844.8, 717.6, 29881-RT, 29877-RT

Incorrect answer. The diagnosis code reported here indicates a current injury rather than degenerative disease. CPT code 29877 is included in the meniscectomy code (29881) and should not be reported separately unless different compartments of the knee are involved per National Correct Coding Initiative edits reported for Medicare patients with HCPCS Level II code G0289.

d. 717.2, 715.96, 29881-RT, 29874-RT

Incorrect answer. The diagnosis code for loose body of the knee was omitted. CPT code 29874 is included in 29881 except when different compartments of the knee are involved per National Correct Coding Initiative edits.

ICD-10-CM Code(s): M23.221, M17.31, M23.41

ICD-10-CM Rationale: The Alphabetic Index main term is Tear, torn, subterm meniscus, old. The coder is directed to see Derangement, knee, meniscus, due to old tear, medial, posterior horn. The coder completes the code using the Tabular List. The main term is Degeneration, degenerative, subterm joint disease. The coder is directed to see Osteoarthritis. Osteoarthritis, subterm knee leads the coder to M17.9, which is completed using the Tabular List. A review of the Tabular List shows that M17.31 is the more accurate code. For the chondral loose bodies, see main term Loose, subterm body, knee. The coder completes the code using the Tabular List.

8.38.   a. 727.1, 735.4, 99242-25, 28202, 28285

Incorrect answer. Diagnosis codes 715.97, 754.52, and 754.59 were omitted. The CPT code 28202 is inappropriate because the tendon repair is included in the other procedure codes, 28299-TA, and 28285-T1.

b. 727.1, 715.97, 754.52, 735.4, 754.59, 28299-TA, 28285-T1

Correct answer.

c. 735.4, 754.52, 28296

Incorrect answer. Diagnosis codes 715.97, 727.1, 735.4, and 754.59 were omitted. CPT code 28299-TA represents the combined procedure (Keller + Austin) and CPT code 28285-T1 was omitted for the hammertoe repair. Note that code 28299 is not an unlisted procedure code but represents a double osteotomy.

d. 727.2, 715.97, 754.52, 735.4, 754.59, 28296-TA and 28292-TA-59, 28285-T1

Incorrect answer. Code 727.2 is the code for specific bursitis, often with occupational origin, rather than the code for a bunion. CPT code 28299 exists for severe cases where combined techniques are needed for correction, so it is not appropriate to assign two bunionectomy codes for the same foot.

ICD-10-CM Code(s): M20.12, M19.90, Q66.2, M20.42, Q66.8

ICD-10-CM Rationale: The Alphabetic Index main term is Deformity with subterms toe, hallux valgus (the main term Bunion refers the coder to Deformity, toe, hallux valgus). The main term is Osteoarthritis. The Alphabetic Index main term is Primus varus. When checking the Tabular List, code Q66.2 appears to be a better code since it references the metatarsus. Another main term is Hammer toe with a note to "See also Deformity, toe, hammer toe." Another main term is Distortion with subterm toe(s). Code Q66.8 refers to other congenital deformity.

8.39. a. 882.1, 817.1, 26418, 26735, 26746, 11012

Incorrect answer. Code 882.1 does not include the tendon involvement that required repair. Code 817.1 is for an open fracture of hand bones, which is not documented in this case. The correct CPT codes are 26418-F1, 26418-F2, 26418-F3, 26418-F5, 11010-F1, and 11012-F4. Failure to report the debridements and duplication of the same procedure on different fingers constitutes underreporting and may result in inappropriately low reimbursement for the surgery. As no fracture reduction is described, only debridement is reported.

b. 842.12, 817.0, 26746-F4, 11010-F1, 11012-F4

Incorrect answer. Code 842.12 is for a sprain, rather than a fracture of the metacarpophalangeal joint. No fracture treatment was rendered except for debridement. The correct codes for the procedure are 26418-F1, 26418-F2, 26418-F3, 26418-F5, 11010-F1, and 11012-F4. Failure to report the duplication of the same procedure on different fingers constitutes under-reporting and may result in inappropriately low reimbursement for the surgery.

c. 842.12, 817.1, 26418-F1, 26418-F2, 26418-F3, 26418-F4

Incorrect answer. Code 842.12 is for a sprain, rather than a fracture of the metacarpophalangeal joint. Code 817.1 is for an open fracture of hand bones, which is not documented in this case. The debridement codes (11010-F1, 11012-F4) were omitted.

d. 882.2, 816.11, 26418-F1, 26418-F2, 26418-F3, 26418-F5, 11010-F1, 11012-F4

Correct answer.

ICD-10-CM Code(s): S61.215A, S61.213A, S61.217A, S56.424A, S56.426A, S56.428A, S62.621A, S62.617A

ICD-10-CM Rationale: The Alphabetic Index main term is Laceration, subterm fingers. The coder should look at the subterms little, ring and middle fingers of the left hand to get the correct code. The injury to the tendon is coded separately. The Alphabetic Index main term Laceration, subterm tendon directs the coder to "See Injury, muscle, by site, laceration." The Alphabetic Index main term is Injury, muscle, finger, little, extensor, laceration. The same path is used for middle (S56.42) and ring (S56.42). The codes are completed using the Tabular List. The Alphabetic Index main term for the fracture is Fracture, subterm finger, index, medial phalanx (S62.62). The coder completes the code using the Tabular List. For the fracture of the little finger it is Fracture, subterm finger, little, proximal (S62.61). The coder completes the code using the Tabular List. All of these codes have a seventh character extension of A to indicate the initial encounter for this injury.

Neoplasms

8.40.   a. 173.31, 11641

Incorrect answer. The total excised diameter of the lesion is 1.0 cm for the lesion plus 0.2 cm (2 mm) inferior margin plus 0.2 cm (2 mm) superior margin, for a total of 1.4 cm. Therefore, the correct CPT code is 11642.

b. 173.31, 11642

Correct answer.

c. 239.2, 11441

Incorrect answer. The postoperative diagnosis is basal cell carcinoma of the skin of forehead. The correct diagnosis code is 173.31 for malignant neoplasm of the skin of forehead. The CPT code category for this lesion removal should be malignant lesions. The total excised diameter of the lesion is 1.0 cm for the lesion plus 0.2 cm (2 mm) inferior margin plus 0.2 cm (2 mm) superior margin, for a total of 1.4 cm. Therefore, the correct CPT code is 11642.

d. 239.2, 11442

Incorrect answer. The correct diagnosis code is 173.31 for malignant neoplasm of the skin of forehead. The CPT code category for this lesion removal should be malignant lesions. The correct CPT code is 11642.

ICD-10-CM Code(s): C44.39

ICD-10-CM Rationale: The Neoplasm Table subterm is skin with subterm face. Basal cell carcinoma refers coder to malignant neoplasm of skin.

8.41.   a. 203.01, 199.1, 38221

Incorrect answer. ICD-9-CM coding guidelines require reporting to the highest degree of specificity at the close of the encounter, and the melanoma has not yet been confirmed. Metastatic disease in the bone has been documented, but there is no confirmation of the primary neoplasm (198.5 for the bone metastases and 199.1 for the unknown primary). The history of breast cancer (V10.3) is known, and the pathologic fractures (733.19), osteoporosis (733.00), and urinary tract infection (599.0 and 041.43) also affect the patient's management and should be coded.

b. 198.5, 199.1, 733.19, 733.00, V10.3, 599.0, 041.43, 38221

Correct answer.

c. 199.0, 27299

Incorrect answer. There is no documentation to support the code for carcinomatosis. ICD-9-CM coding guidelines require reporting to the highest degree of specificity at the close of the encounter. We know that there is metastatic disease in the bone but do not have confirmation of the primary neoplasm (198.5 and 199.1). The history of breast cancer (V10.3) is known, and the pathologic fractures (733.19), osteoporosis (733.00), and urinary tract infection (599.0 and 041.43) also affect the patient's management and should be coded. A bone marrow biopsy was performed and should be coded (38221).

d. 198.5, 203.01, 174.9, 38221

Incorrect answer. If this were an inpatient visit, the diagnosis reported as "suspected" or "rule out" could be coded as if present, but because this is an ambulatory service, this code assignment is inappropriate. Correct reporting is the established bone metastatic disease (198.5) and an additional code for the unknown primary site (199.1). The history of breast cancer (V10.3) is known, and the pathologic fractures (733.19), osteoporosis (733.00), and urinary tract infection (599.0 and 041.43) also affect the patient's management and should be coded.

ICD-10-CM Code(s): C79.51, C80.1, M80.80xA, Z85.3, N39.0, B96.2

ICD-10-CM Rationale: The metastatic bone cancer is coded by reviewing main term Neoplasm, subterm bone, Malignant Secondary column. There is an unknown primary. Main term Neoplasm, subterm unknown site or unspecified. Patient has pathological fractures found at main term Fracture, subterm spontaneous or nontraumatic. These refer the coder to Fracture, pathological. However, there is no such subterm. Main term Pathological tells the coder to "See condition." The coder can go to main term Osteoporosis, subterm specified type, with pathological fracture. The code for the history of breast cancer is found at History, subterm personal, malignant neoplasm, breast. Main term for UTI is Infection, subterm urinary tract. The subterm *Escherichia coli*, as cause of disease classified elsewhere under main term Infection reports the organism involved.

8.42.   a. 153.3, 197.4, 49329

Incorrect answer. Code 197.4 is incorrect. The metastasis is to the abdominal pericolic adipose tissue (198.89). The evaluation of the pericolic lesions is considered a peritoneal biopsy. The appropriate code is 49321. With confirmation from the physician, a case may be made for assigning 49329 because more than just a biopsy was performed (some dissection). The colonoscopy with biopsy must also be reported in this case with 45380.

b. 153.9, 49321-74, 45380-59

Incorrect answer. The first-listed diagnosis is not as specific as possible (report 153.3 for sigmoid colon). The modifiers appended to the CPT codes are not necessary. The procedure was not discontinued before completion, only changed due to the nature of the pathology discovered, so modifier -74 is not correct. Modifier -59 is not necessary because the colonoscopy would not be considered a component of the laparoscopic surgery. The metastases to the abdominal pericolic adipose tissue should also be coded.

c. 197.4, 153.3, 197.7, 49321, 45380

Incorrect answer. An initial diagnosis of cancer generally shows the primary carcinoma code in the first position, unless the diagnosis or treatment was focused on the metastases. The liver metastasis is not yet confirmed and cannot be reported for an outpatient encounter. Code 197.4 is incorrect. The metastasis is to the abdominal pericolic adipose tissue (198.89). The procedure codes are correct.

d. 153.3, 198.89, 49321, 45380

Correct answer.

ICD-10-CM Code(s): C18.7, C79.89

ICD-10-CM Rationale: In the Neoplasm Table the subterm is colon with selection of a code from the Malignant Primary column. Also in the Neoplasm Table, the main term is Specified site NEC (for the pericolic adipose).

8.43. a. 239.5, 250.00, 332.0, 278.00, 57410, 56620

Incorrect answer. Based on the tissue report, the lesion is VIN III or Carcinoma in situ of the vulva, coded as 233.32. The remainder of the diagnoses are correct. Code 57410 for pelvic exam under anesthesia is included in the main procedure of 56620.

b. 624.02, 250.00, 332.0, 278.00, 56630

Incorrect answer. Based on the tissue report, the lesion is VIN III or Carcinoma in situ of the vulva, coded as 233.32. Code 624.02 is for VIN II of the vulva. The procedure performed was a simple, partial vulvectomy based on the definitions in the CPT book. The correct code is 56620.

c. 233.32, 250.00, 57410, 11626, 12042

Incorrect answer. Parkinsonism, 332.0, and obesity, 278.00, should both be reported. The pelvic exam under anesthesia should be coded as part of the major procedure, a simple partial vulvectomy. This lesion was not described as a skin lesion and therefore integumentary codes are not correct. The correct code is 56620.

d. 233.32, 250.00, 332.0, 278.00, 56620

Correct answer.

ICD-10-CM Code(s): D07.1, E11.9, G20, E66.9

ICD-10-CM Rationale: The Alphabetic Index main term is Neoplasm, subterm vulva, Ca in Situ column. The main term is Diabetes, diabetic. The main term is Parkinsonism. The main term is Obesity.

Disorders of the Nervous System and Sense Organs

8.44.   a. 956.5, E920.4, E849.0, 64831, 28200

Incorrect answer. The complicated open wound would be reported as the reason for the visit. Although a digital nerve repair was performed, this also involved a nerve graft, so code 64890 is assigned. The -LT modifier may be assigned to the CPT codes to show that the repair was to the left foot.

b. 892.2, 956.5, E920.4, E849.0, 64891, 28202

Incorrect answer. The nerve was grafted, but the graft did not measure more than 4 mm, so code 64890 is reported. There was no tendon graft, so code 28202 is inappropriate; code 28200 should be assigned. The -LT modifier may be assigned to the CPT codes to show that the repair was to the left foot.

c. 892.2, 956.5, E920.4, E849.0, 64890-LT, 28200-LT

Correct answer.

d. 956.5, 64890-LT, 28200-LT

Incorrect answer. The complicated open wound would be reported as the reason for the visit, so code 892.2 should be reported as the primary diagnosis, with 956.5 as a secondary diagnosis. Codes E920.4 and E849.0 are added to show the cause of the injury.

ICD-10-CM Code(s): S94.8x2A, S96.822A, S91.312A, S91.115A, W27.1xxA, Y92.017, Y93.h2, Y99.8

ICD-10-CM Rationale: The Alphabetic Index main term is Injury with subterms nerve, foot, specified NEC. The main term is Injury with subterms muscle, foot, specified site NEC, laceration. The Tabular List reminds the coder to code also the associated open wound. The Index to External Cause main term is Contact with subterms with, hoe. The Index to External Cause main term is Place of occurrence with subterms yard, single family house. The Index to External Cause main term is Accident with subterm gardening. Another main term in the Index to External Cause is External cause status with subterm specified NEC.

8.45.   ICD-9-CM Code: 337.20

ICD-9-CM Rationale: This condition is located in the Alphabetic Index under Dystrophy, sympathetic. Code 337.20 is all that can be reported without further documentation because no specific site is specified.

CPT Code: 64510

CPT Rationale: The stellate ganglion is a sympathetic nerve, not a peripheral nerve. Code 64510 is the correct code for the stellate ganglion, which is also called the cardiothoracic plexus.

ICD-10-CM Code(s): G90.511

ICD-10-CM Rationale: The Alphabetic Index main term is Dystrophy, subterm reflex. The coder is directed to see Syndrome, pain, complex regional 1, upper limb. The coder completes the code using the Tabular List.

8.46. a. 436, 99284-25, 70450

Incorrect answer. There are documented residuals of the CVA with infarct (434.91), which need to be reported with codes 342.90 and 784.5. Coexisting conditions may impact patient management, so 305.1 should be reported for tobacco use and 250.00 for diabetes. Code V17.1 should be used to show a family history of cerebrovascular disease.

Rationale: The CMS Web site (http://www.cms.gov/manuals) states that modifier -25 should be appended to an evaluation and management code when reported with another procedure on the same day of service. Different fiscal intermediaries may have varying requirements for use of modifier -25.

b. 434.91, 99283, 70470

Incorrect answer. The residual conditions should be coded by assignment of 342.90 and 784.5. Comorbid conditions are reported also with 305.1 for tobacco use and 250.00 for type II diabetes. Code V17.1 should be used to show a family history of cerebrovascular disease. The wrong code is used for the CT scan because no contrast was employed. In this case, code 70450 is appropriate. For facility reporting, the acuity level established by the facility is reported, rather than any use of the key elements of CPT code reporting. Level IV acuity is 99284.

c. 434.91, 342.90, 784.59, 305.1, 250.00, V17.1, 99284-25, 70450

Correct answer.

Rationale: The CMS Web site (http://www.cms.gov/manuals) states that modifier -25 should be appended to an evaluation and management code when reported with another procedure on the same day of service. Different fiscal intermediaries may have varying requirements for use of modifier -25.

d. 436, 342.90, 784.59, 305.1, 250.00, V17.1, 99284, 70470

Incorrect answer. The diagnosis listed is not as specific as it should be. When an infarction is established, code 436 is not used, but a code from category 434 is reported. In this case, we know it is an arterial occlusion with an infarct, so code 434.91 is assigned. The wrong code is used for the CT scan because no contrast was employed. In this case, code 70450 is appropriate.

ICD-10-CM Code(s): I63.422, G81.91, R47.2, F17.210, E11.9, Z82.3

ICD-10-CM Rationale: The Alphabetic Index main term is Occlusion with subterms artery, cerebral, anterior, with infarction due to embolism. The Alphabetic Index main term is Hemiplegia. Another main term is Disturbance, subterm speech. Another main term is Dependence with subterms drug, nicotine, cigarettes. The main term in the Alphabetic Index is Diabetes, diabetic with subterm type 2. Another main term is History with subterms family (of), stroke (cerebrovascular).

8.47. a. 350.1, 64600, 77003

Incorrect answer. The foramen ovale was involved and the use of radiologic monitoring results in code 64610. The other codes are appropriate.

b. 350.1, 64610, 77003

Correct answer.

c. 350.1, 64610

Incorrect answer. For ambulatory reporting, it is important to include radiologic guidance. Per CPT guidelines, code 77003 is appropriate for reporting fluoroscopic guidance in this procedure.

d. 350.1, 64605

Incorrect answer. Code 64610 is required for the procedure described. Per CPT guidelines, code 77003 is appropriate for reporting fluoroscopic guidance in this procedure.

ICD-10-CM Code(s): G50.0

ICD-10-CM Rationale: The Alphabetic Index main term is Neuralgia, subterm trigeminal.

8.48. a. 353.6, V10.81, 62311

Incorrect answer. It is appropriate to use the V49.75 to show that the patient has an absence of the limb. Code 62311 does not reflect an epidural injection using US guidance.

b. 353.6, 729.5, V49.75, V10.81, 62311

Incorrect answer. It is not necessary to code pain in the limb. The code for the phantom pain is the only code needed.

c. 353.6, V49.75, V10.81, 0230T

Correct answer.

d. 353.6, V49.75, 170.7, 0230T

Incorrect answer. The bone malignancy should not be coded. The tumor was removed and the patient completed chemotherapy. It should be coded as a history code.

ICD-10-CM Code(s): G54.6, Z89.51, Z85.830

ICD-10-CM Rationale: The Alphabetic Index main term is Syndrome with subterm phantom limb, with pain. Another main term is Absence with subterms leg, below, knee (acquired). The Alphabetic Index main term is History with subterm personal (of), malignant neoplasm (of), bone.

8.49. CPT Code(s):

61750, Stereotactic biopsy, aspiration, or excision, including burr hole(s), for intracranial lesion; 70450, Computed tomography, head or brain; without contrast material.

Rationale: See *CPT Assistant* (1996, June). When the attachment of the stereotactic frame is a component of a more comprehensive procedure, it is not reported separately. Code 20660 should not be reported because it is considered to be a part of the biopsy procedure.

CT mapping was performed, rather than MRI, so code 70450 would be appropriate. The CT mapping was performed prior to the procedure; therefore, reporting Intraoperative use of CT or MRI guidance (code 61751) is not accurate.

8.50. a. 361.02, 379.23, 364.3, 67108

Correct answer.

b. 361.9, 379.23, 364.3, 67108

Incorrect answer. The body of the operative report states multiple tears of the retina, so this can be classified as 361.02 rather than 361.9 unspecified.

c. 361.02, 364.3, 67108

Incorrect answer. An additional diagnosis code for the vitreous hemorrhage should be assigned.

d. 361.02, 379.23, 364.10, 67107, 67036

Incorrect answer. This is a traumatic iritis, not chronic. Code 67108 includes all the procedures, the repair of the retinal detachment (scleral buckle), and the vitrectomy.

ICD-10-CM Code(s): H33.022, H43.12, H20.00

ICD-10-CM Rationale: The Alphabetic Index main term is Detachment with subterms retina, with retinal: break, multiple. Another main term is Hemorrhage with subterm vitreous (humor) (intraocular). The Alphabetic Index main term is Iritis where there is a note to "see also Iridocyclitis", subterm acute (this was due to blunt trauma).

8.51. a. 470, 478.0, 519.8, 473.0, 473.2, 473.1, 471.8, 31276-50, 31255-50, 30140-50-59, 30520, 31256-50

Correct answer.

b. 470, 478.0, 519.8, 473.0, 473.2, 473.1, 471.8, 31276, 31255, 30140, 30520, 31256

Incorrect answer.

Rationale: CPT codes for sinus endoscopy require modifiers to identify whether the procedure was performed on the left side (LT), right side (RT), or bilaterally (-50). See *CPT Assistant* (2003, April:25).

c. 470, 478.0, 519.8, 461.0, 461.1, 461.2, 471.8, 31276-50, 31255-50, 30520, 31256-50

Incorrect answer. According to CPT coding guidelines, it is inappropriate to report CPT code 30140 in addition to CPT code 31255, since the middle turbinate is part of the ethmoid bone and the approach to access procedures performed in the sphenoid, maxillary, or frontal sinus procedures. Therefore, in this case, the inferior turbinate resection is coded with modifier -59 to show that it is a distinct procedure. In addition, the source document identified the patient's sinusitis as chronic, not acute. See *CPT Assistant* (2003, May:5–6).

d. 470, 478.0, 519.8, 461.0, 461.1, 461.2, 471.8, 31276-50, 31255-50, 30140-50-59, 30520, 31256-50

Incorrect answer.

Rationale: The source document indicates the patient's sinusitis is chronic, not acute.

ICD-10-CM Code(s): J34.2, J34.3, J34.89, J32.1, J32.2, J32.0, J33.8

ICD-10-CM Rationale: The Alphabetic Index main term is Deviation, subterm septal. The Alphabetic Index main term is Hypertrophy, subterm nasal, turbinate. The Alphabetic Index main term is Obstruction, subterm nasal. The Alphabetic Index main term is Sinusitis, frontal (J32.1), ethmoidal (J32.2) and maxillary (J32.0). The Alphabetic Index main term is Polyposis, which directs the coder to main term Polyp, subterm sinus.

Newborn/Congenital Disorders

8.52. a. V53.01, 62230

Incorrect answer. In this situation the physician indicates there is a malfunction of the shunt. Therefore, 996.2 should be reported as the first-listed code for the shunt valve malfunction, followed by the congenital hydrocephalus (742.3), which is not resolved (or the patient would not require the shunt).

b. 996.2, 742.3, 62230

Correct answer.

c. 742.3, V53.01, 62225

Incorrect answer. Aftercare codes are assigned in the secondary position only when aftercare is provided during an episode of care for an unrelated diagnosis. If the patient had presented to a facility for the purpose of aftercare (shunt maintenance) without any additional management or treatment, code V53.01 would be the appropriate code for the reason for the visit. In this case, the patient was evaluated by a consulting physician who concurred with the pediatrician's analysis that the shunt catheter should be replaced with a longer one because the child had grown. Code 62225 is the code for reporting the ventricular catheter rather than the peritoneal catheter and would not include the valve replacement. Code 62230 is the appropriate code.

d. 742.3, 62230

Incorrect answer. The consulting physician found that the shunt valve was malfunctioning. Code 996.2 should be reported as the first-listed code.

ICD-10-CM Code(s): T85.89xA, Q03.9

ICD-10-CM Rationale: The Alphabetic Index main term is Complication, subterm ventricular shunt (device). The main term is Hydrocephalus, subterm congenital (external) (internal).

8.53. a. 770.84, 765.19; 99285

Incorrect answer. The code for prematurity is based on birth weight, not current weight, so code 765.18 is the correct code. An additional code should be assigned for cardiac arrest, which in a newborn is 779.84, with a code from the circulatory system to further describe the specific condition, 427.5. The CPT codes for hospital and physician reporting are incorrect. Both would report code 99291 for services where critical care is provided in the emergency department, regardless of the age of the patient. The hospital would also report the CPR procedure with code 92950.

b. 770.84, 779.85, 427.5, 765.18; 99291, 92950, 31500

Correct answer. Hospitals report only one critical care code, 99291, irrespective of the length of time critical care is rendered. Critical care for outpatient services is reported with 99291 regardless of age of the patient.

c. 770.84, 779.85, 765.18; 99468, 92950

Incorrect answer. The diagnosis of cardiac arrest (427.5) from the circulatory system chapter may be added to the codes for greater specificity behind the perinatal condition codes. CPR is reported with code 92950 (CPR) and 31500 (intubation) because they are not included as bundled services in critical care.

d. 770.84, 779.85, 427.5, 765.18, 99291

Incorrect answer. The CPR procedure (CPT code 92950) and the intubation (31500) are not bundled codes with critical care, so they would be reported separately for both the physician and the hospital. The patient is still considered neonatal, as the age of the infant is 28 days.

ICD-10-CM Code(s): P28.5, P29.81, P07.18, P07.32

ICD-10-CM Rationale: The Alphabetic Index main term is Failure, failed, subterm respiration, newborn. The patient suffered cardiac arrest. The main term is Arrest, subterm cardiac, newborn. The main term is Low, subterm birth weight, with weight of 2000–2499 grams. A note tells the coder to also code the gestational period (P07.32). When both birth weight and gestational age of the newborn are available, both should be coded with birth weight sequenced before gestational age.

Pediatric Conditions

8.54. a. 741.02, 596.54, 564.81, 737.30, 996.2

Incorrect answer. The scoliosis is documented as repaired; therefore, V13.68 should be assigned for personal history of corrected congenital malformations of integument, limbs, and musculoskeletal systems instead of 737.30. The VP shunt is not documented as having a complication. The physician states that Neurology should assess the VP shunt but does not document a complication. V45.2 should be assigned to report the presence of the VP shunt.

b. 741.02, 596.54, 564.81, V45.2, V13.68
Correct answer.

c. 741.90, 596.54, 331.4, 737.30

Incorrect answer. The combination code for thoracic spina bifida with hydrocephalus should have been used rather than 741.90 and 331.4. Code 564.81 should have been reported for neurogenic bowel. The scoliosis is documented as repaired; therefore, V13.68 should be assigned for personal history of corrected congenital malformations of integument, limbs, and musculoskeletal systems instead of 737.30. V45.2 should be assigned to report the presence of the VP shunt.

d. 741.92, 596.54, 564.81, V45.2, V13.68

Incorrect answer. The combination code for thoracic spina bifida with hydrocephalus should have been used rather than 741.92.

ICD-10-CM Code(s): Q05.1, N31.9, K59.2, Z98.2, Z87.76

ICD-10-CM Rationale: The Alphabetic Index main term is Spina bifida, subterms thoracic, with hydrocephalus. The main term is Neurogenic, subterms bladder and bowel NEC. Another main term is Presence, subterm cerebrospinal fluid drainage device. The main term is History, subterms personal (of), congenital malformation, musculoskeletal system.

Conditions of Pregnancy, Childbirth, and the Puerperium

8.55.   ICD-9-CM and CPT Code(s): 635.92, V25.2, V15.82, 59841, 58670-59. The modifier -59 should be appended to the second procedure to show that these procedures were unique and should be coded separately.

ICD-10-CM Code(s): Z33.2, Z30.2, Z87.891

ICD-10-CM Rationale: The Alphabetic Index main term for the elective abortion is Encounter, subterm termination of pregnancy, elective. The main term is Encounter, subterm sterilization. The patient has a history of smoking. The Alphabetic Index main term is History, subterm personal, nicotine dependence.

8.56.   a. 648.81, 250.01, V58.67, 99235

Incorrect answer. The fifth digit of 1 is incorrect because the patient did not deliver during this episode of care. 250.01 is not used for gestational diabetes. Refer to the excludes note at category 250 in the tabular volume of ICD-9-CM. Code 99235 is the correct code if the payer requires evaluation and management codes for observation of patients. The coding professional should always verify payer reporting guidelines.

b. 648.83, 250.81, 99235

Incorrect answer. Codes in category 250 are not used for gestational diabetes. Refer to the excludes note at category 250 in the tabular volume of ICD-9-CM. Code V58.67 should be assigned to indicate the use of insulin. Code 99235 is the correct code if the payer requires evaluation and management codes for observation of patients. The coding professional should always verify payer reporting guidelines.

c. 648.83, V58.67, 99235

Correct answer. Code 99235 is the correct code if the payer requires evaluation and management codes. The coding professional should always verify payer reporting guidelines.

d. 648.83, 790.29, V58.67, 99235

Incorrect answer. 790.29 is not used for gestational diabetes. The excludes note refers the coding professional to code 648.8x. Code 99235 is the correct code if the payer requires evaluation and management codes. The coding professional should always verify payer reporting guidelines.

ICD-10-CM Code(s): O24.424, Z79.4

ICD-10-CM Rationale: The Alphabetic Index main term is Diabetes, diabetic, subterms gestational (in pregnancy), in childbirth, insulin (and diet) controlled. The main term is Long-term (current) drug therapy (use of), subterm insulin.

8.57. ICD-9-CM and CPT Code(s): 640.03, V23.41, 923.11, E819.1

ICD-9-CM Rationale: The patient has a history of pre-term labor and is currently pregnant. Therefore, code V23.41 is assigned. 389.05, unilateral conductive hearing loss, is not coded as it was not treated and has no impact on the care of the patient.

ICD-10-CM Code(s): O20.0, S50.01xA, O09.211, V49.9xxA

ICD-10-CM Rationale: The Alphabetic Index main term is Threatened, subterm abortion. The contusion code is found under Contusion, subterm elbow. The Alphabetic Index main term for the high-risk pregnancy is Pregnancy, subterm supervision, high-risk, due to, pre-term labor. To identify the MVA, the Alphabetic Index main term is Accident, subterm transport, car occupant.

8.58. a. 633.20, 620.2, 59121, 49320

Incorrect answer. The ectopic pregnancy is located at the fimbriated end of the left tube. Code 633.10 is therefore the correct choice. The diagnosis code for peritubular cyst would also be reported (620.8). The CPT code for laparoscopic treatment of an ectopic pregnancy (59150) would be reported rather than 59121, which is the code for reporting an open procedure. Drainage of the ovarian cyst would be reported with CPT code 58662. The diagnostic laparoscopy is included in the surgical laparoscopy (code 59150), so CPT code 49320 would not be reported.

b. 633.10, 620.2, 620.8, 59150, 58662

Correct answer.

c. 633.10, 620.2, 58673, 49320

Incorrect answer. The diagnosis code for peritubular cyst would also be reported (620.8). This is a laparoscopic salpingostomy, but it is for the treatment of an ectopic pregnancy. CPT code 59150 is the correct choice rather than 58673. The diagnostic laparoscopy is included in the surgical laparoscopy (code 59150), so CPT code 49320 would not be reported.

d. 633.20, 654.43, 58673, 58662

Incorrect answer. The ectopic pregnancy is located at the fimbriated end of the left tube. Code 633.10 is therefore the correct choice. The ovarian cyst is not complicating a pregnancy. Code 620.2 is reported rather than 654.43. This is a laparoscopic salpingostomy, but it is for the treatment of an ectopic pregnancy. CPT code 59150 is the correct choice rather than 58673.

ICD-10-CM Code(s): O00.1, N83.20, N83.8, O34.81

ICD-10-CM Rationale: The Alphabetic Index main term is Pregnancy, subterm fallopian tube. The main term is Cyst, subterm ovary, ovarian and fallopian tube. Another main term is Pregnancy, subterm complicated by, abnormal, pelvic organs, specified NEC.

Disorders of the Respiratory System

8.59. ICD-9-CM Diagnosis Codes:

V55.0, Attention to artificial openings, tracheostomy

V46.11, Other dependence on machines, respirator

ICD-9-CM Rationale: This is not a complication of the tracheostomy, such as an infection or a mechanical breakdown of the tube or tracheal stenosis. Code V55.0 is the most appropriate code for scar tissue redundancy. An additional code could be assigned for the respirator dependence because it would affect the evaluation and management of the case.

CPT Code:

31614, Tracheostomy revision, complex, with flap rotation

CPT Rationale: This is a revision of a tracheostomy already established. Flap rotation is supported by documentation. This is not a fenestration procedure.

ICD-10-CM Code(s): Z43.0, Z99.11

ICD-10-CM Rationale: The Alphabetic Index main term is Attention (to) artificial, tracheostomy. The main term is Dependence, subterm respirator.

8.60. a. 784.7, 30901-RT, 30903-RT, 30905-RT, 36430-RT

Incorrect answer. The diagnosis code is correct, but the additional conditions should also be coded (280.0 for the blood loss anemia and 496 for the COPD). Modifier -59 should be appended to the second anterior packing with cauterization and the posterior packing to show that separate and distinct sessions were involved. Normally, these CPT codes would not appear on the same claim. HCPCS Level II codes with the number of units should be added to account for the blood products that were transfused. These codes would generate additional reimbursement under the APC system.

b. 784.7, 280.0, 496, 30901-RT, 30901-RT-76, 30905-RT-77, P9021

Incorrect answer. The procedure codes are incorrect because the second procedure involved the cauterization, and the first was limited to simple packing. Only if both procedures were the same would modifier -76 appear. Also, the -77 would not be needed for code 30905 because there was no other code reported for that number. The number of units would be reported for P9021 to account for the blood product. The transfusion administration code (36430) must be assigned in order for the additional APC to be generated.

c. 784.7, 285.9, 30901-RT, 30903-RT-59, 30905-RT-77, 36430-RT, P9021 (2 units)

Incorrect answer. Blood loss anemia has a specific code, 280.0. COPD may be coded, even if it is mentioned in the history portion of the procedure, according to *Coding Clinic* (1992, 2Q). Modifier -59, rather than -77, should be appended to code 30905, because it is a distinct session from the other procedures and normally the codes would not appear on the same claim.

d. 784.7, 280.0, 496, 30901-RT, 30903-RT-59, 30905-RT-59, 36430-RT, P9021 (2 units)

Correct answer. The appropriate E/M code(s) for the observation service should also be reported if the payer requires evaluation and management codes.

Rationale: Coder may query physician for acute blood loss anemia (285.1) due to clinical indicators and documentation of drop in hematocrit, extensive bleeding, and transfusion.

ICD-10-CM Code(s): R04.0, D50.00, J44.9

ICD-10-CM Rationale: The Alphabetic Index main term is Epistaxis (multiple). Another main term is Anemia, subterm blood loss (chronic). The main term is Disease, diseased, subterms lung, obstructive (chronic).

8.61. a. 486, 692.3, V10.11, E879.2, 71010

Incorrect answer. The pneumonitis is stated as being caused by radiation therapy and is therefore 508.0. The dermatitis is also caused by the radiation therapy and is coded as 692.82. In addition, the atrial fibrillation and long-term use of anti-coagulant should be reported as 427.31 and V58.61. The two-view chest x-ray is coded as 71020.

b. 508.0, 692.82, 427.31, V58.61, V10.11, E879.2, 71020

Correct answer.

c. 508.0, 990, E926.5, 162.4, 427.31, V58.69, 71030

Incorrect answer. This patient has specific complications of radiation therapy. Code 990 is only coded when the documentation does not indicate a specific side effect. Rather, 692.82 should be coded for the radiation dermatitis. The exclusion note under E926.5 refers the coder to E879.2 for abnormal reactions to radiation therapy without mention of a misadventure. The patient has completed the treatment for the lung cancer, and the tumor was eradicated. A history of lung cancer is coded as V10.11. The two-view chest x-ray is coded as 71020.

d. 508.1, 692.82, 162.4, 427.31, V58.69, E926.5, 71020

Incorrect answer. The radiation pneumonitis is coded as 508.0. Code 508.1 describes the condition of radiation fibrosis, which is a long-term complication of radiation therapy with permanent damage to the lungs. The patient has completed the treatment for the lung cancer, and the tumor was eradicated. A history of lung cancer is coded as V10.11. The exclusion note under E926.5 refers the coder to E879.2 for abnormal reactions to radiation therapy without mention of a misadventure.

ICD-10-CM Code(s): J70.0, W88.8xxA, L58.1, I48.0, Z85.118, Z79.01

ICD-10-CM Rationale: The Alphabetic Index main term for the pneumonitis is Pneumonitis, subterm radiation. The coder is directed to use an additional code to identify the external cause. This is found in the Index to External Cause under main term Radiation, subterm ionized, ionizing, other NEC. The main term is Radiodermatitis, subterm chronic. The atrial fibrillation can be found at main term Fibrillation, subterm atrial. Patient has a history of lung cancer. The main term is History, personal (of), malignant neoplasm, lung. The main term is Long-term, subterm anti-coagulant.

8.62.   a. 473.9, 31256-50, 31287

Incorrect answer. The code reported is for unspecified sinusitis. Separate codes should be assigned for the sinusitis to fully describe what areas are involved (473.0, 473.2, and 473.3). The code for polyps (471.8) should also be reported because a polypectomy was described, even though it is included in the more extensive CPT codes. The CPT codes that should be reported are 31255-50, 31267-50, and 31288-50 because tissue removal was described for the maxillary and sphenoid areas, and the physician described the procedure as ethmoidectomy (on both sides), not ethmoidotomy.

b. 473.0, 473.2, 473.3, 471.8, 31256-50, 31287-50

Incorrect answer. The CPT codes reported should be 31255-50, 31267-50, and 31288-50 because tissue removal was described for the maxillary and sphenoid areas, and the physician described the procedure as ethmoidectomy, anterior and posterior (on both sides), not ethmoidotomy. Tissue removal was part of each procedure, so codes 31267 and 31288 are required instead of the codes reported, which are without mention of tissue removal.

c. 473.0, 473.2, 473.3, 471.8, 31255-50, 31267-50, 31288-50

Correct answer.

d. 473.0, 473.2, 473.3, 471.8, 31255, 31267

Incorrect answer. The diagnosis codes are correct and the procedure codes are correct, but modifier -50 must be appended to each procedure to reflect that these were carried out bilaterally. Per the instructional note preceding code 31231, the endoscopic sinus procedures are unilateral in nature. CPT code 31288-50 is also assigned for the sphenoidotomy, with tissue removal.

ICD-10-CM Code(s): J32.0, J32.2, J32.3, J33.8

ICD-10-CM Rationale: The Alphabetic Index main term is Sinusitis, subterms maxillary, ethmoidal and sphenoidal. Another main term is Polyp, polypus, subterm maxillary (sinus).

Trauma and Poisoning

8.63.   a. 805.04, 344.01, E828.2, 99291, 31500

Incorrect answer. For facility reporting, the first hour of critical care is reported. There is a combination code for fracture with spinal cord injury. (See the includes note at code 806.)

b. 805.04, 344.01, E828.2, 99291, 31500

Incorrect answer. There is a combination code for fracture with spinal cord injury. (See the includes note at code 806.)

c. 806.01, E828.2, 99291, 31500

Correct answer.

d. 806.01, E828.2, 99291, 31500, 22305

Incorrect answer. Code 22305 is not reported because fracture care was not performed at this initial visit. The patient was transferred to another hospital for definitive fracture care.

ICD-10-CM Code(s): S12.300A, S14.114A, V80.010A, Y93.52, Y99.8

ICD-10-CM Rationale: The Alphabetic Index main term is Fracture, subterm neck, cervical, vertebra, fourth. The Tabular List directs the coder to code also any associated cervical spinal cord injury (S14-). To identify the cause of the injury, see main term Accident in the Index to External Cause. The subterms are transport, animal-rider, noncollision, specified as horse-rider. All of the injury codes have a seventh character extension of A to indicate that this is the initial encounter for this injury. The activity is horseback riding. The code is found in the Index to External Cause under main term Activity, subterm horseback riding. The external cause code is Y99.8.

8.64.   a. 816.00, 26756-F4, 13131-F4

Incorrect answer. This fracture is documented as an open fracture of the middle phalanx. Therefore, the correct code is 816.11. E codes should be reported for the cause of injury on this case. The appropriate codes are E920.1 for injury with a power hedge cutter and E849.0 for place of occurrence in the home. While the fracture was aligned with a pin, it states that this was done in an open fashion, or by visualizing the fracture site. Code 26756 describes a percutaneous pinning of the fracture, or through the skin at the end of the finger. This is an open repair and the closure code is included in the procedure. The correct CPT code is 26735.

b. 816.01, E920.1, 11012, 26735-F4

Incorrect answer. This fracture is documented as an open fracture of the middle phalanx, not a closed fracture. The correct code is 816.11. The E code for the place of occurrence should be reported as E849.0 for home. The CPT code is correct.

c. 816.11, E920.1, E849.0, 26735-F4

Correct answer.

d. 816.11, E920.1, E849.0, 26756-F4, 26418-F4, 26540-F4, 11012, 13131

Incorrect answer. While the fracture was aligned with a pin, it states that this was done in an open fashion, or by visualizing the fracture site. Code 26756 describes a percutaneous pinning of the fracture, or through the skin at the end of the finger. When the correct CPT code for open repair of the fracture is coded as 26735-F4, all of the other procedures are included in the fracture repair. All of the other codes are included per the NCCI edits.

Rationale: E codes E000.8 and E016.1 would be appropriate to use as well.

ICD-10-CM Code(s): S62.627B, W29.3xxA, Y92.017, Y93.h2, Y99.8

ICD-10-CM Rationale: The Alphabetic Index main term is Fracture, subterms finger, little, medial phalanx. A seventh character extension of B is assigned to this code to indicate an initial encounter for open fracture. The Index to External Cause main term is Contact, subterms with, tool, powered, hedge trimmer. A seventh character extension of A is assigned to this code to indicate an initial encounter for this injury. The Index to External Cause main term is Place of occurrence, subterms residence, house, single family, yard. The main term in the Index to External Cause is Activity, subterm trimming shrubs. Another main term in the Index to External Cause is Status of external cause, subterm specified NEC.

8.65. ICD-9-CM and CPT Code(s): 969.4, 980.0, 873.42, 311, E950.3, E950.9, 43753, 12051

Rationale: The poisoning codes for the Dalmane and the Tranxene are the same so do not need to be reported twice. In addition to the listed codes, an E&M level code to reflect services provided would also be reported.

ICD-10-CM Code(s): T42.4x2A, T51.0x2A, S01.81xA, F53

ICD-10-CM Rationale: The Table of Drugs and Chemicals is used to find the codes for intentional self-harm for Dalmane, Tranxene, and the alcohol. The codes for intentional self-harm using Dalmane and Tranxene are the same so only one is reported. The main term Laceration, subterm forehead gives the code for the laceration. All of the injury codes have a seventh character extension of A to indicate that this is the initial encounter for this injury. The depression is coded by reviewing main term Depression, subterm postpartum.

8.66. ICD-9-CM and CPT Code(s): 813.43, 882.0, 911.0, 916.0, 910.0, E816.3, E849.5, E000.9, 12041, 29065

Rationale: The repair of the laceration on the palm of the hand is coded as an intermediate closure because of the extensive debridement that was done on the wound. Only one code (910.0) is needed for the abrasions on the cheek and on the scalp. The appropriate E&M level code would also be used.

ICD-10-CM Code(s): S52.602A, S30.1xxA, S61.421A, S80.212A, S00.81xA, S00.01xA, V28.1xxA, Y99.8, Y93.89, Y92.488

ICD-10-CM Rationale: The Alphabetic Index main term is Fracture, subterms ulna, lower end. The main term is Contusion, subterms abdomen, abdominal, wall. The main term is Laceration, subterms hand, with foreign body. The main term is Abrasion, subterms knee, cheek, and scalp. The Index to External Cause main term is Accident, subterms transport, passenger, noncollision accident (traffic), nontraffic. Another Index to External Cause main term is Activity, subterm specified NEC. The Index to External Cause main term is Place of occurrence, subterm road. Another main term is External cause status, subterm specified NEC. All of the injury codes have a seventh character extension of A to indicate that this is the initial encounter for this injury.

Chapter 9. Case Studies from Physician-based Health Records

Unless otherwise stated, code set answers given in Chapter 9 are ICD-9-CM, CPT, and/or HCPCS Level II.

Anesthesia Services

9.1.   a. 745.10, 00562-AA-23, 99100

Incorrect answer. The correct anesthesia code is 00561 for procedures on the heart using the pump oxygenator on patients under one year of age. No mention is made of unusual anesthesia circumstances. The infant's physical status was P5. Code 99100 is not to be reported with 00561 per instructional note under 99100: Do not report 00561 in conjunction with 99100.

b. 745.11, 00561-AD-P5, 99140

Incorrect answer. The correct ICD-9-CM code for transposition of the great vessels is 745.10. The appropriate modifier for the anesthesiologist is -AA. There is no mention of emergency circumstances. The qualifying circumstance is 99100 for a patient under one year of age and should not be reported with 00561 per instructional note: Do not report 00561 in conjunction with 99100.

c. 745.10, 00561-AA-P5

Correct answer.

d. 745.19, 00563-AA-P5, 99100, 99140

Incorrect answer. The correct ICD-9-CM code for transposition of the great vessels is 745.10. The correct anesthesia code is 00561 for procedures on the heart using the pump oxygenator, but without mention of systemic hypothermia. There is no mention of emergency circumstances, so qualifying circumstance code 99140 is not appropriate here, and it is inappropriate to report 99100 with 00561.

ICD-10-CM Code(s): Q20.3

ICD-10-CM Rationale: The Alphabetic Index main term is Transposition, subterm great vessels.

9.2.   a. 723.3, 907.3, E929.0, 99201, 64413

Correct answer.

Rationale: The supply code for the medication (J code) for the Marcaine and steroid injection also is reported per payer guidelines.

b. 907.3, 723.3, E929.0, 99242, 64413

Incorrect answer. The residual cervicobrachial syndrome should be sequenced before the late effect code per ICD-9-CM coding guidelines. All three key components of history, physical examination, and medical decision making must be met or exceeded to assign an evaluation and management code. The brief history makes 99201 the appropriate code. The procedure code is correct.

c. 723.3, 907.3, E929.0, 99212, 64415

Incorrect answer. This was not an established patient office visit, but a new patient office visit. Based upon the documentation of history, physical examination, and medical decision making, 99201 is the appropriate evaluation and management code. The injection was of the cervical rather than the brachial plexus, so code 64413 is the correct CPT procedure code.

d. 907.3, E929.0, 99245, 64490

Incorrect answer. The residual cervicobrachial syndrome should be sequenced before the late effect code, per ICD-9-CM coding guidelines. Based upon the documentation of history, physical examination, and medical decision making, 99201 is the appropriate evaluation and management code. The injection was of the cervical rather than the brachial plexus, so code 64413 is the correct CPT procedure code.

ICD-10-CM Code(s): M53.1, S14.2xxS, V44.5xxS

ICD-10-CM Rationale: The Alphabetic Index main term is Syndrome, subterm cervicobrachial (diffuse). Main term is Sequelae (of) where there is a note for the main term injury for the coder to "code to injury with extension S." The main term is now Injury, subterms nerve, spinal, root, cervical. The Index to External Cause main term is Sequelae (of), subterm motor vehicle accident, with a note to "See V00–V99 with seventh character S."

9.3.   a. 354.0, 64719

Incorrect answer. The report specifies the median nerve. The surgeon provided the regional anesthesia, so modifier -47 is reported with code 64721.

b. 354.0, 64722-47

Incorrect answer. The median nerve was specified, so code 64721 is correct. The surgeon provided the regional anesthesia, so modifier -47 is reported with code 64721.

c. 354.0, 64721-47

Correct answer.

d. 354.1, 64721, 01810

Incorrect answer. Carpal tunnel syndrome is reported with ICD-9-CM code 354.0. The regional anesthesia was provided by the surgeon, so modifier -47 is reported with code 64721, rather than reporting a separate anesthesia code.

ICD-10-CM Code(s): G56.00

ICD-10-CM Rationale: The Alphabetic Index main term is Syndrome, subterm carpal tunnel. The coder completes the code using the Tabular List.

Disorders of the Blood and Blood-Forming Organs

9.4.   a. 173.69, 38525

Incorrect answer. The codes for malignant neoplasm of the skin (category 173.X) exclude malignant melanoma, which is reported with a code from category 172.X, in this case, 172.6. A code should also be reported for the injection of the dye (38792).

b. 172.6, 38525, 38792

Correct answer.

c. 172.6, 38525, 38792-51, 78195

Incorrect answer. The lymphoscintigraphy (78195) was performed by the radiologist, and the surgeon should not report the code. Code 38792 is identified in the CPT manual as being exempt from modifier -51 reporting requirements.

d. 172.9, 38525, 38790-51

Incorrect answer. The site of the melanoma is specified (arm), so code 172.9 is incorrect. The dye was injected for identification of sentinel node, so code 38790 is not correct. Refer to the instructional note preceding code 38500, which specifies code 38792 as the appropriate code for injection of dye for identification of sentinel node. Code 38792 is identified in the CPT manual as being exempt from modifier -51 reporting requirements.

ICD-10-CM Code(s): C43.61

ICD-10-CM Rationale: The Alphabetic Index main term is Melanoma, subterm arm.

9.5.   a. 280.0, 792.1, 414.01, 250.00, V45.81

Correct answer.

b. 285.9, 780.79

Incorrect answer. The anemia is specified as due to chronic blood loss, so code 285.9 is not correct. It is also not correct to code the weakness because it is a symptom of the more definitive diagnosis of anemia. The positive hemoccult would be reported because the etiology is still uncertain (792.1). The additional diagnoses of diabetes, ASHD, and status post coronary artery bypass may be coded because they were treated and/or are applicable to the case.

c. 280.0, 578.1, 414.01, 250.00, V45.81

Incorrect answer. It is not correct to assume that the patient had GI bleeding. Occult blood in the stool is reported with code 792.1.

d. 998.11, 285.1, 792.1, 414.01, 250.00, V45.81

Incorrect answer. There is no documentation that the bleeding was a complication of the surgical procedure to substantiate the use of code 998.11. The anemia is specified as severe, but not acute, so code 285.1 would not be used even though the hemoglobin was 5.7. Code 280.0 is appropriate for reporting chronic blood loss anemia.

ICD-10-CM Code(s): D50.0, R19.5, E11.9, I25.10, Z95.1

ICD-10-CM Rationale: The Alphabetic Index main term for the blood loss anemia is Anemia, subterm blood loss. The positive hemoccult is found under Abnormal, subterm stool. The patient is diabetic. The main term is Diabetes. The Alphabetic Index main term is Arteriosclerosis, subterm coronary (artery), native vessel. The CABG is coded by referencing main term Status, aortocoronary bypass.

Disorders of the Cardiovascular System

9.6. a. 972.1, E858.3, 787.01

Incorrect answer. Toxicity from digitalis use is coded as an adverse effect by assigning the codes for the manifestations of the adverse effect (787.01 and 780.79) as the primary diagnoses, followed by the E code that represents the agent in therapeutic use (E942.1). There is no suggestion that the drug was taken inappropriately. Additional codes are assigned for the MI (subsequent episode of care, 410.12) and the CHF (428.0).

b. 410.12, 428.0

Incorrect answer. The treatment in this case was focused on medication management, not the MI or the CHF. Toxicity from digitalis use is coded as an adverse effect by assigning the codes for the manifestations of the adverse effect (787.01 and 780.79) as the primary diagnoses, followed by the E code that represents the agent in therapeutic use (E942.1). There is no suggestion that the drug was taken inappropriately.

c. 787.01, 780.79, E858.3

Incorrect answer. The manifestation codes for the adverse effects of digitalis are correct and are appropriately sequenced as the primary diagnoses, but the E code is that used for a poisoning. The E code that represents the agent in therapeutic use (E942.1) is the appropriate E code. Additional codes are assigned for the MI (subsequent episode of care, 410.12) and the CHF (428.0).

d. 787.01, 780.79, E942.1, 410.12, 428.0

Correct answer.

ICD-10-CM Code(s): R11.2, R53.83, T46.0X5A, I25.2, I50.9

ICD-10-CM Rationale: The Alphabetic Index main term is Nausea, subterm with vomiting. Main term is Fatigue. In the Drug and Chemical Table, the drug Digoxin was referenced and a code was obtained from the Adverse Effect column, cardiotonic glycoside, NEC. Another main term is Old (previous myocardial infarction). The main term is Failure, subterms heart, congestive. In ICD-10-CM, four weeks is the period of time for an acute myocardial infarction.

9.7.   a. 429.9, 424.0, 92961

Incorrect answer. The atrial flutter (427.32) should be assigned as the principal diagnosis. The excludes note at code 424.0 directs the coding professional to category 396 when both mitral and aortic valve disorders are present, whether or not the cause is specified as rheumatic. The cardioversion was external, so CPT code 92960 should be reported.

b. 429.9, 394.1, 33240

Incorrect answer. The atrial flutter (427.32) should be assigned as the principal diagnosis. There is a combination code (396.3) for reporting both mitral and aortic regurgitation. Code 429.9 is reported for the ventricular dysfunction. The procedure was an external cardioversion, not insertion of a pacing cardioverter-defibrillator pulse generator, so code 33240 is not correct. CPT code 92960 is the appropriate code for reporting an external cardioversion.

c. 427.32, 394.1, 429.9, 33211

Incorrect answer. The regurgitation is not specified as rheumatic, and both the mitral and aortic valves are involved, so code 396.3 is correct. The procedure performed was an external cardioversion, not placement of temporary pacemaker, so CPT code 92960 is reported.

d. 427.32, 396.3, 429.9, 92960

Correct answer.

ICD-10-CM Code(s): I48.1, I08.0, I09.9

ICD-10-CM Rationale: The Alphabetic Index main term is Flutter, subterm atrial. The main term Regurgitation directs the coder to Insufficiency, subterm aortic (valve), with mitral (valve) disease. The Alphabetic Index main term is Dysfunction, subterm ventricular. There is an Excludes note that indicates that heart disease specified as rheumatic is coded to (I00–I09). The I09.9 is correct.

9.8.   a. 414.01, 414.05, 410.12, 411.1, 33517, 33533, 33530

Correct answer.

b. 414.01, 414.05, 410.12, 411.1, 33510, 33533

Incorrect answer. The bypass consisted of one venous graft and one mammary (arterial) graft, so codes from 33517–33523 must be used for the venous portion of the bypass per CPT coding guidelines. See instructional note preceding code 33510. The fact that this was a redo procedure should also be coded (33530).

c. 414.00, 414.05, 410.11, 411.1, 33530

Incorrect answer. The coronary atherosclerosis involving the native artery should be coded to 414.01. Code 414.05 for the graft stenosis is correct. The MI was specified as involving the anterior wall (410.12). Code 33530 reports the reoperation only and is an add-on code that should not be reported alone. Codes 33517 and 33533 should be reported in the first two positions for the actual bypass procedure.

d. 414.01, 414.05, 410.12, 412, 33518, 33530

Incorrect answer. The MI was recent (10 days), not old, so code 412 should not be used. The preinfarction angina should also be reported with code 411.1. The bypass was done with one artery and one vein, so the correct codes are 33517 and 33533.

ICD-10-CM Code(s): I25.110, I25.700, I21.01, Z95.1

ICD-10-CM Rationale: The Alphabetic Index main term is Syndrome, subterm intermediate coronary (artery). The Excludes note under I20 excludes "angina with atherosclerotic heart disease—See I25.1." The main term is Arteriosclerosis, arterosclerotic, subterm coronary (artery). Another main term is Arteriosclerosis, with subterms coronary, bypass graft, with, angina pectoris, unstable. Another main term is Infarct, infarction, subterms myocardium, myocardial, ST elevation, anterior. Code I20.01 specifically documents coronary artery so it is used.

9.9.   a. 428.0, 486, 496, 290.0, V49.86

Correct answer.

b. 428.0, 518.4, 486, 496, 290.0

Incorrect answer. According to *Coding Clinic* (1988, 3Q), acute pulmonary edema of cardiac origin is a manifestation of CHF, category 428, and as such is included in the code. The patient is Do Not Resuscitate status, and therefore code V49.86 should be reported.

c. 428.0, 410.91, 486, 496, 290.0, V49.86

Incorrect answer. The MI was ruled out and should not be coded as if present.

d. 518.4, 428.0, 486, 496, 290.0, V49.86

Incorrect answer. According to *Coding Clinic* (1988, 3Q), acute pulmonary edema of cardiac origin is a manifestation of CHF, category 428, and as such is included in the code. The CHF would be assigned alone, and in the principal diagnosis position.

ICD-10-CM Code(s): I50.9, J44.9, J18.9, F03, Z66

ICD-10-CM Rationale: The Alphabetic Index main term is Failure, subterm heart, congestive. The edema is not coded separately. The COPD code is found under main term Disease, subterm pulmonary, chronic obstructive. The main term Pneumonia yields code J18.9. The main term for senile dementia is Dementia, subterm senile. The DNR code is found under main term DNR.

9.10.   a. 33880

Incorrect answer. This code is appropriate for coverage of the left subclavian artery origin. The correct code assignment is 33881.

b. 33779

Incorrect answer. The correct code assignment is 33881.

c. 33881

Correct answer.

d. 33881, 33883, 33884

Incorrect answer. The extensions are included in code 33881 and are not reported separately with 33883 and 33884.

9.11. a. 34900, 37221, 37250

Correct answer.

b. 34900, 37221

Incorrect answer. An additional code needs to be assigned for the endovascular ultrasound, 37250.

c. 37221

Incorrect answer. This code is correct for the stent placement, but additional codes must be assigned for the endovascular graft placement, 34900, and the endovascular ultrasound, 37250.

d. 34825, 37221, 37250

Incorrect answer. Code 34825 is for placement of an extension prosthesis for endovascular aneurysm repair. In this case an ilio-iliac tube was placed, which is code 34900.

9.12. a. 92980-RC, 92981-LC

Correct answer.

b. 92982-RC, 92984-LC, 92980-RC, 92981-LC × 2

Incorrect answer. Codes 92982 and 92984 (angioplasty) are not reported in addition to 92980 and 92981 (stenting) per instructional note listed under codes 92980 and 92981: Coronary angioplasty (92982, 92984) in the same artery is considered part of the stenting procedure and is not reported separately. Stenting in the left circumflex coronary artery reported as 92981-LC × 2 is incorrect as the code is not reported based on the number of stents; it is reported based on the number of vessels stented (add-on code states: each additional vessel).

c. 93455, 92980-RC, 92981-LC

Incorrect answer. The codes for the interventional portions of the procedure are appropriate, but the code for the cardiac catheterization is not.

d. 93455, 92982-RC, 92984-LC, 92980-RC, 92981-LC × 2

Incorrect answer. Code 93454 is the appropriate code when catheters are placed into the coronary arteries for interventional procedures without a concomitant left heart catheterization. Codes 92982 and 92984 (angioplasty) are not reported in addition to 92980 and 92981 (stenting) per instructional note listed under codes 92980 and 92981: Coronary angioplasty (92982, 92984) in the same artery is considered part of the stenting procedure and is not reported separately. Stenting in the left circumflex coronary artery reported as 92981-LC × 2 is incorrect as the code is not reported based on the number of stents; it is reported based on the number of vessels stented (add-on code states: each additional vessel).

9.13. ICD-9-CM Code(s): 786.50, 305.11, 401.9, 365.10, 365.71, V43.65, V11.3, V17.49

Rationale: It is important to review the coding guidelines to determine which of the many problems that the patient presented with would be coded. Although the patient has a hiatal hernia, the condition was not further evaluated or treated. The same is true for the DJD—the physician merely mentioned it but did no evaluation of the condition. These diagnoses would not be coded. The patient came in with chest pains so that is the first-listed diagnosis. The physician noted the smoking as a problem with suggestions for treatment for the smoking so that would be coded. The physician evaluated the knee replacement and made the decision that everything was ok but recommended seeing an orthopedist if the problem continues. A V code would be used to indicate that the patient has had a knee replacement. The hypertension is a chronic condition that would always be coded. The physician also evaluates the patient's glaucoma so that is coded along with a code for the stage of the glaucoma. Finally, the family history of cardiovascular disease is included because it is very pertinent to the problem at hand.

ICD-10-CM Code(s): R07.9, F17.210, I10, H40.10, Z96.651, Z82.49

ICD-10-CM Rationale: The reason for visit is chest pains. The Alphabetic Index main term is Pain, subterm chest. The patient smokes cigarettes so Tobacco, use, see Dependence is used. The Alphabetic Index main term Hypertension yields code I10. The Alphabetic Index main term is Glaucoma, subterm open angle. The knee replacement is coded by reviewing Alphabetic Index main term Presence, subterm knee-joint implant. The coder completes the code using the Tabular List. The family history code is found at History, subterm family, disease, cardiovascular.

9.14. a. 427.41, 427.81, 33202, 33213

Incorrect code: The correct code for the initial insertion of a pacemaker including leads and generator is 33208. Individual codes should not be reported for inserting the leads and then inserting the generator. Code 427.41 is for ventricular fibrillation—the patient had atrial fibrillation. The long-term use of Coumadin (V58.61) should be reported.

b. 427.31, 427.81, 33212, 33217

Incorrect code: The correct code for the initial insertion of a pacemaker including leads and generator is 33208. Individual codes should not be reported for inserting the leads and then inserting the generator. The long-term use of Coumadin (V58.61) should be reported.

c. 427.31, V58.61, 33208

Incorrect code: Two codes are needed, 427.31 and 427.81, to report the atrial fibrillation and the sick sinus syndrome.

d. 427.31, 427.81, V58.61, 33208

Correct code.

ICD-10-CM Code(s): I48.0, I49.5, Z79.01

ICD-10-CM Rationale: The Alphabetic Index main term is Fibrillation, subterm atrial or auricular. Main term is Syndrome, subterms sick, sinus. Another main term is Long-term drug therapy, subterm anticoagulants (Coumadin is classified as an anticoagulant).

Disorders of the Digestive System

9.15.   a. 530.81, 535.40, 43239

Correct code.

b. 530.81, 535.50, 43239

Incorrect code: Code 535.50 is incorrect—there is no indication of perforation.

c. 530.81, 535.40, 43202, 43605, 44010

Incorrect code: The correct CPT code is 43239. Only one code is necessary as all three biopsies were done through the endoscope. In addition, codes 43605 and 44010 are open biopsy codes not through an endoscope.

d. 530.81, 535.40, 43239, 43239, 43239

Incorrect code: Only one CPT code is reported. Code 43239 indicates that it is used for single or multiple biopsies.

ICD-10-CM Code(s): K21.9, K29.60

ICD-10-CM Rationale: The Alphabetic Index main term is Reflux, subterm esophageal. The Alphabetic Index main term is Gastritis, subterm specified NEC.

9.16.   a. 578.0, 285.1, 789.59, 99285, 43752

Incorrect answer. The only key component of history, physical examination, and medical decision making that meets criteria for 99285 is the high-complexity medical decision making. In assigning ED codes, all three elements must be met or exceeded unless there is clear documentation of patient inability to cooperate with history and physical examination, which is not present here. Code 99284 is the correct code. The evaluation and management code should have modifier -25 assigned.

b. 578.0, 789.00, 780.4, 99284-25, 91105

Incorrect answer. The abdominal pain is an integral part of the hematemesis, so code 789.00 should not be assigned. The dizziness and light-headedness are both due to the documented blood loss anemia and also should not be coded. The codes for anemia (285.1) and ascites (789.59) should be reported. The gastric tube was inserted by the emergency department physician and left in place to continue draining stomach contents, so code 43752 should also be reported, rather than 91105.

c. 789.51, 578.0, 280.0, 99284, 43752

Incorrect answer. There is no documentation of malignant ascites, 789.51. The hematemesis is the reason for the patient seeking medical care, so this should be reported as the primary diagnosis. The anemia is due to the current episode of acute blood loss and should be assigned code 285.1. The evaluation and management code should have modifier -25 assigned.

d. 578.0, 285.1, 789.59, 99284-25, 43752

Correct answer.

ICD-10-CM Code(s): K92.0, D62, R18.8

ICD-10-CM Rationale: The Alphabetic Index main term is Hematemesis. The main term is Anemia, subterms blood loss, acute. Another main term is Ascites (abdominal).

9.17. a. 562.12, 211.3, 45385, 45384-51 or 45384-59

Correct answer. Either modifier -59 or -51 may be used, depending upon specific payer requirements.

b. 211.3, 562.10, 578.1, 45384

Incorrect answer. Per *CPT Assistant* (1998, July), both 45384 and 45385 should be coded because two lesions were addressed with two different techniques. The diverticulosis is the cause of the bleeding and should be coded as "with hemorrhage" (562.12). This code should be listed first because it was the cause of the patient's seeking attention and undergoing the procedure. The GI bleeding code is not needed with code 562.12 because it is included in the fifth digit.

c. 562.12, 211.3, 578.9, 45385

Incorrect answer. Per *CPT Assistant* (1998, July), both 45384 and 45385 should be coded because two lesions were addressed with two different techniques. The GI bleeding code is not needed with code 562.12 because it is included in the fifth digit.

d. 562.12, 211.3, 45384

Incorrect answer. Per *CPT Assistant* (1998, July), both 45384 and 45385 should be coded because two lesions were addressed with two different techniques.

ICD-10-CM Code(s): K57.31, D12.3

ICD-10-CM Rationale: The Alphabetic Index main term is Diverticulosis, subterm large intestine, with bleeding. The polyps are coded by accessing main term Polyp, polypus, subterm colon, transverse.

9.18. a. 530.81, 530.85, 47562, 43289-51

Incorrect answer. The documentation states "with esophagitis," so code 530.11 is correct. The chronic cholecystitis should also be coded. CPT code 43280 includes laparoscopic Nissen procedures, so the unlisted procedure code is not appropriate.

b. 530.11, 530.85, 574.10, 43327, 47600-52

Incorrect answer. The cholecystitis is not specified as being calculous, so code 574.10 is not correct. Codes 43327 and 47600 are open procedures. It is never appropriate to assign an open procedure code when a laparoscopic approach is specified.

c. 530.11, 530.89, 575.11, 43326

Incorrect answer. Barrett's esophagus codes to 530.85. The correct procedure code is 43280 because there is no documentation of a gastroplasty being performed. The laparoscopic cholecystectomy should also be reported (47562-51).

d. 530.11, 530.85, 575.11, 43280, 47562-51

Correct answer.

ICD-10-CM Code(s): K21.0, K22.70, K81.1

ICD-10-CM Rationale: The Alphabetic Index main term is Reflux, subterms gastroesophageal, with esophagitis. The main term is Barrett's, subterm esophagus. Another main term is Cholecystitis, subterm chronic.

9.19. a. 44207, 44213

Incorrect answer. Per *CPT Assistant* (2006, April), procedure code 44227 describes the procedure performed in this case, including the mobilization of the splenic flexure. Code 44207 describes the procedure of an initial colectomy with immediate anastomosis of the colon to the rectal area.

b. 44207, 44213, 44620

Incorrect answer. Per *CPT Assistant* (2006, April), procedure code 44227 describes the procedure performed in this case, including the mobilization of the splenic flexure. Code 44207 describes the procedure of an initial colectomy with immediate anastomosis of the colon to the rectal area. The closure of the enterostomy described in code 44620 is an open procedure and this re-anastomosis is a laparoscopic procedure.

c. 44227

Correct answer.

d. 44626

Incorrect answer. Code 44626 describes the procedure using an open approach. The documentation describes the procedure being performed with the use of laparoscopy ports and a pneumoperitoneum. Therefore, code 44227 is the correct code.

9.20. a. 455.2, 46221, 45300-51, 46600-51

Correct answer.

b. 455.2, 46221, 46221-59, 45300

Incorrect answer. Per *CPT Assistant* (1997, Oct.), even though there are multiple ligations done, only one is coded. The anoscopy should also be coded per the same reference, even though some payers may not reimburse for this.

c. 455.0, 46945, 45300

Incorrect answer. The hemorrhoids are documented as prolapsed and bleeding, which constitutes a complication. Code 455.2 is the correct diagnosis code. Per *CPT Assistant* (1997, Oct.), the appropriate CPT code for rubber band ligation of hemorrhoids is 46221. The anoscopy should also be coded per the same reference, even though some payers may not reimburse for this.

d. 455.8, 46083, 45300-51, 46600-51

Incorrect answer. There is documentation that the hemorrhoids were internal; therefore 445.2 is the correct ICD-9-CM diagnosis code. Per *CPT Assistant* (1997, Oct.), the appropriate CPT code for rubber band ligation of hemorrhoids is 46221.

ICD-10-CM Code(s): I84.112, I84.111

ICD-10-CM Rationale: The Alphabetic Index main term is Hemorrhoids, subterms internal, prolapsed. In the Tabular List, code I84.111 indicates the bleeding.

Evaluation and Management (E/M) Services

9.21. a. Surgeon's: 19120-52; PCP: 19120

Incorrect answer. Modifier -52 is used to show a reduced service—the procedure itself was performed as planned. The surgeon simply had no preoperative or postoperative part in the patient's care. The PCP did not perform the surgery so a modifier would have to be attached to code 19120.

b. Surgeon's: 19120-54; PCP: 19120-55-56

Correct code.

c. Surgeon's: 19101-54; PCP: 19120-55-56

Incorrect answer. The surgeon's code was reported incorrectly. This was a removal of a lump, not a biopsy as code 19101 indicates.

d. Surgeon's: 19101-54; PCP: 19120, 99213

Incorrect answer. The surgeon's code was reported incorrectly. This was a removal of a lump, not a biopsy as code 19101 indicates. The PCP's code is incorrect. He or she should report only code 19120. The modifiers -55 and -56 indicate that only pre-op and post-op care was provided.

9.22. a. 99219, 99231, 99217

Incorrect answer. An inpatient code (99231) is not appropriate for the place of service for a hospital outpatient.

b. 99219, 99224, 99217

Correct answer. New CPT codes are used to report services on subsequent days of service.

c. 99283, 99219, 99217

Incorrect answer. The emergency department visit should be bundled into the initial observation day code, and a separate outpatient care code is needed for day two.

d. 99283, 99231, 99217

Incorrect answer. An inpatient code (99231) is not appropriate for the place of service for a hospital outpatient. The emergency department visit should be bundled into the initial observation day code, and a separate outpatient care code is needed for day two.

9.23. a. Dr. Smith: 99315, 99219; Dr. Johnson: 99236

Incorrect answer. No mention is made of discharge from the nursing facility.

b. Dr. Smith: 99219; Dr. Johnson: 99217, 99236

Incorrect answer. Observation discharge is not coded when the patient is admitted and discharged on the same day.

c. Dr. Smith: 99219; Dr. Johnson: 99236

Correct answer.

d. Dr. Smith: 99315, 99222; Dr. Johnson: 99238

Incorrect answer. None of these codes is correct. No mention is made of discharge from the nursing facility, nor was the patient admitted to inpatient status on the first day. Instead of hospital discharge 99238, Dr. Johnson's services require code 99236, Observation or inpatient hospital care, for admission and discharge on the same day.

9.24. a. 99214, 99222, 99239, 99305

Incorrect answer. The office visit should be bundled into the initial hospital care code.

b. 99222, 99239, 99305

Correct answer.

c. 99214, 99235, 99305

Incorrect answer. The patient was not admitted and discharged on the same day. Separate codes are needed for the admission and discharge. The office visit should be bundled into the initial hospital care code.

d. 99222, 99305

Incorrect answer. A code for the hospital discharge day is also needed.

9.25. a. 99204, 99354

Incorrect answer. Because there is documentation that counseling comprised more than 50 percent of the total time of the visit, time may be used as the determining factor, resulting in code 99205. The total time of the visit should be used in calculating the evaluation and management code, not the amount of time spent in counseling.

b. 99205, 99354, 99355

Incorrect answer. The documentation states that 50 minutes was spent counseling and coordinating care for a total of 95 minutes. This does not support the use of an additional 30 minutes of prolonged care.

c. 99205, 99354

Correct answer.

d. 99204

Incorrect answer. Because there is documentation that counseling comprised more than 50 percent of the total time of the visit, time may be used as the determining factor, resulting in code 99205. Because code 99205 suggests a time of approximately 60 minutes, there are an additional 35 minutes to be reported, which should be reflected with the prolonged service code 99354.

9.26. a. V72.31, V76.47, V45.77, 99396; 784.0, 99213-25

Correct answer.

b. V70.9, 99396, 784.0, 99213

Incorrect answer. A vaginal pap smear and pelvic examination were performed, so code V72.31 followed by V76.47 is the best choice for the primary diagnosis. A modifier of -25 is needed on the evaluation and management code for the office visit for evaluation of the headache complaint. Acquired absence of the uterus may also be reported (V45.77).

c. V76.2, V76.47, V45.77, G0101, Q0091; 784.0, 99213-25

Incorrect answer. The patient is 56 years old and is not a Medicare beneficiary. Acquired absence of the uterus may also be reported (V45.77).

d. 784.0, V72.31, V76.47, V45.77, 99214

Incorrect answer. A complete preventative medicine examination was performed as scheduled. The patient had an incidental complaint of headache after she arrived, which was evaluated, and this should be coded as a separately identifiable evaluation and management service with modifier -25.

ICD-10-CM Code(s): Z00.01, R51, Z12.72, Z80.0, Z90.710

ICD-10-CM Rationale: The Alphabetic Index main term is Examination, subterms annual (adult), with abnormal findings. Another main term is Headache. The main term is Screening, subterms neoplasm (malignant) (of), vagina. There is a note that reminds the coder to "Use additional code to identify any family history of malignant neoplasm—Z80." Another main term is Absence (of) (organ or part), subterm cervix (acquired).

9.27. a. 99233

Incorrect answer. Critical care services were rendered, with one hour documented. The correct code is 99291.

b. 99291, 99292

Incorrect answer. Only one hour of critical care is documented. The appropriate code is 99291.

c. 99233, 99354

Incorrect answer. Critical care services were rendered, with one hour documented. The correct code is 99291.

d. 99291

Correct answer.

9.28. a. V20.2, 779.31

Incorrect answer. This newborn is only four days old. Code V20.31 is used to indicate that newborn health supervision was provided for a newborn under eight days old.

b. V20.2, 783.21

Incorrect answer. This newborn is only four days old. Code V20.31 is used to indicate that newborn health supervision was provided for a newborn under eight days old. In addition, failure to thrive is not supported in the documentation. The additional code to be reported in this case is 779.31, feeding problems in newborn.

c. V20.31

Incorrect answer. This answer is incomplete. V20.31 is the correct code for newborn health supervision provided for a newborn under eight days old; however, the additional code to be reported in this case is 779.31, feeding problems in newborn.

d. V20.31, 779.31

Correct answer.

ICD-10-CM Code(s): Z00.110, P92.8

ICD-10-CM Rationale: The Alphabetic Index main term is Newborn, subterms examination, under 8 days old. Another main term is Problem, subterms feeding, newborn, slow.

9.29.   a. 272.4, 278.00, 530.81, 311, 401.9, 99204

Incorrect answer. The physician does document that the patient is severely overweight so the code for morbid obesity is correct. The E&M code is incorrect. This is an established patient as indicated in the record. Code 99214 would be the correct code to assign to this encounter.

b. 272.4, 278.00, 530.81, 311, 401.9, 99214

Incorrect answer. The physician does document that the patient is severely overweight so the code for morbid obesity is correct.

c. 272.4, 278.01, 530.81, 311, 401.9, 99214

Correct answer.

d. 272.4, 278.00, 530.81, 311, 401.9, 99213

Incorrect answer. The physician does document that the patient is severely overweight so the code for morbid obesity is correct. In addition, the selection of code 99214 is supported by the level of history, exam, and MDM. Using code 99213 would be downcoding.

ICD-10-CM Code(s): E78.5, I10, E66.01, K21.9, F32.9, Z56.89

ICD-10-CM Rationale: The Alphabetic Index main term is Hyperlipidemia. For the hypertension the main term is Hypertension. The Alphabetic Index main term is Obesity, subterm morbid, due to excess calories. The main term Reflux, subterm gastroesophageal, leads the coder to K21.9. The main term is Depression. To code the problem at work, the main term is Problem, subterm employment, specified NEC.

Endocrine, Nutritional, and Metabolic Diseases and Immunity Disorders

9.30.   a. First visit: 259.4, 259.0; second visit: 253.3

Incorrect answer. There is no mention made of any type of dwarfism. Short stature should be coded.

b. First visit: 783.43, 259.0; second visit: 253.3

Correct answer.

c. First visit: 259.0; second visit: 253.4

Incorrect answer. Short stature should also be coded for the first visit. Code 253.4 describes "deficiency . . . other than growth hormone." Code 253.3 is the appropriate code.

d. First visit: 259.4; second visit: 253.4

Incorrect answer. There is no mention made of any type of dwarfism. Short stature and delay in sexual development should be coded. Code 253.4 describes "deficiency . . . other than growth hormone." Code 253.3 is the appropriate code.

ICD-10-CM Code(s): First Visit: R62.52, E30.0; Second Visit: E23.0

ICD-10-CM Rationale: First Visit: The Alphabetic Index main term is Short, subterms stature (child) (hereditary) NEC. The main term is Delay, subterm puberty. Second Visit: The Alphabetic Index main term is Deficiency, deficient, subterms hormone, growth.

9.31.   a. 240.9

Incorrect answer. A thyroid nodule is not the same as a goiter. The nodule in the left lobe of the thyroid is coded as 241.0. In addition, codes for the cyst and the hemorrhage of the thyroid should be coded (246.2 and 246.3).

b. 241.0, 246.2

Incorrect answer. In addition, code 246.3 should be reported for the hemorrhage of the thyroid.

c. 241.0, 246.3

Incorrect answer. In addition, code 246.2 should be reported for the cyst of the thyroid.

d. 241.0, 246.2, 246.3

Correct answer.

ICD-10-CM Code(s): E04.1, E07.89

ICD-10-CM Rationale: The Alphabetic Index main term is Cyst, subterm thyroid. Code E04.1 covers both the thyroid cyst and the thyroid nodule. The hemorrhage is coded by reviewing main term Hemorrhage, subterm thyroid.

9.32. a. 227.3, 162.9, V77.1

Incorrect answer. It is unclear whether this tumor was benign or malignant. Code 239.7 is the appropriate neoplasm code when the nature of the tumor has not been determined. The patient will be followed for possible development of diabetes insipidus. No screening was done for diabetes.

b. 194.3, 162.9

Incorrect answer. There is no mention of whether the pituitary tumor was benign or malignant. Code 239.7 is the appropriate neoplasm code when the nature of the tumor has not been determined.

c. 239.7, 162.9, 253.5

Incorrect answer. The patient will be followed for possible development of diabetes insipidus, but it has not yet been diagnosed.

d. 239.7, 162.9

Correct answer. If this is a case where an oncologist is providing care for the lung cancer and an endocrinologist is addressing the pituitary tumor concurrently, it is important for each specialist to report only the specific condition(s) that he or she is following in order to avoid the appearance of duplicate coding and billing.

ICD-10-CM Code(s): D49.7, C34.90

ICD-10-CM Rationale: The Alphabetic Index main term is Tumor which refers the coder to the Neoplasm Table, unspecified behavior, by site. The code listed is for Thyroid, unspecified behavior. In the Neoplasm Table, the subterm is lung. Select a code from the Malignant Primary column.

Disorders of the Genitourinary System

9.33. a. 599.71, 280.0, 344.04, 337.3, 596.54, 599.0, 51700, 36430
Correct answer.

b. 599.71, 285.9, 344.03, 337.3, 596.54, 599.0, 51700, 36430

Incorrect answer. There is no indication of acute blood loss anemia. The patient did have use of his hands so this would be coded as an incomplete injury.

c. 599.71, 280.0, 344.04, 337.3, 596.54, 51700, 51702, 36430

Incorrect answer. Code 51702 should not be used. There is a note below the code that states that 51702 should only be reported if it is done independent of any other procedure.

d. 599.71, 280.0, 344.04, 337.3, 51700, 51702, 36430

Incorrect answer. Code 51702 should not be used. There is a note below the code that states that 51702 should only be reported if it is done independent of any other procedure. The code showing that he has a permanent suprapubic catheter is needed (596.54).

ICD-10-CM Code(s): R31.0, D50.0, G82.54, G90.4, N31.0, N39.0, Z96.89

ICD-10-CM Rationale: The Alphabetic Index main term is Hematuria, subterm gross. Patient has anemia which is reported by finding main term Anemia, subterm blood loss (chronic). The Alphabetic Index main term is Quadriplegia, subterm incomplete, C5–C7. The Alphabetic Index main term is Dysreflexia, subterm autonomic. Dependence on the catheter is coded by Alphabetic Index main term Dysfunction, subterm bladder, neuromuscular. The UTI is coded by accessing main term Infection, subterm urinary (tract). The Alphabetic Index main term is Presence, subterm implanted device, specified NEC.

9.34. a. 233.4, 55875, 52000, 77763, 76965, 76000-59

Incorrect answer. Although the physician states that the cancer is localized, carcinoma in situ would not be assumed without being directly stated as such. The primary malignancy should be reported as the reason for the radiation therapy. Code 77778 would be appropriate, rather than 77763, because the treatment of the prostate would be interstitial rather than intracavitary because the prostate is a solid organ. See the note in the CPT manual with code 55875 instructing the coding professional to use codes 77776–77787 for interstitial radioelement application. According to the NCCI, code 52000 is bundled into procedure code 55875 and is not listed separately. Review of code 55875 in the CPT manual states "with or without cystoscopy," which indicates that whether the cystoscopy was performed or not, the code and reimbursement for 55875 are the same.

b. 185, 55875, 77778, 76965, 76000-59

Correct answer. Modifier -51 may be used if accepted by the payer. Depending upon the physician's arrangements with the cancer center, modifier -26 may be needed.

c. 185, 55875, 77787, 76872, 77790

Incorrect answer. There is a specific code for interstitial radioelement application. Code 77787 is used to report remote application using catheters. Code 77778 is the correct code. The ultrasound code should be 76965, which is the specific code for guidance for interstitial application. The fluoroscopy (76000) should also be reported. The port films would not be coded in this case. This is brachytherapy, not radiation therapy, and there is no documentation of films being performed. Also, the code reported is for each period of five days, and this procedure has a different treatment plan.

d. 185, 52000, 77762

Incorrect answer. We need to report the surgical implantation code (55875) with ultrasonic guidance (76965) and the fluoroscopy (76000) codes. This procedure on the prostate, a solid organ, is an interstitial application rather than an injection (intravenous) or intracavitary insertion, which is used only for hollow organs such as the bladder.

ICD-10-CM Code(s): C61

ICD-10-CM Rationale: The Neoplasm Table subterm is prostate and the coder selects the code from the Malignant Primary column.

9.35.   a. 611.72, 610.1, 19120-50

Incorrect answer. When a definitive diagnosis is known, it is reported, so code 174.9 for the primary malignancy would be the first code reported, followed by the code for the fibrocystic disease, and the breast lump would not be coded. A bilateral modifier of -50 applies only to identical procedures on paired organs. The breasts are paired organs, but the procedures involved here were not the same. HCPCS Level II modifier -RT identifies the 19120 procedure on the right side, while the -LT procedure is appended to CPT codes 19125 and 19290 to report the procedure on the left breast.

b. 174.9, 610.1, 19125-50, 19290-50, 19120-50

Incorrect answer. Appropriate use of the bilateral modifier has it appended to only one CPT code when identical procedures are performed on paired organs. Although identical procedures may be performed on the breasts, the code is reported only once with modifier -50. In the case described in this source document, identical procedures were not performed, so the appropriate modifier assignment in this case is -RT and -LT for the two different procedures. Codes 19120 and 19125 would be mutually exclusive under the NCCI otherwise; therefore, they require an additional modifier of -51 to differentiate that a separate procedure was performed on the right breast from the procedure performed on the left breast.

c. 174.9, 610.1, 19120-RT, 19125-LT-51, 19290-LT-51

Correct answer.

d. 174.9, 610.2, 19120, 19125-59, 19290-59

Incorrect answer. The fibrocystic disease was not stated to be fibroadenosis, so code 610.1 is as specific as the documentation here allows. The use of modifier -59 is not appropriate for this case because HCPCS Level II modifiers -RT and -LT would describe the services more accurately.

ICD-10-CM Code(s): C50.911, N60.12

ICD-10-CM Rationale: The Alphabetic Index main term is Neoplasm, subterm breast, Malignant Primary column. The coder completes the code using the Tabular List. The Alphabetic Index main term Fibrocystic, subterm breast directs the coder to see Mastopathy, cystic. Alphabetic Index main term Mastopathy, subterm cystic directs the coder to N60.1. The coder completes the code using the Tabular List.

9.36.   a. 626.8, 218.1, 58558

Correct answer.

b. 626.8, 218.9, 57800, 58558

Incorrect answer. This patient has intramural fibroids. While intramural is not a subterm listed under Fibroids in the index, it is listed as a specific type of uterine fibroid when you view the index. Therefore, 218.1 for intramural fibroids should be chosen as the code. CPT code 57800 is for dilation of the cervical canal and is a separate procedure. Therefore, this cannot be used with another procedure code and is not correct.

c. 627.0, 218.9, 58558, 58120

Incorrect answer. The physician states that this patient has dysfunctional bleeding but does not link it to a premenopausal state. The physician states that the lab work suggests a perimenopausal state but this does not support the use of this code. CPT code 58120 is not coded separately, as code 58558 states "with or without D&C" in the description.

d. 627.0, 218.1, 58558

Incorrect answer. The physician states that this patient has dysfunctional bleeding but does not link it to a premenopausal state. The physician states that the lab work suggests a perimenopausal state but this does not support the use of this code. The CPT code is correct.

ICD-10-CM Code(s): N93.8, D25.1

ICD-10-CM Rationale: The Alphabetic Index main term is Dysfunction, subterms bleeding, uterus. The main term is Fibroid (tumor), subterm uterus. Because the fibroids are intramural, code D25.1 is selected.

9.37. a. 618.2, 57288

Incorrect answer. It cannot be assumed that the cystocele is causing the stress incontinence. Both diagnoses should be reported. Therefore, code 625.6 should be added. Code 57288 describes only the sling procedure and does not include the anterior culporrhaphy with repair of the cystocele, code 57240.

b. 618.2, 625.6, 57240, 53440

Incorrect answer. The diagnoses are correct; however, code 53440 describes the sling procedure performed on a male patient. This patient is female and therefore code 57288 is correct.

c. 618.2, 625.6, 57240, 57288

Correct answer.

d. 625.6, 57288

Incorrect answer. It cannot be assumed that the cystocele is causing the stress incontinence. Both diagnoses should be reported. Therefore, code 618.2 should be added. Code 57288 describes only the sling procedure and does not include the anterior culporrhaphy with repair of the cystocele, code 57240.

ICD-10-CM Code(s): N81.10, N39.3

ICD-10-CM Rationale: The Alphabetic Index main term is Cystocele, subterm female. The Alphabetic Index main term Incontinence, subterm stress (female) yields a code.

9.38. a. 185, 55700

Incorrect answer. Carcinoma in situ of the prostate is coded 233.4 because the malignancy has not extended into any surrounding tissue and is detected early. CPT codes are required for the placement of the ultrasound probe (76872) and the actual provision of ultrasonic guidance for the biopsy (76942). Stones of the prostate (602.0) should also have a code assigned because they may affect current or future care of the patient.

b. 233.4, 790.93, 55705, 76872

Incorrect answer. The biopsy code in CPT is 55700 because no incision is documented. The placement of the transrectal probe is only one component of the procedure. An additional code (76942) is required for the needle guidance for the prostatic biopsy. Stones of the prostate (602.0) should also have a code assigned because they may affect current or future care of the patient. Abnormal laboratory tests are not assigned an additional code when the etiology has been confirmed by the close of the encounter.

c. 185, 790.93, 602.0, 55700, 76872, 76942

Incorrect answer. The neoplasm is specified as carcinoma in situ of the prostate, so code 233.4 is assigned, rather than the code for a primary malignant neoplasm of the prostate. Abnormal laboratory tests are not assigned an additional code when the etiology has been confirmed by the close of the encounter. The other codes are correct.

d. 233.4, 602.0, 55700, 76872, 76942

Correct answer.

ICD-10-CM Code(s): D07.5, N42.0

ICD-10-CM Rationale: In the Neoplasm Table, the subterm is prostate. Select a code from the "Ca in situ" column. Another main term is Calculus, calculi, calculous, subterm prostate.

Infectious Diseases/Disorders of the Skin and Subcutaneous Tissue

9.39. a. 686.9, V12.04, 250.00, 443.81, 99214, 96372

Incorrect answer. 686.9 is found in the index under Infection, leg. However, the specific disease process is cellulitis. When this is found in the index, the subterm entry of leg provides the code of 682.6. This patient has diabetic peripheral vascular disease and therefore the correct codes are 250.70 for the complicated diabetes and 443.81 as the secondary code to describe the type of complication. The E/M code for this visit is 99215 because only two key components are required and this documentation includes a comprehensive examination and high-level medical decision making (a new problem with risk to life or bodily function). The antibiotic is administered through the IV route and not the intramuscular route. An HCPCS code is required to report the medication and the dosage administered.

b. 682.6, V02.54, 250.70, 443.81, 99214, 96374, S0077

Incorrect answer. The cellulitis code is correct, but the patient has a personal history of MRSA and is not a suspected carrier of MRSA, so V12.04 is the correct code. The E/M code for this visit is 99215 because only two key components are required, and this documentation includes a comprehensive examination and high-level medical decision making (a new problem with risk to life or bodily function). The antibiotic and the administration is coded correctly.

c. 682.6, V12.04, 250.70, 443.81, 99215, 96374, S0077

Correct answer.

d. 891.1, V02.54, 250.70, 443.81, 99215, 96372, J3490

Incorrect answer. Code 891.1 represents a complicated open wound of the leg. While the leg has an open wound, it did not start as an open wound; it started as mild redness. The cellulitis code of 682.6 is the most appropriate code. The patient has a personal history of MRSA and is not a suspected carrier of MRSA, so V12.04 is the correct code. The remainder of the coding is correct.

ICD-10-CM Code(s): L03.116, Z86.19, E11.51

ICD-10-CM Rationale: Patient has cellulitis of left leg. The Alphabetic Index main term is Cellulitis, subterm lower limb. The coder completes the code using the Tabular List. The Alphabetic Index main term is History, subterm personal (of), infection, NEC. The Alphabetic Index main term for the diabetes is Diabetes, subterm type 2, with peripheral angiopathy.

9.40. a. 891.0, 882.0, E920.8, E849.0, E013.9, 12004

Incorrect answer. The left ankle laceration was repaired with a layered closure, which constitutes an intermediate repair. It would not be added to the code for the simple closure. The E code that best describes the activity of the patient is E016.9, Other activity involving property and land maintenance, building and construction. An E code for external cause status is also required.

b. 891.1, 882.0, 12002, 12032-51

Incorrect answer. The repair of the wound of the left ankle, even though it required a layered closure, did not meet the criteria for a complex repair. External cause of injury codes (E codes) may be reported to show how the accident occurred and the place of occurrence for full reporting purposes. The E code that best describes the activity of the patient is E016.9, Other activity involving property and land maintenance, building and construction. An E code for external cause status is also required.

Because of the age of the patient, he is assumed to be a Medicare beneficiary, and an HCPCS Level II code, G0168, is used to report repairs using only tissue adhesive.

c. 894.0, 12032, 12002, supply code for the DERMABOND tissue adhesive

Incorrect answer. The use of the multiple open wound ICD-9-CM diagnosis code is incorrect when specified sites are documented. E codes may be reported to show how the accident occurred for full reporting purposes. The E code that best describes the activity of the patient is E016.9, Other activity involving property and land maintenance, building and construction. An E code for external cause status is also required. Because of the age of the patient, he is assumed to be a Medicare beneficiary, and an HCPCS Level II code, G0168, is used to report repairs using only tissue adhesive. The supply is included in this code.

d. 891.0, 882.0, E920.8, E849.0, E000.8, E013.9, 12032, 12002–51, G0168

Correct answer.

ICD-10-CM Code(s): S91.011A, S61.412A, S91.012A, W01.110A, Y92.019, Y93.h9, Y99.8

ICD-10-CM Rationale: The Alphabetic Index main term is Laceration, subterms ankle, hand. The Index to External Cause main term is Fall, subterms due to, falling, slipping, with subsequent striking against object, sharp object, glass. All injury codes will have a seventh character extension of A to indicate that this is the initial encounter. The main term is Place of occurrence, subterms residence, house, single family. Another main term is Activity, subterms maintenance, exterior building NEC. Another main term is External cause status.

9.41. a. 174.0, 19290, 19301

Incorrect answer. The diagnosis for this case is carcinoma in situ. All carcinoma in situ of the breast is coded to a single code of 233.0. Carcinoma in situ is a specific pathologic finding, which is different from the malignant variety of carcinoma. The lumpectomy is performed after preoperative radiologic marker placement and therefore code 19125 is assigned. The needle localization is completed by the radiologist and this service is not reported by the surgeon.

b. 174.9, 19290, 19125

Incorrect answer. The diagnosis for this case is carcinoma in situ. All carcinoma in situ of the breast is coded to a single code of 233.0. Carcinoma in situ is a specific pathologic finding, which is different from the malignant variety of carcinoma. The needle localization is completed by the radiologist and this service is not reported by the surgeon.

c. 233.0, 19125

Correct answer.

d. 233.0, 19301

Incorrect answer. The lumpectomy is performed after preoperative radiologic marker placement and therefore code 19125 is assigned.

ICD-10-CM Code(s): D05.11

ICD-10-CM Rationale: The Alphabetic Index main term is Neoplasm, subterm breast, "Ca in situ" column. The coder completes the code using the Tabular List.

9.42. a. 15220, 15221-51, 15002-51

Incorrect answer. Codes 15220 and 15221 are incorrect. These are the codes for a full-thickness graft, but the graft documented in this source document was a split-thickness graft. Also, code 15221 is an add-on code and is exempt from modifier -51 use.

b. 15100

Incorrect answer. The preparation of the burn site should also be coded with code 15002 with modifier -51, multiple procedure.

c. 14021, 15002-51

Incorrect answer. Code 14021 is used when a flap of tissue is advanced into the site of the defect but remains attached. This report documents a free graft.

d. 15100, 15002-51

Correct answer.

9.43.   a. 195.0, 15120

Incorrect answer. The neoplasm code is indexed under forehead, and 195.0 is not the most specific code possible. The excision of the lesion should also be coded per CPT guidelines.

b. 173.31, 15120, 11646

Correct answer. The excision of the lesion should also be coded per CPT guidelines.

c. 173.31, 15100, 11646

Incorrect answer. The split thickness autograft was performed on the forehead (face, scalp, eyelids, mouth, neck, ears, orbits, genitalia, hands, feet, or multiple digits, 15120) and not the thigh.

d. 195.0, 15004, 15120

Incorrect answer. The neoplasm code is indexed under forehead, and 195.0 is not the most specific code possible. It is not appropriate to assign code 15004 when an excision of a lesion is performed. The excision of the malignant lesion should be coded instead (11646).

ICD-10-CM Code(s): C44.39

ICD-10-CM Rationale: The Alphabetic Index main term Carcinoma directs the coder to see Neoplasm, skin, malignant. The coder selects subterm face under this site.

9.44.   a. 599.0, 682.5, 780.60, 493.90, 99214-25, 99143, 10061, 99000

Incorrect answer. The symptom of fever is not coded with an established diagnosis of an infective process. The incision and drainage of the abscess should be coded as 10060 because the abscess is not described as complicated and a drain is not left in the wound.

b. 599.0, 682.5, 780.61, 99215, 99143, 10061, 36415, 85025, 85009, 81001

Incorrect answer. The symptom of fever is not coded with an established diagnosis of an infective process. Code 780.61 is used to describe fever when present in conditions where fever establishes the severity of the condition. In this case, fever is integral to an infection and therefore not coded separately. The E/M code of 99215 is not supported by documentation. An encounter with a detailed history, comprehensive exam, and moderate decision making is coded as 99214. In this case, a procedure is performed in addition to a significant, separately identifiable E/M service and therefore a -25 modifier is necessary. The code for a manual differential, 85009, should not be used, as an automated differential is included in the CBC code, 85025.

c. 599.0, 682.2, 493.90, 99214, 99144, 10060, 99000, 36415, 85025, 81003

Incorrect answer. The abscess is of the buttock and not of the trunk; therefore, code 682.5 is correct. The E/M code is correct but requires the addition of a -25 modifier to show that a significant, separately identifiable E/M service was performed. The conscious sedation code should be 99143 because the physician performing the procedure did the conscious sedation with the assistance of a trained staff observer. The urinalysis code should be 81001 because the performance of a microscopy is documented.

d. 599.0, 682.5, 493.90, 99214-25, 99143, 10060, 99000, 36415, 85025, 81001

Correct answer.

ICD-10-CM Code(s): N39.0, L02.31, J45.909

ICD-10-CM Rationale: The Alphabetic Index main term is Infection, subterm urinary (tract). Another main term is Abscess, subterm buttock. The Alphabetic Index main term is Asthma.

9.45.   ICD-9-CM and CPT Code(s): 706.2, 11422

Rationale: No other E&M code can be used in this situation because there was no other significant service provided. The patient came in only for the removal of the cyst on the scalp.

ICD-10-CM Code(s): L72.9

ICD-10-CM Rationale: The Alphabetic Index main term is Cyst, subterm skin.

9.46.   a. 610.1, 289.3, 19120-RT, 38525-LT, 38500-LT

Correct answer.

b. 610.2, 130.9, 19120-RT, 38525-LT, 38500-LT

Incorrect answer. The toxoplasmosis was not confirmed. The diagnosis was fibrocystic disease of the breast and not fibroadenosis.

c. 610.2, 289.3, 19100-RT, 38525-LT

Incorrect answer. Code 19100 is incorrect as it describes an aspiration biopsy of the lump, not an excision. A code for the excision of the superficial nodes (38500) is needed.

d. 610.1, 289.3, 19101-RT, 38525-LT, 38500-LT

Incorrect answer. Code 19101 is used to report an open, incisional biopsy of the breast. In this situation, the lump was removed.

ICD-10-CM Code(s): N60.11, I88.9

ICD-10-CM Rationale: The Alphabetic Index main term is Fibrocystic with a note for the coder who is coding fibrocystic disease of the breast to see Mastopathy, cystic. Another main term is Lymphadenitis.

Behavioral Health Conditions

9.47.   a. 965.1, 780.4, 388.30, E950.0, 99284-25, 43753

Correct answer.

b. 965.1, 780.4, E980.0, 99284

Incorrect answer. Tinnitus is coded as 388.30. A suicide attempt is clearly documented in the source document, and code E950.0 is more appropriate than the undetermined code. The gastric tube insertion should also be coded.

c. 780.4, 388.30, E935.3, 99284-25, 43752

Incorrect answer. This would be the appropriate code assignment for an adverse effect of aspirin therapy. The poisoning code, 965.1, should be primary in this case and the manifestations secondary. The gastric tube insertion was done therapeutically and should be coded with code 43753. Modifier -25—significant, separately identifiable E/M service by same physician on same date of procedure or other service—is added to the E/M code.

d. 780.4, 388.30, 965.1, E935.3, 99284, 43752

Incorrect answer. The poisoning code, 965.1, should be the primary diagnosis and the manifestations secondary. The E code reported here reflects an adverse effect, and code E950.0 is more appropriate with the documented suicide attempt. The gastric tube insertion was done therapeutically and should be coded with code 43753. Modifier -25—significant, separately identifiable E/M service by same physician on same date of procedure or other service—is missing from the E/M code.

ICD-10-CM Code(s): T39.012A, R42, H93.13

ICD-10-CM Rationale: Using the Drug and Chemical Table, the code for Poisoning by aspirin, self-harm is T39.012A. The seventh character extension of A is assigned to indicate that this is the initial encounter. Manifestation is dizziness found at main term Dizziness and Tinnitus. The coder is directed to see subcategory H93.1.

9.48.   a. 303.00, 980.9, 99291, 99292

Incorrect answer. The poisoning code should be the primary diagnosis. Alcoholic beverages were specified, so the correct code is 980.0. There is no documentation of alcoholism in the patient, only acute alcohol intoxication. There is no mention of critical care being performed in the emergency department. An E code is needed for the external cause of injury (E860.0).

b. 980.9, 305.00, 99285-25, 12011

Incorrect answer. The laceration was closed with Steri-Strips, which is not coded as a laceration repair per the instructional note preceding code 12001. CPT guidelines state that a wound closure utilizing adhesive strips as the sole means of repair should be reported with an appropriate evaluation and management code. An E code is needed for the external cause of injury (E860.0).

c. 980.0, 305.00, 873.42, E860.0, 99285

Correct answer.

d. 980.0, 303.00, 99291, 12011

Incorrect answer. There is no documentation of alcoholism in the patient, only acute alcohol intoxication. There is no mention of critical care being performed in the emergency department. An E code is needed for the external cause of injury (E860.0). CPT guidelines state that a wound closure utilizing adhesive strips as the sole means of repair should be reported with an appropriate evaluation and management code.

ICD-10-CM Code(s): T51.0x1A, F10.129, S01.111A, R78.0, Y90.1

ICD-10-CM Rationale: The Alphabetic Index main term is the Table of Drugs and Chemicals, subterms alcohol, beverage. The code in the Poisoning, Accidental (unintentional) column is chosen. Another main term is Alcohol, subterm intoxication. The Alphabetic Index main term is Laceration, subterm eyebrow with a note to code to eyelid. The seventh character extension of A is assigned to the injury codes to indicate that this is the initial encounter. The main term is Finding, abnormal, inconclusive, without diagnosis, subterm alcohol and blood. There is a "Use additional code" for the alcohol level.

9.49. a. 307.1, 314.01, 301.83, 493.90, V17.0, 90801

Correct answer.

b. 301.1, 314.01, 301.83, 276.8, 493.90, 359.3, 90801

Incorrect answer. The hypokalemia is stated as "history of." There is no documented evidence that the patient is currently hypokalemic, so code 276.8 is not reported for this admission. The statement of hypokalemic periodic paralysis "per patient report" would not be reported unless confirmed by the attending physician. The family history of psychiatric conditions may also be reported (V17.0).

c. 307.1, 314.01, 301.83, 493.90, V17.0, 99223

Incorrect answer. This is a psychiatric diagnostic/evaluative interview, also known as an Initial Psychiatric Evaluation (IPE), rather than a hospital admission service. The appropriate code is 90801.

d. 301.1, 314.01, 301.83, 276.8, 493.90, 359.3, 99223

Incorrect answer. This is a psychiatric diagnostic/evaluative interview, also known as an Initial Psychiatric Evaluation (IPE), rather than a hospital admission service. The appropriate code is 90801. The hypokalemia is stated as "history of." There is no documented evidence that the patient is currently hypokalemic, so code 276.8 is not reported for this admission. The statement of hypokalemic periodic paralysis "per patient report" would not be reported unless confirmed by the attending physician. The family history of psychiatric conditions may also be reported (V17.0).

ICD-10-CM Code(s): F50.00, F90.9, F60.3, J45.909, Z81.8

ICD-10-CM Rationale: The Alphabetic Index main term is Anorexia, subterm nervosa. The Alphabetic Index main term for ADHD is Attention, subterm deficit disorder or syndrome, with hyperactivity. The coder is directed to see Disorder, subterm attention-deficit hyperactivity. Patient has borderline personality disorder. See main term Disorder, subterm personality, borderline. Patient has asthma. The Alphabetic Index main term is Asthma. The patient has a family history of mental disorder. The Alphabetic Index main term is History, family, mental disorder.

Disorders of the Musculoskeletal System and Connective Tissue

9.50.   a. 21365-LT

Incorrect answer. Code 21365 only covers the open reduction internal fixation of the comminuted tripod and zygomatic arch fractures. There is also a left lateral orbital wall fracture (21406) and a nasal fracture (21315). The endoscopic exam of the orbital floor with debridement also requires reporting of code 31237.

b. 21315-LT, 21365-LT

Incorrect answer. Code 21365 only covers the open reduction internal fixation of the comminuted tripod and zygomatic arch fractures. There is also a left lateral orbital wall fracture (21406). The endoscopic exam of the orbital floor with debridement also requires reporting of code 31237.

c. 21365-LT, 31292-LT

Incorrect answer. Code 21365 only covers the open reduction internal fixation of the comminuted tripod and zygomatic arch fractures. There is also a left lateral orbital wall fracture (21406) and a nasal fracture (21315). The endoscopic exam of the orbital floor does not involve decompression of an orbital fracture. It involves debridement, which is reported with code 31237.

d. 21315-LT, 21365-LT, 21406-LT, 31237-LT

Correct answer.

9.51.   a. 170.7, 27360, 27447, 35721, 27448, 76000

Incorrect answer. The resection of the femur tumor was considered radical resection because the entire proximal femur was removed. Code 27360 describes removal of small pieces of bone, not the entire proximal femur. Code 27445 describes the hinge prosthesis used in this case, rather than a total knee arthroplasty described in 27447. Fluoroscopy was used but the surgeon should correctly report the professional component only by appending modifier -26 to 76000.

b. 170.7, 27365, 27445, 35721, 27448-59, 76000-26

Correct answer.

c. 238.0, 27329, 27445, 27448-59, 76000-26

Incorrect answer. An osteosarcoma is a malignant bone tumor. The ICD-9-CM index directs the coder to the malignant column in the neoplasm table for code 170.7. CPT code 27329 describes the excision of a tumor of the soft tissue of the thigh or knee, not a bone tumor. Therefore, 27365 is the correct code. The femoral artery was explored during the procedure, and code 35721 must be reported to correctly describe the case.

d. 239.2, 27360, 27447, 27448, 76000

Incorrect answer. An osteosarcoma is a malignant bone tumor. The ICD-9-CM index directs the coder to the malignant column in the neoplasm table for code 170.7. The resection of the femur tumor was considered radical resection because the entire proximal femur was removed. Code 27360 describes removal of small pieces of bone, not the entire proximal femur. Code 27445 describes the hinge prosthesis used in this case, rather than a total knee arthroplasty described in 27447. Fluoroscopy was used but the surgeon should correctly report the professional component only by appending modifier -26 to 76000.

ICD-10-CM Code(s): C40.22

ICD-10-CM Rationale: The Alphabetic Index main term is Neoplasm, subterm bone, femur, malignant. The coder completes the code using the Tabular List.

9.52. a. 722.52, 401.9, 63047

Incorrect answer. The diagnosis code 722.52 reports degenerative disc disease rather than disc displacement. CPT code 63047 is used to report laminectomy, facetectomy, and foraminotomy, rather than the partial facetectomy documented in this source document.

b. 722.73, 401.9, 63030

Incorrect answer. Diagnosis code 722.72 is used to report disc disorder with myelopathy. Although there is disc encroachment upon the nerve root, there is no documentation of compression of the spinal cord, which is required to assign a "with myelopathy" code. The CPT code is correct.

c. 722.10, 63047

Incorrect answer. The ICD-9-CM diagnosis code is correct. CPT code 63047 is used to report laminectomy, facetectomy, and foraminotomy, rather than the partial facetectomy documented in this source document.

d. 722.10, 401.9, 63030

Correct answer.

ICD-10-CM Code(s): M51.27, I10

ICD-10-CM Rationale: The Alphabetic Index main term is Displacement, displaced, subterms intervertebral disc, lumbosacral region. Another main term is Hypertension.

9.53. ICD-9-CM First-Listed Diagnosis: 844.2

ICD-9-CM Additional Diagnoses: 836.1, 836.0

CPT Procedure Code(s): 29888-RT, 29880-RT-51

Rationale: It is appropriate to report code 29880 in addition to code 29888 since the meniscectomy is not considered an integral component of the anterior cruciate ligament repair/reconstruction. Modifier -51 should be appended to the secondary code to report multiple procedures were performed at the same session.

ICD-10-CM Code(s): S83.511A, S83.241A, S83.281A

ICD-10-CM Rationale: The Alphabetic Index main term is Sprain, subterm knee, cruciate ligament, anterior. The coder completes the code using the Tabular List. The Alphabetic Index main term is Tear, torn, subterm meniscus, medial, specified type NEC. The coder completes the code using the Tabular List. The Alphabetic Index main term is Tear, torn, subterm meniscus, lateral, specified type NEC. The coder completes the code using the Tabular List.

9.54. ICD-9-CM and CPT Code(s): 733.42, 733.49, 27130-RT

Rationale: The patient was noted to have avascular necrosis of the hip. Because there is no one ICD-9-CM diagnosis code to identify both components of the hip, two diagnosis codes are needed to identify the bones that comprise the hip (femur and acetabulum).

ICD-10-CM Code(s): M87.051

ICD-10-CM Rationale: The Alphabetic Index main term is Osteonecrosis, subterms idiopathic (aseptic), femur.

Neoplasms

9.55. a. 204.00, 996.62, 780.60, 99284-25, 96374

Incorrect answer. This patient has a central venous catheter. Infections of central venous catheters are coded as 999.31. Code 780.60 is not reported in this case because fever is integral to the infective process. The CPT code for the IV push is not reported as this service was provided by facility nursing staff. In addition, the CPT book states in the notes within this section that these codes are not to be reported by physicians in the facility setting. The -25 modifier is not appropriate because no physician-performed procedure was provided.

b. 204.00, 999.31, E878.2, 99284

Correct answer.

c. 208.00, 996.69, 780.61, 99285

Incorrect answer. Acute lymphocytic leukemia is coded as 204.00 by accessing the index under Leukemia, lymphocytic, and then the subterm of acute. This patient has a central venous catheter. Infections of central venous catheters are coded as 999.31. Code 996.69 is used to report an infection of an unspecific catheter. CPT code 99285 is incorrect because the documentation states that the medical decision making was moderate. This limits the emergency department code to 99284.

d. 208.00, 999.31, 99285-25, 96374

Incorrect answer. Acute lymphocytic leukemia is coded as 204.00 by accessing the index under Leukemia, lymphocytic, and then the subterm of acute. CPT code 99285 is incorrect because the documentation states that the medical decision making was moderate. This limits the emergency department code to 99284. The CPT code for the IV push is not reported as this service was provided by facility nursing staff. In addition, the CPT book states in the notes within this section that these codes are not to be reported by physicians in the facility setting. The -25 modifier is not appropriate because no physician-performed procedure was provided.

ICD-10-CM Code(s): C91.00, T82.7xxA, Y83.1

ICD-10-CM Rationale: The Alphabetic Index main term is Leukemia, leukemic, subterm acute lymphoblastic. The coder completes the code using the Tabular List. The Alphabetic Index main term for the infection is Complication, subterm vascular device or implant, infection or inflammation. The coder completes the code using the Tabular List. The seventh character extension of A is assigned to the complication code to indicate that this is the initial encounter. The Alphabetic Index main term for the cause of the infection is found in the Index to External Cause under Complications, implant, implantation, subterm artificial material or tissue which leads to code Y83.2. A review of the Tabular List, however, shows that Y83.1 is the better code.

9.56. a. 162.9, 32400, 77002

Incorrect answer. The diagnosis code may be further specified in location to the lower lobe with code 162.5. Also, the CPT code reported here reflects a pleural biopsy (surface area) rather than deeper into lung tissue as described. Code 32405 is the appropriate code to describe the procedure performed.

b. 786.09, 786.2, 32405

Incorrect answer. Symptoms are not reported when the etiology is established by the close of the visit. The CPT code is correct, but the coding professional should also add the code for fluoroscopic guidance for the procedure. This is reported with code 76003, which is not included in the code for the needle biopsy.

c. 162.5, 32405, 77002-26

Correct answer. The use of modifier -26 on the fluoroscopic guidance code is appropriate. This code is for the radiological supervision and interpretation only; however, it must be billed with a -26 to show the professional component; the facility bills the same code, 77002, with modifier -TC for technical component (owns the equipment).

d. 162.5, 786.09, 786.2, 32405, 77002-26

Incorrect answer. Symptoms are not reported when the etiology is established by the close of the visit. The remainder of the codes are correct.

ICD-10-CM Code(s): C34.32

ICD-10-CM Rationale: The subterm in the Neoplasm Table is lung.

9.57.   a. 197.3, 199.1, 796.2, 31576, 99144

Correct answer. Because the primary site has not been established, diagnosis code 199.1 may be reported following the code for the confirmed metastatic disease. Though the procedure was discontinued, the planned procedure was carried out, so no modifier is necessary.

b. 161.8, 198.89, 401.9, 31510

Incorrect answer. The pathology report indicates that the laryngeal malignancy is metastatic. If the malignancy were primary to the larynx, this would be the correct diagnosis code. Hypertension cannot be coded on the basis of an elevation of blood pressure, so code 796.2 is assigned to reflect that complication. Code 197.3 is the only code that can be assigned because the esophageal primary has yet to be confirmed. Because the primary site has not been established, diagnosis code 199.1 may be reported following the code for the confirmed metastatic disease. Code 198.89 is not the correct code for thyroid cartilage, which is an anatomic portion of the larynx. Code 197.3 is assigned for metastatic disease in this location. The CPT code is for an indirect laryngoscopy with biopsy rather than the flexible fiberoptic procedure described. Code 31576 is the correct code. IV sedation was administered by the physician and code 31576 does not include moderate (conscious) sedation; therefore, code 99144 is reported for IV sedation.

c. 150.9, 197.3, 197.3, 197.3, 197.3, 997.1, 31576-53

Incorrect answer. Because the primary site has not been confirmed, it is not appropriate to assign the code for primary carcinoma of the esophagus. The metastatic disease would not be coded multiple times for the various sites because ICD-9-CM is a classification system. The correct reporting is 197.3, 199.1, and 796.2 to report the increased blood pressure episode. Code 997.1 is inappropriate in this circumstance because neither the diagnosis of hypertension nor a cause-and-effect relationship between the procedure and the elevated blood pressure reading has been documented. Modifier -53 is not needed for the procedure code because the laryngoscopy and biopsies had been accomplished before the procedure was discontinued. IV sedation was administered by the physician and code 31576 does not include moderate (conscious) sedation; therefore, code 99144 is reported for IV sedation.

d. 150.9, 161.8, 796.2, 31576, 99144, 99145

Incorrect answer. It is rarely appropriate to assign two codes for primary neoplasm in the same case; it would never be appropriate without physician documentation that two primary sites with different morphology were present. In this case, the laryngeal malignancy is stated to be metastatic, with a suspected primary in the esophagus. Because this is an outpatient case, we cannot code any diagnosis that is not confirmed. And in any event, physician-reporting guidelines preclude reporting unconfirmed diagnoses in any setting. The correct diagnosis codes, in addition to the elevated blood pressure reading, are 197.3 and 199.1 for the unknown primary. IV sedation was administered by the physician for 16 minutes and code 99144 includes the first 30 minutes; therefore, code 99145 (each additional 15 minutes) is not reportable based on the documentation.

ICD-10-CM Code(s): C78.39, C80.1, R03.0

ICD-10-CM Rationale: The Alphabetic Index main term is Neoplasm, subterm larynx. The subterms for cartilage (including arytenoid, cricoid, and thyroid) and extrinsic larynx all lead the coder to C78.39. The Malignant Secondary column is used. For the unknown primary, the coder should go to Neoplasm, unknown site or unspecified, Malignant Primary. The Alphabetic Index main term for the increase in blood pressure is High, subterm blood pressure, incidental without diagnosis of hypertension.

9.58. a. 153.2, 45384

Incorrect answer. The procedures involve different sites and have different diagnosis codes. The modified code 45380-59 is assigned to show that separate sites were involved in this case. Code 211.3 should also be reported.

b. 153.2, 211.3, 45384, 45380-59

Correct answer. Modifier -59 is required to show that the biopsy and the polypectomy were performed at different sites.

c. V67.09, V10.05, 153.2, G0105, 45384-59

Incorrect answer. Medicare requires that specific HCPCS Level II codes be used to report screening colonoscopy in a high-risk patient, but the codes are used only when no recurrence of disease is found or no procedure is carried out beyond the description of code 45378. The V code for the reason for visit is also incorrect because a recurrence of the primary neoplasm at the same site is documented, which is assigned the code for the malignancy rather than the V code.

d. 153.9, V10.05, V45.89, 45384, 45380

Incorrect answer. There is more definitive location information available, so code 153.2 may be assigned instead of the unspecified code. The "history of" V code is not assigned as an additional code, but it is assigned in a case where the malignancy has been surgically removed and has not recurred. Addition of the V45.89 code does not add any information, so it is not recommended. The CPT codes are not completely correct because it is appropriate to code both a biopsy and a polypectomy when different sites are involved. To show the payer that these are different sites, modifier -59 should be appended to the lesser procedure (the biopsy).

ICD-10-CM Code(s): C18.6, D12.5

ICD-10-CM Rationale: The subterm in the Neoplasm Table is colon; select a code in the Malignant Primary column and also check other subcategory codes for descending colon. Another main term is Polyp, polypus, subterms colon, sigmoid.

9.59.   a. 170.4, 23182

Incorrect answer. The ICD-9-CM index under osteochondroma directs the coder to See Neoplasm, bone, benign. Therefore, 213.4 is the correct diagnosis code. CPT code 23140 correctly describes the removal of a benign tumor from the scapula.

b. 170.4, 23190

Incorrect answer. The ICD-9-CM index under osteochondroma directs the coder to See Neoplasm, bone, benign. Therefore, 213.4 is the correct diagnosis code. CPT code 23140 correctly describes the removal of a benign tumor from the scapula.

c. 213.4, 23140

Correct answer.

d. 213.4, 23190

Incorrect answer. CPT code 23140 correctly describes the removal of a benign tumor from the scapula.

ICD-10-CM Code(s): D16.01

ICD-10-CM Rationale: The Alphabetic Index main term is Osteochondroma. The coder is directed to see Neoplasm, bone, benign. The Alphabetic Index main term is Neoplasm, subterms bone, scapula, Benign column. The coder completes the code using the Tabular List.

9.60.   a. 199.0, 153.9, 36561, 36556-59

Incorrect answer. Two procedures were actually performed, although the left subclavian VAD placement was aborted before completion. Due to the limited aborted procedure documentation, a physician query is required to determine if the left subclavian vein catheter insertion was nontunneled in order to meet the criteria for code 36556. The venipuncture should be reported with modifier -59 to show that code 36410 is a separate procedure at a different site.

b. 153.9, 36563, 36410-53

Incorrect answer. The disseminated disease should be coded as 199.0, although the sequencing is probably not significant because the reason for the visit is the insertion of the port. The CPT codes must reflect the insertion of the port in the right subclavian, as well as the cannulation of the left subclavian. The code 36563 is for an infusion pump, not a VAD with a port. Modifier -59 is assigned rather than -53 to report that code 36410 is a separate procedure at a different site rather than a discontinued procedure.

c. 199.0, 153.9, 36561, 36410-59

Correct answer. The physician would only report fluoroscopy if he had utilized his own equipment. This procedure is performed at the hospital, so the hospital will report the imaging guidance (likely 77002). Due to the limited aborted procedure documentation, a physician query is required to determine if the left subclavian vein catheter insertion was nontunneled in order to meet the criteria for code 36556.

d. V58.81, 199.0, 153.9, 36561, 12031

Incorrect answer. The code V58.81 is used for removal or replacement of a catheter. The neoplasm is sequenced first when the reason for the visit is initial insertion. The catheterization of the left subclavian may also be reported as 36556-59, with the modifier showing that it was not a component of the VAD procedure but involved a different site. Layered closure (12031) is included in code 36561 and would not be reported separately. The venipuncture should be reported with modifier -59 to show that code 36410 is a separate procedure at a different site.

ICD-10-CM Code(s): C79.9, C18.9

ICD-10-CM Rationale: The subterm in the Neoplasm Table is colon and the code from the Malignant Primary column is used for the primary site. The subterm for the metastatic sites in the Neoplasm Table is unknown site or unspecified.

9.61.   a. 172.7

Correct answer.

b. 232.7

Incorrect answer. This is a melanoma, which is classified to category 172.

c. 232.7, 172.7

Incorrect answer. Only one code for the melanoma is necessary. Code category 172 is for melanoma of the skin, which is the most specific code for this patient.

d. 172.7, 709.9

Incorrect answer. The skin lesion was identified as melanoma. Only a code from category 172 is necessary.

ICD-10-CM Code(s): D03.72

ICD-10-CM Rationale: The Alphabetic Index main term is Melanoma, subterm in situ, leg. The coder completes the code using the Tabular List.

Disorders of the Nervous System and Sense Organs

9.62.   a. 438.11, 438.81, 99203, 96105

Incorrect answer. The evaluation and management service described is a consultation and should be reported with code 99243-25.

b. 784.3, 784.69, 99244

Incorrect answer. When neurological problems remain following a CVA, a code from the late effects section of ICD-9-CM is used. In this case, codes 438.11 and 438.81 are used to reflect the aphasia and apraxia. The consultation code is one level too high, based upon documentation of history, physical examination, and medical decision making; it should be 99243, based upon the low-complexity medical decision making. Modifier -25 is added to show that an assessment reported with code 96105 was also provided on the same date in addition to the evaluation and management service.

c. 438.81, 99243

Incorrect answer. There are actually two residual conditions present that warrant coding: the aphasia and the apraxia. Code 438.11 should be assigned in addition to 438.81. The clinic service described is a consultation service, with an additional neurocognitive test performed, reported with code 96105. Modifier -25 may be helpful with code 99243 for the evaluation and management service to show that both services were provided and are separately identifiable.

d. 438.11, 438.81, 99243-25, 96105

Correct answer.

ICD-10-CM Code(s): I69.320, I69.390

ICD-10-CM Rationale: The Alphabetic Index main term is Sequelae (of) with subterms infarction, cerebral, aphasia and apraxia.

9.63.   a. 437.3, 61700

Incorrect answer. Because of the term "microdissection," the code for use of the operating microscope should be assigned. Additional codes should be reported to reflect the postoperative pneumonia, which would be codes 997.3 and 482.1.

b. 430, 482.1, 61700, 69990-51

Incorrect answer. Code 69990 is exempt from modifier -51 use because the + symbol in the CPT manual signifies an add-on code. Such procedures are never reported alone, so modifier -51 is not used. The aneurysm is not described as ruptured, so code 437.3 is the appropriate code. To show that the pneumonia was documented as due to the surgery, code 997.3 should also be reported.

c. 437.3, 997.3, 482.1, 61700, 69990

Correct answer.

d. 747.81, 997.3, 61703, 69990

Incorrect answer. The procedure code is incorrect. Code 61700 correctly describes the procedure performed. Even though the patient is 35 years old, we cannot presume that the aneurysm is congenital. Code 437.3 is correct with this documentation. Code 997.3 identifies that the pneumonia was due to the procedure, but an additional code of 482.1 should be reported to show the organism (Pseudomonas) responsible.

ICD-10-CM Code(s): I67.1, J95.89, J15.1

ICD-10-CM Rationale: The Alphabetic Index main term is Aneurysm, subterm brain. The post-op pneumonia is found at Complication, subterm post-procedural, specified, respiratory system. The coder is directed to code the specific condition. The Alphabetic Index main term is Pneumonia, subterm Pseudomonas.

9.64. a. 333.1, 728.9, 99244-25, 95925, 95927-51

Correct answer. The modifier -25 may or may not be required to show that both an evaluation and management service and a diagnostic procedure were performed at the same time, depending upon payer reporting requirements. For codes 95925 and 95927, care should be taken to report exactly what the physician does. The use of the -26 or -TC modifiers may be indicated if only the supervision or only the equipment were provided. For a unilateral procedure, use the -52 modifier. Code 95920 may also be reported, if documented.

b. 340, 99245-25, 95927

Incorrect answer. For physician reporting, a diagnosis qualified as "rule out" cannot be assigned a definitive code. The symptoms prompting the service are reported instead: 333.1 for intention tremor, and 728.9 for muscle weakness. An additional CPT code should be reported for the testing on the upper limbs (95925). The evaluation and management consultation code may not be higher than level 4 when moderate medical decision making is documented. Code 99245 requires complex medical decision making.

c. 333.1, 728.9, 99204, 95925, 95927-51

Incorrect answer. Consultation services are assigned to a different category of the evaluation and management section of CPT. Modifier -25 may or may not be required to show that both an evaluation and management service and a diagnostic procedure were performed at the same time, depending upon payer reporting requirements.

d. 728.9, 781.0, 99244-25, 95927

Incorrect answer. The ICD-9-CM code for intention tremor has a code from the nervous system chapter (333.1). Tremor NOS would be assigned the symptom code 781.0. Procedure codes are required for both EMG tests (95925 and 95927).

ICD-10-CM Code(s): G25.2, M62.81

ICD-10-CM Rationale: The Alphabetic Index main term is Tremor(s), subterm intention. Another main term is Weak, weakening, weakness, subterm muscle.

9.65. a. 64449

Incorrect answer. Code 64449 is for continuous administration of a local anesthetic agent through a catheter, not a single injection by a needle approach.

b. 62319

Incorrect answer. Code 62319 is for continuous infusion through a catheter, not a single injection by a needle approach.

c. 62311

Correct answer. A caudal injection is in the lumbosacral region.

d. 62311, 77003

Incorrect answer. Fluoroscopy was not mentioned in this case, so it is not appropriate to report this code. Because many such procedures are performed under fluoroscopy, it may be appropriate to query the physician about this. Also, the physician would only report fluoroscopy if he had utilized his own equipment. This procedure was performed at the hospital, so the hospital would report the fluoroscopy.

9.66.　a. 387.9, 997.1, 427.31, 69661-LT

Correct answer. Medicare probably does not cover this patient, but it is possible. If the payer allows the reporting of HCPCS Level II modifiers, the -LT will indicate which side had surgery. If the payer does not allow the use of the modifier -LT, it should be deleted.

b. 387.9, 69661-LT

Incorrect answer. The patient was admitted to the hospital after the procedure, and the postoperative atrial fibrillation should be reported. Even though the cardiologist will follow the patient, these codes should also be reported to show why the patient was admitted to the hospital and why any additional evaluation and management codes will be submitted for the stay.

c. 387.9, 427.31, 69661-LT

Incorrect answer. Because the physician documented that the atrial fibrillation was due to the surgery, code 997.1 should also be assigned, followed by the 427.31.

d. 387.9, 69660-LT

Incorrect answer. According to the documentation, the footplate was drilled out. Code 69661 is correct for reporting this procedure. The complications requiring admission to the hospital should also be reported.

ICD-10-CM Code(s): H80.92, I97.89, I48.0

ICD-10-CM Rationale: The Alphabetic Index main term is Otosclerosis. Another main term is Complication, subterms circulatory system, postprocedural. Another main term is Fibrillation, subterm atrial or auricular.

9.67.　a. 366.1, 401.9, 496, V15.81, 66984-RT

Incorrect answer. Code 366.1 is incorrect as there is no indication that this is a "senile" cataract.

b. 366.9, 401.9, 496, V15.81, 66984-RT

Correct answer.

c. 366.9, 401.9, 496, V15.81, 66985-RT

Incorrect answer. Code 66985 is correct to use because this is for a cataract extraction without placement of a prosthetic lens. Code 66984 includes the placement of the lens.

d. 366.9, 401.9, 496, 66984-50

Incorrect answer. The cataract extraction was not a bilateral procedure; therefore the modifier -50 is incorrect to use in this situation. Only the right eye was operated on.

ICD-10-CM Code(s): H26.9, I10, J44.9, Z91.14, T46.5x6A

ICD-10-CM Rationale: The Alphabetic Index main term is Cataracts. The Alphabetic Index main term is Hypertension. The Alphabetic Index main term is Disease, diseased, subterm pulmonary, chronic obstructive. The Alphabetic Index main term is Noncompliance, subterm with medication regimen. The coder is directed to code the underdosing of medication. The Drug and Chemical Table is used to review Antihypertensive drug, NEC, Underdosing column. The seventh character extension of A is assigned to indicate that this is the initial encounter.

Newborn/Congenital Disorders

9.68. a. 99460, 99462, 99238

Incorrect answer. The physician's attendance at delivery on 11/20 with initial care to the newborn should also be reported with code 99464.

b. 99460, 99464, 99462, 99238

Correct answer.

c. 99460, 99360, 99233, 99238

Incorrect answer. Physician standby (99360) is reported for prolonged attendance without direct patient contact. In this case, the physician did provide the initial care to the newborn. Code 99464 is reported. Also, subsequent hospital care is reported for the normal newborn (99462) rather than the usual hospital inpatient care (99233).

d. 99464, 99232, 99238

Incorrect answer. Code 99464 is correct; however, 99460 should also be reported on 11/20 because the physician initiated the newborn's diagnostic and treatment plan on that date. Also, subsequent hospital care is reported for the normal newborn (99462) rather than the usual inpatient hospital care (99232).

9.69. a. 381.01, 462, 758.0, V45.89, 99214, 96372, J0561

Correct answer.

b. V20.2, 381.01, 462, 758.0, V45.89, 99392, 99214-25

Incorrect answer. Although the chief complaint in this note indicates routine or "preventative" service, there are symptoms and problems indicated in the history of present illness that actually precipitated the visit. Also, CPT instructions state that when less than the code description for preventative care is provided, the usual evaluation and management codes are reported. With a detailed history and physical examination and moderate-level medical decision making (for example, medication management and review of records), code 99214 may be supported. Without the 99392 code, no modifier is needed. The administration of the injection should be reported with the appropriate materials code. This may be J0561 if the payer accepts HCPCS Level II codes, or 99070 in CPT. Code 96372 may be bundled with the evaluation and management code but is appropriately assigned when performed. Because this is not a "well-child" visit, code V20.2 is not appropriate to report. Reporting both services together would be reserved for an instance in which a preventative examination is scheduled for an asymptomatic patient, and, in the course of the evaluation, a condition is identified that requires significant and separately identifiable physician work that is performed for the identified condition, in addition to completion of the components of the preventative service. In that case, the V code is listed first, followed by the identified condition, and both evaluation and management services are reported, with the preventative service reported first and modifier -25 on the office visit code.

c. 381.01, 462, 99214, 96372

Incorrect answer. The Down syndrome code is important to report because the physician did evaluate development and spent part of the visit counseling the mother about the condition. The code for the ventricular septal defect may not be coded for this visit because it was not evaluated and did not affect management. Code V45.89 could be reported to show that the child was status post surgery. It is important for physician office reporting to capture all services including drugs. Third-party payers differ in their policies of accepting HCPCS Level II codes (J0530 in this case), and some might expect CPT code 99070 to be reported, with a description of the drug injected.

d. 758.0, V45.89, 99213, J0561

Incorrect answer. The child presented with symptoms of otitis media and was also followed for developmental and other health concerns surrounding Down syndrome and the cardiac surgery required for repair of the ventricular septal defect. The otitis media (381.01) and sore throat (462) codes are reported as the reason for visit and to explain the need for antibiotic administration. This should also be reported with CPT code 96372, even though some payers will bundle this service into the evaluation and management code and not allow separate reimbursement. The code for Down syndrome (758.0) and status post surgery (V45.89) should also be reported. The evaluation and management value is one level too low because a detailed history, physical examination, and moderate-level medical decision making are documented, which would allow reporting of 99214.

ICD-10-CM Code(s): H65.193, J02.9, Q90.9, Z87.74, Z98.89

ICD-10-CM Rationale: The Alphabetic Index main term is Otitis, subterm media, nonsuppurative, acute. The coder completes the code using the Tabular List. The Alphabetic Index main term Sore, subterm throat directs the coder to "See also Pharyngitis." The Alphabetic Index main term is Pharyngitis. Patient has Down Syndrome; refer to the Alphabetic Index main term Down Syndrome. The Alphabetic Index main term is History, subterms personal (of), congenital malformation, heart (corrected). The Alphabetic Index main term is History, subterm personal (of), surgery NEC.

9.70. a. 749.04, 42225, 42825

Incorrect answer. It would be important to assign code 474.00 as the reason for the tonsillectomy. The physician would add modifier -51 to the tonsillectomy code to reflect multiple procedures at the same operative session.

b. 749.04, 474.00, 42225

Incorrect answer. The tonsillectomy, although "incidental," is reported with CPT code 42825. See *CPT Assistant* (1997, August). The physician would add modifier -51 to the tonsillectomy code to reflect multiple procedures at the same operative session.

c. 749.04, 474.00, 42225, 42825-51

Correct answer.

d. V50.8, 749.04, 474.00, 42200, 42826-51

Incorrect answer. A diagnosis code from the V50 category is used only to report services where there is no medical necessity for a procedure, but a cosmetic or other elective benefit, such as an encounter for circumcision. Revision palatoplasty procedures have specific codes, and in this case code 42225 is the correct code because a pharyngeal flap was employed. A tonsillectomy would not be an integral part of a palatoplasty and is always reported separately; however, the appropriate code is 42825 because the patient is 10 years old. See *CPT Assistant* (1997, August).

ICD-10-CM Code(s): Q35.3, J35.01

ICD-10-CM Rationale: The Alphabetic Index main term is Cleft, subterm palate. The code Q35.3 represents the soft palate so this code should be chosen. Another main term is Tonsillitis, subterm chronic.

9.71. a. 536.49, 079.99, 530.81, 49440

Incorrect answer. No complication of the gastrostomy is documented. The child pulled the tube out, which is not a complication. Attention to the G tube should have been reported as V55.1. Congenital cytomegalovirus infection is coded as 771.1 and not a nonspecific viral infection code. The code is located in the index under Infection, then Congenital and then cytomegalovirus. This condition will affect the child for his entire life and can be coded even though he is no longer a newborn. Erosion of the esophagus should be coded as 530.89 because this is a complication of gastroesophageal reflux disease, not a symptom. The CPT code should be 49450 to report a replacement of a G tube. Even though the physician did not remove the G tube, the tube is replaced using the same gastrostomy site. See *CPT 2008 Changes: An Insider's View* for the description of this procedure.

b. 536.41, 771.1, 530.81, 530.89, 43760, 76000-26

Incorrect answer. No infection of the gastrostomy is documented. The congenital cytomegalovirus infection is not a localized infection of the

G tube site. Attention to the G tube should have been reported as V55.1. The CPT code should be 49450 to report a replacement of a G tube. Even though the physician did not remove the G tube, the tube is replaced using the same gastrostomy site. See *CPT 2008 Changes: An Insider's View* for the description of this procedure. Fluoroscopic guidance is included in code 49450.

c. V55.1, 530.81, 530.89, 771.1, 49450

Correct answer.

d. V55.1, 530.81, 079.99, 49450, 76000-26

Incorrect answer. Congenital cytomegalovirus infection is coded as 771.1 and not a nonspecific viral infection code. The code is located in the index under Infection, then Congenital and then cytomegalovirus. This condition will affect the child for his entire life and can be coded even though he is no longer a newborn. Erosion of the esophagus should be coded as 530.89 because this is a complication of gastroesophageal reflux disease, not a symptom. The CPT code is correct; however, fluoroscopic guidance is included in code 49450.

ICD-10-CM Code(s): Z43.1, K21.9, K22.10, P35.1

ICD-10-CM Rationale: The Alphabetic Index main term is Attention (to), subterm gastrostomy. The Alphabetic Index main term is Disease, diseased, subterm gastroesophageal. The main term is Erosion, subterm esophagus. The congenital CMV is found under main term Infection, subterm cytomegalovirus, congenital.

Pediatric Conditions

9.72.   a. 99281-25, 31505

Correct answer.

b. 99281-25, 31511

Incorrect answer. The removal of the foreign body could not be completed by the ED physician. The diagnostic scope was completed, so this code would be reported instead.

c. 99282, 31505

Incorrect answer. All three elements of history, physical examination, and medical decision making must be met or exceeded to assign an emergency department code. The documentation met a level 1 (99281) on the basis of a problem-focused physical examination. A -25 modifier should be added to the evaluation and management code.

d. 99281, 31511

Incorrect answer. The removal of the foreign body could not be completed. The diagnostic scope was completed, so this code would be reported instead. A -25 modifier should be added to the evaluation and management code.

9.73. a. 770.83, 079.6, 933.1, E911, 99284

Incorrect answer. This infant is not a newborn. The newborn period extends through the 28th day of life. RSV infection (079.6) and Asphyxia by aspiration (933.1) cannot be coded as they are documented as "rule out" conditions. Documentation for this case supports a level 99285 because the history is comprehensive, the exam is comprehensive, and the medical decision making is high (new problem with risk to life or bodily function).

b. 782.5, 786.03, 799.82, 99285

Correct answer. The tabular instructs the coder to use additional code(s) for associated signs and symptoms.

c. 799.82, 99285

Incorrect answer. The CPT code is correct. The ALTE code is correct; however, the tabular instructs the coder to use additional code(s) for associated signs and symptoms. This means that cyanosis and apnea must also be coded.

d. 782.5, 799.82, 99291

Incorrect answer. Cyanosis and ALTE are correct, but the symptom of apnea must also be coded. Critical care is not provided or documented in this case, and the documentation supports a 99285 service.

ICD-10-CM Code(s): R23.0, R06.81, R68.13

ICD-10-CM Rationale: The Alphabetic Index main term is Cyanosis. The Alphabetic Index main term is Apnea. The code for ALTE is found at Event, subterm apparent life threatening in newborn and infant.

9.74. a. 3/31: 813.43, 25600, A4580

4/1: 813.43, 840.9, 99024

4/2: 813.44, 99024, A4580

Incorrect answer. The cast application on 3/31 was for the purpose of pain management. Restorative treatment had not been determined at that point. Code 29075 is reported for the 3/31 services. The global period had not yet begun, so 99024 is not applied on 4/1. The visit on 4/1 was for treatment of a complication, and the office visit can be reported (99213). The global fracture treatment (25600) begins on 4/2. At this point, restorative treatment is done and a treatment plan is established.

b. 3/31: 813.43, 29075, A4580

4/1: 840.9, 813.43, 99213

4/2: 813.44, 25600, A4580

Correct answer.

c. 3/31: 813.43, 25605, A4580

4/1: 840.9, 813.43, 99213

4/2: 813.44, 29075, A4580

Incorrect answer. The cast application on 3/31 was for the purpose of pain management. Restorative treatment had not been determined at that point. Code 29075 is reported for the 3/31 service. Coding for 4/1 is correct. The global fracture treatment (25600) begins on 4/2. At this point, restorative treatment is done and a treatment plan is established. Code 25600 is the appropriate code because no manipulation (reduction) was done.

    d. 3/31: 813.43, 29075, A4580

        4/1: 840.9, 813.43, 99213

        4/2: 813.44, 25605, A4580

Incorrect answer. The fracture treatment on 4/2 did not include manipulation. Code 25600 is the appropriate code.

ICD-10-CM Code(s): 3/31: S52.615A

ICD-10-CM Rationale: 3/31: The Alphabetic Index main term is Fracture, subterms ulna, lower end.

ICD-10-CM Code(s): 4/1: S46.912D, S52.615D

ICD-10-CM Rationale: The Alphabetic Index main term Tear, torn, subterm muscle refers the coder to main term Strain. The coder is now referred to Injury, muscle, by site, strain. The coder therefore codes main term Injury, subterms arm (referred to shoulder), strain. The same fracture site is coded but the coder needs to use the seventh character "D" to represent the subsequent encounter.

ICD-10-CM Code(s): 4/2: S52.532A, S52.612D

ICD-10-CM Rationale: The Alphabetic Index main term is Fracture, subterms ulna, lower end, styloid pressure, displaced.

9.75.   a. 475, 474.00, 075, 250.01, 99239

Correct answer.

    b. 475, 474.00, 075, 250.81, 99238

Incorrect answer. Hypoglycemia is mentioned in evaluating the laboratory values; however, no definitive diagnosis is documented. The correct code for diabetes is 250.01. The discharge code 99239 would be reported because the physician has documented more than 30 minutes spent in discharging the patient.

    c. 475, 075, 250.01, 99238

Incorrect answer. The chronic tonsillitis is specifically excluded from code 475 and is reported separately with code 474.00. The discharge code 99239 would be reported because the physician has documented more than 30 minutes spent in discharging the patient.

    d. 475, 474.0, 075, 250.81, 99239

Incorrect answer. The correct diagnosis code is 474.00. Hypoglycemia is mentioned in evaluating the laboratory values; however, no definitive diagnosis is documented. The correct code for diabetes is 250.01.

ICD-10-CM Code(s): J35.01, B27.90, E10.9

ICD-10-CM Rationale: The Alphabetic Index main term is Abscess, subterm peritonsillar. The chronic tonsillitis is coded to J35.01, as the excludes directs. The mononucleosis is found at main term Mononucleosis, infectious. The DM code is found at main term Diabetes, diabetic, subterm type 1.

Conditions of Pregnancy, Childbirth, and the Puerperium

9.76.   a. 667.02, 670.02, 664.31, 663.31, V27.0; 648.22, 280.0, 59400, 59160-78

Correct answer.

b. 667.04, 670.02, 664.31, 663.31, V27.0; 648.22, 280.0, 59400, 59300-51, 58120-78

Incorrect answer. The patient delivered during this admission, so a fifth digit of 1 or 2 must be used on the pregnancy codes. Code 667.02 is correct because this is a postpartum complication. The episiotomy and repair are not separately reported. A postpartum curettage is coded 59160.

c. 667.02, 664.31, 663.31, V27.0; 59400, 59300, 59160

Incorrect answer. The endometriosis should be coded. The episiotomy and repair are not separately reported. Modifier -78 should be appended to 59160.

d. 667.04, 670.02, 664.31, V27.0; 59400, 58120

Incorrect answer. The patient delivered during this admission, so a fifth digit of 1 or 2 must be used. Code 667.02 is correct. The documentation also states that there was a nuchal cord. A postpartum curettage is coded 59160, and modifier -78 should be appended.

ICD-10-CM Code(s): O72.2, O99.214, E66.9, O86.12, O70.3, O69.81x0, O90.81, Z37.0

ICD-10-CM Rationale: The Alphabetic Index main term is Delivery, subterms complicated by, retention of secundines, partial. Another subterm under Delivery, complicated by, is obesity. There is a "Use additional code" to identify the type of obesity (E66.9). Another main term is Endometritis, subterm puerperal, postpartum, childbirth. Another main term is Laceration, subterms perineum, female, during delivery, fourth degree. The Alphabetic Index main term is Delivery, subterms complicated by cord (umbilical), around neck, without compression. A seventh character extension of "0" is assigned to represent that this was a single gestation. The main term is Pregnancy, subterms complicated by anemia, postpartum. Main term is Outcome of delivery, subterm single NEC, liveborn.

9.77.   a. 632, 493.90, 59820, 59200-51

Incorrect answer. The excludes note at code 632 directs the coding professional to use either 630 or 631 when there is an abnormal product of conception. This anembryonic gestation would be coded as 631. Procedure codes for the insertion of laminaria would not be reported because that procedure was done prior to this episode of care.

b. 630, 493.90, 59870

Incorrect answer. Although the pathology report shows chorionic villi, which would be consistent with a molar pregnancy, code 630 should not be assigned without the physician's diagnosis. With the diagnosis of anembryonic gestation, code 631 is the correct code. CPT coding guidelines state that if the molar pregnancy is unspecified, code 59820 for treatment of missed abortion is reported. See *CPT Assistant* (1999, February).

c. 631, 59856, 59200

Incorrect answer. Diagnosis code 631 is correct. The asthma should also be reported (493.90). This is not an induced abortion but, rather, treatment for a missed abortion (59820). Procedure codes for the insertion of laminaria would not be reported because that procedure was done prior to this episode of care.

d. 631, 493.90, 59820

Correct answer.

ICD-10-CM Code(s): O02.8, J45.909

ICD-10-CM Rationale: The Alphabetic Index main term is Abnormal, subterm product of conception, specified type. To code the asthma, the coder refers to main term Asthma.

Disorders of the Respiratory System

9.78.   a. 491.21, 518.82, 99214

Incorrect answer. Acute respiratory insufficiency is an integral part of COPD and is not coded separately.

b. 518.81, 491.21, 99213

Incorrect answer. The patient had acute respiratory insufficiency, not acute respiratory failure. Acute respiratory insufficiency is an integral part of COPD and is not coded separately. Because this is an established patient, only two out of three of the components of history, physical examination, and medical decision making must be met to assign an evaluation and management level code. Code 99214 is correct.

c. 518.82, 491.21, 99203

Incorrect answer. Acute respiratory insufficiency is an integral part of COPD and is not coded separately. The CPT code for a new patient visit is incorrect because the patient has been seen many times by this practitioner for this condition.

d. 491.21, 99214

Correct answer.

ICD-10-CM Code(s): J44.1

ICD-10-CM Rationale: The Alphabetic Index main term is Disease, subterms lung, obstructive (chronic), with, acute, exacerbation.

9.79.   a. 473.8, 471.8, 349.81, 31201-50, 31051-50, 31020-50

Correct answer. The excision of the uncinate process is a component of the sinus surgeries and would not be separately reported.

b. 473.8, 471.8, 998.2, E870.0, E849.7, 31201-50, 31051-50, 31020-50

Incorrect answer. The complication code is not appropriate in this case because the surgeon indicated that no instruments were used in this area. The coding professional should not assume that a condition is a "complication" of a procedure. Refer to *Coding Clinic* (1990, 3Q and 1992, 2Q) for more information on coding complications. The cerebrospinal fluid leak is then coded to 349.81.

c. 478.19, 473.8, 31267-50, 31288-50, 31254-50

Incorrect answer. The approach for the procedures is intranasal and not endoscopic, so the CPT codes are incorrect. An additional diagnosis code is assigned for the CSF leak (349.81). Code 471.8 is the appropriate code for polyposis of the sinuses rather than 478.19.

d. 473.8, 471.8, 998.11, 998.2, E870.0, E849.7, 31090-50

Incorrect answer. Neither the CSF leak nor the blood loss should be coded as surgical complications. The surgeon indicated that no instrumentation was used in this area of the CSF leak, and there was no documentation to indicate that the moderate bleeding complicated the surgical procedure. The CPT code used is for a unilateral sinusotomy involving three or more sinuses. Codes 31201, 31051, and 31020 are more descriptive of this complex procedure and may be modified to show that the procedure was bilateral.

ICD-10-CM Code(s): J32.4, J33.8, G96.0

ICD-10-CM Rationale: The Alphabetic Index main term is Pansinusitis. The Alphabetic Index main term is Polyp, polypus, subterm sinus. The CSF leak code is found at main term Leak, leakage, subterm cerebrospinal fluid.

9.80. a. 478.33, 31561, 31600

Incorrect answer. Code 31600 is not reported in addition to 31561 because it is designated as a "separate procedure" in CPT.

b. 478.30, 31560

Incorrect answer. The diagnosis code is not as specific as it could be. Because bilateral partial paralysis is documented, code 478.33 may be reported. The correct procedure code is 31561 because the microscopy was used.

c. 478.33, 31561

Correct answer.

d. 478.33, 31560, 69990

Incorrect answer. There is a combination code for laryngoscopy with use of the operating microscope, 31561, which is reported instead of 31560 and 69990.

ICD-10-CM Code(s): J38.02

ICD-10-CM Rationale: The Alphabetic Index main term is Paralysis, paralytic, subterms vocal cord, bilateral.

9.81. a. 162.5, 31641, 99144

Correct answer. The drug should also be coded. The entire record should be reviewed to identify the drug given and the dosage. If this were a Medicare patient, an HCPCS Level II code could be assigned. If Versed were given, for example, code J2250 would be used and repeated for each mg given.

b. 162.5, 31641, 76001

Incorrect answer. Code 99144 should be reported for the conscious sedation (if criteria for its reporting are met). Code 76001 is not separately reported, per CPT guidelines. CPT codes 31622–31646 include fluoroscopy when performed.

c. 239.1, 31640, 99144-51

Incorrect answer. Carcinoma is a malignant neoplasm of the bronchus and should be reported using code 162.5 for the lower lobe. The CPT code is for excision by forceps, and in this situation a laser probe was used, so code 31641 would be assigned.

d. 239.1, 31641, 99144, 76001

Incorrect answer. Carcinoma is a malignant neoplasm of the bronchus and should be reported using code 162.5 for the lower lobe. Code 76001 is not separately reported, per CPT guidelines. CPT codes 31622–31646 include fluoroscopy when performed.

ICD-10-CM Code(s): C34.31

ICD-10-CM Rationale: The Neoplasm Table should be used to find the site bronchus, lower lobe, Malignant Primary column. The coder completes the code using the Tabular List.

9.82.   a. 239.1, V64.1, 31629, 76000

Incorrect answer. The diagnosis code is too presumptive. All masses are not neoplasms and should not be coded from the neoplasm table unless so stated by the physician. The atrial fibrillation code 427.31 should be added to show a condition that affected patient management. The CPT code is correct but requires a modifier to show that the procedure was terminated before completion. Code 76000 is not assigned because fluoroscopy is always included in this code range when performed.

b. 786.6, 427.31, 31629-52

Incorrect answer. Modifier -53 is correct because the procedure was terminated due to circumstances that threatened the well-being of the patient. Code V64.1 is added to show that the procedure was not carried out because of the contraindication of atrial fibrillation.

c. 786.6, 427.31, V64.1, 31628-53

Incorrect answer. The CPT code reported is for transbronchial lung biopsy, which would be performed with biopsy forceps rather than a needle aspiration process. Code 31629 is the appropriate CPT code.

d. 786.6, 427.31, V64.1, 31629-53

Correct answer. If modifiers are accepted, the -53 will show that the physician terminated the procedure due to extenuating circumstances.

ICD-10-CM Code(s): R91, I48.0, Z53.09

ICD-10-CM Rationale: The Alphabetic Index main term is Lung, subterm mass. The main term is Fibrillation, subterm atrial or auricular. Another main term is Canceled procedure (surgical), subterms because of, contraindication.

9.83.   a. 32480, 32663-53

Correct answer.

b. 32663, 32480

Incorrect answer. The open procedure is listed first, and the converted endoscopic procedure is listed second per *CPT Assistant* (1994, Fall).

c. 32480

Incorrect answer. The open procedure is listed first, and the converted endoscopic procedure is listed second per *CPT Assistant* (1994, Fall).

d. 32484, 32663-52

Incorrect answer. The open procedure is listed as a lobectomy, not a segmentectomy. Code 32480 is correct. The appropriate modifier is -53. Modifier -52 is close, but the procedure was terminated because of extenuating circumstances, not reduced.

9.84.   a. 466.0

Correct answer.

b. 466.0, 519.11

Incorrect answer. The bronchospasm is included in the acute bronchitis and is not coded separately. Refer to the alphabetic index: Bronchitis, acute or subacute, with, bronchospasm—466.0.

c. 519.11

Incorrect answer. A code for acute bronchitis should be assigned, which includes bronchospasm.

d. 466.19

Incorrect answer. This is the code for bronchiolitis; this patient has acute bronchitis.

ICD-10-CM Code(s): J20.9

ICD-10-CM Rationale: The Alphabetic Index main term is Bronchitis, subterm acute or subacute (with bronchospasm or obstruction).

Trauma and Poisoning

9.85.   a. 942.32, 943.29, 948.10, E924.0, E849.0, E015.2, E000.8, 99283-25, 16030

Correct answer.

b. 942.32, 948.00, E924.0, E000.8, 16025

Incorrect answer. The total burned area (both second and third degree) was greater than 10 percent; therefore, 948.10 is correct. An E/M code (99283-25) would be reported for the care provided before the burns are treated. These burns are considered large, and code 16030 is most appropriate. An E code to describe that the patient was involved in the activity of cooking should be reported as well as an E code for the place of occurrence.

c. 942.23, 942.33, E924.0, E015.2, 99284, 16025

Incorrect answer. The burn of the chest was described as full thickness or third degree and should be coded as 942.32. The other burn was a partial-thickness burn of the arm and is coded as 943.29 because of the multiple locations on the same arm. Only code 99283 can be justified by the documentation and requires a -25 modifier. An E code for the place of occurrence should be added.

d. 942.22, 943.20, 948.10, E924.0, 11000, 11001

Incorrect answer. The burn of the chest was described as full thickness or third degree and should be coded as 942.32. The second-degree burn is of both the upper and lower arm and is therefore coded to the multiple location code of 943.29. An E code to describe that the patient was involved in the activity of cooking should be reported, as well as an E code for the place of occurrence. An E/M code (99283-25) would be reported for the care provided before the burns are treated. Codes 11000 and 11001 describe debridement of infected skin and are not appropriate here. The codes for debridement of burn wound should be used, and these burns are considered large, or 16030.

ICD-10-CM Code(s): T21.31xA, T22.391A, T31.11, X12.xxxA, Y92.010, Y93.g3, Y99.8

ICD-10-CM Rationale: The Alphabetic Index main term Burn is used to find the site and extent codes. The main term is Burn, subterm chest wall, third degree. The arm burn is found under Burn, upper limb, multiple sites, right, third degree. The extent is found under Burn, extent. The Index to External Cause is used to find Burn, burned, burning, subterms hot, liquid. The place of occurrence is the kitchen which is found under Place of occurrence, residence, house, kitchen. The activity code is found under Activity, cooking and baking. The External status main term gives us code Y99.8.

9.86.   a. 823.10, E819.2, 27535, 11011-51

Incorrect answer. The orthopedic surgeon performed the fracture reduction. The emergency department physician would report the CPT code 11011 in addition to the appropriate level of evaluation and management service for the medical evaluation of the patient prior to the surgical procedure. Modifier -51 is used only when one physician performs more than one procedure at the same operative session. Two different physicians were involved here, so no modifier is required. Diagnosis codes are correct.

b. 823.12, E819.2, 11043

Incorrect answer. Codes from the range 11010–11012 are assigned for debridement associated with open fractures. The emergency department physician would report the appropriate evaluation and management service code and 11011 for the debridement procedure. The diagnosis is an open fracture of the tibia. There is no mention of fibular fracture, so 823.10 is the correct diagnosis code.

c. 823.10, E819.2, 11011

Correct answer.

d. 823.90, E819.2, 27535, 11043-51

Incorrect answer. The orthopedic surgeon performed the fracture reduction. The emergency department physician performed the debridement, but this code is incorrect. Code 11011 is the appropriate code. Modifier -51 is used only when one physician performs more than one procedure at the same operative session. Two different physicians were involved here, so no modifier is required. A more specific diagnosis code for the fracture of the proximal end of the tibia should be used.

ICD-10-CM Code(s): S82.109B, V29.9xxA

ICD-10-CM Rationale: The Alphabetic Index main term is Fracture, subterm tibia. The seventh character extension of "B" is assigned to indicate this is the initial encounter for an open fracture. The main term in the Index to External Cause is Accident, subterms transport, motorcycle.

9.87. a. 512.0, 821.01, 807.03, E819.3; 99284-25, 32551

Incorrect answer. This is a traumatic pneumothorax; code 860.0 is correct. All three key components for evaluation and management code 99285 were met, so that would be the appropriate code.

b. 860.0, 821.01, 807.03, E819.3; 99285-25, 32551

Correct answer.

c. 860.0, 821.00, 807.09, E819.3; 99285, 32422

Incorrect answer. The femur fracture is specified as midshaft. The final diagnosis indicates multiple rib fractures, but review of the rest of the note reveals that three ribs were fractured. Modifier -25 is needed to report a significant, separately identifiable evaluation and management service. No mention of a thoracentesis is made. The chest tube is coded 32551.

d. 512.0, 821.00, 807.09, E819.3; 99284, 32422

Incorrect answer. This is a traumatic pneumothorax; code 860.0 is correct. All three key components for evaluation and management code 99285 were met, so that would be the appropriate code. The final diagnosis indicates multiple rib fractures, but review of the rest of the note reveals that three ribs were fractured. Modifier -25 is needed to report a significant, separately identifiable evaluation and management service. No mention of a thoracentesis is made. The chest tube is coded 32551.

ICD-10-CM Code(s): S72.309A, S22.49xA, V29.9xxA

ICD-10-CM Rationale: The Alphabetic Index main term is Pneumothorax, subterm traumatic. The Alphabetic Index main term is Fracture, femur, shaft (middle third). The coder completes the code using the Tabular List. The Alphabetic Index main term is Fracture, subterm ribs, multiple. The coder completes the code. The Index to External Cause is used to reference Accident, subterm transport, motorcyclist. It is not possible to code to a more specific code due to the limited documentation. The seventh character extension of A is assigned to the injury codes to indicate that this is the initial encounter.

9.88. a. 965.4, E950.0

Incorrect answer. The patient's suicide attempt involved the use of barbiturates (967.0 and E950.1) as well as acetaminophen.

b. 968.3, E950.4

Incorrect answer. The patient's suicide attempt involved the use of non-anesthestic barbiturates (967.0 and E950.1) and acetaminophen (965.4, E950.0).

c. 969.3, E938.3, 965.4, E950.0

Incorrect answer. The patient's suicide attempt involved the use of non-anesthetic barbiturates (967.0 and E950.1).

d. 967.0, E950.1, 965.4, E950.0

Correct answer.

ICD-10-CM Code(s): T42.3x2A, T39.1x2A

ICD-10-CM Rationale: The Alphabetic Index main term in the Drug and Chemical Table is Barbiturate NEC. The Alphabetic Index main term in the Drug and Chemical Table is Acetaminophen. The seventh character extension of A is assigned to the codes to indicate that this is the initial encounter.

9.89.   a. 99291, 99292, 32160, 31500

Correct answer.

b. 99291, 99292, 32160

Incorrect answer. The intubation is not bundled into critical care and should be separately coded.

c. 99291, 99292, 31500-51

Incorrect answer. The cardiac massage should be coded. In addition, code 31500 is exempt from modifier -51 use.

d. 99291, 32160, 31500

Incorrect answer. According to the table provided in the CPT book: critical care time of 30 to 74 minutes (total time of 1 hr 14 minutes is reported with code 99291; and each additional 30 minutes beyond the first 74 minutes (1 hr and 14 minutes), report 99292 for each additional 30 minute block of time. Therefore, 85 minutes of critical care time in the ER requires add-on code 99292 to be reported with 99291.

9.90.   a. 852.40, 61154

Correct answer.

b. 853.00, 61108

Incorrect answer. This CPT code would be used to report a subdural hematoma evacuated via twist drill hole. This case is an epidural hematoma evacuated via burr hole (61154). The diagnosis code 852.40 is more specific.

c. 852.40, 61156

Incorrect answer. This CPT code would be used for treatment of an intracerebral hematoma. This case is an epidural hematoma.

d. 853.00, 61156

Incorrect answer. This CPT code would be used for treatment of an intracerebral hematoma. This case is an epidural hematoma. The diagnosis code 852.40 is more specific.

ICD-10-CM Code(s): S06.4x0A

ICD-10-CM Rationale: The Alphabetic Index main term is Injury, subterms intracranial, epidural hemorrhage (traumatic).

9.91. a. 945.50, 942.44, 942.43, 11100-59, 15150, 15151, 15152 × 7, 15100, 15101 × 3

Correct answer.

b. 945.50, 942.49, 11100-59, 15150, 15151, 15152 × 7, 15100,

15101 × 3

Incorrect answer. The sites of the burns to the trunk are specified as the buttocks and left flank, so they may be coded separately with specific codes.

c. 945.50, 942.44, 942.43, 11100, 15150, 15151, 15152 × 7, 15100, 15101 × 3

Incorrect answer. A modifier should be added to code 11100 to indicate that this was a distinct procedure that was separate from the others.

d. 945.50, 942.44, 942.43, 11100-59, 15150, 15151, 15152, 15100, 15101 × 3

Incorrect answer. There was 720 sq cm of tissue cultured skin graft. Code 15151 covers the first 25 sq cm and code 15151 indicates there was an additional 75 sq cm, which equals 100 sq cm. Code 15152 needs to be assigned 7 times to get to 720 sq cm.

ICD-10-CM Code(s): T24.302D, T24.301D, T21.35xD, T21.32xD, T31.75

ICD-10-CM Rationale: The Alphabetic Index main term is Burn, lower, limb, left, third degree and right, third degree. The Alphabetic Index main term is Burn, buttocks, third degree and Burn, abdominal wall, third degree. The extent of the burns is coded by referencing Burn, extent, 70–79%, with 50–59% 3rd degree. The seventh character extension of "D" is assigned to the burn codes to indicate that this is a subsequent encounter.

Part IV

Coding Challenge

Chapter 10. Coding Challenge: Nonacute Settings; ICD-10-CM and ICD-10-PCS Code Sets; CPT Modifiers, HCPCS Level II Modifiers

Code set answers given in Chapter 10 pertain to multiple code sets.

Home Health

10.1.   a. V-code for aftercare of surgery

Rationale: Bleeding gastric ulcer is not current and would not be coded. Traumatic wounds are not coded for surgical wounds.

10.2.   c. Diabetes mellitus

Rationale: The diabetes mellitus would be reported in M0240 as a secondary diagnosis. The diverticulitis is not a current condition and would not be reported. The pneumonia is still present and the focus of care, and is reported in M0230 as the primary diagnosis.

10.3.   a. 438.20 (Hemiplegia)

Incorrect answer. This code would be reported in M0240, but it is not the focus of the care.

   b. 153.1 (Ca of transverse colon)

Incorrect answer. Because the focus of care is the result of the patient's recent surgery for cancer, the patient's primary diagnosis is V58.42, Aftercare following surgery for neoplasm. ICD-9-CM coding guidelines stipulate that code V58.42 is sequenced before the malignancy code, if the focus of care is aftercare.

c. V58.42 (Aftercare following surgery for neoplasm)

Correct answer. Because the focus of care is the result of the patient's recent surgery for cancer, the patient's primary diagnosis is V58.42, Aftercare following surgery for neoplasm. ICD-9-CM coding guidelines stipulate that code V58.42 is sequenced before the malignancy code, if the focus of care is aftercare.

d. V58.31 (Attention to surgical wound dressings)

Incorrect answer. This code was also a focus of the care, but code V58.42 was selected in the first position because it provides more detailed information.

10.4.   a. M0230: V58.42; M0240: 154.1, V55.3

Incorrect answer. It appears that most of the care is directed at the colostomy care, so it would be the most specific code to use for the primary.

b. M0230: V55.3; M0240: 154.1, V58.42

Correct answer.

c. M0230: 154.1; M0240: V55.3, V58.42

Incorrect answer. The treatment is directed at the colostomy care.

d. M0230: V55.3; M0240: V10.06, V58.42

Incorrect answer. The cancer has been resected, but according to coding guidelines, if there is treatment directed to it, then it is coded as a current cancer.

10.5.   a. 185

Incorrect answer. It would not be correct to report the cancer code since it has been excised and is not currently being treated.

b. V10.46

Correct answer.

c. V16.42

Incorrect answer. The patient has a personal history, not a family history.

d. The status of the cancer would not be reported.

Incorrect answer. It would be correct to report the status code.

10.6.   a. 998.59

Correct answer.

b. V58.31

Incorrect answer. The patient is having surgical wound dressing changes, but it is not the only focus of care. Treatment appears to be centered around the postoperative wound infection. Use V58.31 in M0240.

c. 879.2

Incorrect answer. It is incorrect to code open wound for surgical wounds.

d. 574.10

Incorrect answer. The gallbladder has been removed, so this is not the appropriate diagnosis.

10.7.   M0230: V54.81; M0240: V43.64, 781.2; M0246: 781.2

Rationale: Assign code V54.81, Aftercare following joint replacement, as the first-listed code for the home health care visit. Codes V43.64, Organ or tissue replaced by other means, Joint hip; and 781.2, Abnormality of gait, should be assigned as additional diagnoses.

Discussion: Code 781.2 is appropriate as an additional diagnosis because it describes the current symptom being addressed. Code 719.7, Difficulty in walking, would not be appropriate because codes in this category describe disorders of the joints. This problem does not represent a disorder of the joint.

Code 717.35 should not be assigned for osteoarthritis in the hip joint that was replaced, since the patient no longer has osteoarthritis in this joint after the hip replacement. If the patient still has osteoarthritis in other joints, such as the other hip, then the appropriate code from category 715 should be assigned. See *Coding Clinic* (2004, 2Q).

10.8.   M0230: 454.0; M0240: 250.80, 707.15, 428.0, 401.9

Rationale: M0230: 454.0, Stasis ulcer of the leg.

M0240: 250.80, Diabetes with other specified manifestations

M0240: 707.15, Diabetic ulcer of toe

M0240: 428.0, Congestive heart failure

M0240: 401.9, Hypertension

There is no need to complete M0246 because the patient's primary diagnosis, 454.0, Stasis ulcer of the leg, is not a V code and is not a case mix diagnosis.

Discussion: The most intensive skilled service is provided to the leg dressing related to the stasis ulcer. The stasis ulcer is the appropriate principal/primary diagnosis rather than the diabetic ulcer, since the documentation indicates the patient has a stasis ulcer. The diabetic toe ulcers are reported using the coding sequence 250.80, 707.15. Edema would not be coded and reported because it is integral to CHF. ICD-9-CM coding guidelines indicate that conditions integral to a diagnosis are not coded separately. The CHF and HTN are mentioned as secondary diagnoses because they contribute to the need for medication and physical therapy.

10.9.   M0230: V58.42; M0240: 174.9, 438.31, V58.31

Rationale: M0230: V58.42, Aftercare following surgery for neoplasm.

M0240: 174.9, Malignant neoplasm of female breast, unspecified

M0240: 438.31, Late effects of cerebrovascular disease, monoplegia of upper limb

M0240: V58.31, Attention to surgical wound dressings

There is no need to complete M0246 because the patient's primary diagnosis, V58.42, Aftercare following surgery for neoplasm, is a V code that is not replacing a case mix diagnosis.

Discussion: The most intensive skilled service that is being provided to this patient is the skilled home health treatment activity for the care of her surgical wound. Since the specific focus of care for this patient is the result of the patient's recent surgery for breast cancer, the patient's primary diagnosis is V58.42, Aftercare following surgery for neoplasm. ICD-9-CM coding guidelines stipulate that code V58.42 is sequenced before the malignancy code if the focus of care is aftercare, which it is in this case. Therefore, 174.9, Malignant neoplasm of the female breast, unspecified, is the patient's secondary diagnosis. Since code 174.9 is not a case mix diagnosis, M0246 does not need to be completed, as a V code is not replacing a case mix diagnosis. In addition, the breast cancer is not resolved, as evidenced by the tamoxifen treatment.

The diagnosis of neoplasm will vary depending on the patient's type of neoplasm; ICD-9-CM code 217 would be indicated if the neoplasm was determined to be benign.

The diagnoses that follow will vary depending on the conditions that coexist at the time the Patient's Plan of Care is established, or that have developed subsequently, or that affect the treatment of care. These diagnoses are listed on the Plan of Care in order to best reflect the seriousness of the patient's condition and to justify the disciplines and services provided. The diagnosis responsible for the patient's inability to perform the wound care, late effect of stroke, is reflected as a secondary diagnosis. The patient may not necessarily have a physical inability to perform the wound care. (If she is incapable of performing the procedure due to a learning deficit or a refusal, this requires documentation of the skilled nurse's attempts to teach and the result of the teaching.) The fifth digit for late effects signifies dominant/nondominant/nonspecified side.

10.10. d. All of the above

Rationale: As explained on the first page of the *Official Coding Guidelines*, all facilities must follow Section I.

10.11. M0230: V58.78; M0240: 250.80, 731.8, 781.2, V58.31; M0246: 250.80, 731.8

Rationale: M0230: V58.78, Aftercare following surgery of the musculoskeletal system, NEC

M0240: 250.80, Diabetes with other specified manifestations

M0240: 731.8, Other bone involvement in diseases classified elsewhere

M0240: 781.2, Abnormality of gait

M0240: V58.31, Attention to surgical dressings and sutures

M0246: 250.80, Diabetes with other specified manifestations

M0246: 731.8, Other bone involvement in diseases classified elsewhere

There is a need to complete M0246 because V58.78 is a V code that is replacing a case mix diagnosis (250.80). In this case, the case mix diagnosis, diabetic osteomyelitis, requires multiple coding (250.80 and 731.8).

Discussion: As you can see from this example, diabetic osteomyelitis is at the root of the patient's current problem, which is the loss of the patient's right foot by amputation. Diabetic osteomyelitis is not a direct cause of the treatment need so it is not the primary diagnosis. The primary diagnosis that is associated with the most intensive skilled service provided to this patient is V58.78, Aftercare following surgery of the musculoskeletal system.

Because an aftercare V code is replacing a case mix diagnosis, the agency would be expected to complete M0246 with the case mix diagnosis, which in this case requires multiple coding (250.80, Diabetes with other specified manifestations, and 731.8, Other bone involvement in diseases classified elsewhere). Therefore, because the case mix diagnosis requires a manifestation code, the home health agency is expected to complete both M0246 codes as stated above.

10.12. M0230: V57.1; M0240: 781.2, V54.13; M0246: 781.2

Rationale: M0230: V57.1, Physical therapy

M0240: 781.2, Abnormality of gait

M0240: V54.13, Aftercare for healing traumatic fracture of hip

M0246: 781.2, Abnormality of gait

There is a need to complete M0246 because the patient's primary diagnosis is a V code (V57.1), which replaces a case mix diagnosis.

Discussion: The most intensive skilled service that is being provided to this patient is the skilled physical therapy services for gait training. Code V57.1, Physical therapy, is selected as this patient's primary diagnosis because his treatment is directed at rehabilitation following his hip fracture and surgery. Coding guidelines stipulate that the acute fracture code may only be used for the initial, acute episode of care. The acute fracture code is no longer appropriate once the patient has been discharged from the hospital to home health care. Abnormality of gait (781.2) was selected as the first secondary diagnosis because it accurately describes this patient's current condition and his need for therapy (technically, he no longer has a hip fracture, which was resolved by the hospital surgical treatment) and because the physician specified gait training.

10.13. a. V58.44

Incorrect answer. Code V58.44 is correct, but the instructional note states to "Use additional code to identify the organ transplanted (V42.0–V42.9). Code V42.0 should also be assigned.

b. V58.44, V42.0

Correct answer. This is correct coding from the provided documentation. If there are any other medical conditions still present, for example in the other kidney, then they should be added as secondary codes. Any dressing change codes or any other applicable codes should also be added. Limited documentation was used here to illustrate the new aftercare code.

c. 585.6

Incorrect answer. There is documentation that there is renal failure. The aftercare code should be listed.

d. V42.0

Incorrect answer. This would be a secondary code according to the note. The aftercare code is listed first.

10.14. a. One

Incorrect answer. There are two categories of skin disorders in the HH-PPS.

b. Two

Correct answer. The two categories are: Skin 1—Traumatic wounds, burns, and post-operative complications; Skin 2—Ulcers and other skin disorders.

c. Three

Incorrect answer. There are two categories of skin disorders in the HH-PPS.

d. Four

Incorrect answer. There are two categories of skin disorders in the HH-PPS.

ICD-10-CM

10.15. b. 4

Rationale: According to the *ICD-10-CM Official Guidelines for Coding and Reporting*, a myocardial infarction is acute for four weeks. In ICD-9-CM, a myocardial infarction is acute for eight weeks.

10.16. d. Emphysema

Rationale: Emphysema is found in category J43.

10.17. a. True

Rationale: ICD-10-CM codes will be utilized by all healthcare settings to assign diagnosis codes. ICD-10-PCS codes will be utilized by inpatient hospital settings to assign procedure codes.

10.18. b. M48.06

Rationale: Index the main term Stenosis, subterms spinal, lumbar region, to assign code M48.06.

10.19. c. E20.9, H28

Rationale: Index the main term Cataract, subterms in (due to), hypopara-thyroidism, to assign codes E20.9, H28. The underlying condition of hypoparathyroidism (E20.9) should be assigned first, followed by the cataract code (H28).

10.20. b. J69.0

Rationale: Index the main term Pneumonia, subterms aspiration, due to, food, to assign code J69.0.

ICD-10-PCS

10.21. a. True

Rationale: All ICD-10-PCS codes contain seven alphanumeric characters. The meaning of each character may differ by section. For example, the 3rd character in the Medical and Surgical section means "root operation," whereas the third character in the Mental Health section means "root type."

10.22. a. 0 (Medical and surgical)

b. 0 (Medical and surgical)

c. F (Physical rehabilitation and diagnostic audiology)

d. B (Imaging)

e. 2 (Placement)

f. 8 (Other procedures)

10.23. a. Y (Transplantation)

b. T (Resection)

c. J (Inspection)

d. F (Fragmentation)

e. D (Extraction)

f. L (Occlusion)

g. A (Alteration)

h. 7 (Dilation)

i. N (Release)

j. W (Revision)

k. 2 (Change)

10.24. a. 3 (Percutaneous)

b. 7 (Via Natural or Artificial Opening)

c. 0 (Open)

d. F (Via Natural or Artificial Opening Endoscopic with Percutaneous Endoscopic Assistance)

e. 4 (Percutaneous Endoscopic)

f. 8 (Via Natural or Artificial Opening Endoscopic)

g. X (External)

10.25. a. 2 (Open)

b. 4 (Percutaneous)

c. 1 (Via Natural or Artificial Opening)

d. 3 (Percutaneous Endoscopic)

10.26. Code 0SRC0JZ

Rationale:

0	Medical and Surgical (section)
S	Lower Joints (body system)
R	Replacement (root operation)
C	Knee Joint, Right (body part)
0	Open (approach)
J	Synthetic Substitute (device)
Z	No qualifier

ICD-10-CM/PCS Application Exercise

10.27. a. I21.01

Rationale: Search the registry by date, looking for the presence of code 410.11 when ICD-9-CM was used and code I21.01 when ICD-10-CM was used.

b. 0FJB0ZZ

Rationale: Search the registry by date, looking for the presence of code 51.51 when ICD-9-CM was used and code 0FJB0ZZ when ICD-10-PCS was used.

10.28. 0HBU0ZX

Rationale: This is considered an excision in ICD-10-PCS. The coder should access Excision, breast, left to get the beginning of the code,—0HBU. It was an open procedure so the 5th character is "0". The 6th character is "Z" and because the test was diagnostic, the 7th character is "X".

10.29. 0VB08ZZ

Rationale: The TURP is considered an excision. Use the main term Excision, subterm prostate to get the first four characters. Referencing this table the coder chooses the 5th digit for an endoscopic approach using a natural or artificial opening. The 6th and 7th characters are "Z".

10.30. 0UL74ZZ

Rationale: This procedure is coded as an occlusion. The coder would access main term Occlusion, subterm fallopian tube, bilateral. The first four characters of the code are given and the tables are accessed to finish the code. The 5th digit is for percutaneous endoscopic and the 6th and 7th are "Z".

10.31. 0BTL0ZZ

Rationale: This is considered a resection because the entire lung was removed. The main term is Resection, subterm lung, left. Referencing the table the coder chooses the open approach (0), and no device or qualifier.

CPT Modifiers

10.32. a. No modifier is necessary because Dr. Raddy interpreted the x-ray under contract with the hospital. The hospital will bill the global and pay Dr. Raddy from the reimbursement.

Incorrect answer. Dr. Raddy should report the chest x-ray code with modifier -26, professional component. If he had performed the service with equipment he owned and staff that he employed, he could have reported the global, but because the hospital assumed the technical overhead, he can only report the professional component.

b. Modifier -26, Professional component

Correct answer.

c. Modifier -TC, Technical component

Incorrect answer. Dr. Raddy performed the professional component of the split service, not the technical component. He should report modifier -26.

d. Modifier -59

Incorrect answer. Modifier -26 is the appropriate modifier to report the professional component of a split service. Modifier -59 is reported only when a specific modifier does not exist.

10.33. a. No modifier is needed for the surgery, although the anesthesiologist might need a modifier.

Incorrect answer. Modifier -63, Procedure performed on infants less than 4 kg, should be reported.

b. Modifier -63 is reported because the baby weighs less than 4 kg and thus is a higher surgical risk than a larger neonate.

Correct answer.

c. No modifier is needed because code 44120 already applies to neonates who are very low weight.

Incorrect answer. Code 44120 is not exempt from the assignment of modifier -63, and this modifier should be assigned.

d. A modifier is optional and may or may not be assigned depending upon the departmental coding guidelines.

Incorrect answer. Modifier -63, Procedure performed on infants less than 4 kg, should be reported in this case.

10.34. a. Modifier -59, to show that these were not duplicate charges but indeed separate incidents.

Incorrect answer. Modifier -91 is specific for repeat laboratory tests.

b. No modifier is necessary for repeat laboratory tests, only for repeat surgical procedures.

Incorrect answer. Modifier -91 is specific for repeat laboratory tests.

c. Modifier -91.

Correct answer.

d. Modifiers -91 and -59 should be reported for the second and third determinations.

Incorrect answer. Only modifier -91 is necessary, as it is specific for repeat laboratory tests.

10.35. a. Modifier -76, Repeat procedure by the same physician, should be reported for each chest tube insertion.

Incorrect answer. Modifier -76 is the appropriate modifier, but it should be appended only to the second procedure. No modifier is needed on the first procedure.

b. Modifier -76 should be reported with the second procedure; no modifier is needed on the first procedure.

Correct answer.

c. Modifier -59 should be reported with the second procedure; no modifier is needed with the first procedure.

Incorrect answer. Modifier -76 is specific for repeat of an identical procedure by the same physician and should be reported with the second procedure.

d. Either modifier -59 or -76 may be reported on the first and second procedures.

Incorrect answer. Modifier -76 is specific for repeat of an identical procedure by the same physician and should be reported with the second procedure. Modifier -59 should be used only when a more specific modifier is not available. No modifier should be reported with the first procedure.

10.36. a. No modifier is needed because the ICD-9-CM diagnosis code and the CPT procedure code clearly identify that this was a procedure not related to the cholecystectomy.

Incorrect answer. Even though the procedure is clearly not related, modifier -79, Unrelated procedure or service by the same physician during the postoperative period, should be reported to make the circumstances completely clear to the payer.

b. Modifier -79, Unrelated procedure or service by the same physician during the postoperative period, should be reported with the appendectomy code.

Correct answer.

c. Modifier -78, Return to the operating room for a related procedure during the postoperative period, should be reported with the appendectomy code.

Incorrect answer. There is nothing to suggest that the acute appendicitis was related to the cholecystectomy. Modifier -79, Unrelated procedure or service by the same physician during the postoperative period, should be reported with the appendectomy code.

d. Modifier -58, Staged or related procedure or service by the same physician during the postoperative period, should be reported with the appendectomy code.

Incorrect answer. This was not a related or stated procedure, but an unrelated procedure for an unrelated diagnosis. Modifier -79, Unrelated procedure or service by the same physician during the postoperative period, should be reported with the appendectomy code.

HCPCS Level II Modifiers

10.37. a. No. If an "inpatient only" procedure is performed on an outpatient basis, the hospital cannot obtain reimbursement under any circumstances.

Incorrect answer. Modifier -CA may be assigned when a patient expires prior to admission when an "inpatient only" procedure is performed on an emergency basis.

b. Modifier -CA, Procedure payable only in the inpatient setting when performed emergently on an outpatient who expires prior to admission, may be appended to the CPT procedure code.

Correct answer.

c. Modifier -ST, Related to trauma or injury, may be appended and a 50 percent reimbursement will be available to the hospital.

Incorrect answer. Modifier -CA may be assigned when a patient expires prior to admission when an "inpatient only" procedure is performed on an emergency basis.

d. Modifier -SC, Medically necessary service or supply, may be appended and a 25 percent reimbursement will be available to the hospital.

Incorrect answer. Modifier -CA may be assigned when a patient expires prior to admission when an "inpatient only" procedure is performed on an emergency basis.

10.38. a. No modifier. By definition, bunionectomy is performed on the big toe.

Incorrect answer. Modifier -T5, Right foot, great toe, is the appropriate modifier.

b. Modifier -T5

Correct answer.

c. Modifier -RT

Incorrect answer. Modifier -T5, right foot, great toe, is the appropriate modifier, as it is more specific.

d. Modifier -TA

Incorrect answer. Modifier -TA reports the left foot, great toe.

10.39. a. Modifier -GW

Correct answer.

b. Modifier -AT

Incorrect answer. Modifier -GW is specific for identifying services not related to a hospice patient's terminal condition.

c. Modifier -GZ

Incorrect answer. Modifier -GW is appropriate for reporting services that are not part of a patient's terminal condition.

d. Modifier -SC

Incorrect answer. Modifier -GW is specific for identifying services not related to a hospice patient's terminal condition.

10.40. a. CPT codes

Incorrect answer. They can be used with both CPT and HCPCS Level II codes.

b. HCPCS Level II codes

Incorrect answer. They can be used with both CPT and HCPCS Level II codes.

c. ICD-9-CM Volume III codes

Incorrect answer. They can be used with both CPT and HCPCS Level II codes, but not with ICD-9-CM procedure codes.

d. Both a and b

Correct answer.

10.41. a. Laboratory tests

Incorrect answer. They are reported with dialysis codes.

b. Dialysis codes

Correct answer.

c. Coronary artery interventional procedures

Incorrect answer. They are reported with dialysis codes.

d. Oxygen therapy

Incorrect answer. They are reported with dialysis codes.

10.42. 1. f
2. g
3. i
4. b
5. j
6. h
7. c
8. a
9. e
10. d

10.43. V2523-VP-H9

Rationale: V2523-VP-H9, Contact lens, hydrophilic, extended wear, per lens; aphakic patient; court ordered. The modifier -VP, Aphakic patient, is the most specific and the most important, so it is placed closest to the procedure code. For a Medicare beneficiary, this information is critical to reimbursement because Medicare will only pay for this service (the hydrophilic contact lens) for aphakic patients.

Long-term Acute Care (LTAC) Coding

10.44. a. 433.00, 438.21, 438.11, 438.82

Incorrect answer. The acute bleed (433.00) is completed, and the patient is admitted for therapy for management of the various late effects—the hemiplegia (438.21), the aphasia (438.11), and the dysphagia (438.82)—which should be sequenced as the principal and secondary diagnoses.

b. V57.89, 438.21, 438.11, 438.82

Correct answer.

c. V58.9, 438.21, 438.11, 438.82

Incorrect answer. The admission conditions are the late effects of the bleed and rehabilitation for the same. No specific aftercare is documented.

d. V57.2, V57.3, V57.89

Incorrect answer. The individual types of rehabilitation need not be reported. Code V57.89 followed by the specific sequelae of the bleed are the appropriate principal and secondary diagnoses.

10.45. a. 707.05, 707.07, 707.22, 250.00, 496, 86.28

Correct answer.

b. V57.89, 707.05, 707.07, 707.22, 250.00, 496, 86.28

Incorrect answer. No specific therapy is documented. The patient is admitted for management of the continued acute condition of the decubitus ulcers, which should be assigned as the principal diagnosis.

c. 707.05, 707.07, 707.22, 86.28

Incorrect answer. Although these codes are appropriate, the codes for the concomitant chronic conditions of diabetes and COPD should also be coded, as they impact the patient's response to treatment.

d. 707.05, 707.07, 707.22, 86.22

Incorrect answer. The diagnosis codes are appropriate, but the procedure code, 86.22, reports excisional debridement, not nonexcisional debridement. Code 86.28 is the appropriate code. As this code assignment impacts MS-DRG grouping, this coding error would constitute a significant compliance issue for the hospital.

10.46. a. 496, 414.00, 250.60, 337.1

Incorrect answer. The patient is specifically admitted for pulmonary rehabilitation. Code V57.89 is the appropriate principal diagnosis in this case. The COPD should be reported as a concomitant secondary diagnosis.

b. V57.0, 496

Incorrect answer. Code V57.0 reports only breathing exercises. Pulmonary rehabilitation is a multidisciplinary rehabilitation involving pulmonary, physician, and occupational therapy and sometimes speech-language therapy. Code V57.89 is the appropriate principal diagnosis. The COPD is appropriately reported as a secondary diagnosis. The ASHD and diabetes with neurological manifestations in the form of peripheral neuropathy should also be reported, as they currently affect the patient's condition. Add codes 414.00, 250.60, and 337.1.

c. V57.89, 496, 414.00, 250.60, 337.1
Correct answer.

d. V57.89

Incorrect answer. The rehabilitation is the appropriate principal diagnosis code, but the underlying pulmonary condition for which the rehabilitation is given (496), as well as the concomitant chronic conditions (414.00, 250.60, 337.1), should also be coded.

10.47. a. V57.89

Incorrect answer. Although the patient may eventually receive therapy, management of the stump infection is the primary focus of her admission. Assign code 997.62 as the principal diagnosis.

b. V52.1

Incorrect answer. Although the patient may eventually be fitted with a prosthesis, the main reason for her admission is to resolve the stump infection. Assign code 997.62 as the principal diagnosis.

c. 904.53

Incorrect answer. Although the injury to the posterior tibial artery precipitated the amputation, this episode of care is over. The patient is admitted to the LTAC for management of the stump infection. Assign code 997.62 as the principal diagnosis.

d. 997.62
Correct answer.

Outpatient Rehabilitation Cases

10.48. V57.1, 343.9, 737.30, 754.31

10.49. V57.1, 728.89

Inpatient Rehabilitation Cases

10.50. a. Admit: 821.00

       Principal: V57.89

       Secondary: V54.13
                       V58.43
                       E929.3
                       427.31
                       317
                       V58.61
                       530.81
                       457.1

      b. Etiology: 820.21

       Comorbidities: E929.3
                       427.31
                       317
                       V58.61
                       530.81
                       457.1

Neurology Rehabilitation H&P for Inpatient Case

10.51. a. Admit: 952.9

       Principal: V57.89

       Secondary: 907.2
                       E929.0
                       596.54
                       564.81
                       344.02

      b. Etiology: 952.03

       Comorbidities: E929.0
                       596.54
                       564.81
                       344.02

10.52. a. Admit: 438.9

       Principal: V57.89

       Secondary: 438.20

                 438.6/781.8

                 438.19

                 438.82

                 438.83

                 250.00

                 272.4

                 427.31

                 276.1

                 278.01

                 414.00

                 715.35

                 V58.61

                 726.10

    b. Etiology: 434.91

       Comorbidities: 781.8

                    787.2

                    784.59

                    427.31

                    250.00

                    272.4

                    278.01

Skilled Nursing Facility (SNF) Cases

10.53. a. V54.25, 198.5, V10.3

Correct answer.

b. 733.14, 198.5, V10.3

Incorrect answer. The pathological fracture treatment was carried out in the acute hospital, and the patient was admitted to the skilled nursing facility for aftercare. Assign a code from the "Aftercare for pathological fracture" series as the principal diagnosis, in this case, V54.25.

c. V57.89, 733.14, 198.5, V10.3

Incorrect answer. The patient is not admitted specifically for rehabilitation; she is nonambulatory and is admitted for continued healing of the fracture. Assign a code from the "Aftercare for pathological fracture" series as the principal diagnosis, in this case, V54.25.

d. V54.15, 821.00

Incorrect answer. Code V54.15 reports aftercare for a healing traumatic fracture, but this is documented as a pathological fracture. In addition, code 821.00 reports a traumatic fracture. Codes V54.25, 198.5, and V10.3 are the correct codes to report for this admission.

10.54. a. 486, 496, 401.9, 414.00

Incorrect answer. The pneumonia had resolved in the acute hospital, and no treatment was needed in the skilled nursing facility. The patient was admitted because of Alzheimer's dementia, which should be sequenced as the principal diagnosis, along with the behavior disturbance manifested as wandering off (331.0, 294.11). The other diagnosis codes (496, 401.9, 414.00) are appropriate, if nonspecific.

b. 331.0, 294.11

Incorrect answer. These are appropriate codes for the principal diagnosis, but the underlying chronic diseases of COPD, hypertension, and ASHD should also be coded, as they affect the patient's management. Add codes 496, 401.9, and 414.00.

c. 331.0, 294.11, 496, 401.9, 414.00

Correct answer.

d. V57.89, 331.0, 294.11, 496, 401.9, 414.00

Incorrect answer. There is no documentation of any therapy being ordered. The patient is essentially custodial. Assign the Alzheimer's dementia with behavioral disturbance as the principal diagnosis and the underlying chronic conditions as secondary diagnoses.

10.55. a. V58.75, 780.79, V10.05

Correct answer.

b. V58.75, 997.99, 780.79, V10.05

Incorrect answer. Although the principal diagnosis code is appropriate, there is no documentation that the weakness was a postoperative complication. Delete code 997.99. The remainder of the codes are correct.

c. V10.05, 780.79

Incorrect answer. The patient was admitted for aftercare following the surgery for the carcinoma, not because she had a history of colon cancer. Assign V58.75 as the principal diagnosis.

d. V58.75, 780.79, 153.1

Incorrect answer. Code 153.1 is not appropriate, as the malignancy has been eradicated by the surgery, and the patient is not receiving any treatment at this time. Change to code V10.05. The rest of the codes are correct.